COMPARATIVE MANAGEMENT of SPINE PATHOLOGY

NEUROSURGERY: CASE MANAGEMENT COMPARISON SERIES

SERIES EDITORS

Kaisorn L. Chaichana, MD, FAANS, FACS

Professor of Neurosurgery
Vice Chair of Education
Director of Brain Tumor Surgery
Director of Skull Base and Minimally Invasive Cranial Surgery
Neurosurgery Residency Program Director
Mayo Clinic
Jacksonville, Florida, United States

Alfredo Quiñones-Hinojosa, MD, FAANS, FACS

William J. and Charles H. Mayo Professor
Monica Flynn Jacoby Chair, Neurologic Surgery
Mayo Clinic
Jacksonville, Florida, United States

ASSOCIATE EDITORS

Kingsley Abode-Iyamah, M.D., FAANS
Associate Professor
Department of Neurologic Surgery
Mayo Clinic
Jacksonville, Florida, United States

Oluwaseun O. Akinduro, MD
Department of Neurologic Surgery
Mayo Clinic
Jacksonville, Florida, United States

William E. Clifton, (Bill) III, M.D.
Department of Neurologic Surgery
Mayo Clinic
Jacksonville, Florida, United States

Fidel Valero-Moreno, MD
Department of Neurologic Surgery
Mayo Clinic
Jacksonville, Florida, United States

ELSEVIER

Elsevier
1600 John F. Kennedy Blvd.
Ste 1800
Philadelphia, PA 19103-2899

COMPARATIVE MANAGEMENT OF SPINE PATHOLOGY

ISBN: 978-0-323-82557-3

Content Strategist: Humayra R. Khan
Content Development Specialist: Ranjana Sharma
Publishing Services Manager: Deepthi Unni
Project Manager: Sindhuraj Thulasingam
Design Direction: Patrick C. Ferguson

Printed in India

Last digit is the print number: 9 8 7 6 5 4 3 2 1

Contributors

Kingsley Abode-Iyamah, MD, FAANS
Associate Professor
Department of Neurologic Surgery
Mayo Clinic
Jacksonville, Florida, United States

Oluwaseun O. Akinduro, MD
Resident Physician
Department of Neurologic Surgery
Mayo Clinic
Jacksonville, Florida, United States

Kaisorn L. Chaichana, MD, FAANS, FACS
Professor of Neurosurgery
Vice Chair of Education
Director of Brain Tumor Surgery
Director of Skull Base and Minimally Invasive Cranial Surgery
Neurosurgery Residency Program Director
Mayo Clinic
Jacksonville, Florida, United States

William E. Clifton, (Bill) III, MD
Department of Neurologic Surgery
Mayo Clinic
Jacksonville, Florida, United States

Kelly Gassie, MD
Resident Physician
Department of Neurologic Surgery
Mayo Clinic
Jacksonville, Florida, United States

Jaime L. Martínez Santos, MD
Resident Physician
Department of Neurosurgery
Medical University of South Carolina
Charleston, South Carolina, United States

Alfredo Quiñones-Hinojosa, MD, FAANS, FACS
William J. and Charles H. Mayo Professor
Monica Flynn Jacoby Chair
Neurologic Surgery
Mayo Clinic
Jacksonville, Florida, United States

Henry J. Ruiz-Garcia, MD
Postdoctoral Research Fellow
Department of Neurologic Surgery
Mayo Clinic
Jacksonville, Florida, United States

Fidel Valero-Moreno, MD
Neurosurgeon
Department of Neurologic Surgery
Mayo Clinic
Jacksonville, Florida, United States

Tito Vivas-Buitrago, MD
Mayo Clinic
Jacksonville, Florida, United States;
Universidad de Santander
UDES Bucaramanga, Colombia

Expert Case Reviewers

Anas Abdallah, MD
Associate Professor of Neurosurgery
Department of Neurosurgery
Osmaniye State
Osmaniye, Turkey

Amro F. Al-Habib, MD, MPH
Professor and Head Neurosurgery Division
King Khalid University Hospital
King Saud University
Riyadh, Saudi Arabia

Rafid Al-Mahfoudh, MBChBh
Neurosurgeon
Brighton and Sussex University Hospitals
Brighton, United Kingdom

Todd J. Albert, MD
Professor of Orthopedic Surgery
Hospital for Special Surgery
Weill Cornell Medical College
New York, New York, United States

Richard Allen, MD, PhD
Associate Professor, Orthopedic Surgery
University of California at San Diego
San Diego, California, United States

Andrés Almendral, MD
Neurosurgeon
Clinica Hospital San Fernando
Panama City, Panama

Ali A. Baaj, MD
Associate Professor of Neurological &
 Orthopedic Surgery
University of Arizona and Banner – University
 Medical Center
Phoenix, Arizona, United States

Carlos Bagley, MD
Professor of Neurological Surgery
UT Southwestern Medical Center
Dallas, Texas

Ahmed S. Barakat, MD, MBBCH, MSc
Orthopedic Surgeon
Department of Orthopedics and Traumatology
University of Cairo
Cairo, Egypt

Ignacio Barrenechea, MD, IFAANS
Chairman, Neurosurgery Department
Hospital Privado de Rosario
Santa Fe, Argentina

Pedro Luis Bazán, MD
Spine Surgeon
HIGA San Martín La Plata (Chief Orthopaedic)
Hospital Italiano La Plata
Instituto de Diagnóstico La Plata
La Plata, Buenos Aires, Argentina

Carlo Bellabarba, MD
Chief of Service, Orthopaedics
Director, Spine Service
University of Washington
Harborview Medical Center
Seattle, Washington, United States

Lorin M. Benneker, MD
Professor of Orthopaedic Surgery
Spine Unit
Sonnenhofspital
Bern, Switzerland

Sigurd Berven, MD
Professor of Orthopaedic Surgery
University of California at San Francisco
San Francisco, California, United States

Nitin N. Bhatia, MD
Professor, Orthopedic Surgery
Chief, Adult and Pediatric Spinal Surgery
Chair, Orthopedic Surgery
University of California at Irvine
Orange, California, United States

Mark H. Bilsky, MD
Professor, Neurological Surgery
Memorial Sloan Kettering Cancer Center
New York, New York, United States

Ciaran Bolger, MD
Professor, Neurosurgery
Head of the Department of Clinical
 Neuroscience RCSI
Beaumont Hospital Dublin
Dublin, Ireland

Stefano Boriani, MD
Professor, Orthopaedic Surgery
IRCCS Istituto Ortopedico Galeazzi
Milan, Italy

Richard J. Bransford, MD
Professor Orthopedic Surgery
Director, UW Orthopaedics Spine Fellowship
 Program
University of Washington
Seattle, Washington, United States

Mohamad Bydon, MD
Professor of Neurosurgery, Orthopedic
 Surgery
Department of Neurosurgery
Mayo Clinic College of Medicine
Rochester, Minnesota, United States

Alvaro Campero, MD PhD, MgCh
Chair Department of Neurosurgery
Hospital Padilla – Tucuman
Universidad Nacional de Tucuman
Tucuman, Argentina

Adrian Casey, MD
Consultant Neurosurgeon
National Hospital for Neurology and
 Neurosurgery
London, United Kingdom

Selby G. Chen, MD
Department of Neurosurgery
Mayo Clinic College of Medicine
Jacksonville, Florida, United States

**Jason Cheung, MBBS, MMedSc, MS,
 PDipMDPath, MD, MEd, FHKAM(orth),
 FRCSEd(orth)**
Clinical Associate Professor of the Department
 of Orthopaedics and Traumatology
Head of Orthopedics Department
The University of Hong Kong
Queen Mary Hospital
Pokfulam, Hong Kong SAR, China

John Chi, MD, MPH
Associate Professor of Neurosurgery
Brigham and Women's Hospital
Brigham and Women's Faulkner Hospital
Boston, Massachusetts, United States

Dean Chou, MD
Professor, Neurological Surgery
UCSF Health-UCSF Medical Center
UCSF Weill Institute for Neurosciences
San Francisco, California, United States

Michelle Clarke, MD
Professor of Neurosurgery, Orthopedics
Department of Neurosurgery
Mayo Clinic College of Medicine
Rochester, Minnesota, United States

Fabio Cofano, MD
Neurosurgery
University of Turin
Spine Surgery Unit
Humanitas Gradenigo Hospital
Turin, Italy

Scott Daffner, MD
Professor, Orthopaedics
West Virginia University
Morgantown, West Virginia, United States

Nicolas Dea, MD, MSc, FRCSC
Clinical Associate Professor Neurosurgery
Vancouver Spine Surgery Institute
Vancouver, Canada

H. Gordon Deen Jr., MD
Professor of Neurosurgery
Mayo Clinic College of Medicine
Jacksonville, Florida, United States

Christopher J. Dewald, MD
Assistant Professor, Director, Section of Spinal
    Deformity
Department of Orthopedic Surgery
Rush University Medical Center
Chicago, Illinois, United States

Luis Rodrigo Diaz Iniguez, MD
Orthopedic Surgeon
Hospital Angeles Lindavista
Mexico City, Mexico

Jeffrey Ehresman, BS
Medical Student
Johns Hopkins University School of Medicine
Baltimore, Maryland, United States

Mohamed El-Fiki, MBBCh, MS, MD
Neurosurgeon
Alexandria University
Alexandria, Egypt

Benjamin Elder, M, Ph
Neurosurgeon
Mayo Clinic College of Medicine
Rochester, Minnesota, United States

Belal Elnady, MD
Orthopedic Surgeon
Assiut University
Assiut, Egypt

Hazem Eltahawy, MD, FACS
Neurosurgeon
DMC Detroit Receiving Hospital
Harper University Hospital
Garden City Hospitals
Livonia, Michigan, United States

Esteban F. Espinoza-Garcia, MD, MSc
Neurosurgeon
Department of Neurosurgery
University of Valparaiso
San Felipe, Chile

Harrison Farber, MD
Neurosurgery Resident
Barrow Neurological Institute
Phoenix, Arizona, United States

Michael G. Fehlings, MD, PhD, FRCSC, FACS
Professor of Neurosurgery
Co-Director of the University of Toronto Spine
    Program
University of Toronto
Toronto, Canada

Brett A. Freedman, MD
Associate Professor Orthopedics
Department of Orthopedics
Mayo Clinic College of Medicine
Rochester, Minnesota, United States

Fabio Frisoli, MD
Neurosurgeon, Saint Barnabas Medical Center
Altair Health Spine and Wellness Center
Morristown, New Jersey, United States

Bhavuk Garg, MD
Associate Professor of Orthopaedics
Department of Orthopaedics
All India Institute of Medical Sciences
New Delhi, India

Ziya Gokaslan, MD, FAANS, FACS
Professor and Chair of the Department of
    Neurosurgery
The Warren Alpert Medical School of Brown
    University
Providence, Rhode Island, United States

Jeff D. Golan, MD
Chief of the Division of Neurosurgery
Jewish General Hospital
McGill University
Montreal, Quebec, Canada

Diego F Gómez, MD, MSc
Neurosurgey
Fundación Santafe de Bogotá
Bogota, Colombia

Jorge Eduardo Guzman Prenk, MD
Neurosurgeon
Pontifica Universidad Javeriana
Bogota, Colombia

Fernando Hakim, MD
Professor of Neurosurgery
Chair, Department of Neurosurgery
Hospital Universitario Fundación Santafe de
    Bogota
Bogota, Colombia

Takeshi Hara, MD
Neurosurgeon
Juntendo University
Hongo, Bunkyo-ku
Tokyo, Japan

James S. Harrop, MD, FACS
Professor, Neurological Surgery and
    Orthopedic Surgery
Division Chief, Spine and Peripheral Nerve
    Surgery
Thomas Jefferson University in Philadelphia
Philadelphia, Pennsylvania, United States

Hamid Hassanzadeh, MD
Orthopaedic Surgeon
University of Virginia
Charlottesville, Virginia, United States

John G. Heller, MD
Professor of Orthopedic Surgery
Emory University
Atlanta, Georgia United States

Sandra Hobson, MD
Assitant Professor Orthopedic Surgery
Mayo Clinic College of Medicine
Rochester, Minnesota, United States

Daniel J. Hoh, MD
Professor of Neurosurgery
University of Florida
Gainesville, Florida, United States

Langston T. Holly, MD
Neurosurgeon
Professor and Co-Vice Chair of Clinical Affairs
    for the Department of Neurosurgery
UCLA Santa Monica Medical Center
Santa Monica, California, United States

Patrick C. Hsieh, MD
Professor of Neurosurgery
Keck Medical Center of USC
Los Angeles, California, United States

Meng Huang, MD
Assistant Professor of Neurosurgery
Houston Methodist
Weill Cornell Medical College
New York, New York, United States

Paul M. Huddleston, III, M
Associate Professor in the Departments of
    Orthopedic Surgery and Neurosurgery
Department of Orthopedic Surgery
Mayo Clinic College of Medicine
Rochester, Minnesota, United States

Eyal Itshayek, M
Professor of Neurosurgery
Department of Neurosurgery
Hadassah Medical Center Ein Kerem
Jerusalem, Israel

George I. Jallo, MD
Professor of Neurosurgery
Vice Dean and Physician-in-Chief at Johns
    Hopkins All Children's Hospital
Tampa General Hospital
Tampa, Florida, United States

Maziyar A. Kalani, MD
Neurosurgeon
Mayo Clinic College of Medicine
Phoenix, Arizona, United States

Ilya Laufer, MD
Associate Professor of Neurological Surgery
Weill Cornell Medicine
New York, New York, United States

Michael T. Lawton, MD
Professor and Chair, Neurosurgery
Chief, Neurovascular Surgery
Barrow Neurological Institute
Phoenix, Arizona, United States

Aron Lazary, MD, PhD
Orthopedic Surgeon
Scientific Director, Spine Surgeon, National
    Center for Spinal Disorders
Buda Health Center
Semmelweis University
Budapest, Hungary

Lawrence G. Lenke, MD
Professor of Orthopedic Surgery
Chief, Division of Spinal Surgery
Director, Spinal Deformity Surgery
Columbia University
New York, New York, United States

Allan D. Levi, MD, PhD, FACS
Professor and Chair of Neurosurgery
University of Miami
UMHC-Sylvester Comprehensive Cancer
    Center
Miami, Florida, United States

**Yingda Li, MBBS, BMEDSC,
    PGDIPSURGANAT, FRACS**
Neurosurgeon
Brain and Spine Centre
Westmead Private Hospital
Westmead, NSW, Australia

Ann Liu, MD
Neurosurgeon
Johns Hopkins University School of Medicine
Baltimore, Maryland, United States

Sheng-Fu Lo, MD, MHS, FAANS
Professor of Neurosurgery
Director of Spinal Oncology
Johns Hopkins University School of Medicine
Baltimore, Maryland, United States

Daniel C. Lu, MD
Professor of Neurosurgery
UCLA Spine Center
UCLA Santa Monica Medical Center
Santa Monica, California, United States

Rory Mayer, MD
Neurosurgeon
Neurotrauma Consultant National Football
    League
Baylor University Medical Center
Dallas, Texas, United States

Tong Meng, MD
Orthopaedic Surgeon
Shanghai General Hospital
Shanghai Jiaotong University
Shanghai, China

Catherine Moran, MD
Consultant Neurosurgeon
Beaumont Hospital Dublin
Dublin, Ireland

Praveen Mummaneni, MD, MBA
Professor of Neurosurgery
UCSF Health-UCSF Medical Center
San Francisco, California, United States

Davide Nasi, MD
Neurosurgeon
Polytechnic University of Marche, Umberto
Ancona, Italy

Rodrigo Navarro-Ramirez, MD
Neurosurgeon
Department of Neurosurgery
McGill University
Montreal, Quebec, Canada

Jorge Navarro Bonnet, MD
Neurosurgeon
Hospital Medica Sur
Mexico City, Mexico

Tianyi Niu, MD
Assistant Professor of Neurosurgery
The Warren Alpert Medical School of Brown
    University
Providence, Rhode Island, United States

Susana Núñez-Pereira, MD, PhD
Orthopaedic Surgery
Hospital Universitario Vall d'Hebron
Barcelona, Spain

Sutipat Pairojboriboon, MD
Orthopaedic Surgeon
Vichaiyut Hospital
Phyathai, Thailand

Brenton Pennicooke, MD
Assistant Professor of Neurosurgery and
    Orthopedic Surgery
Washington University in St. Louis
St Louis, Missouri, United States

Manoj Phalak, MD, MBBS, MCh
Neurosurgery
All India Institute of Medical Sciences
New Delhi, India

Frank M. Phillips, MD
Professor, Director, Section of Minimally
    Invasive Spine Surgery
Director, Division of Spine Surgery
Rush University
Chicago, Illinois, United States

Alugolu Rajesh, MD
Professor of Neurosurgery
Department of Neurosurgery
Nizam's Institute of Medical Sciences
Punjagutta, Hyderbad, India

Juan Fernando Ramon, MD
Neurosurgeon
Department of Neurosurgery
University Hospital Fundacion Santa Fe de
    Bogata
Bogota, Columbia

K. Daniel Riew, MD
Professor, Orthopaedic Surgery
Columbia University
New York, New York, United States

Meic Schmidt, MD, MBA, FAANS, FACS
Professor of Neurosurgery
University of New Mexico Hospitals
Albuquerque, New Mexico

Daniel M. Sciubba, MD
Professor of Neurosurgery, Orthopedic Surgery
Chair & Professor of Neurosurgery at Northwell
    Health/Hofstra
Hempstead, New York, United States

Jakub Sikora, MD
Orthopaedic Surgery
University of California at San Diego
San Diego, California, United States

Justin Smith, MD
Neurosurgeon
Department of Neurosurgery
Charlottesville, Virginia, United States

Mohamed A.R. Soliman, MD, MSc, PhD
Neurosurgery
Cairo University
Cairo, Egypt

Khoi D. Than, MD
Associate Professor of Neurological Surgery
    and Orthopaedics
Duke University
Duke Raleigh Hospital
Raleigh, North Carolina, United States

Nicholas Theodore, M, M
Director, Neurosurgical Spine Center
Professor of Neurosurgery
Johns Hopkins University School of Medicine
Baltimore, Maryland, United States

Yasuaki Tokuhashi, MD
Orthopedic Surgeon
Nihon University
Tokyo, Japan

Alexander R. Vaccaro, MD, PhD, MBA
Richard H. Rothman Professor and Chairman,
    Department of Orthopaedic Surgery
President, Rothman Orthopaedic Institute
Thomas Jefferson University
Philadelphia, Pennsylvania, United States

Anand Veeravagu, MD, FAANS
Assistant Professor of Neurosurgery and
    Orthopedic Surgery
Stanford Health Care
Palo Alto, California, United States

Luiz Roberto Vialle, MD
Orthopedic Surgeon
Pontifical Catholic University of Parana
Curitiba, Brazil

Michael Y. Wang, MD, FACS
Professor of Neurosurgery
Departments of Neurological Surgery and
    Rehabilitation Medicine
University of Miami Hospital
Miami, Florida, United States

Clemens Weber, M, Ph
Consultant Neurosurgeon
Department of Neurosurgery
Stavanger University Hospital
Stavanger, Norway

Timothy Witham, MD
Professor of Neurosurgery and Orthopedic Surgery
Director, the Johns Hopkins Neurosurgery
    Spinal Fusion Laboratory
Johns Hopkins University School of Medicine
Baltimore, Maryland, United States

Jean-Paul Wolinsky, MD
Associate Professor of Neurological Surgery,
    Associate Professor of Oncology
Northwestern Memorial Hospital
Chicago, Illinois, United States

Claudio Yampolsky, MD
Chair, Department of Neurosurgery
Department of Neurosurgery
Hospital Italiano de Buenos Aires
Buenos Aires, Argentina

Jang Yoon, MD, MSc
Assistant Professor of Clinical Neurosurgery
University of Pennsylvania
Philadelphia, Pennsylvania, United States

Baron Zarate Kalfopulos, M
Orthopedic Surgeon,
Instituto Nacional de Rehabilitacion
Medica Sur
Mexico City, Mexico

Preface

The care for patients with spine disease continues to evolve as physician expertise increases, technology improves, resources grow, and access to information continues to evolve around the globe. However, there is no concise body of literature that shows how experts throughout the world in both neurosurgical and orthopedic surgery would manage a similar disease, patient, or case. To our knowledge, this book is the first attempt to evaluate how neurosurgical and orthopedic spine specialists throughout the world would handle the same patient with a specific spinal pathology in order to demonstrate the diversity of experts, ideas, and management styles and to explore how different experts around the world with different resources, technology, and cultural backgrounds would approach a similar patient. This book is part of a neurosurgical series that focuses on the spinal pathology to accompany the previous book on brain and skull base tumors, as well as future books on cerebrovascular, functional and epilepsy, pediatric, trauma, and neurocritical care. Each case is a chapter in which the patient's chief complaint, history of presenting illness, past medical and surgical history, medications and allergies, social and family history, physical examination findings, and spinal imaging are presented. Four international experts are presented with a case and each expert provides information on how he or she would handle that specific case. This will be a reference for any health care provider, trainee, and surgeon treating spinal disease by providing access to the minds of experts from around the world on management of patients despite geographic differences, differences in access to resources and technology, and even cultural differences that can potentially influence management. This book is the first of its kind to show the similarities and differences in the management of spinal cases among international experts in both neurosurgery and orthopedics from preoperative workup to operative approaches to postoperative care. We hope you enjoy it, and we hope to bring you more of these types of series in the years to come.

Kaisorn L. Chaichana
Alfredo Quinones-Hinojosa

Contents

Section 3: Spinal Deformity

Section 4: Spinal Oncology

Section 5: Other

1

Grade 1 spondylolisthesis without instability on flexion/extension and claudication

Kingsley Abode-Iyamah, MD

Introduction

Spondylolisthesis was first described by Herbiniaux, who noted the presence of a lumbar vertebrae ventral to the sacrum causing an obstruction to the progression of labor during a routine pelvic exam.[1] The term "spondylolisthesis," however, was not used until Kilian reported the cause of this condition due to the subluxation of the facet joint.[2] Lumbar spondylolisthesis is described as ventral subluxation of one vertebrae body on the other. It is classified as either congenital/dysplastic, isthmic, degenerative traumatic, or pathological based on the classification of Wiltse-Newman-MacNab, which has become the most widely accepted classification system.[3] The degree of slippage is graded based on the Meyerding, where the scale varies from grade I to V[4] (Table 1.1). Grade I spondylolisthesis is defined as slippage less than 25%, grade II is displacement up to 50%, grade III is displacement up to 75%, grade IV is displacement greater that 75%,

and grade V is defined as a complete subluxation of one body on another and is also referred to as spondyloptosis.

Example case

Chief complaint: leg and back pain

History of present illness: A 77-year-old male with a history of back and leg pain for multiple years. Over the last few months, he has had worsening back pain that radiates to his buttocks and lower extremities. He also has some numbness down his lower extremities. He can stand for an extended period time but is only able to walk around 100 yards. He has tried physical therapy without significant improvement. He also underwent an epidural injection, which gave him 1 week of relief (Fig. 1.1).

Medications: losartan, aspirin 81 mg, amlodipine, tamsulosin, simvastatin

Allergies: penicillin

Past medical and surgical history: hypertension, prostate cancer status post prostatectomy, umbilical hernia repair

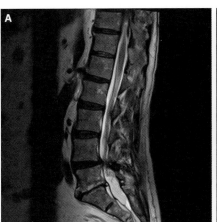 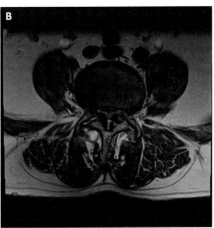

Fig. 1.1 Preoperative MRI. (A) T2 sagittal MRIs and (B) T2 axial MRIs demonstrating L4/5 grade I spondylolisthesis with facet degeneration and canal stenosis.

Family history: noncontributory
Social history: retired engineer, no smoking history, occasional alcohol
Physical exam: Awake, alert, and oriented to person, place, and time; cranial nerves II–XII intact; bilateral deltoids/triceps/ biceps 5/5; interossei 5/5; iliopsoas/knee flexion/knee extension/dorsi; and plantar flexion 5/5
Reflexes: 2+ in bilateral biceps/triceps/brachioradialis with negative Hoffman; 2+ in bilateral patella/ankle and no clonus or Babinski; sensation is intact to light touch

	Rafid Al-Mahfoudh, MBChB Neurosurgery Brighton and Sussex University Hospitals Brighton, United Kingdom	Sigurd Berven, MD Orthopedic Surgery University of California at San Francisco San Francisco, California, United States	Mohamad Bydon, MD Neurosurgery Mayo Clinic Rochester, Minnesota, United States	Sutipat Pairojboriboon, MD Orthopedic Surgery Vichaiyut Hospital Phyathai, Thailand
Preoperative				
Additional tests requested	MRI thoracic and lumbar spine Anesthesia evaluation	Standing AP and lateral lumbar x-rays Possible DEXA	Anesthesia evaluation	CT L-spine Cardiology evaluation Anesthesia evaluation
Surgical approach selected	L4–5 laminectomy	L4–5 TLIF	MIS L4 laminectomy	MIS L4–5 laminectomy
Goal of surgery	Thecal sac and lateral recess decompression	Decompression, stabilization	Nerve root decompression	Decompression, preserving lumbar motion
Perioperative				
Positioning	Prone on Wilson frame	Prone on Wilson frame	Prone	Prone on Jackson table
Surgical equipment	Fluoroscopy Surgical microscope Ultrasonic bone scalpel	Fluoroscopy	Fluoroscopy Surgical microscope Tubular retractors	Fluoroscopy IOM Surgical navigation Surgical microscope Tubular retractors
Medications	Steroids, tranexamic acid	Acetaminophen, gabapentin	None	ERAS protocol (local anesthetic, epidural steroid, short-acting narcotics, NSAIDs)
Anatomical considerations	Thecal sac, facets	Thecal sac, nerve roots	Thecal sac	L4–5 disc space, lamina, medial facets, interlaminar space, ligamentum, thecal sac, bilateral nerve roots
Complications feared with approach chosen	Spinal instability, prolonged hospital stay	Nerve root injury, spinal instability	Nerve root injury, spinal instability	Inadequate decompression, nerve root injury, dural tear
Intraoperative				
Anesthesia	General	General	General	General, ERAS
Exposure	L4	L3–5	L4 hemilamina	L4–5
Levels decompressed	L4	L4–5	L4	L4–5
Levels fused	None	L4–5	None	None

	Rafid Al-Mahfoudh, MBChB Neurosurgery Brighton and Sussex University Hospitals Brighton, United Kingdom	Sigurd Berven, MD Orthopedic Surgery University of California at San Francisco San Francisco, California, United States	Mohamad Bydon, MD Neurosurgery Mayo Clinic Rochester, Minnesota, United States	Sutipat Pairojboriboon, MD Orthopedic Surgery Vichaiyut Hospital Phyathai, Thailand
Surgical narrative	Positioned prone, paramedian needle used to localize operative level, midline incision, unilateral muscle dissection, L4 spinous process osteotomy, McCullouch retractor, x-ray to confirm level, microscope brought in, laminectomy with electric drill, bone is thinned and remainder of lamina removed with upcuts with flavectomy, lateral recess decompression continued with up cuts or ultrasonic bone scalpel, x-ray with instruments at cranial and caudal aspect of decompression, closure in layers	Positioned prone with Wilson frame elevated, expose L3–5 spinous processes, subperiosteal exposure from L3–4 to L4–5 faces with preservation of L3–4 facet, bilateral complete facetectomies at L4–5 including removal of superior articular process to the level of L5 pedicle, place L4–5 pedicle screws with x-ray to check screw placement, TLIF on more symptomatic side with banana-shaped cage for lordosis anteriorly, decorticate L4–5 transverse processes, spinal instability, arthrodesis with local bone with demineralized bone matrix, layered closure	C-arm fluoroscopy for identifying level, sequential dilators are placed over the pin, extend incision as needed, dock tubular retractors on L4 hemilamina, C-arm to confirm level, hemilaminectomy at inferior aspect of L4, removal of yellow ligament, decompression of contralateral side with over the top technique, close in anatomical layers	Positioned prone with Jackson frame, percutaneous reference pin placed on left ilium inferior to PSIS and set up of navigation system, intraoperative CT with O-arm and transfer images to work station, lower edge of L4–5 disc marked, paramedian to midline incision, tubular retractor inserted bluntly, visualize inferior laminar edge, navigation probe to assess area of decompression, thin bone with high-speed drill until insertion zone of yellow ligament reached, switch drill to diamond bur to minimize risk of damage to dura, remove yellow ligament after separating from dura, access ipsilateral lateral recess, begin decompression of nerve root at shoulder, undercut ipsilateral superior and inferior medial facets while using dissector and navigation to evaluate decompression, tilt table away to help decompress contralateral side, retract dura with nerve hook, remove remaining yellow ligament, contralateral recess exposed and decompressed, dissector and navigation to assess adequacy of decompression until passes contralateral inferior pedicle, collagen-sponge soaked steroid applied to nerve roots, standard closure with local anesthetic
Complication avoidance	Hemilaminectomy, thin bone with drill, lateral recess decompression	Preservation of L3–4 facet, remove superior articulating facet to level of the pedicle of L5 to decompress lateral recess and foramen, TLIF on more symptomatic side, anterior placed TLIF	MIS, preserving yellow ligaments, over-the-top technique for bilateral decompression	MIS, surgical navigation, alternating drill bits, decompression of nerve root at shoulder, navigation to help assess decompression, over-the-top technique for bilateral decompression
Postoperative				
Admission	Floor	Floor	Outpatient	Floor
Postop complications feared	CSF leak	Radiculopathy, infection, adjacent segment degeneration	CSF leak, nerve root injury	Inadequate decompression, nerve root injury, dural tear
Anticipated length of stay	1 day	2 days	Same-day discharge	1–2 days
Follow-up testing	Standing flexion-extension x-rays 4–6 weeks after surgery	36-inch standing films prior to discharge, 4 weeks, 3 months, 6 months, 1 year, 2 years after surgery	None	AP and lateral lumbar x-rays 6 months and then annually after surgery
Bracing	None	LSO for comfort	None	None
Follow-up visits	10 days after surgery	4 weeks, 3 months, 6 months, 1 year, 2 years after surgery	6 weeks after surgery	2 weeks, 1 month, 3 month, 6 months, annually after surgery

DEXA, Dual-energy x-ray absorptiometry; ERAS, enhanced recovery after surgery; ESI, epidural spinal injections; IOM, intraoperative monitoring; MIS, minimally invasive surgery; NSAID, nonsteroidal antiinflammatory drug; PSIS, posterior superior iliac spine.

Table 1.1 Meyerding's grading of spondylolisthesis

Grade	Description (%)
1	0–25
2	26–50
3	51–75
4	76–99
5	>100

Table 1.2 Types of spondylolisthesis

Type	Cause
Congenital/dysplastic	Malformed inferior facet
Isthmic	Defect of pars interarticularis
Degenerative	Degeneration of facet
Traumatic	Fracture that typically does not involve the pars
Pathological	Paget disease, hyperthyroidism, osteoporosis, syphilitic changes, infection, and tumor

The different types of spondylolisthesis include the following (Table 1.2):

- *Congenital/dysplastic* is a result of malformed facet joints. It predominately occurs in the lumbosacral junction. A malformed inferior facet joint may lead to enlongation of the facet joint, ultimately leading to a pars defect. Due to this congenital nature, it is commonly associated with spina bifida.[5]
- *Isthmic* is the most common form of spondylolisthesis and results from a defect of the pars interarticularis.[6] This subtype is a result of repeated microfracture and remodeling of the pars.[7–9] This is most common in young athletes who participate in high-impact sports.
- *Degenerative* results from degeneration of the facet joint. Degeneration of the joint space causes abnormal motion. The remodeling that occurs as a result of degeneration causes a more sagittal alignment of the facet, which allows progression of the spondylolisthesis.[10–12] This type is typically associated with both foraminal and canal stenosis.
- *Traumatic* is the result of a fracture that typically does not involve the pars. Over time, slippage of the vertebral body occurs following the injury.[13] This is unique in that healing can occur from simple immobilization. Fractures that are associated with an acute slippage are defined as a fracture dislocation and should be treated accordingly.
- *Pathological* are grouped into two types: generalized and local. Generalized spondylolisthesis is caused by diseases such as Paget disease, hyperthyroidism, osteoporosis, and syphilitic changes.[13, 14] The localized subtype is due to local destruction from tumors and infection. Iatrogenic cause of pathological spondylolisthesis can also be classified as localized spondylolisthesis, although some authors have classified this as its own entity.[13, 15]

Differential diagnosis

- Spondylolisthesis
- Lumbar radiculopathy
- Neurogenic claudication

Important anatomical considerations

This is a case of spondylolisthesis due to degeneration. The patient has developed grade I spondylolisthesis as a result of his degeneration. As noted in the imaging above, he also has far lateral recess stenosis as well as central canal stenosis. There are a few important points to consider in determining the approach in the caring for a patient with spondylolisthesis. All patients undergoing surgical treatment should first exhaust conservative management. This is especially true in older adult patients who have a higher risk of complications with surgical intervention. When determining the best surgical approach for this patient, it is important to take into consideration the patient's back pain. To rule out dynamic instability, it is generally recommended that a flexion-extension x-ray be obtained. Additionally, if considering an instrumented procedure, consideration should be given to obtaining a bone density scan (DEXA) to evaluate for osteoporosis. We further recommend consideration of a computed tomography (CT) scan for bony details. Given the existing spondylolisthesis, the degree of lateral recess stenosis and central stenosis is important to determine how much bony removal can be accomplished without further exacerbating instability at this level. It is been traditionally thought that one-third to half of the facet can be removed without causing instability.[16] Furthermore, the degree of evidence in the literature should also be considered. Multiple recent studies have found that spinal fusion was superior to laminectomy alone.[17, 18]

Approaches to this lesion

The treatment of spondylolisthesis can significantly vary, and this can be separated into open, minimally invasive, and anterior.[19] In the open approach, one can consider a laminectomy alone versus a laminectomy and fusion. With an open laminectomy, the goal is to decompress the stenosis in the central and lateral recesses. Inclusion of fusion with a laminectomy allows one to increase the degree of decompression because instrumented fusion allows stabilization. As above, a minimally invasive approach allows one to accomplish similar results with less destruction of the paraspinal musculature. Both open and minimally invasive instrumentation can be accomplished with interbody fusion; however, in a minimally invasive approach, an interbody fusion is necessary as posterior lateral fusion becomes difficult. Anterior approaches can be accomplished via an anterior lumbar interbody fusion followed by laminectomy or a lateral approach followed by percutaneous pedicle screw placement and decompression. A recent meta-analysis found that although lumbar lordosis, segmental lordosis, and disc height is improved with an anterior approach, there was no statistical difference in postoperative back and leg visual analogue scale (VAS) or Oswestry disability index (ODI) compared with posterior approaches.[19]

What was actually done

In this patient, who had exhausted conservative management, a posterior approach was offered. In addition to the magnetic resonance image (MRI) (Fig. 1.1) that the patient presented with, a flexion-extension x-ray of the lumbar spine was obtained (Fig. 1.2). Although the flexion-extension x-ray did not reveal dynamic instability, given the grade I spondylolisthesis in addition to the back pain, the decision was made to perform a minimally invasive transforaminal interbody fusion with bilateral facetectomy and decompression. Instrumentation was accomplished via two paraspinal 4 cm incision off midline using intraoperative navigation system with O-Arm (Medtronic, Minneapolis, MN 55432). The Nuvasive MAS TLIF pedicle-based retraction system (Nuvasive, San Diego, CA 92121) was used that allowed tissue retraction rostral-caudally as well as medial-laterally. Bilateral facetectomy was performed and central decompression via removal of the hypertrophied ligamentum flavum was accomplished. An interbody fusion was then performed via a transforaminal approach. No intraoperative monitoring was performed during the case. Postoperatively, the patient was given a lumbar corset to use for 6 weeks. The patient tolerated the procedure well with improvement of all symptoms and was discharged on postoperative day 1. During subsequent follow-up, the patient continued to do well with serial imaging showing stable instrumentation (Fig. 1.3).

Commonalities among the experts

There was a wide variability in the requested additional preoperative imaging from our expert teams. One surgeon recommended MRI of the thoracic and lumbar spine, whereas another recommend standing CT, and yet another recommended AP and lateral standing x-rays and possible DEXA scan. The majority of the surgeons recommended a laminectomy alone for this patient, and one surgeon recommended a TLIF. While all agreed that the goal of surgical intervention was decompression, the surgeon favoring a TLIF additionally had the goal of stabilization of the spine at this level. Half of the surgeons planned on an open procedure (one decompression only and one fusion) and the other half planned on a minimally invasive approach (with two preferring decompression only). The major complication feared by most surgeons was nerve root injury, although instability was also frequently mentioned. Most agreed that the patient should be admitted postoperatively with planned discharge after 1 to 2 days, and one surgeon planned same-day discharge after a minimally invasive decompression. Postoperatively, three surgeons recommended postoperative and follow-up x-rays, and only one recommended dynamic imaging.

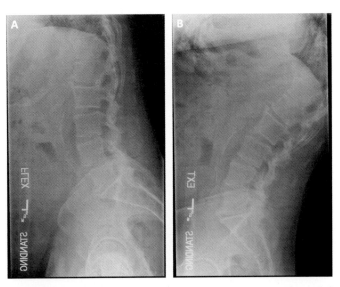

Fig. 1.2 Preoperative x-rays. (A) flexion and (B) extension x-rays showing grade I spondylolisthesis without dynamic instability.

SUMMARY OF QUALITY OF EVIDENCE TO GUIDE SPECIFIC INTERVENTIONS FOR THIS CASE

- Laminectomy versus fusion for degenerative spondylolisthesis: level I
- Anterior versus posterior approach for spondylolisthesis: level II–1

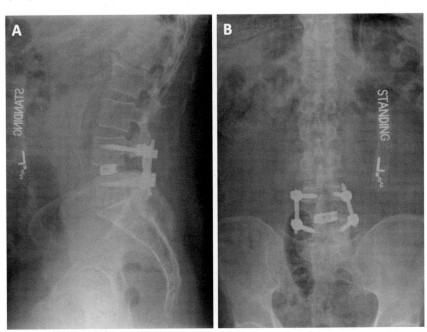

Fig. 1.3 Postoperative standing x-rays. (A) lateral and (B) AP x-rays showing L4–5 fusion.

REFERENCES

1. Neugebauer FI. The classic: A new contribution to the history and etiology of spondyl-olisthesis by F. L. Neugebauer. *Clin Orthop Relat Res*. 1976;117:4–22.
2. McPhee B Spondylolisthesis and Spondylolysis. 1990:2749–84.
3. Wiltse LL, Newman PH, Macnab I. Classification of spondylolisis and spondylolisthesis. *Clin Orthop Relat Res*. 1976;117:23–29.
4. Meyerding HW Spondylolisthesis. *Surg Gynecol Obstet* 1932;54:371–7.
5. Lim THGV. Biomechanical aspects of spondylolisthesis. *Semin Spine Surg*. 1993;5:288–296.
6. Newman PH. Stenosis of the lumbar spine in spondylolisthesis. *Clin Orthop Relat Res*. 1976;115:116–121.
7. Nachemson A, Wiltse LL. Editorial: Spondylolisthesis. *Clin Orthop Relat Res*. 1976;117:2–3.
8. White AAIPM. *Clinical Biomechanics of the Spine*. Philadelphia: JB Lippincott; 1990.
9. Wiltse LL, Jackson DW. Treatment of Spondylolisthesis and Spondylolysis in Children. *Clin Orthop Relat R*. 1976;117:92–100.
10. Grobler JL, Robertson PA, Novotny JE, Pope MH. Etiology of Spondylolisthesis - Assessment of the Role Played by Lumbar Facet Joint Morphology. *Spine*. 1993;18(1):80–91.
11. Grobler LJ, Robertson PA, Novotny JE, Ahern JW. Decompression for Degenerative Spondylolisthesis and Spinal Stenosis at L4-5 - the Effects on Facet Joint Morphology. *Spine*. 1993;18(11):1475–1482.
12. Inoue S, Watanabe T, Goto S, et al. Degenerative spondylolisthesis. Pathophysiology and results of anterior interbody fusion. *Clin Orthop Relat Res*. 1988;227:90–98.
13. Wiltse LLRS. Spondylolisthesis classification diagnosis and natural history. *Semin Spin Surg*. 1993;5:264–280.
14. Elghazawi AK. Clinical syndromes and differential diagnosis of spinal disorders. *Radiol Clin North Am*. 1991;29(4):651–663.
15. Alexander Jr. E, Kelly Jr. DL, Davis Jr. CH, et al. Intact arch spondylolisthesis. A review of 50 cases and description of surgical treatment. *J Neurosurg*. 1985;63(6):840–844.
16. Abumi K, Panjabi MM, Kramer KM, et al. Biomechanical evaluation of lumbar spinal stability after graded facetectomies. *Spine (Phila Pa 1976)*. 1990;15(11):1142–1147.
17. Chan AK, Bisson EF, Bydon M, et al. Laminectomy alone versus fusion for grade 1 lumbar spondylolisthesis in 426 patients from the prospective Quality Outcomes Database. *J Neurosurg Spine*. 2018;30(2):234–241.
18. Ghogawala Z, Dziura J, Butler WE, et al. Laminectomy plus Fusion versus Laminectomy Alone for Lumbar Spondylolisthesis. *N Engl J Med*. 2016;374(15):1424–1434.
19. Cho JY, Goh TS, Son SM, et al. Comparison of Anterior Approach and Posterior Approach to Instrumented Interbody Fusion for Spondylolisthesis: A Meta-analysis. *World Neurosurg*. 2019;129:e286–e293.

2

Lumbar degenerative spondylolisthesis

Jaime L. Martínez Santos, MD

Introduction

Low back pain is prevalent in the United States and the world,[1] and spondylolisthesis is one of the most common causes of back pain with an estimated prevalence of 11.5%.[2,3] Spondylolisthesis refers to the anterior, posterior, or rotational translation of a vertebra relative to another that occurs after an acquired (traumatic fracture, iatrogenic, etc.) or congenital bony defect in the *pars interarticularis* or a facet subluxation (see Chapter 1, Table 2). Degenerative spondylolisthesis (DS) is the most common type and affects the aging population. Patients can develop debilitating instability and neurological deficits from spinal or neuroforaminal stenosis. In this chapter, we utilize an example case to illustrate the clinical presentation and surgical management of lumbar degenerative spondylolisthesis.

Example case

Chief complaint: back pain

History of present illness: The patient is a 66-year-old female with a 3-year history of worsening back pain and no radicular symptoms. She underwent imaging for spondylolisthesis (Figs. 2.1 and 2.2).

Medications: Oxycodone, Aleve

Allergies: no known drug allergies

Past medical and surgical history: obesity with a body mass index (BMI) of 38

Family history: noncontributory

Social history: no smoking; occasional alcohol

Physical exam: awake, alert, and oriented to person, place, and time; cranial nerves II–XII intact; bilateral deltoids/triceps/biceps 5/5; interossei 5/5; iliopsoas/knee flexion/knee extension/dorsi; and plantar flexion 5/5

Reflexes: 2+ in bilateral biceps/triceps/brachioradialis with negative Hoffman; 2+ in bilateral patella/ankle and no clonus or Babinski; sensation is intact to light touch

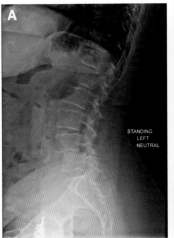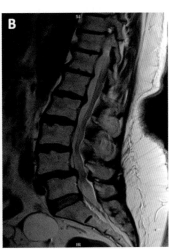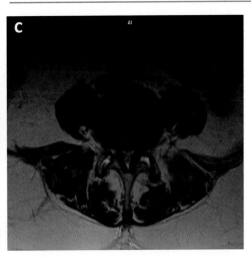

Fig. 2.1 Preoperative imaging. (A) Lateral lumbar spine x-ray. (B) T2 lumbar spine magnetic resonance image. (C) T2 axial magnetic resonance image demonstrating a grade I L4–5 lumbar spondylolisthesis with central and foraminal stenosis.

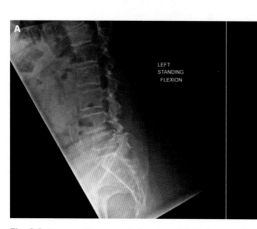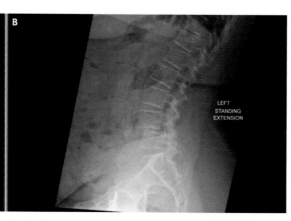

Fig. 2.2 Preoperative dynamic imaging. (A) Flexion and (B) extension lumbar x-rays showing no dynamic instability. Showing grade I spondylolisthesis with minimal dynamic instability.

	Amro F. Al-Habib, MD, MPH Neurosurgery King Khalid University Hospital King Saud University Riyadh, Saudi Arabia	John H. Chi, MD, MPH Neurosurgery Brigham and Women's Hospital Boston, Massachusetts, United States	Bhavuk Garg, MD Orthopedic Surgery All India Institute of Medical Sciences New Delhi, India	Paul M. Huddleston, III, MD Orthopedic Surgery Mayo Clinic Rochester, Minnesota, United States
Preoperative				
Additional tests requested	Scoliosis x-rays DEXA Anesthesia evaluation Sleep study Lower extremity Doppler evaluations Physical therapy	Potentially DEXA Potentially CT L-spine	Complete spine MRI DEXA	DEXA
Surgical approach selected	If physical therapy fails, posterior L4–5 decompression and fusion and TLIF	If conservative measures fail, MIS L4-F TLIF and posterior percutaneous instrumented fusion	L4–5 TLIF with MIS and robotically assisted	L4–5 TLIF
Goal of surgery	Decompression of neural elements and stabilization of segment	Indirect decompression of neural elements, reduction, and stabilization of L4–5	Indirect decompression of neural elements, stabilization	Decompress neural elements, stabilize motion segments, fusion
Perioperative				
Positioning	Prone on Jackson table, no pins	Prone	Prone	Prone on Jackson table, with pins
Surgical equipment	Fluoroscopy Surgical navigation Surgical microscope	Fluoroscopy Surgical navigation O-arm Surgical microscope	Fluoroscopy Surgical navigation O-arm Surgical robot Surgical microscope	Fluoroscopy IOM (EMG) Aquamantys® bipolar
Medications	Steroids	Liposomal bupivacaine	None	Liposomal bupivacaine, tranexamic acid
Anatomical considerations	Facet joint, pedicle, exiting and traversing nerve roots	Thecal sac, pedicles	Exiting and traversing lumbar nerve roots	Exiting and traversing lumbar nerve roots
Complications feared with approach chosen	Weakness namely foot drop, bleeding, wound dehiscence	Wound breakdown, instrument failure, nerve root injury	Nerve root injury	Durotomy, lumbar radiculopathy, wound infection
Intraoperative				
Anesthesia	General	General	General	General
Exposure	L4–5	L4–5	L4–5	L4–5
Levels decompressed	L4–5	L4–5	L4–5	L4–5
Levels fused	L4–5	L4–5	L4–5	L4–5

	Amro F. Al-Habib, MD, MPH Neurosurgery King Khalid University Hospital King Saud University Riyadh, Saudi Arabia	John H. Chi, MD, MPH Neurosurgery Brigham and Women's Hospital Boston, Massachusetts, United States	Bhavuk Garg, MD Orthopedic Surgery All India Institute of Medical Sciences New Delhi, India	Paul M. Huddleston, III, MD Orthopedic Surgery Mayo Clinic Rochester, Minnesota, United States
Surgical narrative	Position prone on Jackson table, level marking using intraoperative navigation, placement of reference frame on L3 spinous process, acquisition of images and connect to navigation system, insert navigation-guided guidewires into the pedicles of L4 and L5 bilaterally using navigated Jamshidi needles, incision of guidewires approximately 3.5 cm off of midline on both sides, confirmation with fluoroscopy, intermuscular dissection reaching right facet joint, right facetectomy under microscope with preserving bone for graft material, identification of right L5 pedicle, decompress both right L5 and L4 nerve roots, L4–5 discectomy and end plate preparation, bone graft application and cage insertion with fluoroscopy, screws are inserted over guidewires and rods are placed with compression, intraoperative O-arm to confirm accuracy of screw insertion, closure in layers, infiltration of subcutaneous Marcaine	Position prone, place reference array on iliac crest, O-arm spin and navigation acquisition, bilateral paramedian incisions, place percutaneous MIS pedicle screws at L4–5, dock MIS tubular retractor over L4–5 facet joint for TLIF, facetectomy under microscope, TLIF and cage placement, placement of auto and allograft, place rods, standard closure	Position prone, intraoperative O-arm and CT, register with surgical robot, MIS percutaneous screw insertion with robotic-assisted, placement of rod on contralateral side, placement of tubular retractor and serially dilate on ipsilateral side, TLIF with microscopic visualization, placement of bullet cage, layered closure	Position prone, x-ray to localize skin incision, posterior midline incision, x-ray to confirm levels, place pedicle screws at L4–5 bilaterally using anatomical approach, check intraoperative x-ray to confirm safe position of implants, use intraoperative EMG to stimulate implants to confirm no nerve root irritation, left facetectomy or symptomatic side of patient's leg pain, isolate exiting nerve root, perform subtotal discectomy through an annulotomy, place interbody cage packed in the interbody space with allograft with femoral head or commercially available allograft, perform manual reduction utilizing rods to fix the spine in place, complete remainder of decompression and the contralateral foramen, dilute betadine irrigation/soak, decorticate contralateral facet and bilateral transverse processes, pack remainder of the bone posteriorly and posterolaterally, final tightening of implants, layered closure without a drain, inject liposomal bupivacaine in the skin and subcutaneous tissue

	Amro F. Al-Habib, MD, MPH Neurosurgery King Khalid University Hospital King Saud University Riyadh, Saudi Arabia	John H. Chi, MD, MPH Neurosurgery Brigham and Women's Hospital Boston, Massachusetts, United States	Bhavuk Garg, MD Orthopedic Surgery All India Institute of Medical Sciences New Delhi, India	Paul M. Huddleston, III, MD Orthopedic Surgery Mayo Clinic Rochester, Minnesota, United States
Complication avoidance	Surgical navigation, minimally invasive approach, placement of cage under fluoroscopy, intraoperative imaging to confirm screw location	Minimally invasive approach in obese patient, surgical navigation, percutaneous pedicle screws	Minimally invasive approach, surgical navigation, robotically assisted, percutaneous pedicle screws	Anatomical placement of pedicle screws, use intraoperative EMG to stimulate implants to confirm no nerve root irritation, facetectomy on symptomatic side, manual reduction with rods
Postoperative				
Admission	Floor	Floor	Floor	Floor
Postoperative complications feared	Weakness namely foot drop from L5 nerve root, infection, medical complications	Instrument failure, nerve root injury	Nerve root injury	Durotomy, lumbar radiculopathy, wound infection
Anticipated length of stay	5–7 days	2 days	1–2 days	3 days
Follow-up testing	L-spine x-ray after surgery Physical therapy	L-spine x-ray 24 hours, 3 months after surgery	L-spine x-rays prior to discharge	L-spine standing AP/lateral/flexion/extension x-rays 3 months after surgery CT L-spine 3 months after surgery Bone stimulator if fusion not appearing at 3 months after surgery
Bracing	None	None	None	Lumbar corset out of bed for 3 months
Follow-up visits	1 month after surgery	4 weeks, 3 months, 12 months after surgery	2 weeks after surgery	2 weeks, 3 months, 12 months after surgery

CT, Computed tomography; DEXA, dual-energy x-ray absorptiometry; ERAS, enhanced recovery after surgery; EMG, electromyography; ESI, epidural spinal injections; IOM, intraoperative monitoring; MIS, minimally invasive surgery; TLIF, transforaminal lumbar interbody fusion.

Differential diagnosis and actual diagnosis

- Spondylolysis
- Congenital or dysplastic spondylolisthesis
- Inflammatory arthritis
- Lumbar stenosis
- Spondylolisthesis

Important anatomical and preoperative considerations

Spondylolisthesis is the slippage, subluxation, or translation of a vertebral body relative to another that occurs secondary to a variety of conditions. Six types can be identified based on the etiology: type I (dysplastic or congenital), type II (isthmic), type III (degenerative), type IV (posttraumatic), type V (pathological), and type VI (postsurgical or iatrogenic)[4] (see Chapter 1, Table 2). Degenerative spondylolisthesis (DS) is one of the most common causes of low back pain in the United States with an estimated prevalence of 11.5%[2] and is more predominant in the older adult population and females (male-to-female ratio of 1:6).[5] DS occurs secondary to spondylosis and facet subluxation in the setting of intact vertebral posterior elements. The most accepted radiographic grading system is by Meyerding,[6] which is based on the degree of anteroposterior slippage of the vertebral body in the sagittal plane: Grade I is <25%, grade II is 25% to 50%, grade III is 50% to 75%, and grade IV is 75% to 100% subluxation (see Chapter 1, Table 1).

The natural history of this condition is poorly understood. Most patients with low-grade DS can be managed nonoperatively. Approximately 75% of all patients with DS will remain asymptomatic.[7] Radiographic and clinical progression occurs in about a third of patients over a 5-year period,[7,8] and patients with preexisting neurological symptoms, lumbosacral deformity,[9] and BMI >30 are more susceptible.[10] Spontaneous symptom relief can occur over time through a process known as "spinal restabilization" characterized by disc space narrowing, ligamentous ossification, osteophyte formation, and subcartilaginous sclerosis that ultimately reduces motion at the involved segment.[7,11]

The various clinical manifestations of degenerative spondylolisthesis are the result of spinal instability, central canal stenosis or neuroforaminal stenosis (from ligamentous and facet hypertrophy, pseudodisc herniation, or both), or nerve root traction or tension. Common presentations include mechanical back pain (especially with extension), referred lumbar facet pain with hamstring tightness, radiculopathy, neurogenic claudication, and sphincter disturbance.[11] Some indications for surgery include failure of conservative management, intolerable pain or instability when upright or with ambulation, spondylolisthesis grade II or higher, or spondylolisthesis grade I with symptomatic spinal stenosis (neurogenic claudication, radiculopathy, or sphincter disturbance) or with proven dynamic instability on flexion-extension x-rays.[5,8,11] Acute neurological deficits or cauda equina syndrome with sphincter disturbance or saddle anesthesia warrant immediate attention.

The surgical management of spondylolisthesis is directed at decompressing the involved spinal canal and neuroforamina, reducing the spondylolisthesis, and stabilizing the spine. The most common technique is a transforaminal lumbar interbody fusion (TLIF), which fuses all three columns of the spine and allows for a thorough direct spinal canal and neuroforaminal decompression via laminotomy or laminectomy, facetectomy and discectomy, indirect neuroforaminal decompression via placement of an intervertebral cage, anatomical reduction of the spondylolisthesis, and spinal stabilization via placement of pedicle screws (in addition to the intervertebral cage). A simple decompression (laminectomy and foraminotomy) can be an effective option in selected patients who are older, poor surgical candidates or poor candidates for spinal fusion (smokers, osteopenia, osteoporosis, etc.), or without hypermobility (no dynamic instability on flexion-extension x-rays).[5,11] Surgery for decompression, fusion, or both can be performed using a traditional "open" approach with a midline incision or smaller paramedian incisions (usually multiple) with a paraspinal muscle-splitting approach or minimally invasive surgery (MIS). MIS techniques have been increasingly used. A meta-analysis comparing open versus MIS approaches in patients with spondylolisthesis showed no significant difference in complication rates or functional or pain outcomes and demonstrated that MIS was associated with reduced intraoperative blood loss and shortened hospitalization.[12] A subgroup analysis of prospective studies showed, however, that MIS was associated with longer operative times,[12] which could represent the learning curve of this newer approach. A more recent study[2] found no significant difference in operative times. Both approaches appear to have similar fusion rates,[13] but long-term data are needed to better assess for this. Neuronavigation can serve as an adjunct for hardware placement and reduces radiation exposure.

What was actually done

The patient's progressive symptoms correlated with the mobile degenerative spondylolisthesis. It was therefore decided to offer an open decompression and fusion via a L4–5 TLIF. She was taken to the operating room and surgery was performed under general anesthesia. The spinal level was confirmed with fluoroscopy, and customary subperiosteal dissection exposed the L4 and L5 posterior elements including the transverse processes. A bilateral L4 laminectomy and a right-sided L4–5 TLIF (facetectomy, microdiscectomy, and placement of lordotic intervertebral body cage) was done. The contralateral (left) L4–5 neuroforamina was thoroughly decompressed with a medial facetectomy. Bilateral L4 and L5 pedicle screws were placed freehand using anatomical landmarks and lateral fluoroscopy guidance. Bilateral rods were locked after reducing the spondylolisthesis. The remaining left L4–5 facet and transverse processes were decorticated, and local and iliac crest autograft and allograft were placed. The wound was closed in anatomical planes. The patient did well postoperatively and reported resolution of back pain. At 3-months' follow-up, the patient remained pain-free and imaging (Fig. 2.3) showed proper spine alignment and no hardware complication.

Commonalities among experts

Most surgeons would obtain a preoperative bone density scan to assess bone mineralization in order to determine candidacy for fusion and need for activity modifications and calcium and vitamin D supplementation. Half advocated for surgery after failing an initial conservative management. All surgeons recommended a single-level unilateral L4–5 TLIF and most preferred an MIS approach with navigated percutaneous pedicle screw placement. The goals of surgery were always nerve decompression first and reduction of spondylolisthesis and spinal stabilization second. Most surgeons would use neuronavigation for screw placement. Half would use local anesthetic (liposomal bupivacaine) as adjuvant for perioperative pain management. Commonly feared complications included nerve injury with postoperative neurological deficit such as foot drop, hardware failure, wound breakdown, and cerebrospinal fluid (CSF) leakage. Most surgeons would obtain immediate postoperative and 3-month standing x-rays. Follow-up is scheduled 2 to 4 weeks postoperatively.

SUMMARY OF QUALITY OF EVIDENCE TO GUIDE SPECIFIC INTERVENTIONS FOR THIS CASE

- Surgical treatment of degenerative lumbar spondylolisthesis offers superior clinical outcomes: level IA.[14]
- A preoperative dynamic lumbosacral flexion-extension x-ray should be obtained in all patients with spondylolisthesis: level IB.
- Surgical treatment of lumbar spondylolisthesis is recommended for grade II and higher and symptomatic grade I: level IC.
- Instrumented fusion is recommended as it may result in superior clinical outcomes and lower reoperation rates: level I.

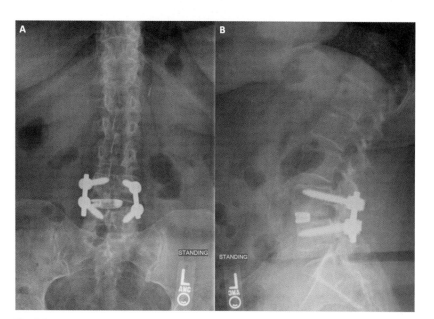

Fig. 2.3 Postoperative standing. (A) anteroposterior and (B) lateral x-rays showing reduction of the spondylolisthesis and good lumbar spine alignment.

REFERENCES

1. Martinez Santos JL, Alshareef M, Kalhorn SP. Back Pain and Radiculopathy from Non-Steroidal Anti-Inflammatory Drug-induced Dorsal Epidural Haematoma. *BMJ Case Reports.* 2019;12(3):e229015.
2. Bisson EF, Mummaneni PV, Virk MS, et al. Open versus minimally invasive decompression for low-grade spondylolisthesis: analysis from the Quality Outcomes Database. *J Neurosurg Spine.* 2020:1–11.
3. Waterman BR, Belmont Jr. PJ, Schoenfeld AJ. Low back pain in the United States: incidence and risk factors for presentation in the emergency setting. *Spine J.* 2012;12(1):63–70.
4. Wiltse LL, Newman PH, Macnab IAN. Classification of Spondyloisis and Spondylolisthesis. *Clinical Orthopaedics and Related Research (1976–2007).* 1976;117:23–29.
5. Bydon M, Alvi MA, Goyal A. Degenerative Lumbar Spondylolisthesis: Definition, Natural History, Conservative Management, and Surgical Treatment. *Neurosurg Clin N Am.* 2019;30(3):299–304.
6. Meyerding HW. Diagnosis and Roentgenologic Evidence in Spondylolisthesis. *Radiology.* 1933;20(2):108–120.
7. Matsunaga S, Sakou T, Morizono Y, et al. Natural history of degenerative spondylolisthesis. Pathogenesis and natural course of the slippage. *Spine (Phila Pa 1976).* 1990;15(11):1204–1210.
8. Karsy M, Bisson EF. Surgical Versus Nonsurgical Treatment of Lumbar Spondylolisthesis. *Neurosurg Clin N Am.* 2019;30(3):333–340.
9. Martinez Santos JL, Dmytriw AA, Fermin S. Neurosurgical management of a large meningocele in Jarcho-Levin syndrome: clinical and radiological pearls. *BMJ case reports.* 2015;2015 bcr2015210240.
10. Cushnie D, Johnstone R, Urquhart JC, et al. Quality of Life and Slip Progression in Degenerative Spondylolisthesis Treated Nonoperatively. *Spine (Phila Pa 1976).* 2018;43(10):E574–E579.
11. Koreckij TD, Fischgrund JS. Degenerative Spondylolisthesis. *J Spinal Disord Tech.* 2015;28(7):236–241.
12. Lu VM, Kerezoudis P, Gilder HE, et al. Minimally Invasive Surgery Versus Open Surgery Spinal Fusion for Spondylolisthesis: A Systematic Review and Meta-analysis. *Spine (Phila Pa 1976).* 2017;42(3):E177–E185.
13. Jin-Tao Q, Yu T, Mei W, et al. Comparison of MIS vs. open PLIF/TLIF with regard to clinical improvement, fusion rate, and incidence of major complication: a meta-analysis. *Eur Spine J.* 2015;24(5):1058–1065.
14. Chan AK, Sharma V, Robinson LC, Mummaneni PV. Summary of Guidelines for the Treatment of Lumbar Spondylolisthesis. *Neurosurg Clin N Am.* 2019;30(3):353–364.

3

Recurrent herniated disc at the same level in a young patient

Kingsley Abode-Iyamah, MD

Introduction

The intervertebral disc allows axial loading that results from an upright posture of the spine. The disc is composed of two components, the outer fibrous annulus fibrosus and the central nucleus pulposus, and originates from the notochord. The nucleus pulposus is composed of proteoglycans and water gels held together by type II collagen and elastin fibers. These acts as a shock absorber that helps distribute forces across the end plates. Degeneration over time causes loss of the water content of the nucleus pulposus as well as weakened annulus fibrosus. There is an increase in disc herniations from the ages of 30 to 50 years that decreases after the age of 50.[1] Although the exact cause leading to degeneration and herniation is not fully understood, it appears that sedentary occupations, previous full-term pregnancy, physical inactivity, increased body mass, tall stature, and smoking act as risk factors.[2]

Disc reherniation following an initial surgery is defined as recurrent herniation ipsilateral or contralateral at a previously operated level with return of symptoms after a 6-month symptom-free interval following the index surgery and is reported to occur 25% of the time.[3, 4] Although surgical techniques have advanced since the initial description of the technique by Mixter and Barr, recurrent disc herniations continue to remain a problem.[5] The incidence of reoperation for recurrent disc herniation continues to remain as high as 18%.[6–18] Although recurrent herniation is common, it should be noted that recurrence of radicular symptoms can also occur from ongoing degeneration, causing foraminal stenosis or excessive epidural scarring resulting in nerve compression. The initial approach to the management of recurrent symptoms due to disc reherniation should remain unchanged from the initial management of disc herniation. This involves physical therapy, nonsteroidal pain management, chiropractic manipulation, and consideration of epidural injection for symptomatic relief. In cases where there is failure of improvement after nonoperative management or when there is neurological deficit, surgical intervention should be considered. The surgical approach following reherniation consists of redo discectomy versus fusion.[19]

Example case

Chief complaint: left leg pain

History of present illness: A 49-year-old female with a history of previous L5-S1 hemilaminectomy and discectomy 3 months prior to presentation (Fig. 3.1). After 2 hours sitting in a car, the patient started having left-sided radicular pain in S1 distribution. She has tried gabapentin and Tylenol with minimal relief. She states that her pain is very severe at this time and is debilitating. She is unable to sleep at night. She presents due to ongoing pain. She notes numbness but denies weakness. She underwent repeat imaging (Fig. 3.2).

Medications: gabapentin, losartan

Allergies: nonsteroidal antiinflammatory drugs

Past medical and surgical history: Hodgkin lymphoma, depression, anxiety, reflux, hypertension, tubal ligation, thymus biopsy, cesarean section (C-section), C5-6 anterior cervical discectomy and fusion, ileostomy

Family history: noncontributory

Social history: teacher, no smoking history, occasional alcohol

Physical exam: awake, alert, and oriented to person, place, and time; cranial nerves II-XII, intact bilateral deltoids/triceps/biceps 5/5; interossei 5/5; iliopsoas/knee flexion/knee extension/dorsi, and plantar flexion 5/5

Reflexes: 2+ in bilateral biceps/triceps/brachioradialis with negative Hoffman; 2+ in bilateral patella/ankle with no clonus or Babinski; sensation decreased in left S1 distribution

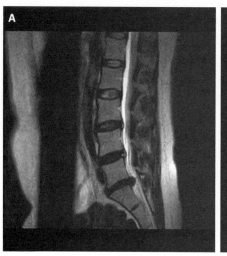
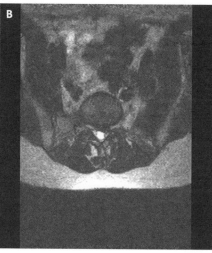

Fig. 3.1 Magnetic resonance images prior to patient's first surgery. (A) T2 sagittal and (B) T2 axial images demonstrating a left L5-S1 disc herniation with lateral recess stenosis.

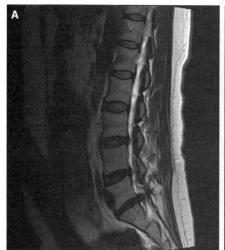
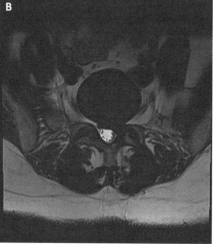

Fig. 3.2 Repeat magnetic resonance images demonstrating reherniation. (A) T2 sagittal and (B) T2 axial images demonstrating a recurrent left L5-S1 disc herniation with lateral recess stenosis.

	Selby Chen, MD Neurosurgery Mayo Clinic Jacksonville, Florida, United States	Christopher J. Dewald, MD Orthopedic Surgery Rush University Medical Center Chicago, Illinois, United States	Bhavuk Garg, MD Orthopedic Surgery All India Institute of Medical Sciences New Delhi, India	Eyal Itshayek, MD Neurosurgery Hadassah Medical Center Jerusalem, Israel
Preoperative				
Additional tests requested	None	Complete history and physical	CT L-spine MRI L-spine DEXA	L5-S1 transforaminal steroid injection MRI L-spine Anesthesia evaluation
Surgical approach selected	Revision left-sided L5-S1 microdiscectomy	Pending above, left L5-S1 TLIF and right L5-S1 percutaneous fusion	L5-S1 TLIF, MIS, and robotically assisted	Revision left-sided L5-S1 laminectomy and microdiscectomy
Goal of surgery	Decompress traversing S1 nerve root	Decompress traversing S1 nerve root, fusion if needed	Decompress traversing S1 nerve root, pain relief	Decompress traversing S1 nerve root

	Selby Chen, MD Neurosurgery Mayo Clinic Jacksonville, Florida, United States	Christopher J. Dewald, MD Orthopedic Surgery Rush University Medical Center Chicago, Illinois, United States	Bhavuk Garg, MD Orthopedic Surgery All India Institute of Medical Sciences New Delhi, India	Eyal Itshayek, MD Neurosurgery Hadassah Medical Center Jerusalem, Israel
Perioperative				
Positioning	Prone	Prone on Jackson table	Prone	Prone on Wilson frame
Surgical equipment	Fluoroscopy Surgical microscope	Fluoroscopy Surgical microscope	Fluoroscopy O-arm Surgical robot Tubular retractors Surgical microscope	Fluoroscopy McCulloch or Taylor retractor set
Medications	Steroids	None	None	None
Anatomical considerations	Thecal sac, medial facet joints	Left S1 nerve roots	Exiting and traversing nerve roots	L5-S1 disc space, lamina, medial facets, thecal sac, left S1 nerve root
Complications feared with approach chosen	Instability	Nerve root injury, CSF leak, pseudoarthrosis, screw malposition	Nerve root injury	Nerve root injury, CSF leak
Intraoperative				
Anesthesia	General	General	General	General
Exposure	L5-S1	L5-S1	L5-S1	L5-S1
Levels decompressed	L5-S1	L5-S1	L5-S1	L5-S1
Levels fused	None	L5-S1	L5-S1	None
Surgical narrative	Position prone, incision over previous lumbosacral incision, identify level using lateral fluoroscopic shot, dissect soft tissue off of remaining L5 lamina on left side in subperiosteal fashion, identify normal landmarks, dissect scar tissue off of bone and dura under microscopic visualization, establish normal anatomical plane between traversing S1 nerve root and medial facet joint, extend hemilaminotomy or medial fasectomy if needed, retract common thecal sac and S1 nerve root medially, incise disc space with 11 blade, remove disc herniation with pituitary rongeur, bone wax to bleeding bone edges, wound closed in anatomical layers	Position prone, x-ray to determine level, posterior slightly extend incision over prior incision if in appropriate location, use Cobb to expose bony lamina adjacent to prior defect, place pedicle screws to distract and open foramen, remove left-sided facet to expose nerve root and disc herniation, decompress nerve root, remove disc material, scrap out disc material and cartilaginous end plates, size intervertebral biomechanical strut device, pack with allograft cancellous bone until firm using interbody impact or to where x-ray looks like it is fused, place bone packed cage (PEEK or titanium) and push toward midbody, place rod on left and compress, percutaneous screws on right with fluoroscopy, place right percutaneous rods, layered closure with drain	Position prone, intraoperative O-arm with CT and robot registration, MIS percutaneous screw insertion using robot, placement of rod on contralateral side, placement of tubular retractor, serially dilate on ipsilateral side, perform TLIF with microscopic visualization, placement of bullet cage, placement of ipsilateral rod, layered closure	Position prone, identify level with x-ray and mark L5-S1 disc, midline incision through previous surgical scar, dissect through scar tissue, look for normal brain anatomy, expose inferior edge of L5 lamina and superior edge of S1 lamina and medial edge of L5-S1 facet, identify borders of previous laminectomy, resect inferior edge of left superior lamina with Kerrison rongeur until normal dura is exposed and entrance to lateral recess revealed, undercut ipsilateral medial facet, decompress nerve roots starting at shoulder of root with Kerrison parallel and just superficial to the root, identify left S1 nerve root, release nerve roots from previous surgery scar tissue and adhesions, mobilize it medially using nerve root retractor to expose disc herniation, confirm adequate decompression verified with Frazier dural dissector via lateral recess to the neural foramen, layered closure

	Selby Chen, MD Neurosurgery Mayo Clinic Jacksonville, Florida, United States	Christopher J. Dewald, MD Orthopedic Surgery Rush University Medical Center Chicago, Illinois, United States	Bhavuk Garg, MD Orthopedic Surgery All India Institute of Medical Sciences New Delhi, India	Eyal Itshayek, MD Neurosurgery Hadassah Medical Center Jerusalem, Israel
Complication avoidance	Identify normal landmarks, extend bone work if needed	Identify normal landmarks, place pedicle screws to distract disc space, significant packing of disc space with allograft bone, decompression from left and placement of right percutaneous pedicle screws	MIS, robotically assisted, percutaneous screws	Look for normal anatomy, decompress nerve roots starting at shoulder of root with Kerrison parallel and just superficial to the root, confirm adequate decompression verified with Frazier dural dissector via lateral recess to the neural foramen
Postoperative				
Admission	Floor	Floor	Floor	Floor
Postoperative complications feared	Wound dehiscence, radiculitis, CSF leak	Nerve root injury, CSF leak, pseudoarthrosis, screw malposition	Nerve root injury, durotomy	Nerve root injury, CSF leak, wound infection
Anticipated length of stay	Overnight	1–2 days	1–2 days	1 day
Follow-up testing	None	L-spine x-rays prior to discharge and 3 weeks after surgery	L-spine x-rays prior to discharge	None
Bracing	None	None	None	None
Follow-up visits	4–6 weeks after surgery	3 weeks after surgery	2 weeks after surgery	6 weeks after surgery

CSF, Cerebrospinal fluid; DEXA, dual-energy x-ray absorptiometry; IOM, intraoperative monitoring; MIS, minimally invasive surgery; PEEK, polyether ether ketone; TLIF, transforaminal lumbar interbody fusion.

Differential diagnosis

- Lumbar disc reherniation
- Spinal instability
- Failed back syndrome

Important anatomical considerations

The above patient presented with reherniation of the disc at the previously operated L5-S1 level. Although the L4-5 location represents the most common level for reherniation due to the increased motion at this level compared with other segments, increased load at L5-S1 may predispose this level for reherniation as well. Important consideration in addressing disc reherniation is to determine how much bone was removed from the initial surgery. Related to this, the surgeon must determine whether there is instability at this level, which may be contributing to the reherniation. For this reason, it is essential to obtain flexion-extension x-rays to look for dynamic movement at the lumbar segment (Fig. 3.3). Reoperation in this location requires identification of the bony elements above and below the previous laminectomy and sharp dissection to identify the dural plane. We advocated additional bony removal if needed to identify a normal dural plane rostrally to allow identification of the scar-dural plane to assist in dissection.

Approaches to this lesion

Redo laminectomy and discectomy for reherniation of a lumbar disc herniation can be accomplished through an open or minimally invasive approach via tubular system. Additionally, one can consider a fusion operation following recurrent disc herniation. Currently, data suggest similar outcomes in patients undergoing redo discectomy after first-time reherniation versus fusion.[20] It is therefore our practice to attempt redo discectomy after the first reherniation followed by a fusion procedure if there is a third episode of herniation. A recent meta-analysis by Tanavalee et al. showed a reoperation rate following discectomy of 9% versus 2% for fusion.[4, 19] Although there was a lower rate of reoperation following fusion operation for reherniation, the main reason for reoperation following a fusion was for hardware removal and adjacent segment disease.[19] In patients who underwent discectomy, the main reason for reoperation was for reherniation, although there was no statistical difference in the rate of reoperation.[19] Additionally, there was no noted difference between the two groups regarding operative time and length of stay.[19]

What was actually done

The patient underwent a flexion-extension x-ray to rule out instability. After it was determined that there was not instability, the patient was offered a minimally invasive discectomy via a tubular approach. A 1.5 cm off midline incision was chosen. Given that the patient underwent a previous open laminectomy and discectomy, care was taken to dock on the rostral remaining laminar to allow dilation for a minimally invasive approach. A small laminotomy was performed. Sharp dissection was performed and the dural edge was identified. Dissection was then carried out caudally. The herniated disc material was identified

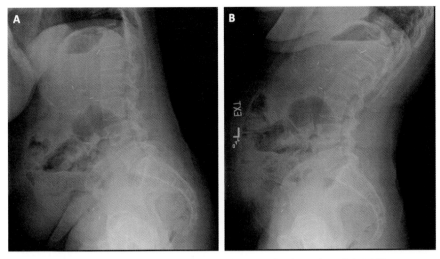

Fig. 3.3 Preoperative x-rays. (A) flexion and (B) extension x-rays showing no dynamic instability.

and removed. The traversing nerve root was identified and completely decompressed. The 2 cm incision was closed. The patient ambulated the same day with a lumbar corset for comfort and discharged on postoperative day 1.

Commonalities among the experts

The approach to this pathology varied significantly among our experts, who were evenly split in their recommendations. Half of our experts recommended additional imaging such as a magnetic resonance image (MRI) and computed tomography (CT), whereas half recommended transforaminal epidural injection. Half of the experts recommended revision laminectomy and microdiscectomy, and the other half recommended a transforaminal lumbar interbody fusion (TLIF) at this level. All recommended a posterior approach with the goals of decompressing the compromised nerve root, with three preferring a minimally invasive approach. While three surgeons were concerned with nerve root injury, spinal instability was a concern for the one surgeon who recommended redo laminectomy and microdiscectomy. All patients were recommended a one- to two-night hospital stay postoperatively, while only those who underwent fusion had planned additional imaging.

SUMMARY OF QUALITY OF EVIDENCE TO GUIDE SPECIFIC INTERVENTIONS FOR THIS CASE

- Redo microdiscectomy versus fusion for disc reherniation: level II–1

REFERENCES

1. Miller JA, Schmatz C, Schultz AB. Lumbar disc degeneration: correlation with age, sex, and spine level in 600 autopsy specimens. *Spine (Phila Pa 1976).* 1988;13(2):173–178.
2. Rajasekaran S, Babu JN, Arun R, et al. ISSLS prize winner: A study of diffusion in human lumbar discs: a serial magnetic resonance imaging study documenting the influence of the endplate on diffusion in normal and degenerate discs. *Spine (Phila Pa 1976).* 2004;29(23):2654–2667.
3. Ambrossi GL, McGirt MJ, Sciubba DM, et al. Recurrent lumbar disc herniation after single-level lumbar discectomy: incidence and health care cost analysis. *Neurosurgery.* 2009;65(3):574–578; discussion 8.
4. Fritzell P, Knutsson B, Sanden B, et al. Recurrent Versus Primary Lumbar Disc Herniation Surgery: Patient-reported Outcomes in the Swedish Spine Register Swespine. *Clin Orthop Relat Res.* 2015;473(6):1978–1984.
5. Mixter WJBJ. Rupture of the intervertebral disc with involvement of the spinal canal. *N Engl J Med.* 1934;211(5):210–215.
6. Carragee EJ, Han MY, Suen PW, Kim D. Clinical outcomes after lumbar discectomy for sciatica: the effects of fragment type and anular competence. *J Bone Joint Surg Am.* 2003;85(1):102–108.
7. Carragee EJ, Spinnickie AO, Alamin TF, Paragioudakis S. A prospective controlled study of limited versus subtotal posterior discectomy: short-term outcomes in patients with herniated lumbar intervertebral discs and large posterior anular defect. *Spine (Phila Pa 1976).* 2006;31(6):653–657.
8. Daneyemez M, Sali A, Kahraman S, et al. Outcome analyses in 1072 surgically treated lumbar disc herniations. *Minim Invasive Neurosurg.* 1999;42(2):63–68.
9. Fountas KN, Kapsalaki EZ, Feltes CH, et al. Correlation of the amount of disc removed in a lumbar microdiscectomy with long-term outcome. *Spine (Phila Pa 1976).* 2004;29(22):2521–2524. discussion 5-6.
10. Henriksen L, Schmidt K, Eskesen V, Jantzen E. A controlled study of microsurgical versus standard lumbar discectomy. *Br J Neurosurg.* 1996;10(3):289–293.
11. Kim CH, Chung CK, Park CS, et al. Reoperation rate after surgery for lumbar herniated intervertebral disc disease: nationwide cohort study. *Spine (Phila Pa 1976).* 2013;38(7):581–590.
12. Leven D, Passias PG, Errico TJ, et al. Risk Factors for Reoperation in Patients Treated Surgically for Intervertebral Disc Herniation: A Subanalysis of Eight-Year SPORT Data. *J Bone Joint Surg Am.* 2015;97(16):1316–1325.
13. Malter AD, McNeney B, Loeser JD, Deyo RA. 5-year reoperation rates after different types of lumbar spine surgery. *Spine (Phila Pa 1976).* 1998;23(7):814–820.
14. Martin BI, Mirza SK, Flum DR, et al. Repeat surgery after lumbar decompression for herniated disc: the quality implications of hospital and surgeon variation. *Spine J.* 2012;12(2):89–97.
15. McGirt MJ, Eustacchio S, Varga P, et al. A prospective cohort study of close interval computed tomography and magnetic resonance imaging after primary lumbar discectomy: factors associated with recurrent disc herniation and disc height loss. *Spine (Phila Pa 1976).* 2009;34(19):2044–2051.
16. Osterman H, Sund R, Seitsalo S, Keskimaki I. Risk of multiple reoperations after lumbar discectomy: a population-based study. *Spine (Phila Pa 1976).* 2003;28(6):621–627.
17. Thome C, Barth M, Scharf J, Schmiedek P. Outcome after lumbar sequestrectomy compared with microdiscectomy: a prospective randomized study. *J Neurosurg Spine.* 2005;2(3):271–278.
18. Weber H. Lumbar disc herniation. A controlled, prospective study with ten years of observation. *Spine (Phila Pa 1976).* 1983;8(2):131–140.

19. Tanavalee CLW, Yingsakmongkol W, Luksanapruksa P, Singhatanadgige W. A comparison between repeat discectomy versus fusion for the treatment of recurrent lumbar disc herniation: Systematic review and meta-analysis. *J Clin Neurosci.* 2019;66:202–208.

20. Kerezoudis P, Goncalves S, Cesare JD, et al. Comparing outcomes of fusion versus repeat discectomy for recurrent lumbar disc herniation: A systematic review and meta-analysis. *Clin Neurol Neurosurg.* 2018;171:70–78.

4

Adjacent segment disease after anterior cervical decompression and fusion

Jaime L. Martínez Santos, MD

Introduction

Anterior cervical decompressions and fusions (ACDFs) are one of the most common spine surgeries worldwide and the gold standard treatment for symptomatic cervical spondylosis.[1] Adjacent segment disease is a very common sequela and occurs in about 26% of all patients within 10 years from surgery[2] requiring reoperation. The best treatment modality is a matter of debate and should be tailored to the patient. In this chapter, we present a case of adjacent segment disease following ACDF.

Example case

Chief complaint: neck pain and hoarseness

History of present illness: The patient is a 62-year-old female with a history of three prior anterior cervical decompressions and fusions (ACDFs) spanning from C3 to C6. She was referred for worsening neck pain over the past 3 months. Her pain was mechanical in nature and there was no accompanying radiculopathy. She denied weakness or difficulty ambulating. She underwent imaging concerning for cervical kyphotic deformity with C5–6 pseudoarthrosis and adjacent segment degeneration at C2–3 and C6-T1, causing spinal cord compression and neuroforaminal stenosis (Fig. 4.1).

Medications: none

Allergies: no known drug allergies

Past medical history: none

Past surgical history: previous three ACDFs (the most recent was 1 year ago)

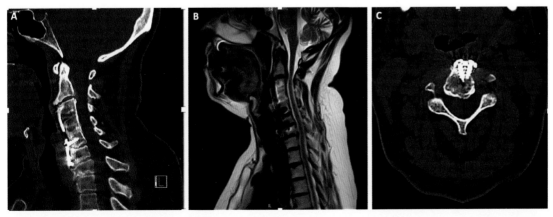

Fig. 4.1 Preoperative imaging. (A and C), Sagittal and axial computed tomography (CT) bone windows demonstrating sagittal malalignment secondary to cervical kyphotic deformity and two separate ACDF plates spanning C3–6 with appropriate fusion from C3 to 5 and incomplete fusion and pseudoarthrosis at C5–6. Note the superior plate overlying the C2–3 disc space resulting in adjacent segment ossification and osteophyte formation. (B) Sagittal T2 magnetic resonance image demonstrating adjacent segment degeneration at C2–3 and C6-T1, causing spinal cord compression and neuroforaminal stenosis.

Family history: noncontributory

Social history: none

Physical exam: awake, alert, and oriented to person, place, and time; cranial nerves II-XII intact, bilateral deltoids, biceps, triceps, grip, and hand intrinsic muscles 5/5; iliopsoas, knee flexion, knee extension, dorsiflexion, plantar flexion 5/5. Reflexes: 2+ in bilateral biceps, triceps, brachioradialis with negative Hoffman; 2+ in bilateral patella and ankle and no clonus or Babinski; sensation is intact to light touch.

	Alvaro Camparo, MD Ramiro Barrera, MD Neurosurgery Hospital Padilla–Tucuman Universidad Nacional de Tucuman Tucuman, Argentina	Scott Daffner, MD Orthopedic Surgery West Virginia University Morgantown, West Virginia, United States	Daniel C. Lu, MD, PhD Neurosurgery University of California at Los Angeles Los Angeles, California, United States	Luiz Robert Vialle, MD Orthopedic Surgery Pontifical Catholic University of Parana Curitiba, Brazil
Preoperative				
Additional tests requested	C-spine dynamic x-ray C-spine dynamic MRI	C-spine upright/AP/lateral/flexion/extension x-ray DEXA Laboratories (CBC/ESR/CRP/vitamin D/calcium)	C-spine flexion-extension x-rays DEXA Endocrinology evaluation Anesthesia evaluation	C-spine MRI axial Dynamic x-rays Vocal cord evaluation
Surgical approach selected	Anterior C2–3 decompression and fusion	Posterior C4-T2 fusion	Posterior C2-T2 fusion with possible C2-C3 laminectomy/decompression	If conservative management fails, anterior C2–3, C5–6, and C6–7 decompression and fusion
Goal of surgery	Decompression, fusion	Treatment of pseudoarthrosis, fusion	Treatment of pseudoarthrosis for pain and spinal cord protection	Decompression, cervical lordosis reconstruction
Perioperative				
Positioning	Supine	Prone, with Mayfield pins	Prone, with Mayfield pins	Supine
Surgical equipment	Fluoroscopy Surgical microscope PEEK implant	IOM (MEP/SSEP) Fluoroscopy	IOM (MEP/SSEP) Fluoroscopy Surgical navigation	Wired endotracheal tube Nasopharyngeal tube
Medications	NSAIDs	Maintain MAP >80	None	None
Anatomical considerations	Carotid sheath, trachea, esophagus	Vertebral artery, nerve roots	Vertebral artery, midline avascular plane	Carotid artery, esophagus, vertebral artery, laryngeal nerve
Complications feared with approach chosen	Dysphagia, recurrent laryngeal nerve palsy, hematoma, esophageal perforation	Wound infection, hematoma, adjacent segment disease	Pseudoarthrosis	Esophageal fistula, dysphonia
Intraoperative				
Anesthesia	General	General	General	General
Exposure	C2–3	C4-T2	C2-T2	C2-C7
Levels decompressed	C2–3	None	None	C2–3, C5–6, C6–7
Levels fused	C2–3	C4-T2	C2-T2	C2-C7

	Alvaro Camparo, MD Ramiro Barrera, MD Neurosurgery Hospital Padilla–Tucuman Universidad Nacional de Tucuman Tucuman, Argentina	Scott Daffner, MD Orthopedic Surgery West Virginia University Morgantown, West Virginia, United States	Daniel C. Lu, MD, PhD Neurosurgery University of California at Los Angeles Los Angeles, California, United States	Luiz Robert Vialle, MD Orthopedic Surgery Pontifical Catholic University of Parana Curitiba, Brazil
Surgical narrative	Position supine, right transverse cervical neck incision, vertical incision in platysma, blunt dissection between sternocleidomastoid and carotid sheath, retract carotid sheath laterally and trachea/esophagus medially, confirmation of space with needle and fluoroscopy, separation of longus colli muscles, discectomy with microscope, percutaneous bone graft extraction with needle biopsy of iliac crest, placement of PEEK with screws in the space, closure with a drain	Baseline IOM, position prone, confirm alignment with x-ray, midline posterior incision, subperiosteal dissection to expose C4–7 lateral masses and proximal transverse processes of T1 and T2, place lateral mass screws from C4–6 and T1–2 pedicle screws bilaterally, possible spinous process wires at C5–6 if poor bone quality, seat rods in screws and apply caps with little extra rod proximally if fusion construct needs to be extended, harvest iliac crest bone graft, irrigate cervical wound, decorticate exposed posterior bone, pack cancellous bone graft over decorticated bone, layered closure with subfascial drain	Position prone in neutral neck position with attention to angle of gaze, mark midline incision based on anatomical landmarks, midline posterior incision, dissect to posterior elements in midline avascular plane, x-ray to localize, expose C2-T2, navigation spin, drill bilateral lateral mass pilot holes from C3-C6 using Magerl technique and likely skip C7, navigate pilot holes and place pedicles screws at C2 and T1-T2, confirm placement of pedicle screws with O-arm spin, place rods, decorticate exposed bony surfaces and pack allograft generously, layered closure with subfascial drain, place vancomycin powder epifascially	Position supine, approach based on vocal cord analyses, remove nasopharyngeal tube to avoid more compression once esophagus is localized, use previous plate without fluoroscopy to determine levels, remove plate, prepare disc spaces as usual using Caspar distractor, cage test and select seize, cages filled with allograft bone—do this at C2–3, C5–6, and C6–7, close with drain
Complication avoidance	Anterior approach	Preflip IOM, skip instrumentation at C7 to facilitate rod placement, possible spinous process wires to augment fusion, leave proximal rod a little longer for potential future surgery	Magerl technique for lateral mass screws, skip instrumentation at C7, surgical navigation for pedicle screws	Anterior approach, side of approach based on vocal cord assessment, have in mind the previous surgery
Postoperative				
Admission	ICU	Floor	Floor	Floor
Postoperative complications feared	Dysphagia, hematoma	Wound infection, hematoma, adjacent segment disease	Hardware failure, pseudoarthrosis, adjacent level disease	Dysphagia, dystonia, hematoma
Anticipated length of stay	2 days	2–3 days	3–4 days	2 days
Follow-up testing	C-spine x-ray after surgery, 1 and 3 months after surgery C-spine CT 6 months after surgery	CT C-spine prior to discharge C-spine x-rays 6 weeks C-spine flexion/extension x-rays at 3 months, 6 months, 12 months, 24 months after surgery Vitamin D levels annually	Cervical and thoracic AP/Lateral X-rays at 2 weeks, 6 weeks, and as needed follow-up	C-spine x-rays after surgery, 1 month, 3 month, and 6 months after surgery
Bracing	Philadelphia collar for 2 weeks	Aspen collar for 6 weeks	None	Soft collar for 3 weeks
Follow-up visits	7 days, 1 month, 3 months, and 6 months after surgery	2 weeks, 6 weeks, 3 months, 6 months, 12 months, 24 months after surgery	2 weeks, 6 weeks, and as needed follow-up after surgery	1 month, 3 months, and 6 months after surgery

CBC, Complete blood count; CRP, C-reactive protein; CT, computed tomography; DEXA, dual-energy x-ray absorptiometry; ESR, erythrocyte sedimentation rate; IOM, intraoperative monitoring; MAP, mean arterial pressure; MEP, motor evoked potential; NSAIDs, nonsteroidal antiinflammatory drugs; PEEK, polyetheretherketone; SSEP, somatosensory evoked potential.

Differential diagnosis

- Adjacent segment disease
- Spinal instability
- Cervical stenosis

Important anatomical and preoperative considerations

Adjacent segment degeneration (or radiological adjacent segment pathology [RASP]) is the accelerated spondylosis or degenerative changes that occur at spinal levels (or mobile segments) that are contiguous to a surgically fused level (or immobile segment). This process can occur, however, in the absence of surgical fusion (i.e., after cervical laminectomies).[3] When symptomatic (radiculopathy or myelopathy), this condition is referred to as adjacent segment disease (or clinical adjacent segment pathology [CASP]). ASD is common and may be the natural history of the preexisting spondylosis or natural aging process of the cervical spine.[4] The reported incidence of adjacent segment disease (ASD) in patients who underwent ACDFs was 3% per year and estimated to be 26% within 10 years of the operation.[2,5] The rates of ASD over a 7-year period appear to be lower with cervical disc arthroplasties (CDAs) compared with plate-construct ACDFs (3.7% vs. 13.6% for one level and 4.4% vs. 11.4% for two levels).[1]

Potentially preventable risk factors include anatomical disruption adjacent to the surgical level[6] (i.e., incorrect needle localization was associated with a threefold increase in odds of having adjacent segment degeneration),[7] adjacent level ossification by disrupting the soft tissue (anterior longitudinal ligament and longus colli muscle) and placing the ACDF plate within 5 mm of the adjacent disc space,[8] increased mechanical stress and intradiscal pressure adjacent to a fused level (which is especially high in neck flexion-extension compared with CDA),[5,9] and postoperative sagittal malalignment and loss of cervical lordosis.[4,5,10] Other risk factors include preexisting yet disregarded neurological compression at the adjacent segment, surgery adjacent to the C5–6 and C6–7 levels, younger age (<60), smoking, female sex, level-treated osteopenia, and coexisting lumbar degenerative disc disease.[1,3,6]

Clinical manifestations result from biomechanical instability or neurological compression and include mechanical neck pain, cervical spine deformity, radiculopathy, and myelopathy. Surgical management is tailored to each patient with the main goals of decompressing the spinal cord and nerve roots, restoring cervical lordotic alignment, and stabilizing the spine across the mobile segments. Whenever possible, the failed hardware should be removed. Single-level ASD can be treated with a second ACDF, CDA, laminoplasty, or posterior cervical decompression and fusion (PCDF). A two-level ASD, like the case presented here, is more challenging especially for having a longer construct (from C3 to C6) and multiple prior operations. Both anterior and posterior approaches are equally effective at treating two-level ASD.[11] Revision surgery using an anterior approach is an option but has its limitations when working through thick scar and doing multiple spine levels and in patients with ossified posterior longitudinal ligament (OPLL). An anterior approach can expose up to C1 and down to T2 in some cases with proper dissection and dynamic retraction. Sometimes a manubriotomy and sternotomy is needed to reach down at T1 and T2.[12,13] However,

this more aggressive exposure and retraction may risk injuring the esophagus and recurrent laryngeal nerve[14] and even the superior laryngeal nerve, hypoglossal nerve, pleura, and thoracic duct. A preoperative laryngoscopy to evaluate vocal cord function should be obtained in all patients with prior neck dissections whenever a contralateral approach is being considered.[15] Additionally, in a study by Cao et al.[11] comparing anterior and posterior reoperations in patients with two-level ASD, the recurrence rate was higher with the anterior approaches (30% vs. 13%). An appealing option is placing stand-alone cages at the diseased levels without revising the existing hardware. However, there is not enough evidence to support this. A case series comparing stand-alone cages with anterior plate constructs in CASP showed lower fusion rate (69% vs. 95%) and higher reoperation rates (14% vs. 0%)[16] with stand-alone cages. Some advantages of a posterior approach include better and easier cranio-caudal exposure, more extensive central and neuroforaminal decompression, and more options for correcting the deformity, restoring the cervical sagittal alignment (i.e., osteotomies), and instrumenting the cervicothoracic spine. Posterior approaches may be associated with higher blood loss and longer hospital stay.[11,17] Complications include spinal cord injury, C5 palsy, cerebrospinal fluid (CSF) leak, wound dehiscence, and vertebral artery injury.

What was actually done

The patient's progressive symptoms correlated with the radiological finding of C5–6 pseudoarthrosis and adjacent level stenosis at C2–3 and C6–7 levels. Important considerations were that the patient had multiple (three) prior anterior neck approaches, bilateral neck scars, and signs of vocal cord abnormality (hoarseness). In this case a posterior approach was chosen. If an anterior approach is to be performed, a preoperative laryngoscopic examination of the vocal cords would be obtained and would dictate the side of the approach (the paralyzed side). The patient was taken to the operating room, placed in Mayfield pins, and flipped prone onto the operating table maintaining anatomical cervical lordosis. Neurophysiologic monitoring baselines were obtained before and after flipping. The patient's mean arterial pressure was maintained ~20% higher than baseline. Decompressive laminectomies were performed at C2, C3, C6, C7, and T1, and the cervicothoracic spine was instrumented from C2 to T2. The bilateral C3–6 lateral mass screws were placed freehand, and the bilateral C2 pars and T1 and T2 pedicle screws were placed with navigation guidance after an O-arm spin. An intraoperative computed tomography (CT) reconstruction confirmed proper hardware placement and restoration of the cervical lordosis. Local autograft, cancellous allograft granules, and recombinant human bone morphogenic protein (rh-BMP) was applied after thorough bone and joint decortication. The patient had an uneventful postoperative course and was discharged on postoperative day 4 with instructions to wear a hard-cervical collar at all times. Symptoms improved and the patient remain neurologically intact. A postoperative CT showed solid C2-T2 fusion (Fig. 4.2).

Commonalities among experts

All surgeons recommended obtaining preoperative flexion-extension x-rays of the cervical spine to assess for dynamic instability. Half of the surgeons advocated for an anterior

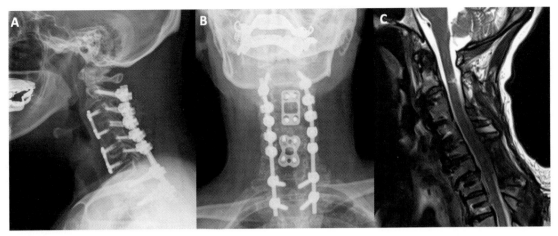

Fig. 4.2 Postoperative imaging. (A and B), X-rays showing the final C2-T2 pedicle screw and rods construct and restoration of cervical lordosis. (C) Sagittal T2 magnetic resonance image showing adequate spinal cord decompression.

approach and half for a posterior approach. The goals of surgery were decompression and stabilization across the pseudoarthrosis. Commonly feared complications were carotid artery, vertebral artery, esophageal and recurrent laryngeal nerve injury with an anterior approach, and wound infection and hardware failure with a posterior approach. All surgeons including those performing ACDFs would place a wound drain. Most surgeons agreed on obtaining an immediate postoperative cervical spine x-ray and a CT in the first 6 months. Half recommended wearing a hard collar postoperatively. Most would schedule follow-up in 1 to 2 weeks and then every 1 to 3 months thereafter.

SUMMARY OF QUALITY OF EVIDENCE TO GUIDE SPECIFIC INTERVENTIONS FOR THIS CASE

- Obtaining dynamic cervical spine flexion-extension x-rays is recommended for all patients with cervical adjacent segment disease: level IB.
- A posterior approach is suggested for patients with multiple prior anterior neck dissections and vocal cord dysfunction, multilevel disease, posterior compression, and OPLL as it may be safer, more versatile, and allow for wider decompression, hardware revision, and more extensive fusion: level III.
- There is no proven benefit of wearing a postoperative cervical collar: level III.

REFERENCES

1. Nunley PD, Kerr 3rd EJ, Cavanaugh DA, et al. Adjacent Segment Pathology After Treatment With Cervical Disc Arthroplasty or Anterior Cervical Discectomy and Fusion, Part 2: Clinical Results at 7-Year Follow-Up. *Int J Spine Surg.* 2020;14(3):278–285.
2. Hilibrand AS, Carlson GD, Palumbo MA, et al. Radiculopathy and myelopathy at segments adjacent to the site of a previous anterior cervical arthrodesis. *J Bone Joint Surg Am.* 1999;81(4):519–528.
3. Hilibrand AS, Robbins M. Adjacent segment degeneration and adjacent segment disease: the consequences of spinal fusion? *Spine J.* 2004;4(6 Suppl):190S–194S.
4. Alhashash M, Shousha M, Boehm H. Adjacent Segment Disease After Cervical Spine Fusion: Evaluation of a 70 Patient Long-Term Follow-Up. *Spine (Phila Pa 1976).* 2018;43(9):605–609.
5. Saavedra-Pozo FM, Deusdara RA, Benzel EC. Adjacent segment disease perspective and review of the literature. *Ochsner J.* 2014;14(1):78–83.
6. Chung JY, Park JB, Seo HY, Kim SK. Adjacent Segment Pathology after Anterior Cervical Fusion. *Asian Spine J.* 2016;10(3):582–592.
7. Nassr A, Lee JY, Bashir RS, et al. Does incorrect level needle localization during anterior cervical discectomy and fusion lead to accelerated disc degeneration? *Spine (Phila Pa 1976).* 2009;34(2):189–192.
8. Kim HJ, Kelly MP, Ely CG, et al. The risk of adjacent-level ossification development after surgery in the cervical spine: are there factors that affect the risk? A systematic review. *Spine (Phila Pa 1976).* 2012;37(22 Suppl):S65–74.
9. Eck JC, Humphreys SC, Lim TH, et al. Biomechanical study on the effect of cervical spine fusion on adjacent-level intradiscal pressure and segmental motion. *Spine (Phila Pa 1976).* 2002;27(22):2431–2434.
10. Hwang SH, Kayanja M, Milks RA, Benzel EC. Biomechanical comparison of adjacent segmental motion after ventral cervical fixation with varying angles of lordosis. *Spine J.* 2007;7(2):216–221.
11. Cao J, Qi C, Yang Y, Lei T, et al. Comparison between repeat anterior and posterior decompression and fusion in the treatment of two-level symptomatic adjacent segment disease after anterior cervical arthrodesis. *J Orthop Surg Res.* 2020;15(1):308.
12. Lee JG, Kim HS, Ju CI, Kim SW. Clinical Features of Herniated Disc at Cervicothoracic Junction Level Treated by Anterior Approach. *Korean J Spine.* 2016;13(2):53–56.
13. Lee J, Paeng SH, Lee WH, et al. Cervicothoracic Junction Approach using Modified Anterior Approach: J-type Manubriotomy and Low Cervical Incision. *Korean J Neurotrauma.* 2019;15(1):43–49.
14. Erwood MS, Hadley MN, Gordon AS, et al. Recurrent laryngeal nerve injury following reoperative anterior cervical discectomy and fusion: a meta-analysis. *J Neurosurg Spine.* 2016;25(2):198–204.
15 Cunningham CJ, Martínez JL. The Wandering Nerve: Positional Variations of the Cervical Vagus Nerve and Neurosurgical Implications. *World Neurosurg.* 2021;156:105–110.
16. Gandhi SD, Fahs AM, Wahlmeier ST, et al. Radiographic Fusion Rates Following a Stand-alone Interbody Cage Versus an Anterior Plate Construct for Adjacent Segment Disease After Anterior Cervical Discectomy and Fusion. *Spine (Phila Pa 1976).* 2020;45(11):713–717.
17. Bydon M, Alvi MA, Goyal A. Degenerative Lumbar Spondylolisthesis: Definition, Natural History, Conservative Management, and Surgical Treatment. *Neurosurg Clin N Am.* 2019;30(3):299–304.

5

Lumbar adjacent segment disease

Jaime L. Martínez Santos, MD

Introduction

Back pain is prevalent in the United States and worldwide. Lumbar arthrodesis techniques are being increasingly used to address congenital, degenerative, and traumatic spinal pathologies. Adjacent segment degeneration continues to be a very common sequela of lumbar arthrodesis occurring in up to 77% of patients[1–3] and resulting in back pain and progressive neurological deficits. The treatment is surgical and should be tailored to the patient. A thorough understanding of the spine anatomy and biomechanics, as well as expertise with the various surgical techniques, is of utmost importance. In this chapter, we utilize a case example to illustrate the clinical presentation and surgical management of lumbar adjacent segment disease.

Example case

Chief complaint: back pain

History of present illness: The patient is a 71-year-old male with history of lumbosacral spondylosis and previous L4-S1 decompression and fusion at an outside institution. He now presents with a 6-month history of back pain and bilateral leg pain when walking. Lumbar spine imaging showed transitional vertebral anatomy with six lumbar vertebrae and adjacent segment degeneration at the L3–4 level with L3–4 disc herniation and ligamentum flavum and facet hypertrophy causing severe canal and neuroforaminal stenosis (Figs. 5.1 and 5.2).

Medications: oxycodone, aspirin 81 mg

Allergies: no known allergies

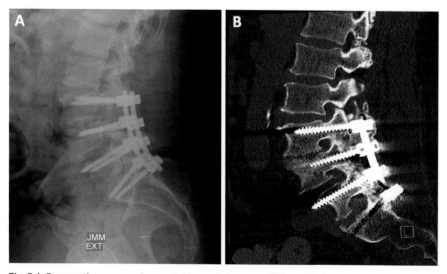

Fig. 5.1 Preoperative x-rays and computed tomography scans. (A) Lateral lumbar spine x-ray. (B) Lateral computed tomography scan demonstrating L3-S1 pedicle screw and rods construct, bicortical purchase and anterior vertebral body breach of one of the L6 screws, and a L4–5 intervertebral cage.

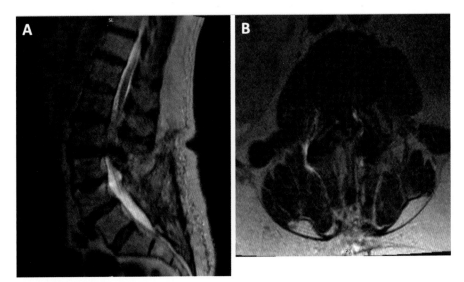

Fig. 5.2 Preoperative magnetic resonance imaging. (A) Sagittal and (B) axial image demonstrating transitional vertebral anatomy with six lumbar vertebrae adjacent segment degeneration at L3–4 with L3–4 disc herniation and ligamentum flavum and facet hypertrophy causing severe canal and neuroforaminal stenosis.

Past medical history: coronary artery disease, benign prostate hyperplasia
Past surgical history: previous L3-S1 fusion and decompression 2 years prior
Family history: no history of malignancies
Social history: no smoking, occasional alcohol
Physical examination: awake, alert, and oriented to person, place, and time; cranial nerves II–XII intact; bilateral deltoids/

triceps/biceps 5/5; interossei 5/5; iliopsoas/knee flexion/knee extension/dorsi, and plantar flexion 5/5
Reflexes: 2+ in bilateral biceps/triceps/brachioradialis with negative Hoffman; 2+ in bilateral patella/ankle and no clonus or Babinski; sensation intact to light touch; negative straight leg raise and hip motion testing
Laboratories: all within normal limits

	Ali A Baaj, MD Neurosurgery Weill Cornell New York, New York, United States	Ahmed S. Barakat, MD Orthopaedic Surgery University of Cairo Cairo, Egypt	Nitin N. Bhatia, MD Orthopaedic Surgery University of California at Irvine Orange, California, United States	Claudio Yampolsky, MD Neurosurgery Hospital Italiano de Buenos Aires Buenos Aires, Argentina
Preoperative				
Additional tests requested	CT L-spine to assess fusion Standing scoliosis x-rays for sagittal and coronal balance DEXA bone scan Physical therapy and/or ESI	MRI L-spine CT L-spine Echocardiogram Cardiac evaluation	Flexion-extension L-spine x-rays Standing full length 36-inch x-rays CT L-spine DEXA bone scan Infection labs (ESR/CRP/EBC)	Flexion-extension L-spine x-rays CT L-spine
Surgical approach selected	L2–3 laminectomy and extension of prior fusion L2-S1	L2–3 TLIF and extension of prior fusion L2-S1	L2–3 laminectomy with bilateral facetectomy, L2–3 TLIF, exploration of L3-S1 fusion with revision fusion if needed	If clear evidence of compression, L2–3 XLIF or DLIF and L2-S1 fusion
Goal of surgery	Decompression of the adjacent segment, stabilization	Decompression, stabilization	Decompression, fusion	Decompression, stabilization
Perioperative				
Positioning	Prone	Prone	Prone with four-post spine frame	Lateral, then prone
Surgical equipment	IOM Surgical microscope	Cell saver	IOM Fluoroscopy	IOM Fluoroscopy Surgical navigation
Medications	Antibiotics	Tranexamic acid	Perioperative pain regimen	None

	Ali A Baaj, MD Neurosurgery Weill Cornell New York, New York, United States	Ahmed S. Barakat, MD Orthopaedic Surgery University of Cairo Cairo, Egypt	Nitin N. Bhatia, MD Orthopaedic Surgery University of California at Irvine Orange, California, United States	Claudio Yampolsky, MD Neurosurgery Hospital Italiano de Buenos Aires Buenos Aires, Argentina
Anatomical considerations	Traversing and exiting nerve roots, central canal	Nerve root, dura	Previously decompressed spinal canal	Psoas muscle, lumbar plexus, vasculature, kidneys
Complications feared with approach chosen	Pseudoarthrosis, CSF leak, residual stenosis	Pseudoarthrosis, pedicle fracture, endplate fracture, neurological injury	CSF leak, neurological injury	Vascular injury, lumbar plexus injury, infection
Intraoperative				
Anesthesia	General, ERAS	General	General	General
Exposure	L2-S1	L2-S1	L2-S1	L2–3
Levels decompressed	L2–3	L2–3	L2–3	L2–3
Levels fused	L2-S1	L2-S1	L2-S1	L2-S1
Surgical narrative	Incision opened and extended, previous hardware identified and removed, new hardware placed from L2-S1 with consideration for possible L2–3 only if fusion is good, L2–3 laminectomy, interbody or posterolateral fusion, plastic surgery closure	Prone position, midline incision from L2-S1, evaluate previous hardware, replace loose screws with larger diameter screws, place L2 pedicle screws, L2–3 TLIF, connect screws with larger stiff rod, vancomycin powder in the incision, closure with subfascial drain	Prone position, midline posterior incision utilizing previous incision, residual L2–3 spinous process will be identified along with scar from previous decompression, dissection carried laterally to identify L2–3 facet joint/L2 traverse process/previous instrumentation, remove previous caps and rods removed, hardware and fusion examined, replace hardware if loose with larger diameter and length hardware based on preoperative CT, leave hardware if fusion is solid, place pedicle screws at L2, decompress L2–3 with bilateral hemilaminectomies with subtotal vs. total facetectomies, interbody fusion with cage application with attention toward maintaining sagittal and coronal alignment, place new rods and caps, posterolateral fusion by connecting L2 transverse process to previous fusion mass using auto and allograft, vancomycin powder in surgical cavity, wound closed in layers with subfascial drain	Lateral decubitus position, lateral incision after confirming with x-ray, minimal dissection, retractor placement over psoas muscle, monitoring of psoas muscle, annulotomy over confirmed disc space, discectomy, placement of cage with bone graft placement, reposition prone, extend fusion to L2, layered closure
Complication avoidance	Limited to level of stenosis, plastic surgery closure	Replace loose screws with larger diameter screws	Evaluate previous hardware intraoperatively, bilateral hemilaminectomies	Lateral approach, psoas monitoring, posterior supplementation
Postoperative				
Admission	Floor	Intermediate care	Floor	Floor
Postoperative complications feared	Hematoma, new radiculopathy	Neurological injury, wound healing	Hematoma, CSF leak, hardware malposition, neuropraxia	Vascular injury, lumbar plexus injury, infection
Anticipated length of stay	2–3 days	4 days	2–4 days	2–3 days
Follow-up testing	Upright AP/lateral L-spine x-rays after surgery	AP/lateral lumbar x-rays 2 days after surgery	Standing x-rays within 48 hours, 6 weeks, 3 months, 6 months, 1 year, and 2 years after surgery	L-spine AP/lateral x-rays within 48 hours, 30 days after surgery MRI L-spine 3 months after surgery CT L-spine 3 months after surgery

	Ali A Baaj, MD Neurosurgery Weill Cornell New York, New York, United States	Ahmed S. Barakat, MD Orthopaedic Surgery University of Cairo Cairo, Egypt	Nitin N. Bhatia, MD Orthopaedic Surgery University of California at Irvine Orange, California, United States	Claudio Yampolsky, MD Neurosurgery Hospital Italiano de Buenos Aires Buenos Aires, Argentina
Bracing	None	None	None	None
Follow-up visits	2 weeks for wound check; 3, 12, and 24 months	2 weeks, 3 months, 6 months, 12 months after surgery	2–3 weeks, 6 weeks, 3 months, 6 months, 1 year, and 2 years after surgery	7 days, 3 months after surgery

AP, Anteroposterior; CRP, C-reactive protein; CSF, cerebrospinal fluid; CT, computed tomography; ERAS, enhanced recovery after surgery; ESI, epidural spinal injections; ESR, erythrocyte sedimentation rate; IOM, intraoperative monitoring; MRI, magnetic resonance imaging; WBC, white blood cell count.

Differential diagnosis

- Lumbar facet syndrome
- Lumbar stenosis
- Lumbar adjacent segment disease
- Metastasis
- Primary extradural spine tumor

Important anatomical and preoperative considerations

Although the anatomy and biomechanics of the lumbar spine are different from the cervical spine, the disease process of chronic adjacent segment degeneration is similar. The basic definitions of adjacent segment degeneration (also called radiographic adjacent segment pathology) and disease (or clinical adjacent segment pathology) are discussed in Chapter 4.

There are many more options for stabilizing the lumbar spine, and consequently the reported incidence of lumbar adjacent segment degeneration and adjacent segment disease ranges widely from 5% to 77% and 0% to 27%, respectively,[1–3] with an annual risk of 2% to 3%.[4] The etiology is multifactorial, but as with the cervical spine (see Chapter 4), this chronic degenerative process could be the result of natural aging of the spine and not necessarily a direct complication of spine arthrodesis. The cumulative risk of developing adjacent segment disease in patients that underwent lumbar decompressions without fusion is 10% over 4 years.[5] Proposed risk factors specific to the lumbar spine include older age, genetic factors (proinflammatory single nucleotide pleomorphisms in the *IL18RAP* gene were associated with lower adjacent disc space height), high body mass index (BMI ≥25), preexisting adjacent segment stenosis, laminectomy at the level adjacent to a fusion, multilevel instrumentation, malalignment with excessive distraction or insufficient lumbar lordosis, "floating fusion" or constructs ending at L5 and not including the sacrum, coronal wedging of the L5-S1 disc, posterior tilting of the pelvis, and osteoporosis.[2] General recommendations for preventing adjacent segment disease are avoiding unnecessary anatomical disruption (facet capsules, posterior tension band) and preserving or restoring anatomical alignment and maintaining lumbar lordosis.[6,7] Techniques aimed specifically at restoring lumbar motion, such as disc arthroplasty, were developed to reduce the biomechanical stresses at the adjacent level and have shown promising results and lower rates of adjacent segment disease.[2,3]

The clinical presentation for adjacent segment disease includes mechanical low back pain, radiculopathy, neurogenic claudication, cauda equina syndrome, or sphincter disturbance. The treatment is surgical and tailored to the patient with the goals of nerve root decompression, restoration of spine alignment, lumbar lordosis, and spinal stabilization. The preoperative workup and surgical planning should include a standing scoliosis x-ray, a dynamic flexion-extension x-ray, a bone density scan and a lumbosacral spine computed tomography (CT), and a magnetic resonance imaging (MRI) or CT myelogram (if an MRI is contraindicated). Various options include posterior (posterior lumbar interbody fusion [PLIF]), posterolateral (transforaminal lumbar interbody fusion [TLIF]), anterior (anterior lumbar interbody fusion [ALIF]), and lateral (lateral lumbar interbody fusion [LLIF] or extreme lateral lumbar interbody fusion [XLIF]). Posterior and posterolateral techniques are overall more versatile and therefore used more commonly as they allow for hardware revision and replacement, more thorough decompression via laminectomy, foraminotomy, and discectomy, deformity correction through various means including osteotomies, and more extensive instrumentation. Some advantages of using anterior (ALIF) or lateral (XLIF) techniques are ease of exposing a "virgin" anatomy, obviating the need of dissecting through scar tissue and thus reducing the risk of durotomy and cerebrospinal fluid (CSF) leak. These approaches are, however, associated with other complications such as postoperative thigh pain and hip flexion weakness (usually transient)[8,9]; visceral, vascular, and lumbar plexus injury; and retrograde ejaculation.[10] Indirect neuroforaminal decompression can be achieved by increasing the disc space height using large interbody grafts cautiously not to precipitate subsidence. The hardware revision approach is usually dictated by the approach utilized in the index procedure. If minimally invasive surgery (MIS) techniques are utilized, patients can be kept in lateral decubitus (or placed prone) and the hardware revised and extended as needed using percutaneous MIS technique.

What was actually done

The patient was taken to the operating room for L3–4 decompression and hardware revision with extension of fusion up to L3. Surgery was done under general anesthesia and neurophysiologic monitoring. All of the existing hardware was removed, including the pedicle screws, and the track probed to confirm no bony breach. All pedicle screws were upsized

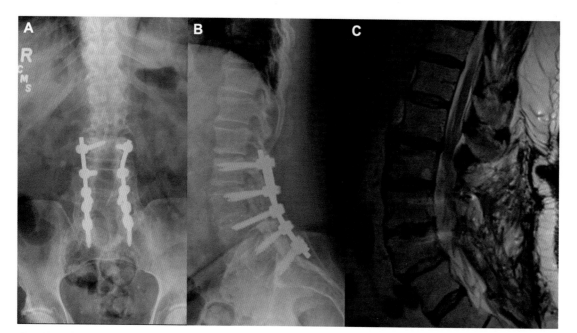

Fig. 5.3 Postoperative images. (A and B) Standing x-rays showing the final L3-S1 pedicle screw and rods construct with good restoration of lumbar lordosis. (C) Sagittal T2 magnetic resonance image showing adequate nerve root decompression.

by 1 mm (except for the L6, which were too long and had breached anteriorly) to optimize the likelihood of solid long-term fusion. The lamina of L3 and bilateral medial L3–4 facets were removed with rongeurs and high-speed drill attaining posterior central and neuroforaminal decompression. New rods were locked bilaterally in anatomical lumbar lordosis. Fluoroscopy was used to verify proper hardware placement and spine alignment. The wound was thoroughly irrigated with antibiotic solution and then the bone was thoroughly decorticated. Local autograft, iliac crest autograft, corticocancellous allograft, and recombinant human bone morphogenic protein 2 (rhBMP-2) were applied away from the dura. A subfascial wound drain was placed. The patient did well postoperatively and was discharged home on postoperative day 3 with instructions to wear a thoracolumbosacral ortosis (TLSO) when out of bed. His pain improved and he was weaned off of his long-term narcotic medications. Postoperative imaging showed adequate decompression, spine alignment, and strong fusion (Fig. 5.3). He reported no issues 2 years after surgery.

Commonalities among experts

All surgeons would obtain lumbar spine CT scans for hardware assessment and preoperative planning. Most agreed on having standing films to assess dynamic instability either with a dedicated 36-inch scoliosis x-ray or with flexion-extension x-rays. All surgeons would extend the fusion up a level and most advocated for doing a thorough decompression with facetectomies and TLIF at that level, although one surgeon advocated for a lateral interbody fusion (XLIF). Most surgeons used intraoperative neurophysiologic monitoring. Commonly feared complications included neurological injury (nerve root with a posterior approach and lumbosacral plexus with a lateral approach), durotomy, hematoma, hardware failure, and pseudoarthrosis. Most surgeons would replace all the screws and half commented on upsizing the diameter and length for a stronger fixation. Subfascial wound drainage and a layered wound closure were common practices. Most surgeons would

obtain lumbar x-rays in the immediate postoperative period. Follow-up was scheduled in 2 to 3 weeks and then 3 months postoperatively.

SUMMARY OF QUALITY OF EVIDENCE TO GUIDE SPECIFIC INTERVENTIONS FOR THIS CASE

- Obtaining dynamic lumbosacral flexion-extension x-rays is recommended for all patients with lumbar adjacent segment disease: level IB.
- Postoperative lumbar bracing did not correlate with outcome improvement in patients with degenerative lumbar spine disease: level II.[11]
- A posterior approach is suggested for patients presenting with neurological compression as it may be more versatile and allow for wider direct circumferential decompression, hardware revision, and fusion extension: level III.

REFERENCES

1. Xia XP, Chen HL, Cheng HB. Prevalence of adjacent segment degeneration after spine surgery: a systematic review and meta-analysis. *Spine (Phila Pa 1976).* 2013;38(7):597–608.
2. Hashimoto K, Aizawa T, Kanno H, Itoi E. Adjacent segment degeneration after fusion spinal surgery-a systematic review. *Int Orthop.* 2019;43(4):987–993.
3. Harrop JS, Youssef JA, Maltenfort M, et al. Lumbar adjacent segment degeneration and disease after arthrodesis and total disc arthroplasty. *Spine (Phila Pa 1976).* 2008;33(15):1701–1707.
4. Radcliff KE, Kepler CK, Jakoi A, et al. Adjacent segment disease in the lumbar spine following different treatment interventions. *Spine J.* 2013;13(10):1339–1349.
5. Bydon M, Macki M, De la Garza-Ramos R, et al. Incidence of Adjacent Segment Disease Requiring Reoperation After Lumbar Laminectomy Without Fusion: A Study of 398 Patients. *Neurosurgery.* 2016;78(2):192–199.

6. Saavedra-Pozo FM, Deusdara RA, Benzel EC. Adjacent segment disease perspective and review of the literature. *Ochsner J.* 2014; 14(1):78–83.

7. Kim SI, Min HK, Ha KY, et al. Effects of Restoration of Sagittal Alignment on Adjacent Segment Degeneration in Instrumented Lumbar Fusions. *Spine (Phila Pa 1976).* 2020

8. Louie PK, Haws BE, Khan JM, et al. Comparison of Stand-alone Lateral Lumbar Interbody Fusion Versus Open Laminectomy and Posterolateral Instrumented Fusion in the Treatment of Adjacent Segment Disease Following Previous Lumbar Fusion Surgery. *Spine (Phila Pa 1976).* 2019;44(24):E1461–E1469.

9. Louie PK, Varthi AG, Narain AS, et al. Stand-alone lateral lumbar interbody fusion for the treatment of symptomatic adjacent segment degeneration following previous lumbar fusion. *Spine J.* 2018;18(11):2025–2032.

10. Xu DS, Walker CT, Godzik J, et al. Minimally invasive anterior, lateral, and oblique lumbar interbody fusion: a literature review. *Ann Transl Med.* 2018;6(6):104.

11. Nasi D, Dobran M, Pavesi G. The efficacy of postoperative bracing after spine surgery for lumbar degenerative diseases: a systematic review. *Eur Spine J.* 2020;29(2):321–331.

6

Recurrent stenosis after laminectomy

Jaime L. Martínez Santos, MD

Introduction

Lumbar spinal stenosis is one of the most common diagnoses in the United States and worldwide that predominantly affects the aging population, with reported prevalence estimates up to 47%.[1-3] Advanced disease results in back pain and neurological compression. Lumbar laminectomy is the gold standard treatment with overall good outcomes and symptom relief. However, up to 33% of patients in some reports[4] can develop symptomatic restenosis that requires a reoperation. Oftentimes, a preexisting spinal malalignment is the culprit, which can be easily overlooked. In this chapter, we utilize a case example to illustrate the clinical presentation, preoperative workup, and surgical management of recurrent stenosis after lumbar laminectomy.

Example case

Chief complaint: leg and back pain

History of present illness: The patient is a 54-year-old male with history of L4–5 laminectomy a year ago for neurogenic claudication who presents with a 3-month history of back pain that radiates down the posterior aspect of his thighs and legs to his ankles. His symptoms are leg-predominant and worse with Valsalva maneuvers. He also reports imbalance and fear of falling when walking but does not need assistance. Lumbar spine imaging (Figs. 6.1 and 6.2) showed diffuse lumbar spondylosis most prominent at the L3–4 and L4–5 levels with disc desiccation and narrowing, L3–4 canal and neuroforaminal stenosis from herniated intervertebral disc, and ligamentum flavum and facet arthropathy with hypertrophy and joint effusion. Anteroposterior x-rays (Fig. 6.1A) showed mild dextrorotatory curvature, and

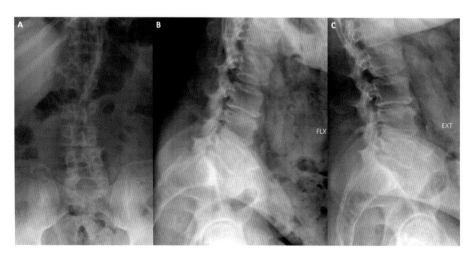

Fig. 6.1 Preoperative standing x-rays. (A) Anteroposterior x-ray demonstrating diffuse lumbar spondylosis, mild dextrorotatory curvature, and coronal wedging on the left L3–4. **(B)** Lateral flexion and **(C)** extension lumbosacral x-rays showing diffuse lumbar spondylosis most prominent at the L3–4 and L4–5 levels with disc narrowing and zygapophyseal arthropathy with widened (radiolucent) facet joints predominantly at L4–5. There is also mild L3–4 retrolisthesis with extension.

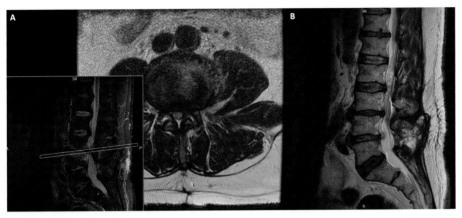

Fig. 6.2 Preoperative magnetic resonance images. (A) Axial and (B) sagittal T2 images demonstrating L3–4 canal and neuroforaminal stenosis from herniated intervertebral disc and ligamentum flavum and zygapophyseal arthropathy with hypertrophy and effusion (evidenced by increased T2 signal intensity).

dynamic flexion-extension x-rays showed mild L3–4 retrolisthesis with extension (Fig. 6.1B and 6.1C).
Medications: acetaminophen
Allergies: no known drug allergies
Past medical history: atrial fibrillation, coronary artery disease, deep vein thrombosis
Past surgical history: previous L4–5 laminectomy
Family history: no history of malignancies
Social history: smoking (one pack per day), occasional alcohol

Physical examination: awake, alert, and oriented to person, place, and time; cranial nerves II–XII intact; bilateral deltoids/triceps/biceps 5/5; interossei 5/5; iliopsoas/knee flexion/knee extension/dorsi, and plantar flexion 5/5
Reflexes: 2+ in bilateral biceps/triceps/brachioradialis with negative Hoffman; 2+ in bilateral patella/ankle and no clonus or Babinski; sensation intact to light touch; negative straight leg raise and hip motion testing
Laboratories: all within normal limits

	Richard Allen, MD, PhD Jakub Sikora, MD Orthopaedic Surgery University of California at San Diego San Diego, California, United States	Juan Fernando Ramon, MD Neurosurgery University Hospital Fundacion Santa Fe de Bogata Bogota, Columbia	Susana Núñez-Pereira, MD, PhD Orthopaedic Surgery Hospital Universitario Vall d'Hebron, Barcelona, Spain	Michael Y. Wang, MD Yingda Li, MBBS Neurosurgery University of Miami Miami, Florida, United States
Preoperative				
Additional tests requested	Flexion/extension L-spine x-rays	Flexion/extension L-spine x-rays Medicine evaluation	Full body AP/lateral x-rays to evaluate sagittal alignment	Pain drawing Standing AP/lateral L-spine x-rays Anesthesia evaluation
Surgical approach selected	L3–4 bilateral hemilaminal foraminotomies, partial facetectomies	L3–4 laminectomy, facetectomy, foraminotomy, L2–5 posterior fusion	L3–4 laminectomy and posterior fusion +/- TLIF (based on spinopelvic parameters)	L3–4 lateral MIS lumbar interbody fusion
Goal of surgery	Decompression of central/subarticular/foraminal stenosis	Decompression, stabilization	Decompression, stabilization	Indirect decompression, stabilization, and fusion to relieve neurogenic claudication and mechanical back pain
Perioperative				
Positioning	Prone on Jackson table with Wilson frame	Prone	Prone, on Jackson table	Lateral
Surgical equipment	Fluoroscopy Osteotomes	Fluoroscopy O-arm	Fluoroscopy	IOM (MEP, SSEP, EMGs) Fluoroscopy Cell saver Retractor system with light source Allograft BMP

	Richard Allen, MD, PhD Jakub Sikora, MD Orthopaedic Surgery University of California at San Diego San Diego, California, United States	Juan Fernando Ramon, MD Neurosurgery University Hospital Fundacion Santa Fe de Bogata Bogota, Columbia	Susana Núñez-Pereira, MD, PhD Orthopaedic Surgery Hospital Universitario Vall d'Hebron, Barcelona, Spain	Michael Y. Wang, MD Yingda Li, MBBS Neurosurgery University of Miami Miami, Florida, United States
Medications	None	None	None	Preoperative bowel prep
Anatomical considerations	Spinous process, interspinous ligaments, lamina, inferior articular facets	Facets, transverse apophysis, L3 lamina, foramen, dura	L3–4 nerve roots	Ilioinguinal and iliohypogastric nerves, retroperitoneal viscera, lumbar plexus, anterior longitudinal ligament, abdominal aorta and vena cava
Complications feared with approach chosen	Instability	CSF leak, nerve root injury	Instability	Epidural scar, CSF leak, paraspinal musculature compromise, spinal instability
Intraoperative				
Anesthesia	General	General	General	General
Exposure	L3–4	L2–5	L3–4	Lateral L3–4
Levels decompressed	L3–4	L3–4	L3–4	L3–4
Levels fused	None	L2–5	L3–4	L3–4
Surgical narrative	Position prone, midline incision over L3–4 down to lamina and spinous process of L3 and L4, place McCullough retractor, lateral x-ray to verify level, Leksell rongeur then matchstick bur to demarcate area of resection, thin lamina down to ligamentum flavum, feel out pars to confirm remaining bone with Epstein curette, decompress and find epidural tissue plane, release leigmaentum flavum, perform bilaterally to expose thecal sac, finalize hemilaminectomy at L3 bilaterally and at L4, go down onto superior articular processes and release any capsule and ligamentum flavum, remove this process and all compressive tissue underneath, walk out each neural foramina and decompress foramens, layered closure	Position prone, midline incision from L3-L5, open fascia, muscle dissection from top of incision to locate L3 lamina, L3 laminectomy with high-speed drill, open ligamentum flavum, full facetectomy and foramen decompression with Kerrison rongeur, revise inferior level decompression, place L2–5 pedicle screws with fluoroscopy, decorticate exposed bone surfaces, pack autograft into decorticated areas, layered closure with subfascial drain	Position prone, incision planned on bony landmarks and previous scar, subperiosteal dissection until posterior arch of L3 identified, scar tissue below and lack of spinous process of L4 help to confirm level, confirm with fluoroscopy, L3–4 facetectomy with chisel, insert poly axial pedicle screws L3–4 bilaterally with freehand technique and fluoroscopic control, careful dissection of lower limit of L3 lamina and bony removal with small chisel/gouge/Kerrison until reaching ligamentum flavum, minimize drill for arthrodesis, flavectomy and decompression bilaterally until wide decompression fo thecal sac is achieved and nerve roots identified without compression, check L3–4 foramina and decompress further if needed, TLIF symptomatic side, remove superior articular process of L4 with gentle dissection of foramen to isolate nerve root, protect thecal sac and remove L3–4 disc, insert cage filled with autologous bone graft with maximal possible height, insert rods, x-ray to confirm hardware placement, close rod-screw system, layered closure with drain	Position lateral with most symptomatic side up, table break at iliac crest, fluoroscopy to confirm orthogonal position, two incision technique, entry into retroperitoneum, sweep away retroperitoneal viscera, guide initial dilator to disc space with finger, intradiscal Kirschner wire and retractor positioning with light source under fluoroscopic visualization, Kittner to dissect psoas off of disc, discectomy avoiding end plate and/or ALL violation, Cobb across contralateral annulus, trial then final implant filled with autograft and BMP under fluoroscopy, antibiotic irrigation, removal of retractors, layered closure
Complication avoidance	Feel out pars to confirm remaining bone, remove superior articular processes to access foramens	Full facetectomy to open up space, revise inferior level decompression	Identify normal anatomy, free-hand technique for pedicle screws, minimize drill for arthrodesis, TLIF symptomatic side, care to protect exposed thecal sac	Lateral position, fluoroscopy for localization/placement of dilators and retractor/ insertion of graft, maintaining end plates and ALL

	Richard Allen, MD, PhD Jakub Sikora, MD Orthopaedic Surgery University of California at San Diego San Diego, California, United States	Juan Fernando Ramon, MD Neurosurgery University Hospital Fundacion Santa Fe de Bogata Bogota, Columbia	Susana Núñez-Pereira, MD, PhD Orthopaedic Surgery Hospital Universitario Vall d'Hebron, Barcelona, Spain	Michael Y. Wang, MD Yingda Li, MBBS Neurosurgery University of Miami Miami, Florida, United States
Postoperative				
Admission	Outpatient	Floor	Floor	Floor
Postoperative complications feared	Infection, instability	Infection, CSF leak, neurological injury	Infection, CSF leak, nerve root irritation, residual pain	Anterior thigh pain/dysesthesia, hip flexion weakness, lumbar plexopathy, abdominal wall pseudo hernia, visceral or vascular injury, hematoma, instability, subsidence, pseudoarthrosis
Anticipated length of stay	Same day	4–5 days	4–5 days	1–2 days
Follow-up testing	L-spine x-ray 6 weeks after surgery	L-spine x-rays within 24 hours, 1 month, 3 months, 6 months after surgery	L-spine standing x-ray after drain removal	Standing flexion extension x-rays at 3 months after surgery Physical therapy as needed
Bracing	None	TLSO for 2 months	None	Lumbar orthosis
Follow-up visits	2 weeks, 6 weeks, 6 months, 12 months after surgery	10 days, 1 month, 3 months, 6 months after surgery	2 weeks, 6 weeks and then 6 and 12 months after surgery	2 weeks and 3 months after surgery

ALL, Anterior longitudinal ligament; AP, anteroposterior; BMP, bone morphogenic protein; CSF, cerebrospinal fluid; EMG, electromyography; IOM, intraoperative monitoring; MEP, motor evoked potentials; MIS, minimally invasive surgery; SSEP, somatosensory evoked potentials; TLIF, transforaminal lumbar interbody fusion; TLSO, thoracic lumbar sacral orthosis.

Differential diagnosis

- Lumbar facet syndrome
- Lumbar restenosis
- Adjacent level restenosis
- Lumbar adjacent segment disease

Important anatomical and preoperative considerations

Lumbar spinal stenosis is a common cause of back pain and affects over 200,000 adults in the United States.[5] Reported prevalence estimates range widely from 6% to 47% with increased prevalence in the aging population.[1–3] Advanced disease is associated with central canal and neuroforaminal neurological compression with low back pain, radiculopathy, neurogenic claudication, sphincter disturbance, or cauda equina syndrome. Treatment has not been standardized and various surgical techniques can be used to decompress, stabilize or both—based mostly on the surgeon's preference.[2] In fact, there is a global trend of surgical treatment of lumbar stenosis.[6] In the United States, for example, there has been a 45% increase in lumbar decompressions and 60% increase in lumbar fusions only between 2004 to 2009.[7] Lumbar laminectomy via an open or a minimally invasive surgery (MIS) approach is the most common modality of treatment with success rates around 70%.[8] Postoperative pain is not uncommon and it is of utmost importance to distinguish persisting or returning preoperative symptoms from the development of new postlaminectomy pain that could result from immediate postoperative complications such as hematoma or neurological injury, intermediate complications such as infections or spinal instability, or delayed complications such as natural progression of the degenerative process or even a condition termed postdecompressive neuropathy (PDN). PDN may result from neurapraxia and is characterized by a delayed-onset lower extremity neuropathic pain and paresthesia in a nondermatomal distribution without weakness that resolves within 3 to 6 months with only supportive treatment.[9] Lumbar canal or neuroforaminal restenosis can occur in about 5% to 33% of patients after a decompression[4] at the same level or at an adjacent level.

Risk factors associated with restenosis include preexisting or iatrogenic postoperative spine malignment from coronal imbalance (scoliosis)[10] or sagittal imbalance with loss (or unrestored) lumbar lordosis.[4] Progressive disc degeneration with decreased disc height and increased coronal wedging, as well as lateral instability by disrupting the facet capsules, pars interarticularis, and perhaps transverse-spinous muscles and ligaments on the concave side of the coronal deformity may predispose to deformity progression and accelerated neuroforaminal stenosis.[4] Additionally, laminectomies can predispose to adjacent segment stenosis (see Chapter 5) or spondylolisthesis. The latter may occur after laminectomies in patients whose adjacent zygapophyseal joints are oriented more parallel to the sagittal plane (which normally occurs at higher lumbar levels).[11]

Besides a lumbar spine magnetic resonance imaging, the diagnostic and preoperative workup should always include a dedicated standing scoliosis x-ray to assess for spine malalignment, lateral flexion-extension x-rays of the lumbosacral spine to assess for dynamic instability, a computed tomography (CT) of the lumbosacral spine (also used for planning the instrumentation), and an electromyogram and nerve conduction study. Symptomatic restenosis with neurological compression resulting in radiculopathy, neurogenic claudication, cauda equina syndrome, or sphincter disturbance are typically managed surgically. The goals of surgery are twofold: (1) neurological decompression and (2) maintenance of spinal alignment or correction of any preexisting spinal malalignment with instrumented fusion. The main surgical approaches to the lumbar spine are posterior, lateral, or anterior using either open or MIS techniques. Lateral approaches, such as lateral lumbar interbody fusion (LLIF), obviate the need of dissecting a thick posterior scar and working near and around the spinal canal, dura, and nerve roots, thus reducing the risk of durotomy and cerebrospinal fluid (CSF) leak. Anterior and lateral approach-related complications include visceral, neurological (lumbosacral and hypogastric plexus), and vascular injuries.[12] An indirect neuroforaminal decompression can be achieved by distracting the vertebral bodies with a large intervertebral graft cautiously to not cause subsidence. Lateral approaches may be effective at improving disc height and segmental lordosis.[13,14] Posterior approaches utilize the old midline scar and are more versatile as they allow for a more thorough direct decompression with laminectomies, foraminotomies, and facetectomies; more options for deformity correction (i.e., osteotomies); and ease of extensive instrumentation. Posterior approaches can be done using both open and MIS techniques. A single-level MIS transforaminal lumbar interbody fusion (TLIF) is another good option if there is dynamic instability, spondylolisthesis, advanced facet arthropathy, or severe neuroforaminal and far-lateral stenosis at that level.

What was actually done

The patient was taken to the operating room for L2 and L3 laminectomies and instrumented fusion from L2 to pelvis. Spinal levels were localized using fluoroscopy. Their prior posterior midline incision was extended, and the paraspinal musculature was dissected off the posterior elements of L2 to S1 in subperiosteal fashion exposing bilateral facets and transverse processes. Bilateral L2–5 pedicle screws were placed using freehand technique using anatomical landmarks and fluoroscopy for guidance. An O-arm spin was obtained for navigating the S1 and iliac screws. Adequate screw placement was confirmed with an intraoperative O-arm CT reconstruction and triggered electromyography. Then bilateral L2 and L3 laminectomies and foraminotomies were performed with high-speed drill and rongeurs, thoroughly decompressing the central canal and neuroforaminae. Bilateral prebent rods were locked in place preserving good lumbar lordosis. The wound was thoroughly irrigated with antibiotic solution. The remaining bone, facets, and transverse processes were thoroughly decorticated, and local and iliac crest autograft and allograft were placed. Vancomycin powder was sprinkled in the wound and two subfascial drains placed. The patient did well postoperatively and reported resolution of back pain. At 3 months' follow up, the patient remained pain-free and imaging (Fig. 6.3) showed proper spine alignment and no hardware complication.

Commonalities among experts

All experts agreed on obtaining preoperative standing x-rays to assess for dynamic stability and sagittal alignment. The goal of surgery was always neurological decompression. However, the selected approaches were completely different. Most surgeons selected a posterior approach while only one selected a LLIF with indirect decompression. Commonly feared complications included instability and CSF leak. All surgeons would decompress L3–4 and half would fuse only those levels. One surgeon advocated for a more extensive L2–5 decompression. Most surgeons would obtain standing x-rays in the immediate postoperative period and then

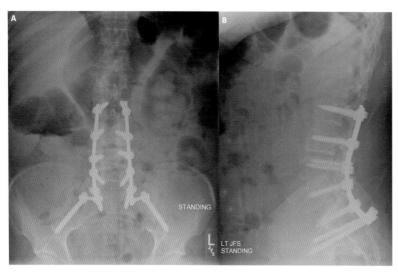

Fig. 6.3 Postoperative standing x-rays. (A) Anteroposterior and **(B)** lateral standing lumbosacral x-rays demonstrating good alignment and no hardware complication.

in 1 to 3 months. Outpatient follow up was scheduled in 2 weeks then 1 to 3 months thereafter.

REFERENCES

1. Jensen RK, Jensen TS, Koes B, Hartvigsen J. Prevalence of lumbar spinal stenosis in general and clinical populations: a systematic review and meta-analysis. *Eur Spine J.* 2020;29(9):2143–2163.
2. Munting E, Roder C, Sobottke R, et al. Patient outcomes after laminotomy, hemilaminectomy, laminectomy and laminectomy with instrumented fusion for spinal canal stenosis: a propensity score-based study from the Spine Tango registry. *Eur Spine J.* 2015;24(2):358–368.
3. Hart LG, Deyo RA, Cherkin DC. Physician office visits for low back pain. Frequency, clinical evaluation, and treatment patterns from a U.S. national survey. *Spine (Phila Pa 1976).* 1995;20(1):11–19.
4. Haimoto S, Nishimura Y, Hara M, et al. Clinical and Radiological Outcomes of Microscopic Lumbar Foraminal Decompression: A Pilot Analysis of Possible Risk Factors for Restenosis. *Neurol Med Chir (Tokyo).* 2018;58(1):49–58.
5. Lurie J, Tomkins-Lane C. Management of lumbar spinal stenosis. *BMJ.* 2016;352:h6234.
6. Deyo RA, Mirza SK, Martin BI, et al. Trends, major medical complications, and charges associated with surgery for lumbar spinal stenosis in older adults. *JAMA.* 2010;303(13):1259–1265.
7. Bae HW, Rajaee SS, Kanim LE. Nationwide trends in the surgical management of lumbar spinal stenosis. *Spine (Phila Pa 1976).* 2013;38(11):916–926.
8. Phan K, Mobbs RJ. Minimally Invasive Versus Open Laminectomy for Lumbar Stenosis: A Systematic Review and Meta-Analysis. *Spine (Phila Pa 1976).* 2016;41(2):E91–E100.
9. Boakye LAT, Fourman MS, Spina NT, et al. "Post-Decompressive Neuropathy": New-Onset Post-Laminectomy Lower Extremity Neuropathic Pain Different from the Preoperative Complaint. *Asian Spine J.* 2018;12(6):1043–1052.
10. Yamada K, Matsuda H, Cho H, et al. Clinical and radiological outcomes of microscopic partial pediculectomy for degenerative lumbar foraminal stenosis. *Spine (Phila Pa 1976).* 2013;38(12):E723–731.
11. Hikata T, Kamata M, Furukawa M. Risk factors for adjacent segment disease after posterior lumbar interbody fusion and efficacy of simultaneous decompression surgery for symptomatic adjacent segment disease. *J Spinal Disord Tech.* 2014;27(2):70–75.
12. Xu DS, Walker CT, Godzik J, et al. Minimally invasive anterior, lateral, and oblique lumbar interbody fusion: a literature review. *Ann Transl Med.* 2018;6(6):104.
13. Louie PK, Haws BE, Khan JM, et al. Comparison of Stand-alone Lateral Lumbar Interbody Fusion Versus Open Laminectomy and Posterolateral Instrumented Fusion in the Treatment of Adjacent Segment Disease Following Previous Lumbar Fusion Surgery. *Spine (Phila Pa 1976).* 2019;44(24):E1461–E1469.
14. Louie PK, Varthi AG, Narain AS, et al. Stand-alone lateral lumbar interbody fusion for the treatment of symptomatic adjacent segment degeneration following previous lumbar fusion. *Spine J.* 2018;18(11):2025–2032.

7

Multilevel cervical stenosis from ossified posterior longitudinal ligaments

Kingsley Abode-Iyamah, MD

Introduction

Ossification of the posterior longitudinal ligament (OPLL) is one of many conditions classified as enthesopathies, which result from progressive inflammation of the tendons and ligaments of the spine followed by degeneration and calcification. Other examples of enthesopathies include ossification of the anterior longitudinal ligament, ossification of the ligamentum flavum, diffuse idiopathic skeletal hypertrophy, and ankylosing spondylitis. Since it was first recognized in 1838, there have been many identified genetic factors predisposing to OPLL. Some of these include association with human leukocyte antigen (HLA) haplotype and collagen 6A1 gene (COLA1).[1–3] Epidemiological studies suggest OPLL tends to be a frequent cause of cervical myelopathy in the Japanese population and is therefore thought be common in those of Asian descent.[4] However, the frequency of OPLL in those of non-Asian descent may be more common than previously believed. OPLL can be divided into four categories depending on the continuity of the ossification. The subtypes include continuous, segmental, mixed, and localized. The OPLL leads to compression of the spinal cord resulting in cervical myelopathy. The progression of symptoms, severity of symptoms, and recovery can be somewhat variable. In addition to known factors such a kyphosis, cord signal change, length of symptoms, and number of level of compression, there is increasing evidence that genetic factors may play a role in cervical myelopathy.[5–8]

Example case

Chief complaint: gait instability

History of present illness: A 67-year-old male with a history of numbness in his lower extremity and a gait instability for approximately 5 years has similar symptoms that worsened over the past 6 months. He has also had difficulty with dexterity in his hands. He also notes urinary urgency but denies incontinence. He also has an increasing frequency of falls (Figs. 7.1 and 7.2).

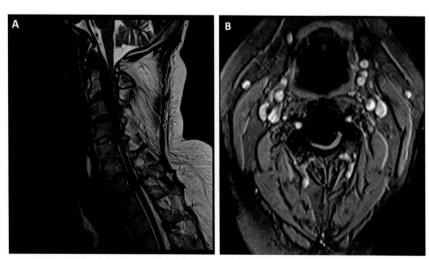

Fig. 7.1 Preoperative magnetic resonance imaging. (A) T2 sagittal and **(B)** T2 axial images demonstrating large mass causing a ventral compression and flattening of the spinal cord with noted cord signal change.

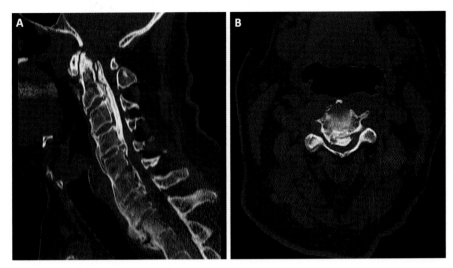

Fig. 7.2 **Preoperative computed tomography scans. (A)** sagittal and **(B)** axial images showing large ossified mass extending from C1-C5.

Medications: amlodipine, bethanechol, bupropion, carvedilol, fluoxetine, glimepiride, hydrocholorthiazide, synthroid, losartan, metformin, omeprazole, simvastatin
Allergies: vancomycin
Past medical and surgical history: chronic kidney disease, hypertension, diabetes, obesity, liver cirrhosis, obstructive sleep apnea, hypothyroidism
Family history: noncontributory

Social history: no smoking history, occasional alcohol
Physical examination: awake, alert, and oriented to person, place, and time; cranial nerves II–XII intact; bilateral deltoids/triceps/biceps 5/5; interossei 5/5; iliopsoas/knee flexion/knee extension/dorsi, and plantar flexion 5/5
Reflexes: 2+ in bilateral biceps/triceps/brachioradialis; 3+ in bilateral patella/ankle with no clonus or Babinski; negative Hoffman; sensation intact to light touch

	Anas Abdallah, MD Neurosurgery Osmaniye State Hospital Osmaniye, Turkey	Nitin N. Bhatia, MD Orthopaedic Surgery University of California at Irvine Orange, California, United States	Praveen Mummaneni, MD Brenton Pennicooke, MD Neurosurgery University of California at San Francisco San Francisco, California, United States	Manoj Phalak, MCh Neurosurgery All India Institute of Medical Sciences New Delhi, India
Preoperative				
Additional tests requested	MRI brain MRI T- and L-spine CT cervical spine Cervical flexion-extension x-rays CTA Anesthesia evaluation	MRI T- and L-spine CTA cervical spine Flexion-extension cervical x-rays Anesthesia evaluation	None	CTA C-spine DEXA Anesthesia evaluation
Surgical approach selected	C2–5 open-door laminoplasty	Posterior C1–5 decompression and instrumented fusion with possible extension to occiput	C1-T2 posterior instrumentation, C1–7 laminectomy	C1–5 laminectomy and C2–5 fusion
Goal of surgery	Decompression of spinal cord	Decompression of areas affected by OPLL, preservation of neurological function	Decompression of spinal cord	Decompression of spinal cord, rapid procedure
Perioperative				
Positioning	Prone with Mayfield pins	Prone on four-post frame with Mayfield pins	Prone on Jackson table, with Mayfield pins	Prone on horseshoe headrest
Surgical equipment	IOM (MEP/SSEP) Surgical microscope Laminoplasty plate and screws	Fluoroscopy Surgical navigation	IOM (MEP/SSEP/EMG) Fluoroscopy Surgical navigation Intraoperative CT	IOM (MEP/SSEP) O-arm Surgical navigation Ultrasonic bone scalpel

	Anas Abdallah, MD Neurosurgery Osmaniye State Hospital Osmaniye, Turkey	Nitin N. Bhatia, MD Orthopaedic Surgery University of California at Irvine Orange, California, United States	Praveen Mummaneni, MD Brenton Pennicooke, MD Neurosurgery University of California at San Francisco San Francisco, California, United States	Manoj Phalak, MCh Neurosurgery All India Institute of Medical Sciences New Delhi, India
Medications	Steroids, maintain MAP	None	None	None
Anatomical considerations	Spinal cord, nerve roots, dura	Vertebral arteries, thecal sac, C2 nerve root	Spinal cord, vertebral arteries	Vertebral arteries
Complications feared with approach chosen	Facet joint fusion, motor deficit, CSF leak	CSF leak	Spinal cord injury	C5 palsy, CSF leak, vertebral artery injury, violation of C1–2 joints
Intraoperative				
Anesthesia	General	General	General	General
Exposure	C2–5	Occiput-C5	C1-T2	Occiput-C5
Levels decompressed	C2–5	C1-C5	C1–7	C1–5
Levels fused	C2–5	Occiput-C5	C1-T2	C2–5
Surgical narrative	Positioned prone with Mayfield pins with slight flexion, vertical midline posterior incision from C2–5, central splitting of nuchal ligament to spinous process, subperiosteal dissection with preservation of semispinalis attachments to C2 spinous process, shorten spinous process to use as autograft spacers, gutter created on right side because narrowest along lamina-facet interface from C2–5, open lamina bilaterally with diamond bit drill and Kerrison rongeurs, open lamina-facet interface down to ligamentum flavum with preservation of interspinous ligament, a hinge is created on the left side in the same way, ligamentum flavum at upper and lower ends transversely cut, lamina elevated on right side (open-door), autografts can be used to increase anterior-posterior diameter, autografts are placed between lamina and facets to keep hinge open, place laminoplasty plate and screws, nonabsorbable sutures are used to fix cranial and caudal interspinal ligaments and along left side, reconnect semispinalis to C2 spinous process with nonabsorbable suture, layered closure with drain	Fiberoptic intubation, position prone with no hyperextension, positioned confirmed by fluoroscopy, midline posterior incision, place C1 lateral mass screws/C2 pars vs. translaminar vs. pedicle based on preoperative imaging, place C3–5 lateral mass screws, decompress from C1–5, contour rods to reduce motion around open canal, place rods and set screws, place vancomycin powder in cavity, closure in layers with deep drain, focus on fascial layer closure	Position prone, lateral x-ray to plan incision, midline posterior incision, expose from C1-C6, navigation array on T1 spinous process, obtain intraoperative CT and register with navigation system, plan entry points for C3-T1 using navigation, decorticate entry points/drill screw tracks/and place lateral mass screws from C3-C7 and T1 pedicle screws bilaterally, ligate C2 nerve roots proximal to ganglion and section, attach navigation array to skull clamp, obtain intraoperative CT and register while checking C3-T1 screws, place C1 lateral mass and C2 pars screws under navigation, C1-T1 laminectomy and care to minimize traction according to the spinal cord, MEP after laminectomy, obtain another intraoperative CT to confirm C1–2 screw placement, placement of rods connecting screws, cap and final tighten once hardware confirmed in good location, place local bone autograft from laminectomies along decorticated surfaces lateral to screw heads, layered closure with subfascial drains	Awake fiberoptic intubation with avoiding neck manipulation, baseline IOM preflip, log-roll with collar on horseshoe head rest, keep neutral position, postflip IOM, midline incision, subperiosteal dissection exposing occiput down to C5, O-arm spine, place C2 pars screws and C3–5 lateral mass screws, C1–5 laminectomy with bone scalpel and high-speed drill, look for posterior displacement of thecal sac and normal pulsations, O-arm to evaluate position of screws, place rods, layered closure

	Anas Abdallah, MD Neurosurgery Osmaniye State Hospital Osmaniye, Turkey	Nitin N. Bhatia, MD Orthopaedic Surgery University of California at Irvine Orange, California, United States	Praveen Mummaneni, MD Brenton Pennicooke, MD Neurosurgery University of California at San Francisco San Francisco, California, United States	Manoj Phalak, MCh Neurosurgery All India Institute of Medical Sciences New Delhi, India
Complication avoidance	Preserve semispinalis attachments to C1 spinous process to minimize postoperative kyphosis, spinous processes used as autograft spacers, open-door laminoplasty, reattach semispinalis to C2 spinous process	Confirm position with fluoroscopy, C2 screw type based on preoperative imaging, limit motions around open canal	Surgical navigation, expose C1 lateral mass by ligating and sectioning C2 nerve roots, repeated intraoperative CT to confirm hardware location, minimize traction on spinal cord	Pre- and postflip IOM, O-arm and surgical navigation, look for posterior displacement of thecal sac and normal pulsations to evaluate adequacy of decompression
Postoperative				
Admission	Floor	Floor	Floor	ICU
Postoperative complications feared	Hematoma, CSF leak, nerve palsy, neck pain, kyphotic deformity, displacement of lamina, restricted neck motion from facet joint fusion	Hematoma, CSF leak, neurological deterioration, instrument malposition, vertebral artery injury	C5 palsy	C5 palsy, CSF leak, vertebral artery injury, violation of C1–2 joints
Anticipated length of stay	3 days	3–4 days	3 days	3–5 days
Follow-up testing	CT C-spine within 24 hours and 3 months after surgery	Standing x-rays within 48 hours of surgery, 6 weeks, 3 months, 6 months, 1 year, and 2 years after surgery	AP and lateral C-spine x-rays prior to discharge, 6 weeks, 3 months, 6 months, 1 year, and 2 years after surgery	C-spine x-ray within 24 hours, and 3 months after surgery
Bracing	Rigid neck collar for 4–6 weeks	Aspen or Miami J for comfort for maximum of 6 weeks	Miami J for 6 weeks	Philadelphia collar for 6 weeks
Follow-up visits	2 weeks, 6 weeks, 3 months, 6 months, and 12 months after surgery	2–3 weeks, 6 weeks, 3 months, 6 months, 1 year, and 2 years after surgery	3 weeks, 6 weeks, 3 months, 6 months, 1 year, and 2 years after surgery	10 days and 3 months after surgery

AP, Anteroposterior; CSF, cerebrospinal fluid; CT, computed tomography; CTA, computed tomography angiography; DEXA, dual-energy x-ray absorptiometry; EMG, electromyogram; ICU, intensive care unit; IOM, intraoperative monitoring; MAP, mean arterial pressure; MEP, motor evoked potential; MRI, magnetic resonance imaging; OPLL, ossified posterior longitudinal ligament; PLL, posterior longitudinal ligament; SSEP, somatosensory evoked potential.

Differential diagnosis

- OPLL
- Diffuse idiopathic skeletal hyperostosis
- Ankylosing spondylitis

Important anatomical considerations

As previously discussed above, OPLL can be divided into four subtypes: continuous, segmental, mixed, and localized. The continuous subtype consist of a contiguous ossified ligament spanning multiple vertebrae. The segmental subtype is the most common and is found behind vertebral bodies but does not cross the disc space. The mixed subtype is a combination of the continuous and segmental subtype. The localized subtype is localized to the disc spaces and is rarely found. A computed tomography (CT) scan of the cervical spine is critical in defining the extent of ossification

in these cases. Additionally, magnetic resonance imaging (MRI) should be obtained to determine the degree of stenosis. Furthermore, there is often significant attachment of the ossification to the dura often leading to significant dural tears and cerebral spinal fluid leak when an anterior approach is taken. As in the presented case, the ossification can also extend to the C2 vertebrae, leading to compression at the occipital cervical junction. Although intraoperative monitoring remains controversial, this should be given consideration in patients with OPLL and severe compression.[9–15] Furthermore, as it relates to trauma, a low threshold should be maintained to obtain an MRI when there is neck pain in the absence of a fracture on CT scan.

Approaches to this lesion

Conservative management for OPLL is only advised for those who are asymptomatic. However, asymptomatic patients should continue to be followed closely looking for early signs of long track symptoms. The modified

Table 7.1 Nurick score of cervical myelopathy

Grade	Description
0	Root symptoms only or normal
1	Signs of cord compression; normal gait
2	Gait difficulties but fully employed
3	Gait difficulties prevent employment, walks unassisted
4	Unable to walk without assistance
5	Wheelchair or bedbound

Table 7.2 Modified Japanese Orthopaedic Association (mJOA) score of cervical myelopathy

	Score
Motor dysfunction score of upper extremities	
Inability to move hands	0
Inability to eat with spoon, able to move hands	1
Inability to button shirt, able to eat with spoon	2
Able to button shirt with great difficulty	3
Able to button shirt with some difficulty	4
No dysfunction	5
Motor dysfunction score of lower extremities	
Complete loss of motor and sensory function	0
Sensory preservation without ability to move legs	1
Able to move legs but unable to walk	2
Able to walk on flat floor with a walking aid	3
Able to walk up and/or down stairs with rail	4
Moderate to significant lack of stability but able to walk up and/or down stairs with great difficulty	5
Mild lack of stability but walk unaided with smooth reciprocation	6
No dysfunction	7
Sensation	
Complete loss of hand sensation	0
Severe sensory loss or pain	1
Mild sensory loss	2
No sensory loss	3
Sphincter dysfunction	
Unable to micturate voluntarily	0
Marked difficulty in micturition	1
Mild-to-moderate difficulty in micturition	2
Normal micturition	3

Japanese Orthopaedic Association (mJOA) (Table 7.1) and Nurick score (Table 7.2) can also be maintained on patients to determine their progression of symptoms. For those patients with any degree of symptoms, surgical intervention should be considered. Early intervention should be considered at the earliest sign of symptoms to prevent irreversible damage. As with any cervical spine pathology, the approach to these lesions can be anterior or posterior. Anterior approach includes both direct decompression via resection of the ossified lesion and floating decompression without complete removal of the lesion. An anterior approach involves cervical corpectomy, although care must be taken given the risk of cerebral spinal fluid leak and epidural hematoma. There have been good outcomes reported with an anterior approach corpectomy; however, this approach has also been associated with more reoperations and complications.[16–20] Posterior approaches include laminectomy, laminoplasty, and laminectomy with fusion. A recent meta-analysis by Youssef et al. found significant improvement of posterior fusion and decompression with low rates of reoperations and complications.[21–23]

What was actually done

The patient was first assessed with CT and MRI to determine the extent of the ossification. Flexion-extension x-rays were also obtained to determine whether there was instability. Given that the ossification extended to C2 with compression at the level of the posterior arch of C1, the patient was offered a C1 to C7 laminectomy and C1 to T2 posterior cervical fusion. This was accomplished with the patient in a Mayfield headpin for stabilization of the head on an OSI table. Prepositioning intraoperative monitoring was obtained and continued after the positioning. Additionally, the mean arterial pressure (MAP) was maintained greater than 85 during the induction and throughout the case. The patient was also given a one-time dose of 10 mg of dexamethasone at the beginning of the case. The instrumentation was completed prior to the laminectomy. The laminectomy at C1 was completed last. Postoperatively the patient was admitted to the surgical intensive care unit on bed rest and placed on MAP goals of >85, and postoperative x-rays showed good location of the hardware (Fig. 7.3). He was mobilized on postoperative day 1 and discharged on postoperative day 4.

Commonalities among the experts

There was a consensus among our experts that this patient was best served with a posterior approach, although the levels and whether fusion was necessary varied. The majority recommended obtaining a computed tomography angiography (CTA) to evaluate the vertebral arteries, and half also recommended obtaining MRI of the thoracic and lumbar spine. One of the experts also recommended an MRI of the brain along with the MRI of the thoracic and lumbar spine. Half recommended flexion-extension x-rays, while only one did not recommend further imaging. While the majority of our experts recommended a decompression and fusion, only one surgeon recommended a laminoplasty alone from C2–5. Of those that recommend laminectomy and fusion, there was consensus that decompression needed to include C1, and one surgeon recommended laminectomy from C1–7. Two experts recommended fusion only to C5, and one surgeon recommended beginning at C2 and the other recommended C1–5 instrumentation. The one expert who recommended laminectomy from C1–7 also recommended instrumented fusion from C1-T2. The majority also recommended intraoperative monitoring and surgical navigation for placement of instrumentation. The most common concern was a cerebrospinal fluid leak, although spinal cord injury and C5 palsy were also mentioned. The majority planned admission to the floor with planned discharged 3 to 5 days after surgery.

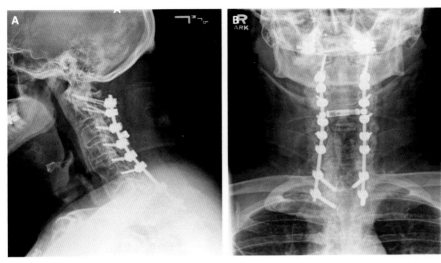

Fig. 7.3 Postoperative x-rays. (A) Lateral and **(B)** anteroposterior (AP) x-rays showing postoperative changes following C1-T2 instrumentation.

SUMMARY OF QUALITY OF EVIDENCE TO GUIDE SPECIFIC INTERVENTIONS FOR THIS CASE

- Anterior versus posterior approach for OPLL: level II.1
- Laminectomy versus laminoplasty and fusion for OPLL: level II.1
- Intraoperative monitoring for spine surgery: level II.1
- Intraoperative blood pressure of >80 for cervical myelopathy: level II.2

REFERENCES

1. Koga H, Sakou T, Taketomi E, et al. Genetic mapping of ossification of the posterior longitudinal ligament of the spine. *Am J Hum Genet*. 1998;62(6):1460–1467.
2. Liu Y, Zhao Y, Chen Y, et al. RUNX2 polymorphisms associated with OPLL and OLF in the Han population. *Clin Orthop Relat Res*. 2010;468(12):3333–3341.
3. Terayama K. Genetic studies on ossification of the posterior longitudinal ligament of the spine. *Spine (Phila Pa 1976)*. 1989;14(11):1184–1191.
4. Epstein N. Diagnosis and surgical management of cervical ossification of the posterior longitudinal ligament. *Spine J*. 2002;2(6):436–449.
5. Abode-Iyamah KO, Stoner KE, Grossbach AJ, et al. Effects of brain derived neurotrophic factor Val66Met polymorphism in patients with cervical spondylotic myelopathy. *J Clin Neurosci*. 2016;24:117–121.
6. Setzer M, Vrionis FD, Hermann EJ, et al. Effect of apolipoprotein E genotype on the outcome after anterior cervical decompression and fusion in patients with cervical spondylotic myelopathy. *J Neurosurg Spine*. 2009;11(6):659–666.
7. Wang D, Liu W, Cao Y, et al. BMP-4 polymorphisms in the susceptibility of cervical spondylotic myelopathy and its outcome after anterior cervical corpectomy and fusion. *Cell Physiol Biochem*. 2013;32(1):210–217.
8. Wang ZC, Hou XW, Shao J, et al. HIF-1alpha polymorphism in the susceptibility of cervical spondylotic myelopathy and its outcome after anterior cervical corpectomy and fusion treatment. *PLoS One*. 2014;9(11):e110862.
9. Costa P, Bruno A, Bonzanino M, et al. Somatosensory- and motor-evoked potential monitoring during spine and spinal cord surgery. *Spinal Cord*. 2007;45(1):86–91.
10. Fehlings MG, Brodke DS, Norvell DC, Dettori JR. The evidence for intraoperative neurophysiological monitoring in spine surgery: does it make a difference? *Spine (Phila Pa 1976)*. 2010;35(9 Suppl): S37–S46.
11. Hilibrand ASSD, Sethuraman V, Vaccaro AR, Albert TJ. Comparison of transcranial electrical motor and somatosensory evoked potential monitoring during cervical spine surgery. *J Bone Joint Surg*. 2004;86A:1248–1253.
12. Langeloo DD, Lelivelt A, Louis Journee H, et al. Transcranial electrical motor-evoked potential monitoring during surgery for spinal deformity: a study of 145 patients. *Spine (Phila Pa 1976)*. 2003;28(10):1043–1050.
13. Sutter M, Eggspuehler A, Grob D, et al. The validity of multimodal intraoperative monitoring (MIOM) in surgery of 109 spine and spinal cord tumors. *Eur Spine J*. 2007;16(Suppl 2):S197–S208.
14. Traynelis VC, Abode-Iyamah KO, Leick KM, et al. Cervical decompression and reconstruction without intraoperative neurophysiological monitoring. *J Neurosurg Spine*. 2012;16(2):107–113.
15. Weinzierl MR, Reinacher P, Gilsbach JM, Rohde V. Combined motor and somatosensory evoked potentials for intraoperative monitoring: intra- and postoperative data in a series of 69 operations. *Neurosurg Rev*. 2007;30(2):109–116; discussion 16.
16. Kato S, Nouri A, Wu D, et al. Comparison of Anterior and Posterior Surgery for Degenerative Cervical Myelopathy: An MRI-Based Propensity-Score-Matched Analysis Using Data from the Prospective Multicenter AOSpine CSM North America and International Studies. *J Bone Joint Surg Am*. 2017;99(12):1013–1021.
17. Kim DH, Lee CH, Ko YS, et al. The Clinical Implications and Complications of Anterior Versus Posterior Surgery for Multilevel Cervical Ossification of the Posterior Longitudinal Ligament; An Updated Systematic Review and Meta-Analysis. *Neurospine*. 2019;16(3):530–541.
18. Qin R, Chen X, Zhou P, et al. Anterior cervical corpectomy and fusion versus posterior laminoplasty for the treatment of oppressive myelopathy owing to cervical ossification of posterior longitudinal ligament: a meta-analysis. *Eur Spine J*. 2018;27(6):1375–1387.
19. Sarkar S, Rajshekhar V. Long-Term Sustainability of Functional Improvement Following Central Corpectomy for Cervical Spondylotic Myelopathy and Ossification of Posterior Longitudinal Ligament. *Spine (Phila Pa 1976)*. 2018;43(12):E703–E711.
20. Yang H, Sun J, Shi J, et al. Anterior Controllable Antedisplacement Fusion (ACAF) for Severe Cervical Ossification of the Posterior Longitudinal Ligament: Comparison with Anterior Cervical Corpectomy with Fusion (ACCF). *World Neurosurg*. 2018;115:e428–e436.
21. Lee CH, Sohn MJ, Lee CH, et al. Are There Differences in the Progression of Ossification of the Posterior Longitudinal Ligament Following Laminoplasty Versus Fusion?: A Meta-Analysis. *Spine (Phila Pa 1976)*. 2017;42(12):887–894.
22. Youssef JA, Heiner AD, Montgomery JR, et al. Outcomes of posterior cervical fusion and decompression: a systematic review and meta-analysis. *Spine J*. 2019;19(10):1714–1729.
23. Lebl DR, Bono CM. Update on the Diagnosis and Management of Cervical Spondylotic Myelopathy. *J Am Acad Orthop Surg*. 2015;23(11): 648–660.

8

Thoracic disc herniation

Jaime L. Martínez Santos, MD

Introduction

Thoracic disc herniations (TDHs) are commonly found on imaging and occur in up to 37% of asymptomatic individuals.[1] A large proportion of TDHs are giant (occupying >40% of the spinal canal) and calcified[2] with tendencies to adhere and erode through the dura[3] and cause progressive neurological decline requiring surgical treatment. There is no established gold standard treatment. Thoracic discectomies are challenging and historically have been associated with poor surgical outcomes and high neurological morbidity.

In this chapter we utilize a case example to illustrate the clinical presentation and surgical management of a giant calcified TDH.

Case Example

Chief complaint: back pain and lower extremity pain and weakness

History of present illness: The patient is a 74-year-old male with history of severe low thoracic back pain radiating to above his umbilicus and progressive lower extremity weakness. He also reports difficulty ambulating over the past month. Thoracic spine imaging (Figs. 8.1 and 8.2) revealed a sizable T9–10 calcified thoracic disc compressing and displacing the spinal cord to the left.

Medications: diuretics, ASA 325 mg

Allergies: no known drug allergies

Past medical history: congestive heart failure and coronary artery disease

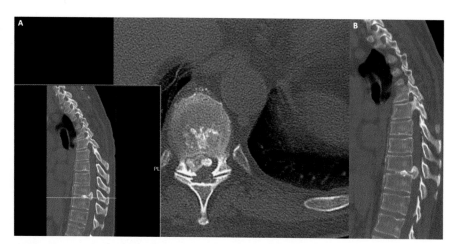

Fig. 8.1 **Preoperative axial (A) and sagittal (B) computed tomography bone windows showing a sizable calcified thoracic disc herniation occupying more than 40% of the anteroposterior spinal canal.** Note that the nucleus pulposus is also abnormally calcified.

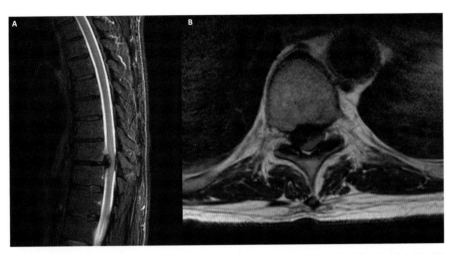

Fig. 8.2 Preoperative sagittal (A) and axial (B) thoracic spine MRI redemonstrating this giant herniated thoracic disc causing spinal cord compression (note the high T2 signal within the spinal cord cranial to the disc) (A) and displacing the spinal cord to the left (B).

Past surgical history: none

Family history: none

Social history: none

Physical examination: awake, alert, and oriented to person, place, and time; cranial nerves II–XII intact, full strength in the upper extremities: bilateral deltoids/triceps/biceps/grip/interossei 5/5; weak lower extremities: hip flexors 3/5, knee extensors 3/5, ankle dorsiflexion 4/5, long toe extensor and ankle plantar flexion 5/5.

Reflexes: 2+ response in bilateral biceps/triceps/brachioradialis with negative Hoffman and lower extremity hyperreflexia and clonus with 3+ response in bilateral patella and Achilles tendons; abnormal lower extremity light touch and proprioception with T10 sensory level

Laboratories: all within normal limits

	Jorge Eduardo Guzman Prenk, MD Neurosurgery Pontifica Universidad Javeriana Bogota, Colombia	Langston Holly, MD Neurosurgery University of California at Los Angeles Los Angeles, California, United States	Sutipat Pairojboriboon, MD Orthopaedic Surgery Vichaiyut Hospital Phyathai, Thailand	Frank M. Phillips, MD Orthopaedic Surgery Rush University Chicago, Illinois, United States
Preoperative				
Additional tests requested	MRI T-spine SSEP/MEP	MRI T-spine T-spine AP and lateral x-rays Medicine evaluation	MRI T-spine Angiogram Cardiology evaluation Anesthesia evaluation	MRI T-spine Standing x-rays
Surgical approach selected	T9–10 MIS laminectomy, foraminotomy	T9–10 transpedicular costotransversectomy for partial corpectomy and discectomy, laminectomy, right facetectomy	T9–10 costotransversectomy discectomy, posterolateral T7-L1 fusion	T9–10 laminectomy, transpedicular discectomy, and fusion
Goal of surgery	Decompress spinal cord	Decompress spinal cord	Decompress spinal cord, neurological preservation	Decompress spinal cord
Perioperative				
Positioning	Left lateral decubitus	Prone on Jackson table	Prone on Jackson table	Prone
Surgical equipment Surgical microscope Hi Speed Drill With diamond tip burrs	Fluoroscopy IOM (MEP/SSEP) Tubular retractor	IOM (MEP/SSEP) Fluoroscopy Surgical microscope Surgical navigation	Fluoroscopy IOM (MEP/SSEP/EMG) Ultrasonic bone scalpel Surgical microscope Ultrasound	Fluoroscopy IOM
Medications	None	None	Steroids, MAPs >80	Maintain MAP

	Jorge Eduardo Guzman Prenk, MD Neurosurgery Pontifica Universidad Javeriana Bogota, Colombia	Langston Holly, MD Neurosurgery University of California at Los Angeles Los Angeles, California, United States	Sutipat Pairojboriboon, MD Orthopaedic Surgery Vichaiyut Hospital Phyathai, Thailand	Frank M. Phillips, MD Orthopaedic Surgery Rush University Chicago, Illinois, United States
Anatomical considerations	Pedicles, facets, dura, nerve root	Spinal cord, nerve roots, segmental artery	Artery of Adamkiewicz, segmental artery, spinal cord	Spinal cord
Complications feared with approach chosen	Instability	CSF leak, spinal cord injury, hardware-related problems	Ventral dural tear, arterial injury, inadequate discectomy	Neural injury, CSF leak
Intraoperative				
Anesthesia	General	General	General	General
Exposure	T9–10	T9–10	T7-L1	T9–10
Levels decompressed	T9–10	T9–10	T9–10	T9–10
Levels fused	None	None	T7-L1	T9–10
Surgical narrative	Position left lateral decubitus, fluoroscopy in AP projection to identify right T9–10 facet and ipsilateral pedicle, right paramedian incision, sequentially place tubes using Seldinger technique with entry point on the superior lateral quadrant of the pedicle, place and fix tubular system, drill T9 right lamina and partial right inferior facet and T10 right superior facet, right T9–10 foraminotomy, drill calcified disc in lateral to medial and inside-out manner if possible, send samples to pathology, withdraw tubular system once hemostasis confirmed, layered closure	Position prone on Jackson table, localize incision using AP fluoroscopy, midline posterior incision, T9–10 laminectomy, right facetectomy, place reference frame, O-arm spin, register with navigation, potentially remove rib head if needed to increase working angle, perform partial transpedicular corpectomy to create space to displace disc away from cord, sacrifice nerve root, incise disc herniation and remove, palpate to confirm decompression, additional O-arm to confirm decompression, layered closure with drain	Position prone on Jackson table, count spinal levels and ribs or pre and intraoperative x-rays, midline skin incision, expose lamina and transverse process, T9–10 laminectomy, remove right facet/transverse process/ribs using ultrasonic bone scalpel or drill, rib removal with care to avoid tearing underlying pleura, identify and follow right T10 nerve root medially to foramen, suture and ligate nerve root, use nerve root for gentle traction, drill down right pedicle, discectomy under surgical microscope, incise PLL and disc annulus, clear disc space with curettes and drill if necessary, send specimen to pathology, separate ventral thecal sac from calcified disc and push disc ventrally into working cavity, ultrasound to evaluate disc morphology and adequacy of decompression, pedicle screw placement three levels above and below and left pedicle at index level, intraoperative O-arm to assess instrumentation, connect rods, local and allograft bone grafts in posterolateral gutters, antibiotic irrigation and vancomycin powder, standard closure with drains	Position prone, laminectomy above and below index level, wide laminectomy at index level without instrument intrusion into spinal canal, resect facet and pedicle as needed adjacent to calcified intracanal material, approach calcified material from far lateral, thin calcified material with drill from inside-out creating thin shell of material adjacent to cord, collapse remaining bony shell away from cord with micro and reverse angle curettes, instrument and fuse level destabilized by wide decompression and facetectomy, layered closure
Complication avoidance	AP fluoroscopy to identify level, minimally invasive approach, drill in lateral to medial and inside-out manner to avoid dural injury	AP fluoroscopy to identify surgical level, potentially remove rib head to increase working angle, surgical navigation, partial corpectomy to displace disc away from cord, sacrifice nerve root, O-arm spin to confirm decompression	Count levels based on spinal level and ribs, costotransversectomy with care to protect pleura, suture and ligate T10 nerve root, use nerve root for gentle traction, removal of T10 pedicle, separate disc from thecal sac, ultrasound to assess disc and decompression, intraoperative O-arm to assess instrumentation	Resect pedicle as need adjacent to calcified intracanal material, approach calcified material from far lateral, eggshell calcified material, remove remaining bone away from cord

	Jorge Eduardo Guzman Prenk, MD Neurosurgery Pontifica Universidad Javeriana Bogota, Colombia	Langston Holly, MD Neurosurgery University of California at Los Angeles Los Angeles, California, United States	Sutipat Pairojboriboon, MD Orthopaedic Surgery Vichaiyut Hospital Phyathai, Thailand	Frank M. Phillips, MD Orthopaedic Surgery Rush University Chicago, Illinois, United States
Postoperative				
Admission	Outpatient	Floor	ICU	Floor
Postoperative complications feared	CSF leak, epidural hematoma, wound infection	Neurological deficit, CSF leak, spinal instability	Inadequate decompression, intercostal neuralgia, dural tear	Neural injury, CSF leak
Anticipated length of stay	Same day	3 days	4–5 days	2–3 days
Follow-up testing	CT T-spine 4 months after surgery MEP/SSEP 4 months after surgery if results unsatisfactory	None	T–L spine x-rays at each follow-up visit	T–L spine x-rays 6 weeks, 3 months, 6 months, 1 year after surgery
Bracing	None	None	None	None
Follow-up visits	10 days, 4 months after surgery	2 weeks, 6 weeks, 3 months, 6 months, 1 year after surgery	2 weeks, every 3 months until 1 year after surgery	2 weeks, 6 weeks, 3 months, 6 months, 1 year after surgery

AP, Anteroposterior; CSF, cerebrospinal fluid; CT, computed tomography; EMG, electromyography; ICU, intensive care unit; IOM, intraoperative monitoring; MAP, mean arterial pressure; MEP, motor evoked potential; MRI, magnetic resonance imaging; PLL, posterior longitudinal ligament; SSEP, somatosensory evoked potential.

Differential diagnosis

- Metastasis
- Tuberculosis
- Fungal infection
- Thoracic stenosis

Important anatomical and preoperative considerations

TDHs are common and can be found in up to 37% of asymptomatic individuals[1] and commonly occur at caudal levels below T7.[4] Although their natural history has not been fully elucidated, TDHs behave differently than cervical and lumbar spine herniations and have a higher tendency to calcify (~42%)[2] and to adhere to the dura and erode into the intradural space.[3]

The most common clinical presentation of TDHs is pain (~92%), which can be localized to the back or radiate as intercostal neuralgia, followed by myelopathy with neurological deficits (~60%), which are usually slow and progressive (~89%) with weakness, ataxia, or sphincter disturbance.[2,3] Acute paraparesis, paraplegia, or Brown-Sequard syndrome can occur in ~11%. Rare cases of transient or permanent anterior spinal cord syndrome from occlusion of the anterior spinal artery have been reported.[5]

The thoracic spinal cord is more vulnerable to compression injury (especially ventral) for the following reasons: (1) the thoracic spinal canal is narrower, (2) the thecal sac and spinal cord is displaced ventrally by the natural thoracic kyphosis and the dentate ligaments anchor the spinal cord preventing major displacements, and (3) the thoracic spinal cord has watershed territories with reduced vascularization.[3,6] "Giant" TDHs occupy more than 40% of the anteroposterior diameter of the spinal canal and almost universally (95%–97%) present with myelopathy.[6–8] These lesions pose a real surgical challenge as most TDHs are calcified (76%–95%)[6,9] and approximately 31% to 75% extend intradurally.[6–8]

Indications for surgery include symptomatic TDHs or TDHs causing high T2 signals on magnetic resonance imaging. Thoracic discectomies are one of the most technically challenging spine surgeries and historically have been associated with high neurological morbidity. The diagnostic and preoperative workup often includes vascular imaging with a formal spinal angiogram or a magnetic resonance angiogram to locate and protect the artery of Adamkiewicz.[3] A computed tomography–guided pedicle marker is often placed preoperatively for intraoperative localization.

Available surgical techniques for thoracic discectomy utilize the following approaches: posterior (laminectomy only, transfacet pedicle-sparing, or transpedicular), posterolateral (transpedicular, costotransversectomy, and lateral extracavitary approach), lateral (open or miniopen MIS retropleural approach), and anterior (via open thoracotomy, thoracoscopic, or minithoracotomy). Selection of the surgical approach is dictated by the location (spinal level and central vs. lateral), size, and type (soft vs. calcified) of the TDH and patient-specific characteristics such as weight, medical history, and pulmonary function.

Anterior approaches are associated with a lower rate of neurological decline, subarachnoid-pleural cerebrospinal fluid (CSF) fistula, and reoperation but greater rate of postthoracotomy pain syndrome (up to 50%),[10] pulmonary complications (atelectasis, pneumonia, and pleural effusion), and extended hospital stay.[3,6] Patients should be able to tolerate single lung ventilation. Anterior approaches provide a wider exposure that could be advantageous for central TDH and giant TDHs with transdural components allowing for circumferential microdissection ventral to the spinal cord and dural reconstruction. Lateral retropleural approaches provide a wider view and allow for removal of centrally located discs while avoiding lung-related complications of the anterior transpleural approaches. However, incidental pleural injuries occur in about 30%, requiring chest tube placement.[3,11] Posterior and posterolateral approaches are perhaps more versatile and may have low complications rates. Posterior approaches are advantageous for smaller and laterally located TDHs with no intradural component and in patients with poor respiratory function.[6] Disadvantages are having to retract the dura (and the spinal cord) in almost all cases, limited visualization of the ventral epidural space and spinal cord, and difficulty repairing ventral dural defects primarily. A transdural approach may be utilized, through this route, to remove stubborn herniations. The dorsal dural incision is closed primarily with suture while the ventral defect is repaired with an onlay dural substitute that usually heals well as a contained pseudomeningocele if there is no violation to the parietal pleura.[12]

The surgical outcomes of thoracic discectomies have improved significantly over the past few decades with about 69% of patients showing neurological improvement and less than 5% having permanent neurological deficits.[6] Reported complication rates range from 20% to 30% and appear to be higher with anterior approaches.[3,13] Postoperative neurological deficits occur in about 2% to 5% and risk factors include giant, calcified, or transdural TDHs, preexisting intramedullary T2 signal change on magnetic resonance imaging, preexisting preoperative neurological deficit, and angle of kyphosis at the TDH level.[6,9] Postoperative intercostal neuralgia occurs in about 30% of thoracotomies but can be prevented with careful dissection of the intercostal neurovascular bundle prior to removing the rib.[3] CSF leaks can occur with transthoracic approaches in up to 15% of cases and giant calcified TDHs have a higher risk.[14] A feared complication is a subarachnoid-pleural fistula, which invariably requires a surgical repair given the negative intrathoracic pressure.

Nowadays, a spinal instrumented fusion can be avoided in most cases. For anterior and lateral approaches, resecting the rib head, pedicle, and edges of adjacent vertebral bodies does not destabilize the spine[15] because the anterior and posterior columns of Denis are maintained. Fusion is required if more than 50% of the vertebral body is removed.[3,4,15] For posterior approaches, a laminectomy with unilateral pedicle-sparing partial facetectomy achieves a good lateral corridor for most TDHs and does not require fusion. Bilateral facet or extensive facet and pedicle removal require fusion.[3]

What was actually done

The patient was taken to the operating room for a lateral transthoracic retropleural approach and T9–10 discectomy. Surgery was performed under general anesthesia and the patient's mean arterial pressures (MAPs) were maintained 10% to 20% higher than his baseline. Somatosensory evoked potentials (SSEPs), motor evoked potentials (MEPs), and electromyography (EMG) were monitored. The patient was positioned in left lateral decubitus on a bean bag with proper axillary padding for a right thoracotomy. Ideally the patient's body is in slight lateral flexion. The thoracotomy approach

was performed by our cardiothoracic surgery colleagues. The T9–10 spinal level and calcified disc were readily localized using fluoroscopy. The tenth rib was initially divided to gain access to the T9–10 disc space; however, the exposure was somewhat limited, and thus it was decided to also divide the eighth and 9th ribs. The endothoracic fascia was incised to expose the parietal pleura, which was bluntly swept and reflected anteriorly and out of the way. Exposure was maintained using malleable self-retaining retractors. The T9–10 space was again localized with fluoroscopy. The operative microscope was brought in and the endothoracic fascia was incised with monopolar to expose the rib head. The rib head was carefully removed with rongeurs and a high-speed drill, leaving its inferior rim to protect the intercostal neurovascular bundle and radicular artery and exposing the intervertebral disc, pedicle, and neuroforamen. The posterolateral T9 and T10 end plates were drilled down and disc fragments were removed in the usual fashion. This created a cavity ventral to the calcified disc. The posterior longitudinal ligament was exposed cranial and caudal to the herniated disc and then removed piecemeal to expose the dura. The intraoperative ultrasound is useful for a real-time assessment of the relationships between the herniated disc and the dura and spinal cord.[16,17] The calcified disc was gently dissected off the ventral dura with microdissection and mobilized toward the cavity created ventrally with Epstein curettes and a right-angle blunt hook. The vector of force was always directed away from the spinal cord and always preventing any recoils from the instrument. Once the disc was removed, the dura was relaxed, pulsatile, and intact. Valsalva maneuvers confirmed no durotomy. A chest tube was placed in the retropleural space, the ribs were plated, and the wound closed in planes.

The patient did well postoperatively; the chest tube was removed on day 3 and he was discharged home on day 5. Postoperative imaging showed good decompression of the thecal sac (Fig. 8.3). His preoperative symptoms resolved; however, he developed a right postthoracotomy intercostal neuralgia that required additional doses of analgesics.

Commonalities among experts

Half of the surgeons would obtain a preoperative evaluation and surgical risk assessment by a medical service. While most surgeons would utilize a posterior approach, all techniques were different. Most surgeons selected open approaches and one surgeon selected a lateral MIS retropleural approach without fusion. Half of the surgeons would perform a T9–10 costotransversectomy with or without fusion and only one surgeon selected the more traditional T9–10 transpedicular microdiscectomy and fusion. It is a standard of care utilizing intraoperative neurophysiologic monitoring during thoracic microdiscectomies. Commonly feared complications include spinal cord injury, occlusion of a major radicular branch supplying the spinal cord, vascular injury, and CSF leak. All surgeons emphasized using meticulous microdissection along the interface between the calcified disc and the dura, creating a space or cavity ventral to the disc, removing the disc piecemeal with drill or using an ultrasonic bone cutter, and then mobilizing the disc toward the ventral cavity and away from the spinal cord. Only half advocated for instrumented fusion on that level (T9–10) or the adjacent three levels (T7-L1). Most surgeons pointed out the importance of carefully localizing the correct spinal level to avoid wrong

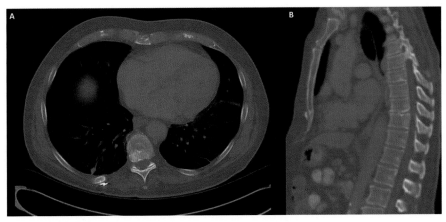

Fig. 8.3 Postoperative axial (A) and sagittal (B) computed tomography scans showing removal of the calcified disc with good decompression of the thecal sac.

level surgery as it is more common in the thoracic spine. Most surgeons would obtain either a plain x-ray or a thoracic computed tomography at some point 1 to 4 months out of surgery. Follow up was scheduled at 2 weeks and then every 3 months.

SUMMARY OF QUALITY OF EVIDENCE TO GUIDE SPECIFIC INTERVENTIONS FOR THIS CASE

- Intraoperative neurophysiologic monitoring is recommended for all thoracic discectomy cases: level IC.
- A lateral approach is suggested for thoracic discectomy as it may be associated with less major postoperative complications[18]: level III.

REFERENCES

1. Wood KB, Garvey TA, Gundry C, Heithoff KB. Magnetic resonance imaging of the thoracic spine. Evaluation of asymptomatic individuals. *J Bone Joint Surg Am.* 1995;77(11):1631–1638.
2. Quint U, Bordon G, Preissl I, et al. Thoracoscopic treatment for single level symptomatic thoracic disc herniation: a prospective followed cohort study in a group of 167 consecutive cases. *Eur Spine J.* 2012;21(4):637–645.
3. Court C, Mansour E, Bouthors C. Thoracic disc herniation: Surgical treatment. *Orthop Traumatol Surg Res.* 2018;104(1S):S31–S40.
4. Quraishi NA, Khurana A, Tsegaye MM, et al. Calcified giant thoracic disc herniations: considerations and treatment strategies. *Eur Spine J.* 2014;23(Suppl 1):S76–83.
5. Guest JD, Griesdale DE, Marotta T. Thoracic disc herniation presenting with transient anterior spinal artery syndrome. A case report. *Interv Neuroradiol.* 2000;6(4):327–331.
6. Gong M, Liu G, Guan Q, et al. Surgery for Giant Calcified Herniated Thoracic Discs: A Systematic Review. *World Neurosurg.* 2018;118:109–117.
7. Hott JS, Feiz-Erfan I, Kenny K, Dickman CA. Surgical management of giant herniated thoracic discs: analysis of 20 cases. *J Neurosurg Spine.* 2005;3(3):191–197.
8. Kapoor S, Amarouche M, Al-Obeidi F, et al. Giant thoracic discs: treatment, outcome, and follow-up of 33 patients in a single centre. *Eur Spine J.* 2018;27(7):1555–1566.
9. Cornips EM, Janssen ML, Beuls EA. Thoracic disc herniation and acute myelopathy: clinical presentation, neuroimaging findings, surgical considerations, and outcome. *J Neurosurg Spine.* 2011;14(4):520–528.
10. Karmakar MK, Ho AM. Postthoracotomy pain syndrome. *Thorac Surg Clin.* 2004;14(3):345–352.
11. Foreman PM, Naftel RP, Moore 2nd TA, Hadley MN. The lateral extracavitary approach to the thoracolumbar spine: a case series and systematic review. *J Neurosurg Spine.* 2016;24(4):570–579.
12. Lowe SR, Alshareef MA, Kellogg RT, et al. A Novel Surgical Technique for Management of Giant Central Calcified Thoracic Disk Herniations: A Dual Corridor Method Involving Tubular Transthoracic/Retropleural Approach Followed by a Posterior Transdural Diskectomy. *Oper Neurosurg (Hagerstown).* 2019;16(5):626–632.
13. Brotis AG, Tasiou A, Paterakis K, et al. Complications Associated with Surgery for Thoracic Disc Herniation: A Systematic Review and Network Meta-Analysis. *World Neurosurg.* 2019;132:334–342.
14. McCormick WE, Will SF, Benzel EC. Surgery for thoracic disc disease. Complication avoidance: overview and management. *Neurosurg Focus.* 2000;9(4):e13.
15. Krauss WE, Edwards DA, Cohen-Gadol AA. Transthoracic discectomy without interbody fusion. *Surg Neurol.* 2005;63(5):403–408. discussion 408-409.
16. Martinez Santos JL, Alshareef M, Kalhorn SP. Back Pain and Radiculopathy from Non-Steroidal Anti-Inflammatory Drug-induced Dorsal Epidural Haematoma. *BMJ Case Reports.* 2019;12(3):e229015.
17. Martinez Santos JLWJE, Kalhorn SP. Microsurgical Management of a Primary Neuroendocrine Tumor of the Filum Terminale: A Surgical Technique. *Cureus.* 2020;12(8):e10080.
18. Kerezoudis P, Rajjoub KR, Goncalves S, et al. Anterior versus posterior approaches for thoracic disc herniation: Association with postoperative complications. *Clin Neurol Neurosurg.* 2018;167:17–23.

9

Cervical spondylotic radiculopathy and myelopathy from facet and uncovertebral hypertrophy

Jaime L. Martínez Santos, MD

Introduction

Cervical spondylotic myelopathy (CSM) is the most common type of spinal cord dysfunction in adults.[1,2] This chronic spinal degeneration is characterized by intervertebral disc herniations, abnormal ligament and joint hypertrophy, and ossification. It almost invariably results in progressive neurological decline. Surgery is the only proven treatment to halt disease progression and restore neurological functioning. The surgical treatment of CSM can be challenging, especially in the setting of ossification of the posterior longitudinal ligament (OPLL) and multilevel disease involving both anterior and posterior spinal cord compressions. In this chapter, we utilize a case example to illustrate the clinical presentation and surgical management of a case with multilevel CSM with anterior and posterior spinal cord compression from OPLL, intervertebral disc herniation, and interlaminar ligament, uncinate, and facet hypertrophy and ossification.

Case Example

Chief complaint: pain in neck and right arm
History of present illness: The patient is a 69-year-old male with a 1-year history of worsening neck pain and right arm pain in a C7 root distribution. He also reports progressive difficulty ambulating. Cervical spine imaging (Figs. 9.1 and 9.2) shows severe cervical spondylosis with left-sided posterolateral spinal cord compression by facet (zygapophyseal) and interlaminar ligament hypertrophy and ossification at C4–5 and right-sided ventrolateral spinal cord and neuroforaminal compression by uncovertebral and disc-osteophyte hypertrophy and ossification at C6–7.
Medications: aspirin 81 mg
Allergies: no known drug allergies
Past medical history: none
Past surgical history: cholecystectomy
Family history: noncontributory
Social history: no smoking and occasional alcohol

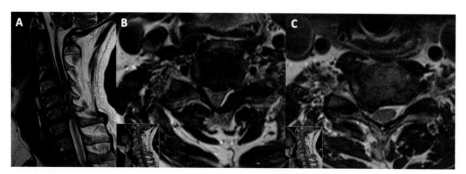

Fig. 9.1 Preoperative T2-weighted magnetic resonance imaging (MRI). (A) Midline sagittal MRI demonstrating loss of cervical lordosis, diffuse cervical spondylosis, intervertebral disc desiccation, and reduced and bulging at C4–5, C5–6, and C6–7 levels. (B) Axial MRI at C4–5 level demonstrating severe posterolateral spinal cord compression from ligamentum flavum and facet hypertrophy and ossification. (C) Axial MRI at the C6–7 level demonstrating severe ventrolateral and neuroforaminal compression from uncovertebral joint hypertrophy and intervertebral disc herniation.

Physical examination: awake, alert, and oriented to person, place, and time; cranial nerves II–XII intact; bilateral deltoids/triceps/biceps 5/5; interossei 5/5; iliopsoas/knee flexion/knee extension/dorsi, and plantar flexion 5/5.

Reflexes: bilateral upper extremity hyperreflexia with 3+ response in bilateral biceps/triceps/brachioradialis and Hoffman's present bilaterally; ataxic gait
Laboratories: all within normal limits

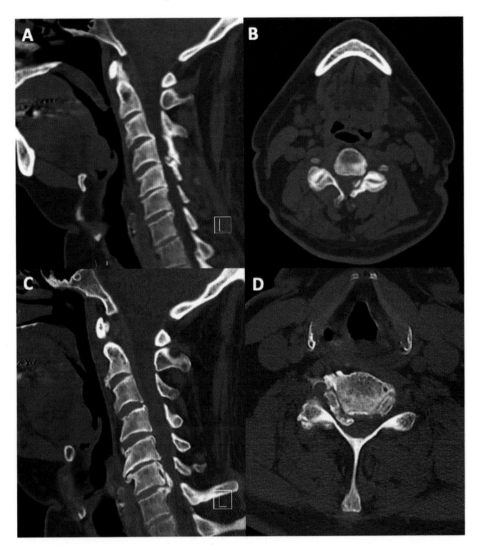

Fig. 9.2 Preoperative computed tomography bone windows. (A) Left paramedian sagittal and (B) axial sections demonstrating hypertrophied facets and calcified interlaminar ligament at the C4–5 level. (C) Midline and (D) axial sections demonstrating ossified posterior longitudinal ligament and prominent osteophytes and uncovertebral joints at the left C6–7 level.

Pedro Luis Bazán, MD Spine Surgeon HIGA San Martín La Plata (Chief Orthopaedic) Hospital Italiano La Plata Instituto de Diagnóstico La Plata La Plata, Buenos Aires, Argentina	Esteban F. Espinoza-García, MD, MSc University of Valparaíso San Felipe, Chile	Brett A. Freedman, MD Sandra Hobson, MD Orthopaedic Surgery Mayo Clinic Rochester, Minnesota, United States	Meic H. Schmidt, MD, MBA Neurosurgery University of New Mexico Albuquerque, New Mexico, United States

Preoperative			
Additional tests requested	C-spine flexion-extension x-ray Neurology evaluation EMG	EMG/NCS MRI brain	C-spine upright AP, lateral, flexion/extension x-rays BMD scans Additional physical exam	Swallow evaluation Vocal cord function assessment Anesthesia clearance

	Pedro Luis Bazán, MD Spine Surgeon HIGA San Martín La Plata (Chief Orthopaedic) Hospital Italiano La Plata Instituto de Diagnóstico La Plata La Plata, Buenos Aires, Argentina	Esteban F. Espinoza-García, MD, MSc University of Valparaíso San Felipe, Chile	Brett A. Freedman, MD Sandra Hobson, MD Orthopaedic Surgery Mayo Clinic Rochester, Minnesota, United States	Meic H. Schmidt, MD, MBA Neurosurgery University of New Mexico Albuquerque, New Mexico, United States
Surgical approach selected	MIS C6–7 foraminotomy	C4–5 laminectomy, C6–7 foraminotomy	C2-T2 posterior instrumented fusion, C4–7 decompression, right C6–7 foraminotomy	C4–5, C5–6, C6–7 ACDF
Goal of surgery	Nerve root decompression	Spinal cord and nerve root decompression	Spinal cord decompression, right C7 nerve root decompression, stabilization	Spinal cord decompression
Perioperative				
Positioning	Prone	Prone without pins	Prone on Jackson table with Mayfield pins	Supine with cervical traction
Surgical equipment	Fluoroscopy Endoscope	Fluoroscopy	IOM (MEP/SSEP/EMG) Surgical navigation O-arm Surgical microscope	IOM Surgical microscope Fluoroscopy Allograft spacer Dynamic plate
Medications	Maintain MAP	Steroids, maintain MAP	Tranexamic acid	Steroids
Anatomical considerations	Surgical level, facet	Dura	Vertebral artery, anterior ossification at right C6–7	Esophagus, carotid artery, spinal cord
Complications feared with approach chosen	Spinal instability	Durotomy, CSF leak	Inadequate decompression	Spinal cord injury from hypotension, dysphagia, vocal cord paralysis, CSF leak
Intraoperative				
Anesthesia	General	General	General	General
Exposure	Right C6–7	C4–7	C2-T2	C4-C7
Levels decompressed	Right C6–7	C4–5, right C6–7	C4–7	C4–5, C5–6, C6–7
Levels fused	None	None	C2-T2	C4–5, C5–6, C6–7

	Pedro Luis Bazán, MD Spine Surgeon HIGA San Martín La Plata (Chief Orthopaedic) Hospital Italiano La Plata Instituto de Diagnóstico La Plata La Plata, Buenos Aires, Argentina	Esteban F. Espinoza-García, MD, MSc University of Valparaíso San Felipe, Chile	Brett A. Freedman, MD Sandra Hobson, MD Orthopaedic Surgery Mayo Clinic Rochester, Minnesota, United States	Meic H. Schmidt, MD, MBA Neurosurgery University of New Mexico Albuquerque, New Mexico, United States
Surgical narrative	Position prone, x-ray to confirm level, posterior midline incision, dissect down onto right C6–7 lamina under exoscopic visualization, foraminotomy, confirm decompression of nerve root, layered closure	Position prone on foam headrest, localizing x-ray, midline incision, bilateral subperiosteal dissection from C4–7, x-ray confirmation of levels, C4–5 laminectomy, yellow ligament removal until dura visualized, localize C6–7 segment, right C6–7 hemilaminectomy and foraminotomy	Preflip signals, apply pin and position prone, postflip IOM after positioning, midline prone incision, dissect down through subcutaneous fat to level of nuchal ligament and deep dorsal fascia, subperiosteal dissection down over and preserving facet joints, x-ray to confirm level, complete exposure from C2–3 facet down to T1–2 facet, decorticate dorsal bone and facets, C3–6 lateral mass screws (start hole in inferior-medial quadrant and aimed up and out) and T1/2 pedicle screws based on anatomical landmarks and stereotactic navigation, skip C7, pack facets and posterolateral bone with bone graft prior to final insertion of screws, C3–6 laminectomy as well inferior C2 and superior C7 with microscope, elevate and resect ligamentum flavum, general right C6–7 foraminotomy by resecting portions of the inferior and superior articulating processes with a bur and curettes and Kerrison rongeurs, repeat on left, confirm head and heck are in preferred posture/ alignment, place appropriate rods and final tighten set screws except for bottom screws, gently compress and final tighten bottom screws, place residual graft, final x-rays, wound filled with dilute povidone solution, removed and vancomycin powder placed, layered closure with drain, incisional VAC placed	Position supine with roll behind shoulder and neck, mild Holter traction with baseline MEP and SSEP, horizontal incision with fluoroscopy aid, dissection, cervical traction, ET tube balloon deflated and reinflated, confirm levels based on fluoroscopy, Caspar pins at all levels, microscopic discectomies and placement of grafts starting at top, dynamic plate placement, subplatysmal drain
Complication avoidance	No fusion, endoscopic MIS	No fusion	Preflip IOM, decorticate bone and facet prior to screw placement, exclude C7 lateral mass screw, surgical navigation for pedicle screws, compress on lower screws before final tightening, VAC placement	Traction to aid exposure, IOM, cuff deflation/inflation
Postoperative				
Admission	Floor	Floor	Floor	ICU
Postoperative complications feared	Nerve root injury, spinal instability	CSF leak, spinal instability	C5 palsy, wound healing issues, continued neck pain	Dysphagia, vocal cord paralysis, CSF leak, esophageal injury, spinal cord injury
Anticipated length of stay	1–2 days	2 days	2–3 days	2–3 days
Follow-up testing	C-spine CT within 24 hours after surgery C-spine flexion-extension x-rays 1 month after surgery	C-spine CT 1 day and 3 months after surgery	C-spine upright AP and lateral x-rays prior to discharge, 3 months, 6 months after surgery CT C-spine 6 months after surgery ESR/CRP while inpatient	L-spine upright AP/ lateral x-rays Outpatient physical therapy
Bracing	None	Philadelphia collar for 3 months	Aspen collar for 3 months	None
Follow-up visits	2 weeks after surgery	3 weeks after surgery	2 weeks, 3 months, 6 months after surgery	3, 6, 12, and 24 months with x-rays CT at 12 months

AP, Anteroposterior; BMD, bone mineral density; CRP, C-reactive protein; CSF, cerebrospinal fluid; CT, computed tomography; EMG, electromyography; ESR, erythrocyte sedimentation rate; ICU, intensive care unit; IOM, intraoperative monitoring; MAP, mean arterial pressure; MEP, motor evoked potentials; MIS, minimally invasive surgery; MRI, magnetic resonance imaging; NCS, nerve conduction study; SSEP, somatosensory evoked potentials; VAC, vacuum-assisted closure.

Differential diagnosis

- Cervical disc herniation
- Amyotrophic lateral sclerosis
- Diffuse idiopathy skeletal hyperostosis (DISH)
- Tuberculosis
- Fungal infection
- Metastasis
- Primary bone tumor

Important anatomical and preoperative considerations

Cervical spondylosis is a chronic and progressive degenerative spine disease that involves abnormal OPLL and ligamentum flavum, arthropathy with hypertrophy and abnormal ossification of zygapophyseal and uncovertebral joints, and degenerative disc disease (disc herniation and osteophyte formation). All of these ultimately result in neck pain, radiculopathy, muscle weakness (usually affecting hand intrinsics and triceps initially), decline in fine motor skills, gait disturbance, paresthesia, sensory loss, and sphincter dysfunction.[3] CSM is the most common type of spinal cord dysfunction in adults worldwide and accounts for 54% of all nontraumatic myelopathies in North America with an incidence of 76 per million population/year.[1,4] The natural history of CSM is variable and not fully understood. Young patients with mild symptoms may improve or remain stable with conservative treatment.[5] Nevertheless, a progressive neurological decline occurs in about 20% to 62% of patients,[3] and there may be a higher risk of acute myelopathy and central spinal cord syndrome with minor traumas.

The pathophysiology of CSM is multifactorial and may involve static compression from spinal stenosis, dynamic compression and "microtrauma" from dynamic instability or segmental hypermobility, ventral spinal cord displacement against the vertebral bodies and axial spinal cord traction or tension from spinal malalignment, and the cascade of events resulting from chronic spinal cord ischemia (e.g., increased neuroinflammation from microglial activation and disruption of blood-spinal cord barrier, and demyelination).[6] Early surgical decompression has shown to halt disease progression and to recover neurological functioning with expected quality of life improvements in up to 70% of patients.[3,7] In contrast to most spinal disorders, there are some established clinical practice guidelines for CSM.[2] There is strong evidence supporting surgery for patients with moderate (defined as a modified Japanese Orthopaedic Association [mJOA] score of 12 to 14) and severe (mJOA <11) myelopathy (see Chapter 7, Table 2). However, the management of patients with mild disease (mJOA 15–17) or radiological spinal cord compression without clinical myelopathy is less straightforward. Surgical intervention or a trial of physical therapy and rehabilitation under close supervision is suggested for patients with mild myelopathy. Prophylactic surgery should not be offered initially to patients with asymptomatic radiographic compression; however, these patients should be educated on the signs and symptoms of myelopathy, counseled on the risks of progression, and followed closely. Neurophysiologic monitoring with motor and somatosensory evoked potentials may play a role in detecting mild spinal cord dysfunction in asymptomatic patients and monitoring disease evolution in patients with mild myelopathy.[8] Other indications for surgery may include high spinal cord T2 signal on magnetic resonance imaging at the level of radiological compression, refractory radiculopathy, symptomatic deformity, and dynamic instability.[9] Some recognized predictors of surgical outcome include patient's age (worse if >65), smoking history and medical comorbidities, duration of neurological symptoms (worse if >12 months), preoperative neurological function (worse if mJOA <12), and presence of OPLL.[3,8,10]

The goals of surgery are neurological decompression, maintenance or restoration of disc height, cervical spine alignment and lordosis, and spine stabilization. Cervical spine surgeries can be divided into anterior and posterior approaches and are usually supplemented by instrumented fusion. The surgical approach is usually dictated by the patient's clinical presentation, the location of the most compressive element (i.e., anterior approaches for disc herniations and posterior approaches for ligamentum flavum hypertrophy), the number of levels to address, and the presence of OPLL. Anterior approaches are advantageous for ventral compressions preferably involving three or less adjacent levels. Anterior techniques include anterior cervical decompressions and fusions (ACDFs) for direct decompression by performing a discectomy and a ventral foraminotomy and indirect decompression by placing a large intervertebral graft (cautiously so as not to cause subsidence) with or without uncinectomy, anterior corpectomies and fusion, and anterior decompression-only with partial discectomy and uncinectomy for ventral neuroforaminal decompression. Posterior approaches are perhaps more versatile and allow for wider decompressions (central and lateral neuroforaminal), deformity correction, and more extensive instrumentation with more options (lateral mass screws, pedicle screws, laminar screws, occipital plating, condyle screws, and C1–2 fusion, etc.). Posterior techniques include posterior cervical decompressions and fusions, laminoplasties, and decompression-only techniques such as laminectomies, foraminotomies, or both using open or minimally invasive surgery (MIS) techniques. The overall reported complication rates of common procedures used to address CSM are 15.6% after ACDF, 29.2% after posterior cervical decompressions and fusion (PCDF), 41.1% after combined anterior and posterior approaches, and 22.4% after laminoplasty.[3]

As mentioned before, the presence of OPLL is associated with worse surgical outcomes and longer operation time and hospital stay.[3] Anterior approaches may be associated with better clinical outcomes at final follow-up compared with posterior approaches, but CSF leak and disastrous complications such as postoperative paraplegia and quadriplegia were more common.[11] A posterior approach has shown to be safe and effective and is therefore usually preferred for treating multilevel CSM with OPLL.[11] Mild to moderate compression from OPLL should be addressed with a posterior decompression, but more severe OPLL may require an anterior approach, usually with a corpectomy and stepwise technique involving careful piecemeal "egg shelling" of the OPLL with an ultrasonic aspirator, prior to disconnecting it from its attachment, to minimize as much as possible the transmission of vibrations to the spinal cord, then thoroughly decompressing the ventral epidural space cranial and caudal to the OPLL and leaving a small "loose" fragment at the vertex cemented to the ventral dura. Alternatively, this piece can be removed with microdissection, which commonly results in dural violation and requires a primary dural repair or placement of a muscle flap or dural substitute followed by cerebrospinal fluid diversion with a lumbar drain.

What was actually done

The patient was taken to the operating room for a C3–7 posterior cervical decompression and fusion. Somatosensory and motor evoked potentials were monitored during the case and the patient's mean arterial pressures (MAPs) were maintained 10% to 20% higher than his baseline. Through a midline posterior incision and subperiosteal paraspinal muscle dissection, the laminae and lateral masses of C3 to C7 were exposed. Correct levels were verified with anatomy and confirmed with fluoroscopy. Lateral mass screws were placed in the usual fashion and the lamina of C3, C4, C5, C6, and C7 were drilled down to the interlaminar ligament (ligamentum flavum) using high-speed drill medial to the lateral masses. The interlaminar ligament was entered and removed piecemeal using Kerrison rongeurs. As noted in the preoperative imaging (Fig. 9.2), the interlaminar ligament on the left C4–5 level was hypertrophied and calcified and had to be carefully dissected off the dura. The thecal sac was nice and pulsatile. Then bilateral C7 pedicles screws were placed free hand while palpating their medial wall with a Woodson dissector. There were no changes on neurophysiologic monitoring. Slightly bent rods were locked to the screws bilaterally. A subfascial closed suction drain was tunneled out within the sterile field and complete epidural and paraspinal hemostasis was achieved with thrombin and bipolar electrocautery. The wound was thoroughly irrigated with antibiotic solution. The bone and facets were decorticated, and local bone autograft and allograft was placed away from the dura for fusion. The patient did well postoperatively and was discharged home on day 6 with a rigid cervical collar. Postoperative imaging (Fig. 9.3) showed no hardware complication.

Commonalities among experts

Half of the surgeons would obtain a preoperative electromyogram and nerve conduction study to identify the injured roots. Half would obtain flexion-extension x-rays to rule out dynamic instability. Most surgeons selected a posterior approach, but their procedures were different. Half of the surgeons would perform decompression-only procedures, one with a right C6–7 MIS foraminotomy and another one with a right C6–7 open foraminotomy and C4 laminectomy. The surgeon who selected a three-level anterior cervical decompression and fusion would obtain a preoperative swallow study and laryngoscopy for vocal cord function evaluation. The goals of surgery were nerve root and spinal cord decompression. Each of the following were advocated by half of the surgeons: use of intraoperative neurophysiologic monitoring, maintaining higher MAPs, and use of intraoperative steroids. Feared complications included spinal cord injury, incomplete decompressions, spinal instability, C5 palsy, and cerebrospinal fluid leak. Surgeons performing decompression-only procedures would obtain an immediate postoperative computed tomography (CT) while the rest would obtain an immediate postoperative plain x-ray and a CT within 6 months. Half of the surgeons recommend wearing a rigid cervical collar postoperatively. Follow-ups were scheduled within 2 to 3 weeks and then every 3 to 6 months.

> SUMMARY OF QUALITY OF EVIDENCE TO GUIDE SPECIFIC INTERVENTIONS FOR THIS CASE

- Surgery is recommended for patients with severe (mJOA <11) and moderate (mJOA 12–14) CSM: level IB.[2]
- An individualized approach is recommended accounting for pathoanatomical variations. A posterior approach is favored in the presence of posterior compression, three or more stenotic levels, maintained cervical lordosis, and presence of OPLL: level IC.[12,13]

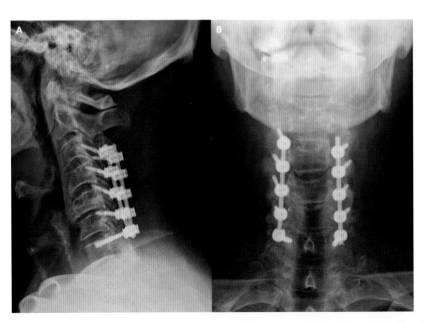

Fig. 9.3 Postoperative x-rays. (A) Lateral and (B) anteroposterior x-rays demonstrating good position of lateral mass screws from C3–6 and C7 pedicle screws.

REFERENCES

1. New PW, Cripps RA, Bonne Lee B. Global maps of non-traumatic spinal cord injury epidemiology: towards a living data repository. *Spinal Cord*. 2014;52(2):97–109.
2. Fehlings MG, Tetreault LA, Riew KD, et al. A Clinical Practice Guideline for the Management of Patients With Degenerative Cervical Myelopathy: Recommendations for Patients With Mild, Moderate, and Severe Disease and Nonmyelopathic Patients With Evidence of Cord Compression. *Global Spine J*. 2017;7(3 Suppl):70S–83S.
3. Veeravagu A, Connolly ID, Lamsam L, et al. Surgical outcomes of cervical spondylotic myelopathy: an analysis of a national, administrative, longitudinal database. *Neurosurg Focus*. 2016; 40(6):E11.
4. Fehlings MG, Tetreault LA, Riew KD, et al. A Clinical Practice Guideline for the Management of Degenerative Cervical Myelopathy: Introduction, Rationale, and Scope. *Global Spine J*. 2017;7(3 Suppl):21S–27S.
5. Yarbrough CK, Murphy RK, Ray WZ, Stewart TJ. The natural history and clinical presentation of cervical spondylotic myelopathy. *Adv Orthop*. 2012;2012:480643.
6. Nouri A, Tetreault L, Singh A, et al. Degenerative Cervical Myelopathy: Epidemiology, Genetics, and Pathogenesis. *Spine (Phila Pa 1976)*. 2015;40(12):E675–693.
7. Al-Tamimi YZ, Guilfoyle M, Seeley H, Laing RJ. Measurement of long-term outcome in patients with cervical spondylotic myelopathy treated surgically. *Eur Spine J*. 2013;22(11):2552–2557.
8. Jannelli G, Nouri A, Molliqaj G, et al. Degenerative Cervical Myelopathy: Review of Surgical Outcome Predictors and Need for Multimodal Approach. *World Neurosurg*. 2020;140:541–547.
9. Pepke W, Almansour H, Richter M, Akbar M. [Spondylotic cervical myelopathy: Indication of surgical treatment]. *Orthopade*. 2018; 47(6):474–482.
10. Iyer A, Azad TD, Tharin S. Cervical Spondylotic Myelopathy. *Clin Spine Surg*. 2016;29(10):408–414.
11. Kim DH, Lee CH, Ko YS, et al. The Clinical Implications and Complications of Anterior Versus Posterior Surgery for Multilevel Cervical Ossification of the Posterior Longitudinal Ligament; An Updated Systematic Review and Meta-Analysis. *Neurospine*. 2019;16(3):530–541.
12. Lawrence BD, Jacobs WB, Norvell DC, et al. Anterior versus posterior approach for treatment of cervical spondylotic myelopathy: a systematic review. *Spine (Phila Pa 1976)*. 2013;38(22 Suppl 1):S173–182.
13. Wilson JR, Tetreault LA, Kim J, et al. State of the Art in Degenerative Cervical Myelopathy: An Update on Current Clinical Evidence. *Neurosurgery*. 2017;80(3S):S33–S45.

10

One level cervical radiculopathy from a herniated disc

Kingsley Abode-Iyamah, MD

Introduction

The cervical spine is composed of seven vertebrae. With the exception of the first cervical vertebrae, each vertebra has an associated nerve that exits the foramen above the named vertebrae. Additionally, the vertebral artery enters the foramen transversarium typically at the sixth cervical vertebrae and exits at C1 prior to entering the foramen magnum. Cervical radiculopathy is pain or sensorimotor deficit resulting from compression of the cervical nerve root.[1-4] Cervical radiculopathy can be caused by degenerative changes or more acute causes such as a disc herniation. While degenerative changes can lead to disc-osteophyte complex formations that cause nerve compression in older adult patients, disc herniation is more commonly found in younger patient populations. The compression of the nerve leads to inflammatory process, which is cytokine-mediated, resulting in demyelination of large-diameter axons. This results in radicular pain, numbness/tingling, or motor deficits typically in a characteristic distribution of the compressed nerve root. The usual first step in the treatment of cervical radiculopathy is conservative management with physical therapy, steroid injection, and nonsteroidal pain medications, as up to 90% will improve without surgical intervention; however, some may warrant surgical intervention.[5, 6]

Example case

Chief complaint: right arm pain

History of present illness: A 61-year-old male presents a history of radiculopathy in the C7 distribution for approximately 3 months. He rates the pain as approximately 8/10 but is now improved to about 5/10. The pain is constant and worse at certain times. He also has weakness in his right upper extremity. He has tried physical therapy and gabapentin without improvement. This led to imaging of his cervical spine (Figs. 10.1 and 10.2).

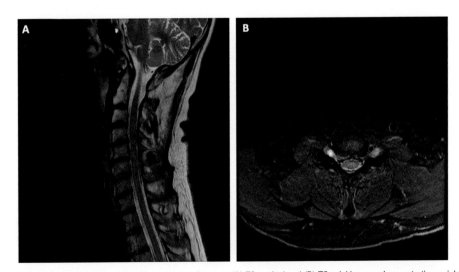

Fig. 10.1 Preoperative magnetic resonance images. (A) T2 sagittal and (B) T2 axial images demonstrating a right C6–7 disc herniation with compression of the exiting nerve.

Medications: Eliquis, amlodipine, lisinopril, tramadol
Allergies: no known drug allergies
Past medical and surgical history: atrial fibrillation status post ablation and cardioversion, hypertension, knee arthroscopy
Family history: noncontributory
Social history: construction worker, no smoking history, occasional alcohol

Physical examination: awake, alert, and oriented to person, place, and time; cranial nerves II–XII intact; bilateral deltoids/biceps 5/5; interossei, 5/5 left triceps, 4/5 right triceps; iliopsoas/knee flexion/knee extension/dorsi, and plantar flexion 5/5
Reflexes: 2+ in bilateral biceps/triceps/brachioradialis; 2+ in bilateral patella/ankle; no clonus or Babinski; negative Hoffman; sensation intact to light touch

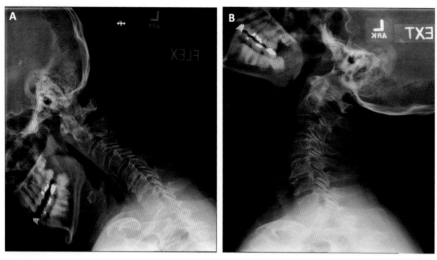

Fig. 10.2 Preoperative x-ray. (A) Flexion and (B) extension x-rays showing no evidence of dynamic instability.

	Lorin M. Benneker, MD Orthopaedic Surgery Spine Unit, Sonnenhofspital, Bern Switzerland Bern, Switzerland	Paul M. Huddleston, III, MD Orthopaedic Surgery Mayo Clinic Rochester, Minnesota, United States	Justin S. Smith, MD, PhD Neurosurgery University of Virginia Charlottesville, Virginia, United States	Clemens Weber, MD, PhD Neurosurgery Stavanager University Hospital Stavanager, Norway
Preoperative				
Additional tests requested	MRI C-spine for better assessment of foramen Periradicular right C6–7 steroid injection	CT C-spine DEXA EMG Right C7 nerve root steroid/local anesthetic block	MRI C-spine for better assessment of foramen EMG/NCS of upper extremities Selective nerve block	Cardiology evaluation
Surgical approach selected	If temporary improvement with steroid injection, C6–7 ACDA and right C6–7 foraminotomy	If not responsive to steroid injection and EMG confirms level, right C6–7 posterior keyhole lamino-foraminotomy	Conservative approach first Right C6–7 foraminotomy	C6–7 ACDF
Goal of surgery	Decompress C7 nerve root, preserve segmental mobility	Decompress C7 nerve root, preserve segmental mobility	Decompress C7 nerve root	Decompress C7 nerve roots
Perioperative				
Positioning	Supine, with Gardner-Wells tongs	Prone in Jackson table, with pins	Prone, with pins	Supine, no pins
Surgical equipment	Surgical microscope Fluoroscopy	IOM (MEP/SSEP/EMG) Fluoroscopy Surgical microscope	Fluoroscopy	Fluoroscopy Surgical microscope
Medications	None	Tranexamic acid, steroids, Toradol, liposomal bupivacaine	None	None

	Lorin M. Benneker, MD Orthopaedic Surgery Spine Unit, Sonnenhofspital, Bern Switzerland Bern, Switzerland	Paul M. Huddleston, III, MD Orthopaedic Surgery Mayo Clinic Rochester, Minnesota, United States	Justin S. Smith, MD, PhD Neurosurgery University of Virginia Charlottesville, Virginia, United States	Clemens Weber, MD, PhD Neurosurgery Stavanager University Hospital Stavanager, Norway
Anatomical considerations	ICA, recurrent laryngeal nerve	Dura, exiting nerve root, vertebral artery	Spinal cord, nerve root, vertebral artery	ICA, esophagus
Complications feared with approach chosen	Recurrent laryngeal palsy	Instability, CSF leak, neuropraxia, C5 palsy	Bleeding, instability	Bleeding, nerve root injury
Intraoperative				
Anesthesia	General	General	General	General
Exposure	C6–7	C6–7	C6–7	C6–7
Levels decompressed	C6–7	C6–7	C6–7	C6–7
Levels fused	C6–7	None	None	C6–7
Surgical narrative	Position supine, left-sided oblique incision, blunt dissection to expose C6–7 disc, confirm correct level with x-ray, place Caspar pin in C6 and C7, discectomy, slight distraction, right foraminotomy, placement of trials, placement of final prosthesis, x-ray control, layered closure	Position prone with Mayfield pins after IOM, postflip IOM, x-ray to localize level, subperiosteal dissection, confirm level with x-ray, right C6–7 laminoforaminotomy under microscopic visualization, identify thecal sac and exiting C7 nerve root, decompress nerve root removing bony spurs and ligamentum while preserved facet capsule, irrigate with dilute betadine and saline, layered closure with liposomal bupivacaine, apply cervical collar	Position prone with Mayfield pins, fluoroscopy to mark midline posterior incision at C6–7 level, expose right C6–7, confirm level with fluoroscopy, right C6–7 foraminotomy with drill and Kerrison punch, close wound in layers	Position supine, right-sided neck dissection to C6–7 level, blunt dissection between vessels and trachea/esophagus, confirm level with fluoroscopy, black belt retractor, microscopic visualization, incision and removal of disc, identify uncus bilaterally, open PLL, decompression of nerve roots, insertion of titanium cage with no plate, no drain
Complication avoidance	Left-sided approach to access right foramen, slight distraction, arthroplasty to preserve segment motion	Pre- and postflip IOM, preserve facet capsule	Right foraminotomy, only expose right side	Blunt dissection between vessels and trachea/esophagus
Postoperative				
Admission	Floor	Outpatient	Floor	Outpatient
Postoperative complications feared	Recurrent laryngeal nerve injury	Instability, CSF leak, neuropraxia, C5 palsy	Bleeding, instability	Nerve root injury, hoarseness, dysphagia
Anticipated length of stay	1–2 days	Same day	Overnight	6 hours
Follow-up testing	C-spine x-ray within 48 hours, 6–8 weeks after surgery	C-spine flexion/extension x-rays 3 months after surgery	MRI in 12 months if symptoms do not improve	Physical therapy 6 weeks after surgery No follow-up imaging unless needed
Bracing	Soft collar for sleep for 2 weeks	Soft collar for 2 weeks	None	None
Follow-up visits	6–8 weeks after surgery	2 weeks, 3 months, 12 months after surgery	10–14 days, 6 weeks, 6 months, and 1 year after surgery	3 months after surgery

BMP, Bone morphogenic protein; DEXA, dual-energy x-ray absorptiometry; EMG, electromyogram; ICA, internal carotid artery; ICU; intensive care unit; IOM, intraoperative monitoring; MEP, motor evoked potentials; MIS, minimally invasive surgery; MRI, magnetic resonance imaging; NCS, nerve conduction study; PLL, posterior longitudinal ligament; SSEP, somatosensory evoked potentials.

Differential diagnosis

- Cervical radiculopathy
- Radial nerve neuropathy
- Brachial plexus injury

Important anatomical considerations

The cervical spine is composed of seven vertebrae. With the exception of the first cervical vertebrae, each vertebra has an associated nerve which exits the foramen above the named vertebrae. Additionally, the vertebral artery enters the foramen transversarium typically at the sixth cervical vertebrae and exits at C1 prior to entering the foramen magnum. It is important to identify the cause of the compression as this will affect the surgical decision. Degeneration leading to foraminal stenosis, especially when there is associated facet degeneration, would eliminate arthroplasty as a viable surgical option. Additionally, those with disc herniations are more likely to improve with conservative management or have a good outcome from a posterior approach without the need for fusion. When significant weakness is present along the distribution of the compressed nerve, earlier intervention is recommend in order to prevent irreversible damage.[7–9]

Approaches to this lesion

The surgical treatment for cervical radiculopathy is decompression of the affected nerve. Decompression can be accomplished via an anterior or posterior approach. Anterior cervical decompression is accomplished via an anterior cervical discectomy with or without fusion. Anterior cervical decompression and fusion (ACDF) is one of the most common procedures performed by the spine surgeon. It is a safe procedure with minimal complications. There is a high fusion rate especially with a single-level ACDF. As with any fusion surgery, ACDF does carry a risk of adjacent segment degeneration requiring additional surgery.[10] Recently, anterior cervical arthroplasty has been popularized due to its motion-preserving characteristics.[11–16] A recent meta-analysis comparing ACDF to arthroplasty found increased reoperation rates, increased adjacent segment disease, and decreased motion in the ACDF group compared with arthroplasty group.[17] Like arthroplasty, posterior approach is motion preserving. This includes posterior discectomy and cervical foraminotomy. Both of these procedures can be done with a minimally invasive approach, improving the postoperative pain management. While a recent study found no difference in improvement of symptoms at 5 years, there was a higher frequency of restenosis in the cervical foraminotomy group compared with the ACDF group without a difference in the frequency of adjacent segment disease.[18]

What was actually done

Given the patient's weakness and failed conservative therapy, the patient was offered surgical intervention. The options of both an anterior and posterior approach were discussed. There was significant facet degeneration noted; therefore he was not offered an arthroplasty. The patient elected for an ACDF. He underwent an anterior cervical discectomy and fusion with placement of a titanium interbody and a cervical plate placement. No monitoring was used during the case and a drain was not used because thorough hemostasis was achieved. A cervical collar was not used as long as it was a single-level fusion and the patient had good bone quality. The patient was discharged on postoperative day 1 and at follow-up had significant improvement in his arm pain and weakness. Postoperative x-rays showed good location of the hardware (Fig. 10.3).

Commonalities among the experts

There was consensus among all the experts that the patient's symptoms were a result of C7 nerve root compression that would benefit from surgical intervention if conservative management failed. Half recommended electromyography and nerve conduction studies to help identify the radiculopathy, and the majority favored additional injections at that location. Half offered a posterior noninstrumented foraminotomy and the other half recommended an anterior approach with fusion. The majority did not require the use of intraoperative monitoring. Of the individuals who chose to pursue a foramiontomy, the commonly feared complication was instability, and those recommending an anterior approach were mainly concerned about recurrent

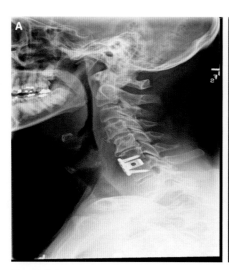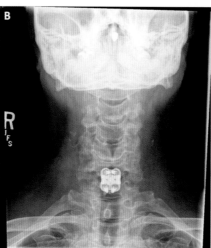

Fig. 10.3 Postoperative x-ray. (A) Lateral and (B) anteroposterior x-rays showing postoperative changes of a C6–7 anterior cervical discectomy and fusion.

laryngeal injury and bleeding. Half recommended x-rays postoperatively.

SUMMARY OF QUALITY OF EVIDENCE TO GUIDE SPECIFIC INTERVENTIONS FOR THIS CASE

- Intraoperative monitoring for spine surgery: level II.1.
- Cervical foraminotomy versus ACDF for cervical radiculopathy: level II.2.

REFERENCES

1. Carette S, Fehlings MG. Clinical practice. Cervical radiculopathy. *N Engl J Med*. 2005;353(4):392–399.
2. Ellenberg MR, Honet JC, Treanor WJ. Cervical radiculopathy. *Arch Phys Med Rehabil*. 1994;75(3):342–352.
3. Fouyas IP, Statham PF, Sandercock PA. Cochrane review on the role of surgery in cervical spondylotic radiculomyelopathy. *Spine (Phila Pa 1976)*. 2002;27(7):736–747.
4. Humphreys SC, Chase J, Patwardhan A, et al. Flexion and traction effect on C5-C6 foraminal space. *Arch Phys Med Rehabil*. 1998;79(9): 1105–1109.
5. Radhakrishnan K, Litchy WJ, O'Fallon WM, Kurland LT. Epidemiology of cervical radiculopathy. A population-based study from Rochester, Minnesota, 1976 through 1990. *Brain*. 1994;117(Pt 2): 325–335.
6. Sampath P, Bendebba M, Davis JD, Ducker T. Outcome in patients with cervical radiculopathy. Prospective, multicenter study with independent clinical review. *Spine (Phila Pa 1976)*. 1999;24(6): 591–597.
7. Aarabi B, Alexander M, Mirvis SE, et al. Predictors of outcome in acute traumatic central cord syndrome due to spinal stenosis. *J Neurosurg Spine*. 2011;14(1):122–130.
8. Fehlings MG, Rabin D, Sears W, et al. Current practice in the timing of surgical intervention in spinal cord injury. *Spine (Phila Pa 1976)*. 2010;35(21 Suppl):S166–S173.
9. Lenehan B, Fisher CG, Vaccaro A, et al. The urgency of surgical decompression in acute central cord injuries with spondylosis and without instability. *Spine (Phila Pa 1976)*. 2010;35(21 Suppl): S180–S186.
10. DiAngelo DJ, Foley KT, Vossel KA, et al. Anterior cervical plating reverses load transfer through multilevel strut-grafts. *Spine (Phila Pa 1976)*. 2000;25(7):783–795.
11. Buchowski JM, Anderson PA, Sekhon L, Riew KD. Cervical disc arthroplasty compared with arthrodesis for the treatment of myelopathy. Surgical technique. *J Bone Joint Surg Am*. 2009;91 (Suppl 2):223–232.
12. Goffin J, Van Calenbergh F, van Loon J, et al. Intermediate follow-up after treatment of degenerative disc disease with the Bryan Cervical Disc Prosthesis: single-level and bi-level. *Spine (Phila Pa 1976)*. 2003;28(24):2673–2678.
13. Gornet MF, Burkus JK, Shaffrey ME, et al. Cervical disc arthroplasty with PRESTIGE LP disc versus anterior cervical discectomy and fusion: a prospective, multicenter investigational device exemption study. *J Neurosurg Spine*. 2015;23(5):558–573.
14. Heller JG, Sasso RC, Papadopoulos SM, et al. Comparison of BRYAN cervical disc arthroplasty with anterior cervical decompression and fusion: clinical and radiographic results of a randomized, controlled, clinical trial. *Spine (Phila Pa 1976)*. 2009;34(2):101–107.
15. Luo J, Gong M, Huang S, et al. Incidence of adjacent segment degeneration in cervical disc arthroplasty versus anterior cervical decompression and fusion meta-analysis of prospective studies. *Arch Orthop Trauma Surg*. 2015;135(2):155–160.
16. Wigfield C, Gill S, Nelson R, et al. Influence of an artificial cervical joint compared with fusion on adjacent-level motion in the treatment of degenerative cervical disc disease. *J Neurosurg*. 2002;96(1 Suppl):17–21.
17. Zou S, Gao J, Xu B, et al. Anterior cervical discectomy and fusion (ACDF) versus cervical disc arthroplasty (CDA) for two contiguous levels cervical disc degenerative disease: a meta-analysis of randomized controlled trials. *Eur Spine J*. 2017;26 (4):985–997.
18. MacDowall A, Heary RF, Holy M, et al. Posterior foraminotomy versus anterior decompression and fusion in patients with cervical degenerative disc disease with radiculopathy: up to 5 years of outcome from the national Swedish Spine Register. *J Neurosurg Spine*. 2019:1–9.

11

Lumbar pseudoarthrosis

Kingsley Abode-Iyamah, MD

Introduction

Pseudoarthrosis is a common complication following fusion operations. It can be found in both instrumented and noninstrumented fusions but more commonly occurs following noninstrumented fusion. Pseudoarthrosis is defined as symptomatic nonunion after 1 year of a fusion surgery. The symptoms can vary from mechanical back pain, radicular pain, or focal deformity due to construct failure. Pseudoarthrosis can also be identified radiographically in asymptomatic patients. Additionally, the rate of pseudoarthrosis also varies depending on the number of fused levels.[1-3] There are known risk factors that increase the risk of pseudoarthrosis and include osteoporosis, smoking, malnutrition, rheumatoid arthritis, age, radiation therapy, and the use of immunosuppressants.[4-6] Pseudoarthrosis can also lead to failure at the bone-metal interface causing haloing of the pedicle as well as hardware

failure. For cases of lumbar spinal pseudoarthrosis requiring reoperation, fusion adjuncts such as bone morphogenetic protein have been found to increase rate of fusion.[7,8] Additionally, reduction of the modifiable risk factors predisposing to pseudoarthrosis should be attempted to improve the likelihood of fusion following revision.

Example Case

Chief complaint: back pain and leg pain

History of present illness: A 29-year-old male presents with a history of back pain and left leg numbness. He underwent a L5-S1 decompression and fusion at that time. He had improvement of the leg pain but no change in his back pain. He underwent revision a year later with a spinous process device to help his back pain. Immediately postoperatively, he had pain in L5 distribution down his left leg. He presented with back pain and burning leg pain and imaging was done (Fig. 11.1).

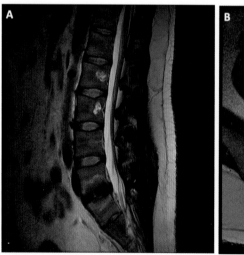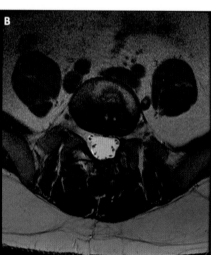

Fig. 11.1 Preoperative magnetic resonance images. (A) T2 sagittal and (B) T2 axial images demonstrating hyperintensity of the L5-S1 disc space, L5-S1 vertebral edema, and left L5-S1 foraminal stenosis.

Medications: hydrocodone, tizanidine

Allergies: no known drug allergies

Past medical and surgical history: L5-S1 fusion x 2

Family history: noncontributory

Social history: engineer, no smoking history, occasional alcohol

Physical examination: awake, alert, and oriented to person, place, and time; cranial nerves II–XII intact; bilateral deltoids/ biceps/triceps 5/5; interossei 5/5; iliopsoas/knee flexion/ knee extension/dorsi, and plantar flexion 5/5

Reflexes: 2+ in bilateral biceps/triceps/brachioradialis; 2+ in bilateral patella/ankle; no clonus or Babinski; negative Hoffman; sensation intact to light touch

	Belal Elnady, MD Orthopaedic Surgery Assiut University Assiut, Egypt	Mohamed El-Fiki, MBBCh, MS, MD Neurosurgery Alexandria University Alexandria, Egypt	John G. Heller, MD Orthopaedic Surgery Emory University Atlanta, Georgia, United States	Langston Holly, MD Neurosurgery University of California at Los Angeles Los Angeles, California, United States
Preoperative				
Additional tests requested	L-spine flexion-extension x-rays Laboratory studies (ESR, CRP, CBC)	L-spine flexion-extension x-rays CT L-spine high resolution Complete electrodiagnostic study Lower extremity dopplers	None	Flexion-extension lumbar x-rays
Surgical approach selected	L5-S1 TLIF	If instability demonstrated, Stage 1: L5-S1 OLIF Stage 2: L5-S1 percutaneous posterior fusion	Stage 1: L5-S1 ALIF and removal of TLIF Stage 2: Left L5-S1 foraminotomy, L5-S1 instrumented posterolateral fusion	If convinced symptoms are due to the pseudoarthrosis, L5-S1 MIS posterolateral fusion
Goal of surgery	Stabilize spine	Stabilize spine, decompress foramina	Stabilize spine, decompress left L5-S1 nerve roots	Stabilize spine, treat pseudoarthrosis
Perioperative				
Positioning	Prone, no pins	Stage 1: lateral Stage 2: prone	Stage 1: supine Stage 2: prone, no pins	Prone, no pins
Surgical equipment	Fluoroscopy	IOM Fluoroscopy Endoscope Tubular retractor Surgical navigation	Fluoroscopy	Fluoroscopy Surgical navigation Surgical microscope
Medications	None	None	None	None
Anatomical considerations	Dura, nerve root	Abdominal viscera, great vessels, segmental radicular artery	Common iliac vessels namely left common iliac vein, posterior annular defect, left L5-S1 nerve roots	Thecal sac, spinal nerves, pedicles
Complications feared with approach chosen	Dural tear, CSF leak	Lumbar plexus injury, durotomy, end plate fracture, psoas weakness, retroperitoneal hematoma	Persistent left leg pain, nerve injury, infection	Retrograde ejaculation with ALIF, CSF leak, nerve root injury
Intraoperative				
Anesthesia	General	General	General	General
Exposure	L5-S1	Stage 1: L5-S1 Stage 2: L5-S1	Stage 1: L5-S1 Stage 2: L5-S1	L5-S1
Levels decompressed	L5-S1	Stage 1: L5-S1 Stage 2: L5-S1	Stage 1: L5-S1 Stage 2: L5-S1	L5-S1
Levels fused	L5-S1	Stage 1: L5-S1 Stage 2: L5-S1	Stage 1: L5-S1 Stage 2: L5-S1	L5-S1

	Belal Elnady, MD Orthopaedic Surgery Assiut University Assiut, Egypt	Mohamed El-Fiki, MBBCh, MS, MD Neurosurgery Alexandria University Alexandria, Egypt	John G. Heller, MD Orthopaedic Surgery Emory University Atlanta, Georgia, United States	Langston Holly, MD Neurosurgery University of California at Los Angeles Los Angeles, California, United States
Surgical narrative	Position prone, posterior midline incision, subperiosteal dissection, removal of interspinous implant, decortication of the posterolateral elements, pedicle screw insertion at L5-S1, fascetectomy and transforaminal discectomy, removal of loose interbody cage, good debridement of the disc space and remove all fibrous tissue until bleeding cancellous bone seen, insertion of new interbody cage filled with bone graft, gentle compression over pedicle screws to stabilize cage, insertion of bone graft in the posterolateral gutter to achieve 360-degree fusion, closure of wound in layers	Stage 1: position right lateral with left side up, mild flexion of left hip nad mild flexion of table, x-ray to mark (anterior, posterior, midpoint) L5-S1 disc, traverse skin incision, dissect bluntly external and internal obliques and transversus muscles, dissect transversalis fascia as laterally as possible to avoid peritoneum, place tubular retractor toward midline after identifying retroperitoneal fat until anterior psoas border and intervertebral space is felt, release adhesions between peritoneum and anterior border of psoas muscle, medial limit is lateral border of ALL, direct tubular retractor obliquely centered on L5-S1 disc posterior to lumbar plexus, repeated fluoroscopy during annulus release and end plate preparation, remove old prosthesis, place interbody. Stage 2 (same day): position prone, placement of percutaneous L5-S1 pedicle screws using x-rays, placement of rods, layered closure	Stage 1: position supine, transverse left anterior incision to access retroperitoneal space, identify left ureter and mobilize across midline with peritoneal contents, medial border of left iliac vein exposed, ligate medial branches off of vein to allow tension-free retraction to the left, ligate median sacral vessels, bluntly dissect across to the right side of L5-S1 disc, mobilize right iliac vessels, place right Brau blade, place left iliac vein retractor making sure to not tear vein at bifurcation, L5-S1 complete discectomy with removal of lower portion of L5 and upper portion of S1 to remove TLIF cage, prepare surfaces for fusion, place cage that is assembled in situ and actively distracts segments to normal height and lordotic angle, place BMP. Stage 2 (same day): position prone, midline incision, subperiosteal dissection, fully expose and decorticate left L5 transverse process and sacral ala, place pedicle screws bilaterally at L5-S1, use combination of local bone and iliac crest bone graft, layered closure with subfascial drain	Position prone, place percutaneous dynamic reference frame, use navigated probe to create two separate 1-inch incisions over L5 and S1 pedicle screw entry sites, dissect through muscle and fascia and using the bovie, expose L5 transverse process and sacral ala using microscope bilaterally, harvest iliac crest autograft, decorticate L5 transverse process/facet complex/sacral ala, place autograft bone over it, place navigated percutaneous pedicle screws, confirm accuracy with O-arm, lock rods, standard closure
Complication avoidance	Good debridement of disc space, gentle compression over pedicles to compress screws, attempt to achieve 360-degree fusion	Mild flexion of left hip to relax left psoas, be aware of nerves under internal oblique muscle, avoid extended muscular dissections, use anatomical corridors around disc with anterior border of psoas and left lateral border of aorta or left iliac artery with minimal retraction of psoas not beyond coronal plane to avoid injury to genitofemoral nerve	Two-staged approach, ligate medial branches off of left iliac vein, ligate median sacral vessels, remove lower portion of L5 and upper portion of S1 to allow removal of TLIF cage, place cage that distracts to provide indirect decompression, standard closure, BMP	Surgical navigation, minimally invasive approach, iliac crest autograft
Postoperative				
Admission	Intermediate care	Floor	Floor	Floor
Postoperative complications feared	CSF leak, wound infection	End plate fracture, psoas weakness, injury to segmental radicular artery, nerve root injury, major vessel injury	Persistent left leg pain, nerve injury, infection	Screw misplacement, pseudoarthrosis
Anticipated length of stay	2 days	1–3 days	3–4 days	3 days

	Belal Elnady, MD Orthopaedic Surgery Assiut University Assiut, Egypt	Mohamed El-Fiki, MBBCh, MS, MD Neurosurgery Alexandria University Alexandria, Egypt	John G. Heller, MD Orthopaedic Surgery Emory University Atlanta, Georgia, United States	Langston Holly, MD Neurosurgery University of California at Los Angeles Los Angeles, California, United States
Follow-up testing	L-spine x-rays 2 months, 6 months, 1 year after surgery	L-spine x-rays immediately after surgery, 1 day, 1 month, every 3 months until adequate fusion assured after surgery CT L-spine every 3 months until fusion assured ESR/CRP until normalization	L-spine AP and lateral 6 weeks, 3 months, 6 months, 12 months after surgery CT L-spine 6 or 12 months after surgery	L-spine AP/lateral x-rays after surgery, 6 weeks, 3 months, 6 months, 1 year, 2 years after surgery Bone stimulator
Bracing	None	None	None	LSO brace for 3 months
Follow-up visits	2 weeks, 2 months, 6 months, 1 year after surgery	10 days, 1 month, every 3 months until fusion after surgery	6 weeks, 3 months, 6 months, 12 months after surgery	2 weeks, 6 weeks, 3 months, 6 months, 1 year, 2 years after surgery

AP, Anteroposterior; ALIF, anterior lumbar interbody fusion; ALL, anterior longitudinal ligament; BMP, bone morphogenic protein; CBC, complete blood count; CRP, C-reactive protein; CSF, cerebrospinal fluid; CT, computed tomography; ESR, erythrocyte sedimentation rate; IOM, intraoperative monitoring; LSO, lumbar-sacral orthosis; MIS, minimally invasive surgery; OLIF, oblique lateral interbody fusion; TLIF, transforaminal lumbar interbody fusion.

Differential diagnosis

- Pseudoarthrosis
- Discitis
- Osteomyelitis

Important anatomical considerations

Following an instrumented fusion procedure, the instrumentation acts as a strut until bony growth can occur over the instrumented area. This construct is subject to the stress of movement and, without fusion, can lead to failure of the instrumentation or failure at the bone-instrument interface. A computed tomography (CT) scan is necessary to identify fusion following an instrumented fusion, which is expected to take 6 to 18 months in most individuals (Fig. 11.2).[9] Additionally, inadequate decortication prior to placement of grafting can also affect fusion across the facets and transverse processes. Furthermore, other factors such as osteoporosis, smoking, malnutrition, rheumatoid arthritis, older age,

radiation therapy, and the use of immunosuppressants drastically reduce the rate of boney fusion.[4–6]

When it is determined that a patient requires revision surgery due to pseudoarthrosis, a number of factors must be taken into account. The ultimate goal is to identify new bony real estate in which a new arthrodesis can be performed. First, it is important to identify whether there was an interbody fusion performed in the previous surgery. In addition, it is important to identify whether prior arthrodesis of the transverse processes was attempted. Furthermore, the state of the facet joint is important as it is a potential area for arthrodesis. Finally, the integrity of the prior instrumentation and, more specifically, the bone-instrument interface should be identified to determine whether new additional levels should be added to improve the construct and allow fusion to occur.

Recombinant human bone morphogenetic protein (rhBMP) is a synthetic protein first discovered in 1984. It has the ability to promote bone formation and increase fusion rate in the cervical and lumbar spine with a failure rate of 14.5% versus 39% for rhBMP versus autologous bone graft in the setting of

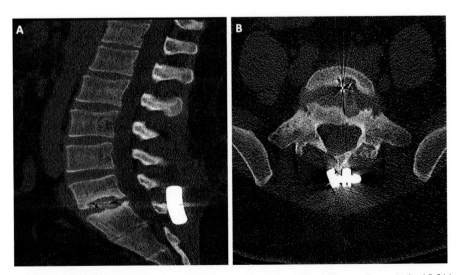

Fig. 11.2 Preoperative computed tomography scans. (A) Sagittal and (B) axial images demonstrating L5-S1 interbody fusion with subsidence of the interbody graft. No bony fusion is present.

revision posterolateral spinal fusion, respectively.[10, 11] For this reason, its use has steadily increased since its approval by the U.S. Food and Drug Administration (FDA) for anterior interbody fusion and revision posterolateral fusion.

Approaches to this lesion

The options for these cases are limited given that this is a case of pseudoarthrosis; however, a number of options can be considered depending on what was previously done. In very limited circumstances, an anterior-only approach can be considered. This is recommended in cases where there is pseudoarthrosis due to failure from prior transforaminal interbody or posterior lumbar interbody where failure is in the disc space. In these cases, salvage anterior lumber interbody fusion with removal of prior instrumentation can be performed. This technique has been shown to resolve the presenting symptoms and is also associated with good fusion rates.[12] In cases where there is either failure of the instrumentation due to rod fracture and/or failure at the bone-instrument interface, an anterior and posterior approach can be considered.

In cases where no prior interbody was performed or hardware failure is also present, a posterior only-approach can be

considered. When only a posterior-lateral fusion was initially performed, the addition of an interbody has been shown to increase the fusion rate.[13] Additionally, the prior instrumentation should be interrogated to determine its integrity. When there is hardware loosening, replacement of the pedicle screws with larger diameter screw should be considered. Furthermore, obtaining better bony purchase with the addition of one level above and below the prior instrumentation should be considered.

What was actually done

This is a young patient who underwent a prior decompression and interbody fusion with a spinous process device, which was again revised when he returned with back pain (Fig. 11.3). Following the second procedure, the patient developed radicular pain and was found to have pseudoarthrosis. Given his failed fusion and recurrent symptoms, it was determined that he would benefit from surgical intervention. The patient did not have prior attempted posterior lateral fusion or pedicle screw placement, so the decision was made to perform posterior lateral fusion with pedicle screw placement at L5 and S1. The interspinous device was removed (Fig. 11.4). The previously placed

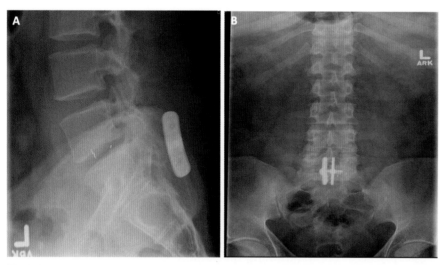

Fig. 11.3 Preoperative x-rays. (A) Lateral x-ray. (B) Anteroposterior (AP) x-rays demonstrating L5-S1 interbody fusion with a spinous process device.

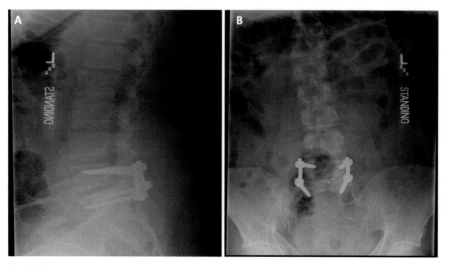

Fig. 11.4 Postoperative x-rays. (A) Lateral and (B) AP x-rays showing postoperative instrumentation at L5-S1.

interbody was not removed and a posterior-only approach was thought most appropriate for this patient given his age. The local autograft was harvested for grafting in addition to allograft, and a small kit of rhBMP was used to improve fusion rate. The patient tolerated the procedure well with resolution of his prior symptoms.

Commonalities among the experts

There was some variability in what our experts recommended for treatment in this case. The majority recommended additional imaging with flexion-extension x-rays, while only one recommended additional laboratory work (erythrocyte sedimentation rate, C-reactive protein, complete blood count) to rule out an infection. Additionally, one expert recommended preoperative CT. While half recommended a posterior-only approach, the other half recommended an anterior-posterior reconstruction. Of those recommending a posterior approach, a minimally invasive transforaminal lumbar interbody fusion (TLIF) was suggested by one surgeon and the other recommended posterior instrumentation alone. The two anterior approaches that were suggested were an anterior lumbar interbody fusion (ALIF) with removal of prior interbody and an oblique lateral approach with placement of an additional interbody. All aimed to stabilize the spine, with half also recommending decompression of the exiting nerve root at this location. While half planned on navigated screw placement, all used intraoperative fluoroscopy. For those recommending a posterior approach, the main concern was dural tear, persistent pain, nerve injury, and infection. Those who recommended an anterior approach were mainly concerned about lumbar plexus injury, end plate fracture, psoas weakness (with oblique lateral interbody fusion), and retrograde ejaculation (with ALIF). Only one expert recommended the use of bone morphogenic protein (BMP) in this case, and another suggested iliac crest harvest. The expected hospital stay varied from 1 to 4 days with only one expert recommending postoperative bracing.

SUMMARY OF QUALITY OF EVIDENCE TO GUIDE SPECIFIC INTERVENTIONS FOR THIS CASE

- BMP for revision of posterior lateral fusion: level II.2.
- ALIF versus TLIF for interbody fusion: level II.2.

REFERENCES

1. Glassman SD, Minkow RE, Dimar JR, et al. Effect of prior lumbar discectomy on outcome of lumbar fusion: a prospective analysis using the SF-36 measure. *J Spinal Disord*. 1998;11(5):383–388.
2. Lee KB, Johnson JS, Song KJ, et al. Use of autogenous bone graft compared with RhBMP in high-risk patients: a comparison of fusion rates and time to fusion. *J Spinal Disord Tech*. 2013;26(5):233–238.
3. Narayan P, Haid RW, Subach BR, et al. Effect of spinal disease on successful arthrodesis in lumbar pedicle screw fixation. *J Neurosurg*. 2002;97(3 Suppl):277–280.
4. Glassman SD, Dimar 3rd JR, Burkus K, et al. The efficacy of rhBMP-2 for posterolateral lumbar fusion in smokers. *Spine (Phila Pa 1976)*. 2007;32(15):1693–1698.
5. Kim YJ, Bridwell KH, Lenke LG, et al. Pseudarthrosis in long adult spinal deformity instrumentation and fusion to the sacrum: prevalence and risk factor analysis of 144 cases. *Spine (Phila Pa 1976)*. 2006;31(20):2329–2336.
6. Li G, Patil CG, Lad SP, et al. Effects of age and comorbidities on complication rates and adverse outcomes after lumbar laminectomy in elderly patients. *Spine (Phila Pa 1976)*. 2008;33(11):1250–1255.
7. Bodalia PN, Balaji V, Kaila R, Wilson L. Effectiveness and safety of recombinant human bone morphogenetic protein-2 for adults with lumbar spine pseudarthrosis following spinal fusion surgery: A systematic review. *Bone Joint Res*. 2016;5(4):145–152.
8. Taghavi CE, Lee KB, Keorochana G, et al. Bone morphogenetic protein-2 and bone marrow aspirate with allograft as alternatives to autograft in instrumented revision posterolateral lumbar spinal fusion: a minimum 2-year follow-up study. *Spine (Phila Pa 1976)*. 2010;35(11):1144–1150.
9. Tuli SK, Tuli J, Chen P, Woodard EJ. Fusion rate: a time-to-event phenomenon. *J Neurosurg Spine*. 2004;1(1):47–51.
10. Lindley TE, Dahdaleh NS, Menezes AH, Abode-Iyamah KO. Complications associated with recombinant human bone morphogenetic protein use in pediatric craniocervical arthrodesis. *J Neurosurg Pediatr*. 2011;7(5):468–474.
11. Papakostidis C, Kontakis G, Bhandari M, Giannoudis PV. Efficacy of autologous iliac crest bone graft and bone morphogenetic proteins for posterolateral fusion of lumbar spine: a meta-analysis of the results. *Spine (Phila Pa 1976)*. 2008;33(19):E680–E692.
12. Yun DJ, Yu JW, Jeon SH, et al. Salvage Anterior Lumbar Interbody Fusion for Pseudoarthrosis After Posterior or Transforaminal Lumbar Interbody Fusion: A Review of 10 Patients. *World Neurosurg*. 2018;111:e746–e755.
13. Macki M, Bydon M, Weingart R, et al. Posterolateral fusion with interbody for lumbar spondylolisthesis is associated with less repeat surgery than posterolateral fusion alone. *Clin Neurol Neurosurg*. 2015;138:117–123.

12

Anterior C1-C2 pannus

Fidel Valero-Moreno, MD and Henry Ruiz-Garcia, MD

Introduction

C1-C2 pannus most commonly results from both chronic instability of the atlanto-axial segment and an inflammatory process of the atlanto-axial joint (AAJ).[1,2] These degenerative processes are typically associated with rheumatoid arthritis (RA) and cause ligamentous structural destruction.[2,3] RA affects an estimated 1% to 2% of the adult population.[4,5] Although RA spares the axial skeleton, the cervical spine is an important exception, being involved in up to 86% of all patients with this condition.[3,4,6] Cervical inflammatory disease usually manifests as atlanto-axial subluxation (AAS), cranial settling (CS), and subaxial subluxation (SAS).[3,4] Interestingly, spinal involvement is commonly described as a late manifestation of the condition.[6] Moreover, 50% of the patients who suffered from RA for at least 7 years may develop craniocervical complications.[2] Neurological symptoms are reported in 7% to 34% of all the patients,[3] where neck pain is the most common symptom.[3,5] Other notable symptoms radiculopathy, myelopathy, and cranial nerve dysfunction,[7] where the presence of multiple cranial neuropathies strongly suggests the presence of a cervical pannus.[8] Pannus develops from the inflamed synovial lining surrounding the odontoid and is typically located between the dens and the anterior arch of C1.[1,2,4] Pannus involving the AAJ leads to further instability and may cause progressive compression of the cervico-medullary junction.[1,7] The prevalence of a C1-C2 pannus ranges from 32% to 93%.[9] Standard radiography is considered the first-line imaging method of choice and is indicated as a routine evaluation for patients with RA.[5,9] Magnetic resonance imaging (MRI) is the best modality to assess the C1-C2 pannus, dens erosions, and neurological impact of the rheumatoid lesions.[9] Patients with persistent neck or suboccipital pain and neurological impairment should undergo surgical treatment.[2,5,7,10] Arthrodesis and posterior stabilization of the atlanto-axial segment remain the preferred techniques in cases of RA with cervical articular degeneration and pannus.[2,5,7,10] Direct mass removal is not advocated as retrodental pannus significantly diminishes after immobilization.[5,10]

Example Case

Chief complaint: neck pain, upper limb weakness

History of present illness: An 81-year-old male patient presents with progressive neck pain for a year, and he has a 6-month history of difficulty using his hands and lifting his arms. The patient underwent a computed tomography (CT) scan and x-rays as part of his evaluation (Fig. 12.1).

Medications: warfarin, oxycodone

Allergies: no known drug allergies

Past medical and surgical history: atrial fibrillation, coronary artery disease, deep vein thrombosis

Family history: none

Social history: smoking, occasional alcohol

Physical examination: awake, alert, and oriented to person, place, and time; cranial nerves II–XII intact; bilateral deltoids/triceps/biceps 5/5; right interossei 4/5; left interossei 5/5; iliopsoas/knee, flexion/knee extension/dorsi, and plantar flexion 5/5

Reflexes: 3+ in bilateral biceps/triceps/brachioradialis with positive Hoffman; 3+ in bilateral patella/ankle; three beats of ankle clonus and positive Babinski; sensation intact to light touch

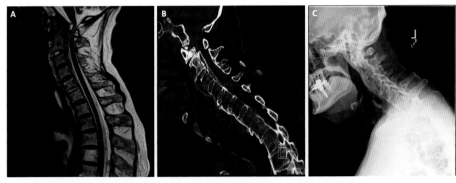

Fig. 12.1 Preoperative imaging. (A) Sagittal T2-weighted imaging and (B) sagittal computed tomography scan demonstrating severe C1-C2 central canal stenosis resulting from hypertrophic synovial tissue from the atlanto-odontoid joint (pannus). There is severe compression of the spinal cord with increased cord signal. The odontoid process appears irregular due to the presence of erosion. The atlanto-dental distance shows mild widening. There is also C2-C7 ankylosis secondary to diffuse idiopathic skeletal hyperostosis. (C) Lateral x-rays demonstrating osteopenia with prominent osteophytes along the upper cervical spine with slightly milder changes inferiorly. The motion was limited but there was no dynamic instability.

	James S. Harrop, MD Neurosurgery Jefferson University Philadelphia, Pennsylvania, United States	John G. Heller, MD Orthopaedic Surgery Emory University Atlanta, Georgia, United States	Manoj Phalak, MCh Neurosurgery All India Institute of Medical Sciences New Delhi, India	Mohamed A.R. Soliman, MD, MSc, PhD Neurosurgery Cairo University Cairo, Egypt
Preoperative				
Additional tests requested	C-spine flexion-extension x-rays CT C-spine	C-spine lateral flexion-extension x-rays Standing full-length AP/lateral spine x-rays CTA C-spine Urine nicotine test Medicine evaluation	MRI complete spine and craniovertebral junction Standing full-length AP/lateral spine x-rays PET Cardiology evaluation Anesthesia evaluation	CT head and C-spine spine CTA head and C-spine spine MRI C-spine with flexion-extension DEXA Lower extremity Dopplers Medicine, anesthesia, rheumatology evaluation
Surgical approach selected	C1–4 laminectomy and C1–5 posterior fusion	C1 laminectomy, C1–2 instrumented fusion, with possible extension to the occiput	Confirm no malignancy, C1–2 laminectomy	C1 and foramen magnum decompression and C1–2 posterior fusion
Goal of surgery	Decompress spinal cord, stabilize C1–2	Decompress spinal cord, stabilize C1–2, reduce C1–2 subluxation	Decompress spinal cord	Decompress medulla and spinal cord, stabilize C1–2
Perioperative				
Positioning	Prone with neck neutral and Mayfield pins	Prone with Mayfield pins	Prone on horseshoe headrest	Prone with Mayfield pins on Jackson table
Surgical equipment	Fluoroscopy IOM (MEP/SSEP, BAERs)	Fluoroscopy IOM (MEP/SSEP)	Fluoroscopy Ultrasonic bone scalpel	Fluoroscopy IOM Surgical navigation Ultrasound Surgical microscope
Medications	Steroids	Maintain MAP	None	Steroids, maintain MAP
Anatomical considerations	Occipital bone, vertebral arteries	C2 nerve roots, venous plexus, spinal cord, vertebral arteries	Dura, vertebral artery	Vertebral artery, neural structures, C1–2 bony anatomy
Complications feared with approach chosen	Spinal cord injury, CSF leak, vertebral artery injury	Spinal cord injury, vertebral artery injury, nonunion, pseudoarthrosis	Spinal instability, vertebral artery injury, medical complications	Vertebral artery injury, stroke, brainstem and spinal cord injury

	James S. Harrop, MD Neurosurgery Jefferson University Philadelphia, Pennsylvania, United States	John G. Heller, MD Orthopaedic Surgery Emory University Atlanta, Georgia, United States	Manoj Phalak, MCh Neurosurgery All India Institute of Medical Sciences New Delhi, India	Mohamed A.R. Soliman, MD, MSc, PhD Neurosurgery Cairo University Cairo, Egypt
Intraoperative				
Anesthesia	General	General	General	General
Exposure	C1–5	C1–2	C1–2	Occiput-C2
Levels decompressed	C1–4	C1	C1–2	Occiput-C1
Levels fused	C1–4/5	C1–2	None	C1–2
Surgical narrative	Intubated with fiberoptic, head fixed in Mayfield pins, baseline IOM, prone position with neutral neck, stable IOM, midline incision, expose C1–5, C-arm to identify levels, bilateral C1 lateral mass/C2 pars screws, C3–5 lateral mass screws, drill off C1 and C2 lamina, en bloc laminectomy of C3–5, subfascial drain	Intubated with head/neck in neutral position, preflip IOM, position prone adjusting brow-chin angle to desired position, lateral x-ray document C1–2 relationship and brow-chin angle, postflip IOM, standard midline posterior exposure of C1 and C2, detach extensor insertions into the spinous processes and lamina of C2, C1 laminectomy avoiding ventral manipulation of lamina, section C2 nerve proximal to dorsal root ganglia on one or both sides in order to provide more bony surface for fusion/venous control of plexus/removal of some pseudopannus, screws in C1 articular mass and C2 pars or pedicle depending on local anatomy, pack cancellous iliac crest autograft into decorticated C1–2 joint posteriorly and filling void between exposed remaining portions of C1 arch and C2 pars, add BMP inside the joints before bone graft, bur hole in C2 spinous process and repair muscle attachments with nonabsorbable suture, layered closure	Fiberoptic intubation avoiding neck manipulation, position prone on horseshoe headrest with collar, avoid IOM and monopolar cautery because of pacemaker, midline incision, subperiosteal dissection exposing C1 posterior arch up to 1.5 cm from midline on either side, maintain C2 attachments, confirm level with x-ray, C1 laminectomy using bone scalpel or high-speed drill with partial drilling of superior C2 lamina, look for posterior displacement of thecal sac and pulsation, layered closure	Intubated with fiberoptic intubation avoiding neck extension and/or manipulation, baseline IOM check, patient positioned prone with head in neutral position, intraoperative fluoroscopy to confirm good alignment, attach surgical navigation, incision made from inion to 3 cm below C2, dissect in avascular plane of ligamentum nuchae, subperiosteal dissection of neck muscles from spinous process of C2/lamina of C1, expose lateral mass of C1 and C2, register navigation, identify boundaries of C1 lateral mass, retract C2 nerve root downward, place C1 lateral mass with Goel technique and place C2 pedicle screw, use preoperative CT to estimate length and width of screws, another intraoperative spin to confirm screw position, decorticate lateral mass and joints, place slightly lordotic rod, decompress foramen magnum using high-speed drill and C1 laminectomy with Kerrison rongeurs, confirm decompression with ultrasound, place autograft on decorticated bone, closure in layers
Complication avoidance	Avoid occipital screws, baseline IOM	Pre- and postflip IOM, section C2 nerve root to facilitate fusion/hemostasis/pseudopanns removal, iliac crest bone graft and BMP, repair muscle attachments to C2 spinous process through bur hole	Avoid IOM and monopolar cautery because of pacemaker, expose C1 posterior arch up to 1.5 cm from midline on either side, maintain C2 attachments, look for posterior displacement of spinal cord and normal pulsations to assess adequacy of decompression	Baseline IOM, surgical navigation, ultrasound to assess decompression
Postoperative				
Admission	Spine unit	ICU	ICU	Floor
Postoperative complications feared	Dysphagia, spinal cord injury, CSF leak	Hematoma, stroke, loss of fixation, nonunion, malpositioning of head	Spinal instability, vertebral artery injury, medical complications	Worsening neurological function, CSF leak, pseudoarthrosis

	James S. Harrop, MD Neurosurgery Jefferson University Philadelphia, Pennsylvania, United States	John G. Heller, MD Orthopaedic Surgery Emory University Atlanta, Georgia, United States	Manoj Phalak, MCh Neurosurgery All India Institute of Medical Sciences New Delhi, India	Mohamed A.R. Soliman, MD, MSc, PhD Neurosurgery Cairo University Cairo, Egypt
Anticipated length of stay	2–3 days then rehab	5–7 days	5–7 days	3–4 days
Follow-up testing	Standing x-ray	C-spine x-rays 6 weeks, 3 months, 6 months, 12 months after surgery CT C-spine 6 or 12 months after surgery	C-spine flexion-extension x-rays prior to discharge and 3 months after surgery	CT head and cervical spine within 24 hours of surgery and 6 months after surgery MRI brain and cervical spine within 3 days of surgery
Bracing	6 weeks	Rigid collar for 12 weeks when out of bed	Philadelphia collar for 6 weeks	None
Follow-up visits	2 weeks with APP, 6 weeks	6 weeks, 3 months, 6 months, 12 months after surgery	10 days and 3 months after surgery	10–14 days, 4 weeks, 3 months, 6 months, 1 year after surgery

APP, Advanced practice provider; BAERs, brainstem auditory evoked responses; BMP, bone morphogenic protein; CSF, cerebrospinal fluid; CT, computed tomography; CTA, computed tomography angiography; DEXA, dual-energy x-ray absorptiometry; ICU, intensive care unit; IOM, intraoperative monitoring; MAP, mean arterial pressure; MEP, motor evoked potentials; MRI, magnetic resonance imaging; SSEP, somatosensory evoked potentials.

Differential diagnosis

- Cervicomedullary junction tumor
- Retro-odontoid synovial cyst
- Epidural hematoma
- Calcium pyrophosphate arthropathy
- Basilar invagination

Important anatomical and preoperative considerations

The cervical spine is constituted by two parts: the upper cervical spine (C1–C2 with the atlanto-axial, atlanto-odontoid, and atlantooccipital joints), and the lower cervical spine (C3–C7).[11] The occipital-AAJ is involved in most of the rotational movement of the neck and is supported just by ligamentous structures without any interlocking bone.[3,11] The C1-C2 complex is responsible for 60 degrees of axial rotation.[4] The ligaments and articulations of this complex control mobility and restriction of movement. Therefore, loosening of these structures could lead to instability and dislocation in any direction.[3,4] Moreover, the cervical spine is particularly susceptible to RA due to the large number of articulations and their mobility.[7] The ring of C1 articulates with the occipital condyles at the base of the skull and is restrained by the tectorial membrane, which is a continuation of the posterior longitudinal ligament.[4] The anterior atlanto-occipital membrane connects the anterior arch of C1 to the anterior-inferior margin of the foramen magnum. This structure is a prolongation of the anterior longitudinal ligament and limits the extension of the atlanto-occipital joint.[4] Additionally, the posterior arch of C1 is linked to the posterior edge of the foramen magnum through the posterior atlanto-occipital membrane, which is continuous inferiorly with the ligamentum flavum.[4] Additionally, C1 forms important articulations with axis (C2). The anterior arch of C1 establishes an important synovial joint with the odontoid process of C2, which is stabilized by the transverse ligament, preventing anterior translation of C1 relative to C2.[4,11] RA is characterized by an inflammatory synovial proliferation resulting in deterioration of ligaments, tendinous tissue, and bone erosion, hence allowing sliding motion between the atlas and axis and consequently atlanto-axial instability.[3,5,7] Defined as an atlanto-dental distance of 3 mm or more on lateral radiographs in flexion or neutral position, AAS represents the most common form of instability of the AAJ. Furthermore, spinal cord compression may occur when this distance exceeds 9 mm.[5,6] Continuity loss of the transverse ligament plays a fundamental role in the development of this disorder.[2,5,11]

The development of pannus is caused by chronic instability, hypermobility of the cervical spine, amd persistent inflammation that generates accumulation of granulation tissue around the dens.[2] Neural elements compression can originate as a dynamic process caused by instability or secondary mass effect produced by significant pannus formation.[7] Due to the critical location of pannus, the potential neurological signs and symptoms are vast and diverse, including craniocervical pain (69%), radiculopathy (58%), myelopathy (58%), cranial neuropathy (20%), or a combination.[4,5] Severe neurological morbidity, such as compression of the medulla oblongata, hydrocephalus, sudden death, or stroke/vertebrobasilar insufficiency, is not uncommon.[4,5]

Conventional radiographs are traditionally used as the initial assessment and screening of asymptomatic patients with RA. X-rays are useful to evaluate alignment, osteopenia, and erosion of the odontoid process, as well as the major patterns of instability (flexion-extension).[5,7] Cervical CT scans provide a more detailed evaluation of the bone anatomy and represent a fundamental tool for diagnosis and surgical planning, including evaluation of bone and facet joints erosion, dens fractures, or pseudoarthrosis.[5,7] In addition, a preoperative computed tomography angrography (CTA) to evaluate the position of the vertebral arteries is typically advocated.[7] For the assessment of soft tissue, pannus, nerve compression, and myelopathy, MRI is the study of choice.[5,7]

Patients with RA and craniocervical instability who develop persistent pain, myelopathy, or progressive neurological deficit typically require surgical intervention.[2,7,11] Rheumatoid cervical disease is invariably a progressive condition and may lead to permanent neurological impairment or even death if left untreated.[4] Surgical techniques vary across studies[11]; however, atlanto-axial fusion via C1-C2 arthrodesis remains the most commonly employed method for attaining posterior stabilization and motion reduction to decrease pannus.[2,4,5,7,10,11] Atlanto-axial transarticular screw fixation improves fusion rates and has been considered the gold standard to achieve satisfactory C1-C2 fixation.[5,7] Nevertheless, the use of C1 lateral mass and C2 pedicle screws represents an alternative and safe technique to reduce the risk of vascular injury.[12] Direct excision of pannus compressing the spinal cord is not usually advocated, as the size of the mass significantly recedes after immobilization of the atlanto-axial segment.[5,10] Trans oral dens resection is indicated in cases of cranial migration of the dens and failure of pannus regression after posterior fixation. However, this is a challenging procedure that carries a high risk of infection and usually requires a second operation due to the postoperative instability.[5,7,10,11]

What was actually done

Given the severe C1–2 cervical stenosis and rapidly progressive myelopathy, surgery was recommended. The patient was taken to the operating room and placed under general anesthesia. Intraoperative monitoring including motor evoked potentials (MEPs) and somatosensory evoked potentials (SSEPs) were stablished before positioning the patient prone. Signals in extremities were very poor for both sensory and motor monitoring, which was clearer distally. The head was fixed in a Mayfield head holder and kept in a neutral position. A midline incision was made from the inion to approximately C7. Intraoperative x-rays confirmed the correct levels. Following subperiosteal dissection of the dorsal spine, monitoring signals had significantly decreased. In consequence,

the C1 lamina and the superior aspect of the C2 lamina were removed immediately for decompression. Mean arterial pressure was increased to 100 mm Hg, and steroids were provided. SSEP and MEP signals gradually improved over the next 20 to 30 minutes while this pressure was maintained throughout the entire procedure. Then, the instrumentation started with screw placement at C2 pedicles and C3-C6 lateral masses bilaterally. An occipital plate was then placed, followed by the fixation with two bilateral longitudinal members after previous confirmation of adequate instrumentation with the C-arm. A right cortical cancellous iliac crest autograft was harvested. The occiput lateral arches of C1 and C2 were then heavily decorticated. Both autografts were then placed in the posterolateral gutters from the occiput to C2 beneath the rods. Notably, the patient was auto fused from C2 to his upper thoracic spine. A deep Hemovac was placed, and vancomycin was distributed within the wound. The wound was then closed in anatomical layers. The patient woke up with worsened right-sided weakness in the upper and lower extremities, which gradually improved during recovery. A CT scan showed no postoperative hematoma or other complications, and cervical radiographs showed good location of the posterior instrumentation (Fig. 12.2). They were discharged to rehabilitation on postoperative day 5 and returned to baseline strength at last follow-up.

Commonalities among the experts

Half of the surgeons opted for a cervical spine flexion-extension radiographs and CT angiography as part of the additional preoperative studies. The rest of the surgeons requested studies considerably varied. The majority advocated for a posterior stabilization and fusion of the upper cervical spine. One of the surgeons favored the inclusion of the occipital bone, and one suggested decompression alone. All aimed for upper cervical decompression of the spinal cord. All were aware of the vertebral arteries. The most feared complications were spinal cord and vertebral artery injury. Surgery was generally pursued with fluoroscopy and intraoperative monitoring. Half of the physicians recommended preoperative steroids. Surgical nuances varied,

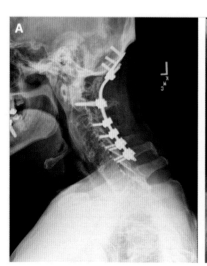
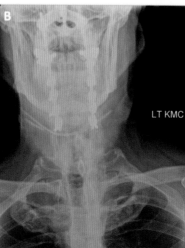

Fig. 12.2 Postoperative x-rays. (A) Lateral and (B) anteroposterior (AP) x-rays demonstrating adequate posterior instrumentation extending from the occiput to C6 with paired rods and screw fixation. Hardware appears intact.

but most agreed on the importance of attaining posterior decompression and stability. After surgery, half admitted their patients to the intensive care unit and the rest to the floor. Postoperative testing and follow-up recommendations widely varied. Use of collar was advocated by half of the experts, and one surgeon selected bracing.

SUMMARY OF QUALITY OF EVIDENCE TO GUIDE SPECIFIC INTERVENTIONS FOR THIS CASE

- Patients with spinal cord compression, persistent/intractable pain, neurological impairment, and major radiological dislocation need surgical treatment: level II.1.
- Atlanto-axial transarticular screw improves fusion rates and attains stabilization: level III.

REFERENCES

1. Joyce AA, Williams JN, Shi J, et al. Atlanto-axial Pannus in Patients with and without Rheumatoid Arthritis. *J Rheumatol.* 2019;46(11): 1431–1437.
2. Landi A, Marotta N, Morselli C, Marongiu A, Delfini R. Pannus regression after posterior decompression and occipito-cervical fixation in occipito-atlanto-axial instability due to rheumatoid arthritis: case report and literature review. *Clin Neurol Neurosurg.* 2013;115(2):111–116.
3. Chung J, Bak KH, Yi HJ, et al. Upper Cervical Subluxation and Cervicomedullary Junction Compression in Patients with Rheumatoid Arthritis. *J Korean Neurosurg Soc.* 2019;62(6):661–670.
4. Gillick JL, Wainwright J, Das K. Rheumatoid Arthritis and the Cervical Spine: A Review on the Role of Surgery. *Int J Rheumatol.* 2015;2015:252456.
5. Janssen I, Nouri A, Tessitore E, Meyer B. Cervical Myelopathy in Patients Suffering from Rheumatoid Arthritis-A Case Series of 9 Patients and A Review of the Literature. *J Clin Med.* 2020;9(3).
6. Del Grande M, Del Grande F, Carrino J, Bingham CO, 3rd, Louie GH. Cervical spine involvement early in the course of rheumatoid arthritis. *Semin Arthritis Rheum.* 2014;43(6):738–744.
7. Kolen ER, Schmidt MH. Rheumatoid arthritis of the cervical spine. *Semin Neurol.* 2002;22(2):179–186.
8. Weerasinghe D, Cordato D, Kuan J, Sturgess A. Teaching NeuroImages: Rheumatoid pannus of the cervical spine: An unusual cause of multiple cranial nerve palsies. *Neurology.* 2017;88(6):e51.
9. Younes M, Belghali S, Kriâa S, et al. Compared imaging of the rheumatoid cervical spine: prevalence study and associated factors. *Joint Bone Spine.* 2009;76(4):361–368.
10. Grob D, Würsch R, Grauer W, Sturzenegger J, Dvorak J. Atlantoaxial fusion and retrodental pannus in rheumatoid arthritis. *Spine (Phila Pa 1976).* 1997;22(14):1580–1583. discussion 1584.
11. Bouchaud-Chabot A, Lioté F. Cervical spine involvement in rheumatoid arthritis. A review. *Joint Bone Spine.* 2002;69(2):141–154.
12. Ryu JI, Bak KH, Kim JM, Chun HJ. Comparison of Transarticular Screw Fixation and C1 Lateral Mass-C2 Pedicle Screw Fixation in Patients with Rheumatoid Arthritis with Atlantoaxial Instability. *World Neurosurg.* 2017;99:179–185.

13

High lumbar stenosis (thoracolumbar junction)

Kingsley Abode-Iyamah, MD

Introduction

Stenosis of the lumbar spine can occur at different areas of the lumbar spine. Stenosis of the lumbar spine is most common at L4-5 level but can also occur at L3-4, L2-3, L5-S1, and L1-2 in decreasing frequency.[1] Stenosis can result from a number of causes such as hypertrophy of the ligamentum flavum. Ossification of the ligamentum flavum can also result in stenosis. Additionally, broad-based disc or rarely calcification of the posterior longitudinal ligament can also contribute to stenosis. Other factors that may lead to stenosis are congenital stenosis of the spine combined with degenerative changes and facet hypertrophy. These changes may be the result of degenerative changes or can be attributed to micro-instability at the location of the stenosis.[2] This can be especially true for stenosis due to adjacent segment disease from a prior surgical fusion.[3–11] Symptoms vary significantly for those with stenosis and can include symptoms of neurogenic claudication, radiculopathy, sensation loss, weakness, and even incontinence.

The management consideration becomes more complex when the stenosis is in the high lumbar spine region. This is especially so when there is a prior instrumentation at this location, which can be further destabilized from further bony removal. Further consideration for destabilization is when the stenosis is in thoracolumbar junction, as the combination of decompression with the high mobility in this location can also lead to destabilization.[12] In this case we review the important factors to consider in thoracolumbar stenosis.

Example Case

Chief complaint: back pain and leg pain

History of present illness: A 66-year-old male with a history of motor vehicle accident 1 year prior. Since that time, he has had progressively worsening gait issues as well as back pain. His gait instability has progressively worsened over the last 6 to 8 weeks. He states that he has gone from ambulating freely to using a cane and now using a walker. He also reports some issues with urgency but denies incontinence. Imaging was done and there was concern for stenosis (Figs. 13.1–13.3).

Medications: lisinopril-hydrochlorothiazide

Allergies: no known drug allergies

Past medical and surgical history: hepatitis C, hypertension, cervical fusion, lumbar laminectomy, appendectomy

Family history: noncontributory

Social history: no smoking history, occasional alcohol

Physical examination: awake, alert, and oriented to person, place, and time; cranial nerves II–XII intact; bilateral deltoids/biceps/triceps 5/5; interossei 5/5; iliopsoas/knee flexion/knee extension/dorsi, and plantar flexion 5/5

Reflexes: 2+ in bilateral biceps/triceps/brachioradialis; 3+ in bilateral patella/ankle; no clonus, positive Babinski on the left, negative Hoffman; sensation decreased in bilateral lower extremities

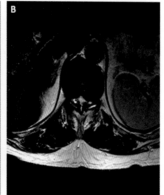

Fig. 13.1 Preoperative magnetic resonance images. (A) T2 sagittal and (B) T2 axial images demonstrating T11-12 ligamentum hypertrophy with cord compression and T2 cord signal change at this location.

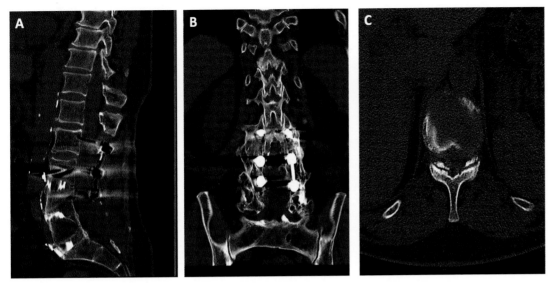

Fig. 13.2 Preoperative computed tomography scans. (A) Sagittal, (B) coronal, and (C) axial images demonstrating previous instrumentation at L2-5 with solid bony fusion.

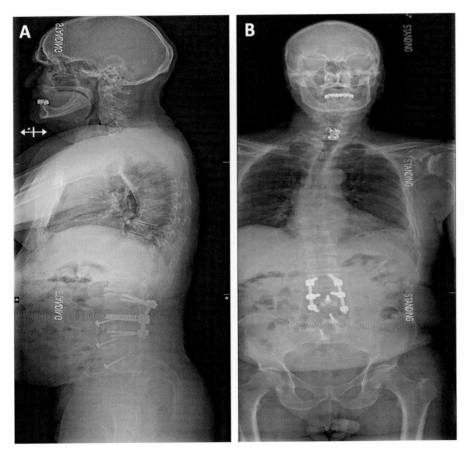

Fig. 13.3 Preoperative x-rays. (A) Lateral and (B) AP x-rays demonstrating L5-S1 interbody fusion with spinous process device.

	Jeff D. Golan, MD Neurosurgery McGill University Montreal, Quebec, Canada	Patrick C. Hsieh, MD Neurosurgery University of Southern California Los Angeles, California, United States	Paul M. Huddleston, III, MD Orthopaedic Surgery Mayo Clinic Rochester, Minnesota, United States	Peter Jarzem, MD Orthopaedic Surgery McGill University Montreal General Hospital Montreal, Canada
Preoperative				
Additional tests requested	None	Hepatology evaluation	DEXA L-spine flexion-extension x-rays CT myelogram	Complete spine MRI DEXA Hepatology evaluation
Surgical approach selected	T11-12 MIS laminectomy	T11-12 laminectomy and facetectomy and excision of synovial cyst and T11-12 posterior fusion	T11-12 laminectomy	T11-12 laminectomy with interbody and fascectomy and domino to previous fusion with vertebroplasty
Goal of surgery	Decompress cord	Decompress cord, spinal stability, and fusion to prevent facet arthropathy	Decompress cord	Decompress cord, stabilization of scoliotic deformity, prevent kyphosis
Perioperative				
Positioning	Prone on Jackson table, no pins	Prone on Jackson table, no pins	Prone on Jackson table, with Mayfield pins	Prone on Jackson table, no pins
Surgical equipment	IOM Fluoroscopy Surgical microscope	IOM (MEP/SSEP) Fluoroscopy O-arm Ultrasound Ultrasonic bone scalpel	IOM (MEP/SSEP/EMG) Surgical microscope Cell saver	IOM (MEP) Fluoroscopy
Medications	None	Steroids, maintain MAP >85, liposomal bupivacaine	Tranexamic acid, liposomal bupivacaine	Steroids, tranexamic acid
Anatomical considerations	T11-12 facets	Spinal cord, T12 nerve roots, pedicle orientation, sagittal alignment	Spinal cord, T11-12 facets	Spinal cord, nerve roots
Complications feared with approach chosen	Inadequate decompression, spinal cord injury, nerve root injury, mechanical back pain from overaggressive facetectomy	Wrong level surgery, CSF leak, spinal cord injury, screw or cage malposition	Instability, infection	CSF leak, spinal cord injury, nerve root irritation
Intraoperative				
Anesthesia	General	General	General	General
Exposure	T11-12	T11-12	T10-L3	T11-L3
Levels decompressed	T11-12	T11-12	T10-L2	T11-12
Levels fused	None	T11-12	None	T11-L3

	Jeff D. Golan, MD Neurosurgery McGill University Montreal, Quebec, Canada	Patrick C. Hsieh, MD Neurosurgery University of Southern California Los Angeles, California, United States	Paul M. Huddleston, III, MD Orthopaedic Surgery Mayo Clinic Rochester, Minnesota, United States	Peter Jarzem, MD Orthopaedic Surgery McGill University Montreal General Hospital Montreal, Canada
Surgical narrative	Position prone, confirm level, 3 cm incision 1 cm off midline on left side (left facet appears more horizontal than right), incise through skin and thoracolumbar fascia, finger dissect through muscle onto base of T11 spinous process and medial lamina, x-ray to confirm level, sequentially dilate to 19 mm tube and dock with final tube, use microscope to define anatomy and dissect residual muscle and periosteum with Bovie to expose base of T11-12 spinous process and caudal portion of T11 and rostral T12 lamina, drill ipsilateral T11 lamina until yellow ligament is freed, drill on underside of spinous process and inner portion of contralateral lamina leaving yellow ligament for now, drill until T12 superior face identified and move laterally until flush with medial portion of pedicle, free yellow ligament and decompress underlying thecal sac, remove ligament on ipsilateral side and in midline using curettes and micro rongeurs, assure adequate bony decompression on contralateral side using curette to feel subarticular space, drill more lamina if needed, identify and recognize contralateral T11 and T12 roots, cord should be free of bony contact and roots well visualized, withdraw tube, close thoracolumbar and Scarpa's fascia, standard closure	Preposition MEP/SSEP, position prone and postflip MEP/SSEP, expose T11-12 level and confirm with x-ray or O-arm, prep pedicle screws T11-12, T11-12 laminectomy and facetectomy with at least 50% facet joint removal to decompress spinal cord, excise synovial cyst, decompress from pedicle to pedicle, completely remove all ligamentum flavum at T11-12, check adequacy of decompression with ultrasound, complete facetectomy and costotransversectomy for discectomy if there is still ventral compression, place T11-12 pedicle screws and rods, check implant with O-arm, arthrodesis and placement of bone graft at T11-12, vancomycin and tobramycin in cavity, closure in layers with drain	Position prone after preflip IOM, postflip IOM, x-ray to guide incision, midline incision, subperiosteal dissection, confirm level with biplanar x-ray and compare with preoperative x-rays to confirm level as well as long x-ray to count from lumbosacral junction, microscope brought into the field hemilaminectomy removing inferior third of T10, central lamina of T11-L1, remove central ligamentum flavum/epidural fat/overgrown facet capsules/lateral recess until flush with medial wall of L2 pedicles, identify L1 nerve roots, foraminotomy of bilateral L1 roots, irrigate with saline and dilute betadine, layered wound closure without a drain, liposomal bupivacaine throughout	Position prone, posterior approach through midline, expose previous hardware, remove topmost screws, add fenestrated screws above compression, complete facet osteotomy at all compressed levels, perform TLIF, check position of hardware with fluoroscopy, place vertebroplasty cannula at level above screws, cement fenestrated screws at vertebral level above the screws under fluoroscopy, domino to previous hardware, close wound over drain
Complication avoidance	MIS, tubular-assisted left-sided approach, limit pressure on dura and underlying cord when using Kerrison rongeur, decompress ipsilateral side to provide contralateral working corridor	Preflip IOM, remove facet to allow access, wide decompression, complete facetectomy and costotransversectomy for discectomy if residual compression on ultrasound	Preflip IOM, confirm level by comparing with preoperative x-ray	Use fenestrated screws above compression, facetectomy at compressed levels, vertebroplasty
Postoperative				
Admission	Floor	Floor	Floor	Floor
Postoperative complications feared	Inadequate decompression, spinal cord injury, nerve root injury, mechanical back pain from overaggressive facetectomy	Pain, hematoma, implant malposition, adjacent segment disease, kyphosis	Instability, infection	Spinal cord injury, CSF leak, wound infection, hardware malplacement
Anticipated length of stay	1 day	2–3 days	1–2 days	3–4 days

| | Jeff D. Golan, MD
Neurosurgery
McGill University
Montreal, Quebec, Canada | Patrick C. Hsieh, MD
Neurosurgery
University of Southern California
Los Angeles, California, United States | Paul M. Huddleston, III, MD
Orthopaedic Surgery
Mayo Clinic
Rochester, Minnesota, United States | Peter Jarzem, MD
Orthopaedic Surgery
McGill University
Montreal General Hospital
Montreal, Canada |
|---|---|---|---|---|
| Follow-up testing | L-spine standing x-rays before discharge

MRI L-spine 3–6 months after surgery | L-spine AP and lateral standing x-rays before discharge and 3 months, 6 months, 1 year, 2 years after surgery | Upright scoliosis x-rays 3 months after surgery

T-L spine flexion-extension 3 months after surgery | T-L spine x-ray after surgery |
| Bracing | None | None | TLSO brace for 6 weeks | None |
| Follow-up visits | 2–4 weeks, 3–4 months, 9–12 months after surgery | 2–3 weeks, 6 weeks, 3 months, 6 months, 12 months, annually after surgery | 2 weeks, 3 months after surgery | 2 weeks after surgery |

AP, Anteroposterior; CSF, cerebrospinal fluid; DEXA, dual-energy x-ray absorptiometry; IOM, intraoperative monitoring; MAP, mean arterial pressure; MEP, motor evoked potential; MIS, minimally invasive surgery; MRI, magnetic resonance imaging; SSEP, somatosensory evoked potential; TLSO, thoracic lumbar sacral orthosis.

Differential diagnosis

- Spinal stenosis
- Facet hypertrophy
- Ligamentum flavum hypertrophy

Important anatomical considerations

The thoracolumbar junction is from T11 to L1. It represents a transition zone of the stiffer thoracic spine and more mobile lumbar spine. The thoracic spine contains rib attachment, although the last two ribs at T11 and T12 are typically floating ribs. The rib cage and its attachment to the sternum increases the stiffness of the thoracic spine and has been referred to as the fourth column. Additionally, the spine facet changes from a more coronally oriented thoracic spine to more sagittal oriented facet joints in the lumbar spine, allowing flexion and extension. The transition from a more stiff spinal segment to a more mobile segment predisposes the thoracolumbar junction to increased mechanical movement, which can predispose this location to not only injury but also destabilization.[13,14] While gross destabilization may not be apparent on dynamic x-rays, pneumatization of the disc space on flexion-extension films may represent microinstability.[15]

Stenosis in this location can result from hypertrophy of the ligamentum flavum, ossification of the ligamentum flavum, broad-based disc, or (rarely) calcification of the posterior longitudinal ligament. Depending on the location of the compression and where the spinal cord ends in the patient, symptoms can vary from neurogenic claudication, radiculopathy, conus medullaris syndrome, or even myelopathic symptoms. When there is a low lying conus, cord signal change and cavitation should be evaluated on magnetic resonance imaging (MRI) as well.

Approaches to this lesion

The approach to thoracolumbar stenosis is posterior in nature. While the argument can be made for a transthoracic approach for a calcified disc in this location, the majority of these cases, even when there is a calcified disc, can be managed safely from a posterior approach. The area of contention lies in whether decompression alone is sufficient in these patients. While some advocate for laminectomy alone,[16] others believe that ligamentum hypertrophy represents the body's attempt to stabilize an already unstable segment. Therefore, a laminectomy alone may further destabilize these patients. Thus, some authors advocate instrumentation when decompressing in the thoracolumbar spine.[15] Additionally, some authors suggest a better outcome in those individuals who have undergone decompressive fusion compared with a laminectomy alone.[15,17]

What was actually done

This patient is unique, having had a previous L2 to S1 fusion. While there was mild degeneration at the adjacent segment, the patient's compression causing his symptoms was in the T11-12 location. There was compression of the spinal cord at this location with cord signal change. Given the concern for the increase in motion at the thoracolumbar junction and the already increased stiffness at the fused level at the level below L2, the decision was made to perform a T11 laminectomy with instrumentation and connection to the previous instrumentation. In this particular patient, there was concern for focal instrumentation further increasing the motion between the two fused segments leading to further degeneration. Additionally, given that there was grade I spondylolisthesis at the T11-12 location already, a laminectomy alone was not entertained. The patient underwent T10 to L1 instrumentation with connection to the previous rod and had good improvement of the preoperative symptoms. The patient was discharged on postoperative day 6, and x-rays showed good position of the instrumentation (Fig. 13.4).

Commonalities among the experts

The response of our experts significantly differed from what was actually done for this patient. One expert recommended hepatology evaluation for the patient preoperatively, and another recommended obtaining additional imaging

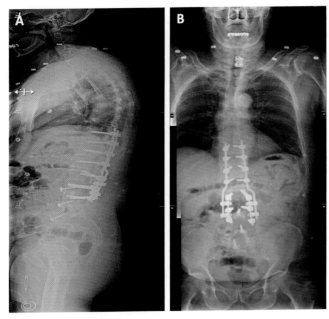

Fig. 13.4 Postoperative x-rays. (A) Lateral and (B) AP x-rays demonstrating postoperative instrumentation at T10 to L1 with rod connection to previous instrumentation.

(dual-energy x-ray absorptiometry, flexion-extension x-rays, and a computed tomography myelogram). Although all experts agreed on a posterior approach as performed for the above case, the need for instrumentation was not agreed upon by all. Some recommended a laminectomy at T11-12, while another recommended a T11-12 laminectomy and instrumentation of only T11-12. The common goal of surgery was decompression of the spinal cord, but one surgeon also included stabilization and prevention of facet arthropathy. Intraoperative monitoring was recommended by all experts with the use of microscope for decompression recommend by two. There was an expected 1- to 3-day hospitalization, and all experts agreed on postoperative x-rays and one recommended follow-up MRI at 3 to 6 months postoperative.

SUMMARY OF QUALITY OF EVIDENCE TO GUIDE SPECIFIC INTERVENTIONS FOR THIS CASE

- Intraoperative monitoring for myelopathy surgery: level II.1
- Fusion versus laminectomy alone for thoracic stenosis: level II.2

REFERENCES

1. Wessberg P, Frennered K. Central lumbar spinal stenosis: natural history of non-surgical patients. *Eur Spine J.* 2017;26(10):2536–2542.
2. Panjabi MM, Goel VK, Takata K. Physiologic strains in the lumbar spinal ligaments. An in vitro biomechanical study 1981 Volvo Award in Biomechanics. *Spine (Phila Pa 1976).* 1982;7(3):192–203.
3. Bastian L, Lange U, Knop C, Tusch G, Blauth M. Evaluation of the mobility of adjacent segments after posterior thoracolumbar fixation: a biomechanical study. *Eur Spine J.* 2001;10(4):295–300.
4. Chow DH, Luk KD, Evans JH, Leong JC. Effects of short anterior lumbar interbody fusion on biomechanics of neighboring unfused segments. *Spine (Phila Pa 1976).* 1996;21(5):549–555.
5. Esses SI, Doherty BJ, Crawford MJ, Dreyzin V. Kinematic evaluation of lumbar fusion techniques. *Spine (Phila Pa 1976).* 1996;21(6):676–684.
6. Fehlings MG, Tetreault L, Nater A, Choma T, Harrop J, Mroz T, et al. The Aging of the Global Population: The Changing Epidemiology of Disease and Spinal Disorders. *Neurosurgery.* 2015;77(Suppl 4):S1–S5.
7. Ha KY, Schendel MJ, Lewis JL, Ogilvie JW. Effect of immobilization and configuration on lumbar adjacent-segment biomechanics. *J Spinal Disord.* 1993;6(2):99–105.
8. Lee CK, Langrana NA. Lumbosacral spinal fusion. A biomechanical study. *Spine (Phila Pa 1976).* 1984;9(6):574–581.
9. Nagata H, Schendel MJ, Transfeldt EE, Lewis JL. The effects of immobilization of long segments of the spine on the adjacent and distal facet force and lumbosacral motion. *Spine (Phila Pa 1976).* 1993;18(16):2471–2479.
10. Quinnell RC, Stockdale HR. Some experimental observations of the influence of a single lumbar floating fusion on the remaining lumbar spine. *Spine (Phila Pa 1976).* 1981;6(3):263–267.
11. Virk SS, Niedermeier S, Yu E, Khan SN. Adjacent segment disease. *Orthopedics.* 2014;37(8):547–555.
12. Yoganandan N, Maiman DJ, Pintar FA, Bennett GJ, Larson SJ. Biomechanical effects of laminectomy on thoracic spine stability. *Neurosurgery.* 1993;32(4):604–610.
13. Flouty O, Abode-Iyamah K, Ahmed R, Wilson S, Menezes AH. Junctional susceptibility of the pediatric spine: a case report. *Childs Nerv Syst.* 2015;31(5):797–800.
14. Jacobs RR, Asher MA, Snider RK. Thoracolumbar spinal injuries. A comparative study of recumbent and operative treatment in 100 patients. *Spine (Phila Pa 1976).* 1980;5(5):463–477.
15. Hitchon PW, Abode-Iyamah K, Dahdaleh NS, Grossbach AJ, El Tecle NE, Noeller J, et al. Risk factors and outcomes in thoracic stenosis with myelopathy: A single center experience. *Clin Neurol Neurosurg.* 201;147:84–89.
16. Osman NS, Cheung ZB, Hussain AK, Phan K, Arvind V, Vig KS, et al. Outcomes and Complications Following Laminectomy Alone for Thoracic Mylopathy due to Ossified Ligamentum Flavum: A Systematic Review and Meta-Analysis. *Spine (Phila Pa 1976).* 2018;43(14):E842–E848.
17. Onishi E, Yasuda T, Yamamoto H, Iwaki K, Ota S. Outcomes of Surgical Treatment for Thoracic Myelopathy: A Single-institutional Study of 73 Patients. *Spine (Phila Pa 1976).* 2016;41(22):E1356–E1363.

14

Cervical stenosis with preservation of lordosis

Kingsley Abode-Iyamah, MD

Introduction

Although first described in 1952 by Brian et al.,[1] cervical spondylotic myelopathy (CSM) continues to be a frequently misdiagnosed pathology. The insidious onset is often mistaken as part of the normal aging process, while patients often have progressive and debilitating neurological deficits. In fact, CSM is the leading cause of spinal cord–related disability in older adults. This results from degenerative changes of the cervical spine, which leads to narrowing of the spinal canal and chronic compression of the cervical spinal cord. The chronic compression leads to ischemia of the spinal cord, demyelination, axonal loss, and, in severe cases, neuronal loss. This leads to the cavitation often seen on magnetic resonance imaging. There is believed to be components of both static and dynamic compression, which contributes to ongoing damage to the spinal cord.

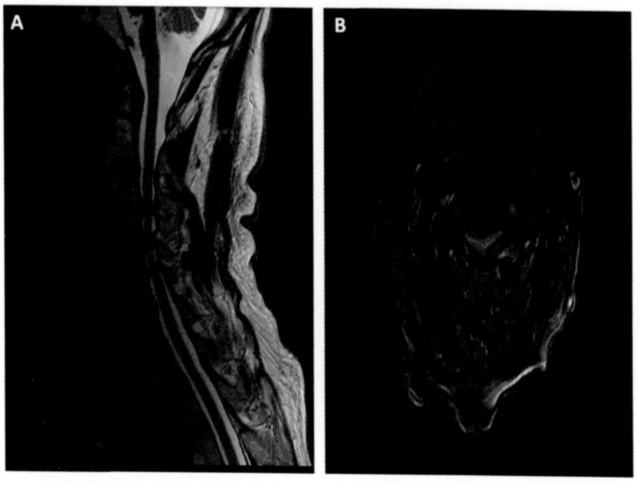

Fig. 14.1 Preoperative magnetic resonance imaging. (A) T2 sagittal and (B) T2 axial images demonstrating a disc, posterior osteophyte, and ligamentum flavum hypertrophy causing circumferential compression of the spinal cord from C3-6 with cord signal change.

This leads to symptoms such as gait instability, weakness, paresthesia, loss of dexterity, and urinary dysfunction. The degree of compression at which a patient presents with symptoms is highly variable, as is the rate of symptomatic progression. There are many factors that may contribute to spondylosis leading to canal stenosis such as genetics, smoking, trauma, heavy labor, and congenital spinal anomalies. Likewise, there are a number of factors that affect the progression of symptoms, and there has been increasing interest in how genetics play into this process.[2]

Example case

Chief complaint: gait imbalance

History of present illness: A 77-year-old male with a history of increasing difficulty with balance. He recently suffered a fall, fracturing his hip. The patient has also had increasing difficulty with his dexterity including difficulty buttoning his shirt and fine motor movement. He denies any bowel bladder dysfunction. He was not using any assistive device before his fall but is now using a wheelchair when out and a walker at home. He underwent imaging and this was concerning for cervical stenosis (Figs. 14.1–14.2).

Medications: amlodipine, aspirin 81 mg, pravastatin, sertraline, tacrolimus, tamsulosin

Allergies: lorazepam

Past medical and surgical history: alcoholic cirrhosis, early-stage dementia, hypertension, hyperlipidemia, depression, skin cancer, cervical myelopathy, liver transplant

Family history: noncontributory

Social history: retired professor, previous alcohol dependency, remote history of smoking

Physical examination: awake, alert, and oriented to person, place, and time; cranial nerves II–XII intact; bilateral deltoids/biceps/triceps 5/5; interossei 5/5; iliopsoas/knee flexion/knee extension/dorsi, and plantar flexion 5/5

Reflexes: 3+ in bilateral biceps/triceps/brachioradialis; 3+ in bilateral patella/ankle no clonus or Babinski, left Hoffman; sensation increased in bilateral lower extremities

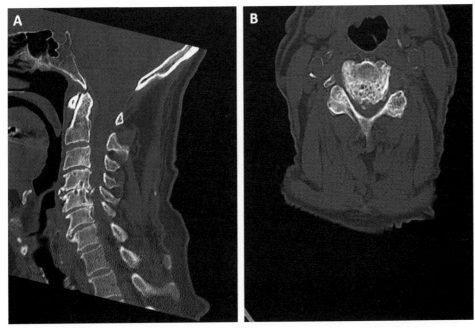

Fig. 14.2 Preoperative computed tomgoraphy scans. (A) Sagittal, and (B) axial images demonstrating degenerative changes of the cervical spine with osteophyte at C4-5. The cervical lordosis is maintained.

	Todd J. Albert, MD Orthopaedic Surgery Hospital for Special Surgery Weill Cornell Medical College New York, New York, United States	Belal Elnady, MD Orthopaedic Surgery Assiut University Assiut, Egypt	Esteban F. Espinoza-García, MD, MSc University of Valparaíso San Felipe, Chile	Langston Holly, MD Neurosurgery University of California at Los Angeles Los Angeles, California, United States
Preoperative				
Additional tests requested	AP, lateral, flexion-extension C-spine x-rays EOS spine imaging	C-spine x-rays Liver function tests	Flexion-extension C-spine x-rays MRI brain Anesthesia evaluation	AP, lateral, flexion-extension C-spine x-rays Medicine evaluation
Surgical approach selected	C3-7 laminoplasty	C3-4, C4-5, C5-6 ACDF	C3-5 laminectomy	C3-7 laminectomy
Goal of surgery	Spinal cord decompression	Spinal cord decompression, fusion	Spinal cord decompression	Spinal cord decompression
Perioperative				
Positioning	Prone with Gardner-Wells tongs on Jackson table with 10–15 lb of traction	Supine, no pins	Prone with Mayfield pins	Prone with Mayfield pins
Surgical equipment	IOM (MEP/SSEP/EMG) Laminoplasty plates Cell saver	IOM (SSEP/EMG) Fluoroscopy Surgical microscope	Fluoroscopy	Fluoroscopy
Medications	Tranexamic acid, steroids, MAPs 85–90	None	Steroids, maintain MAP	None
Anatomical considerations	Spinal cord, C5 nerve roots, insertion of spinal extensors	Spinal cord	Dura, vertebral arteries	Spinal cord, facets
Complications feared with approach chosen	Pseudoarthrosis, incomplete decompression, junctional segment compression, hardware failure, dysphagia	Durotomy, CSF leak	Durotomy, CSF leak, vertebral artery injury	Durotomy, CSF leak, spinal instability, dysphagia

	Todd J. Albert, MD Orthopaedic Surgery Hospital for Special Surgery Weill Cornell Medical College New York, New York, United States	Belal Elnady, MD Orthopaedic Surgery Assiut University Assiut, Egypt	Esteban F. Espinoza-García, MD, MSc University of Valparaíso San Felipe, Chile	Langston Holly, MD Neurosurgery University of California at Los Angeles Los Angeles, California, United States
Intraoperative				
Anesthesia	General	General	General	General
Exposure	C3-7	C3-6	C2-6	C3-7
Levels decompressed	C3-7	C3-6	C3-5	C3-7
Levels fused	None	C3-6	None	None
Surgical narrative	Position prone with Gardner-Wells tongs, keep head neutral to flexed with bivector traction robes, expose C3-7 lateral masses bilaterally, partial laminectomy at caudal end of C3 and rostral end of C7, full trough bilaterally at C4-6 on opening side that is more symptomatic and compression, thin contralateral side trough C4-6, open full trough side, place plates and fixed lamina then spinous process, apply hemostatic agent and steroids on cord, bur down dominant spinous process, five-layer closure	Intubated, supine position, fluoroscopy to identify correct level, right transverse neck incision, incise platysma, work between trachea and esophagus medially and carotid sheath laterally, expose C3-6, start at top level and remove disk, curette disc space, open PLL, use blunt nerve hook behind disc space to ensure adequate decompression, insert PEEK, repeat at C4-5 and C5-6, insert plate, AP and lateral x-rays to confirm good location of interbody grafts and plate, standard closure with subplatysmal drain	Intubated, x-ray to confirm level, midline incision, subperiosteal bilateral exposure of C2-6, C3-5 laminectomy, yellow ligament removal until dural visualized	GlideScope intubation, supine SSEP/MEP, position prone with pins in head neutral, confirm baseline IOM, exposure spine, confirm levels based on lateral fluoroscopy, open ligamentum flavum at C2-3 and C7-T1, drill troughs at C3-7 lamina-facet junction, open ligamentum flavum in the troughs with a 1 mm Kerrison rongeur, lift C3-7 lamina away from spine in one piece, confirm spinal levels with fluoroscopy, layered closure with drain
Complication avoidance	Laminoplasty, opening side of laminoplasty on more symptomatic side, bur down spinous processes	Anterior approach, right side to avoid recurrent laryngeal nerve injury, preserve lordosis, x-ray to confirm	No fusion	Preflip IOM, en bloc laminectomy, no fusion
Postoperative				
Admission	Stepdown unit vs. floor	ICU	ICU	Floor
Postoperative complications feared	C5 palsy	Neurological deterioration	CSF leak, spinal instability, vertebral artery injury, medical complications	C5 nerve palsy, hematoma, CSF leak, medical complication
Anticipated length of stay	1–3 days	2 days	5 days	3 days
Follow-up testing	Cervical AP/lateral x-rays 3 weeks after surgery Cervical flexion-extension/AP/lateral x-rays 3 months after surgery	Cervical x-rays 2 months, 6 months, 12 months after surgery	C-spine CT 1 day, 3 months after surgery, C-spine MRI 3 months after surgery	None
Bracing	Soft collar for 2 weeks	Soft collar for 6 weeks	Philadelphia collar for 3 months	None
Follow-up visits	2–3 weeks after surgery	2 weeks, 2 months, 6 months, 12 months after surgery	3 weeks after discharge	2 weeks, 6 weeks, 3 months, 6 months, 1 year after surgery

ACDF, Anterior cervical decompression and fusion; AP, anteroposterior; CSF, cerebrospinal fluid; EMG, Electromyogram; ESI, epidural spinal injections; ICU, intensive care unit; IOM, intraoperative monitoring; MAP, mean arterial pressure; MEP, motor evoked potentials; MRI, magnetic resonance imaging; PEEK, polyetheretherketone; PLL, posterior longitudinal ligament; SSEP, somatosensory evoked potentials.

Differential diagnosis

- Cervical myelopathy
- Transverse myelitis
- Multiple sclerosis

Important anatomical considerations

The cervical spine is composed of seven vertebrae. With the exception of the first cervical vertebrae, each vertebra has an associated nerve that exits the foramen above the above-named vertebrae. Additionally, the vertebral artery enters the foramen transversarium typically at the sixth cervical vertebrae and exits at C1 prior to entering the foramen magnum. The spinal cord transitions from the lower brainstem to the cervical spinal cord where it runs in the spinal canal. The anterior two-thirds of the spinal cord is supplied by the anterior spinal arteries, which originate from the two vertebral arteries. The posterior spinal artery supplies the posterior one-third of the cervical spinal cord and is supplied by the radicular arteries.

Compression of the spinal cord can occur from different spondylotic processes, which ultimately narrows the spinal canal. These include disc herniation (found more commonly in the younger population), disc-osteophyte complex, spondylolisthesis, ossification of the posterior longitudinal ligament, hypertrophy of the ligamentum flavum, ossification of the ligamentum flavum, and diffuse idiopathic skeletal hyperostosis (may be found more commonly in the older population). Addressing the area from which the compression is originating typically allows the best decompression approach, although there are several factors that can influence this, as described below.

Approaches to this lesion

In general, CSM is best approached through the route that best addresses the compressive lesion, although there are numerous factors that may influence this decision. Decompression of the cervical spinal cord can best be addressed through either an anterior approach or posterior approach depending on the location of the compressive lesion. In a few instances, there may be a need to perform a posterior approach even in the setting of anterior cervical compression, such as in the setting of ossification of the posterior longitudinal ligament.[3,4] Additionally, when there is evidence of kyphosis of the cervical spine on neutral x-rays, there is need for an anterior approach to return the normal lordotic curvature the spinal cord, as this has been found to play a role in recovery. The K-line is a well-recognized decision tool that allows one to determine the best approach, especially in ossification of the posterior longitudinal ligament.[5] This is also a useful tool in determining whether an anterior and/or posterior approach is needed in other pathologies leading to cervical kyphosis.

The anterior approach to the cervical spine for CSM includes both an anterior cervical discectomy and fusion as well as anterior cervical corpectomy. The decision on whether an adequate decompression can be accomplished through a discectomy versus a corpectomy depends on the location of the disc and whether it is calcified. For this reason, in addition to the magnetic resonance images of the cervical spine, a computed tomography scan of the cervical spine is recommended, especially when a large anterior mass is identified. When there is an anterior osteophyte, a corpectomy with anterior cervical fusion may be better, as an anterior cervical decompression and fusion (ACDF) may not adequately remove osteophytes that are rostral and caudal to the disc space.

Posterior approaches can include a laminectomy alone, laminoplasty or laminectomy, and fusion. When there is maintenance of the cervical lordosis, cervical laminectomy or laminoplasty can be achieved with reduced concern for post-surgical kyphosis. This is not advised when there is kyphosis or concerns for instability. Additionally, given that CSM is believed to be a result of both static and dynamic compression, some advocate for fusion for better postoperative outcomes,[6–8] while others argue an equivalent outcome.[9, 10] The use of intraoperative neuromonitoring has remained contentious, with some suggesting its benefit and others contending that it serves no benefit.[11–13]

What was actually done

This patient had a number of comorbidities, which played a role in ultimately deciding on the surgical approach. The patient had both an active squamous cell cancer that needed to be addressed and some baseline dementia. Given the dementia, the goal was to limit the patient's exposure to general anesthesia and overall surgical time. Additionally, given that the patient had open squamous cell cancer that needed surgical intervention, the goal was to avoid instrumentation to minimize the risk of postoperative infection. This patient had good maintenance of his cervical lordosis, increased age, and the issues mentioned above, leading us to posterior laminectomy alone. The patient was taken to the operating room and position Orthopedic System Inc (OSI) table with the head secured in a Mayfield headrest in pins. A C3-5 laminectomy was performed. Mean arterial pressure was maintained greater than 85 during the procedure, and the patient received a one-time dose of 10 mg of dexamethasone intraoperatively. A drain was left in place and removed when output decreased to less than 30 mL per shift. The patient was able to discharge home. Postoperative x-rays showed good maintenance of range of motion (Fig. 14.3).

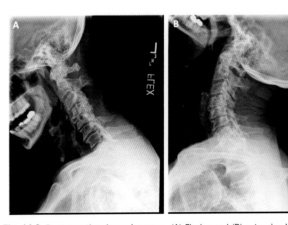

Fig. 14.3 Postoperative dynamic x-rays. (A) Flexion and (B) extension lateral x-rays of the cervical spine without dynamic instability and maintained range of movement.

Commonalities among the experts

The majority requested additional testing prior to surgical intervention. All agreed that dynamic x-rays were needed, while others recommended liver function tests. The majority recommended posterior decompression by laminectomy versus laminoplasty, and one surgeon recommended an anterior cervical discectomy and fusion from C3-6 all with the goal of decompression the spinal cord. Half recommended the use of intraoperative monitoring, while fluoroscopy was used by all. Additionally, half recommended intraoperative steroid use with elevated mean arterial pressure goals. The most common concern for complication was cerebrospinal fluid leak and dysphagia, and some included vertebral artery injury and incomplete decompression. Half recommended admission to the intensive care unit postoperatively, but overall the expected hospital stay was 1 to 5 days. The majority recommended a collar in some form with imaging during the follow-up period.

SUMMARY OF QUALITY OF EVIDENCE TO GUIDE SPECIFIC INTERVENTIONS FOR THIS CASE

- Anterior versus posterior approach CSM: level II.1
- Laminectomy/laminoplasty versus laminectomy and fusion: level II.1
- Intraoperative monitoring for spine surgery: level II.1
- Intraoperative mean arterial blood pressure of >80 for CSM: level II.2

REFERENCES

1. Brain WR, Northfield D, Wilkinson M. The neurological manifestations of cervical spondylosis. *Brain.* 1952;75(2): 187–225.
2. Abode-Iyamah KO, Stoner KE, Grossbach AJ, Viljoen SV, McHenry CL, Petrie MA, et al. Effects of brain derived neurotrophic factor Val66Met polymorphism in patients with cervical spondylotic myelopathy. *J Clin Neurosci.* 2016;24:117–121.
3. Lee CH, Sohn MJ, Lee CH, Choi CY, Han SR, Choi BW. Are There Differences in the Progression of Ossification of the Posterior Longitudinal Ligament Following Laminoplasty Versus Fusion?: A Meta-Analysis. *Spine (Phila Pa 1976).* 2017;42(12):887–894.
4. Youssef JA, Heiner AD, Montgomery JR, Tender GC, Lorio MP, Morreale JM, et al. Outcomes of posterior cervical fusion and decompression: a systematic review and meta-analysis. *Spine J.* 2019;19(10):1714–1729.
5. Fujiyoshi T, Yamazaki M, Kawabe J, Endo T, Furuya T, Koda M, et al. A new concept for making decisions regarding the surgical approach for cervical ossification of the posterior longitudinal ligament: the K-line. *Spine (Phila Pa 1976).* 2008;33(26):E990–E993.
6. Barnes MP, Saunders M. The effect of cervical mobility on the natural history of cervical spondylotic myelopathy. *J Neurol Neurosurg Psychiatry.* 1984;47(1):17–20.
7. Baron EM, Young WF. Cervical spondylotic myelopathy: a brief review of its pathophysiology, clinical course, and diagnosis. *Neurosurgery.* 2007;60(1 Suppl 1):S35–S41.
8. Hattou L, Morandi X, Le Reste PJ, Guillin R, Riffaud L, Henaux PL. Dynamic cervical myelopathy in young adults. *Eur Spine J.* 2014;23(7):1515–1522.
9. Manzano GR, Casella G, Wang MY, Vanni S, Levi AD. A prospective, randomized trial comparing expansile cervical laminoplasty and cervical laminectomy and fusion for multilevel cervical myelopathy. *Neurosurgery.* 2012;70(2):264–277.
10. Phan K, Scherman DB, Xu J, Leung V, Virk S, Mobbs RJ. Laminectomy and fusion vs laminoplasty for multi-level cervical myelopathy: a systematic review and meta-analysis. *Eur Spine J.* 2017;26(1):94–103.
11. Chang SH, Park YG, Kim DH, Yoon SY. Monitoring of Motor and Somatosensory Evoked Potentials During Spine Surgery: Intraoperative Changes and Postoperative Outcomes. *Ann Rehabil Med.* 2016;40(3):470–480.
12. Devlin VJ, Anderson PA, Schwartz DM, Vaughan R. Intraoperative neurophysiologic monitoring: focus on cervical myelopathy and related issues. *Spine J.* 2006;6(6 Suppl):212S–224SS.
13. Traynelis VC, Abode-Iyamah KO, Leick KM, Bender SM, Greenlee JD. Cervical decompression and reconstruction without intraoperative neurophysiological monitoring. *J Neurosurg Spine.* 2012;16(2):107–113.

15

Single level disc disease with back pain

Kingsley Abode-Iyamah, MD

Introduction

Low back pain is one of the leading causes of emergency visits in the United States, leading to billions of dollars in loss of productivity each year. Most Americans will experience back pain during their lifetime, and a majority of these are self-limiting and never require additional treatment. Others may improve with conservative management such as nonsteroidal antiinflammatory drugs and physical therapy, while others may need additional treatment. The exact mechanism leading to back pain is unclear, although the degenerative process is thought to play a role in many cases requiring advanced treatment.[1-3] Diagnostic evaluation for back pain without any red flags (i.e., fever, weight loss, weakness, bowel/bladder incontinence, numbness) should be started after attempted conservative management if the symptoms do not abate. The diagnostic imaging should include magnetic resonance imaging (MRI) and flexion-extension x-rays. Additional imaging studies may be required to determine the cause of the back pain in some cases. The diagnosis is made after the exclusion of radicular pain, spinal deformity, instability, and neural tension signs.[4] It should be noted that there are also nonanatomical causes of pain that should also be considered when determining the cause of axial back pain (i.e., depression).

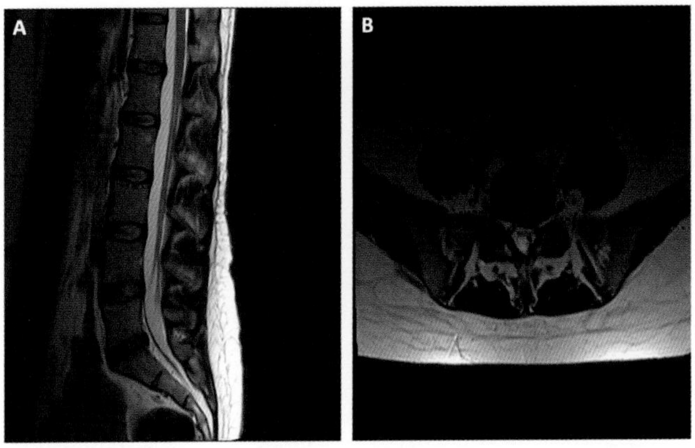

Example Case

Chief complaint: lower back pain

History of present illness: A 43-year-old female with a history lumbosacral back pain after working out. She has worsening pain with activity, which is improved by rest. This includes prolonged sitting, lifting, and repetitive motions. She has done physical therapy, injections, and ablations with minimal improvement. Imaging was done and there was concern for lumbar disc disease (Figs. 15.1–15.3).

Medications: spironolactone, trazodone, ibuprofen, acetaminophen

Allergies: no known drug allergies

Past medical and surgical history: none

Family history: noncontributory

Social history: teacher, no smoking history, occasional alcohol

Physical examination: awake, alert, and oriented to person, place, and time; cranial nerves II–XII intact; bilateral deltoids/biceps/triceps 5/5; interossei 5/5; iliopsoas/knee flexion/knee extension/dorsi, and plantar flexion 5/5

Reflexes: 2+ in bilateral biceps/triceps/brachioradialis; 2+ in bilateral patella/ankle; no clonus or Babinski; no Hoffman; sensation is intact

Fig. 15.1 Preoperative magnetic resonance images. (A) T2 sagittal and (B) T2 axial images demonstrating disc degeneration at L5-S1.

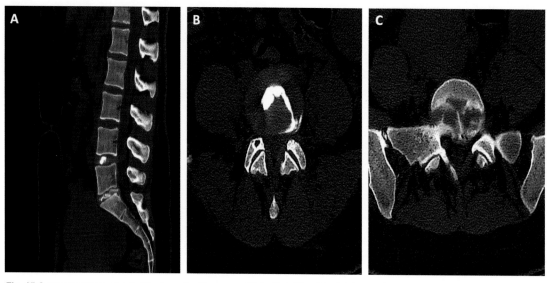

Fig. 15.2 Preoperative computed tomography discogram. (A) Sagittal, (B) axial at L4-5, and (C) axial at L5-S1 images demonstrating normal nuclear morphology at L4-5 but with advanced degenerative disc degeneration with full-thickness posterior annular fissure and filling of a broad-based posterior disc protrusion at L5-S1.

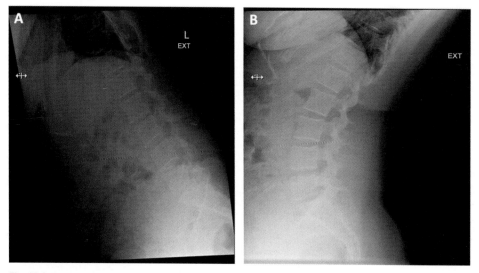

Fig. 15.3 Preoperative x-rays. (A) Flexion and (B) extension x-rays demonstrating no dynamic instability with normal range of movement of the lumbar spine.

	Mohamad Bydon, MD Neurosurgery Mayo Clinic Rochester, Minnesota, United States	Frank M. Phillips, MD Orthopaedic Surgery Rush University Chicago, Illinois, United States	Alugolu Rajesh, MD Neurosurgery Nizam's Institute of Medical Sciences Punjagutta, Hyderbad, India	Yasuaki Tokuhashi, MD Orthopaedic Surgery Nihon University Oyaguchi Kamicho, Itabashi- ku, Tokyo, Japan
Preoperative				
Additional Tests Requested	Pain rehabilitation evaluation	None	Straight leg test F18 bone scan Anesthesiology evaluation	Discogram Disc injection Psychological testing
Surgical Approach selected	Conservative management. However, if worsening and surgical approach becomes necessary, L5-S1 TLIF	Would advise against surgery because of unpredictable outcomes, but, if pursued, L5-S1 ALIF	Left L5-S1 discectomy and foraminotomy	L4-5 positive: L4-5 OLIF with percutaneous pedicle screws L5-S1 positive: microendoscopic discectomy
Goal of Surgery	Decompression and Stabilization	Stabilize spine	Decompression of neural elements	L4-5 positive: spinal stability L5-S1 positive: decrease intradiscal pressure

	Mohamad Bydon, MD Neurosurgery Mayo Clinic Rochester, Minnesota, United States	Frank M. Phillips, MD Orthopaedic Surgery Rush University Chicago, Illinois, United States	Alugolu Rajesh, MD Neurosurgery Nizam's Institute of Medical Sciences Punjagutta, Hyderbad, India	Yasuaki Tokuhashi, MD Orthopaedic Surgery Nihon University Oyaguchi Kamicho, Itabashi- ku, Tokyo, Japan
Perioperative				
Positioning	Prone	Supine	Prone	L4-5 positive: right decubitus, then prone on Hall frame L5-S1 positive: prone on Hall frame
Surgical Equipment	Fluoroscopy Intraoperative Neuromonitoring (SSEPs)	Fluoroscopy Vascular repair instrument on standby	Fluoroscopy IOM (SSEP)	Fluoroscopy Microendoscopic discectomy system
Medications	None	None	None	None
Anatomical considerations	Nerve roots, dura, musculature, bony structures	Great vessels, sympathetic plexus in males	Dura, nerve roots	Bone/muscle/neural structures, major vessels, ureter
Complications feared with approach chosen	Incidental durotomy, nerve root injury, wrong level surgery, vascular injury	Vascular injury	Durotomy, nerve root injury	Wrong level surgery, neurological injury
Intraoperative				
Anesthesia	General	General	General	General
Exposure	L5-S1	L5-S1	L5-S1	L4-5 positive: L4-5 L5-S1 positive: L5-S1
Levels decompressed	L5-S1	L5-S1	L5-S1	L4-5 positive: L4-5 L5-S1 positive: None
Levels fused	L5-S1	L5-S1	None	L4-5 positive: L4-5 L5-S1 positive: None
Surgical Narrative	Prone position, localize appropriate level using fluoroscopy, create 2-3 cm incision immediately lateral to pedicle of L5-S1, perform exposure and visualization using a Jamshidi needle and Kirschner guide wire, insert tubular retractor and endoscope, perform L5-S1 laminectomy with facetectomy, remove ligamentum flavum with curved microcurette, perform micro discectomy and prepare endplates, perform trial of interbody cage as appropriate (to restore appropriate lumbar lordosis, anterior third to maximize lordosis), place percutaneous pedicle screws and rod, standard closure	Position supine, x-ray to guide incision to L5-S1 disc, anterior retroperitoneal approach, mobilize and retract great vessels, bipolar cautery dissection only over anterior spine, identify midline, thorough wide discectomy back to PLL, good end plate preparation, size ALIF cage ensuring good fit with appropriate lordosis and posterior disc space distraction, cage and screw placement, layered closure	Position prone, place trunk on bolsters to create flexion at L5-S1, identify L5-S1, midline skin incision, subperiosteal dissection of paraspinal muscles on left side preserving tissue around facets, cut ligamentum flavum and detach from lower border of L5, left L5-S1 foraminotomy performed with undercutting facet, retract root medially and identify disc space, incise disc space sharply, complete disc decompression, pull loose fragments out, layered wound closure	L4-5 positive: stage 1 for L4-5 OLIF, right lateral decubitus position, check level with fluoroscopy and mark L4-5 vertebral body, 5–7 cm incision at 6 cm anterior vertebral marking, dissect abdominal muscles and expose retroperitoneal exposure, retract psoas to expose L4-5 disc, curettage disc, insertion of lateral lumbar interbody cage with graft bone, closure with drain; stage 2 for percutaneous screws, position prone, mark L4 and L5 pedicles under fluoroscopy, 3 cm longitudinal incision and 2 cm transverse incision on the pedicles, L4-5 pedicle screw insertion under fluoroscopy, rod insertion, fix with compression force between screws L5-S1 positive: position prone, 2 cm incision on L5-S1 interlaminar space under fluoroscopy, insert 16 mm tubular retractor and endoscope, resect yellow ligament and L5-S1 herniotomy, standard closure with drain

	Mohamad Bydon, MD Neurosurgery Mayo Clinic Rochester, Minnesota, United States	Frank M. Phillips, MD Orthopaedic Surgery Rush University Chicago, Illinois, United States	Alugolu Rajesh, MD Neurosurgery Nizam's Institute of Medical Sciences Punjagutta, Hyderbad, India	Yasuaki Tokuhashi, MD Orthopaedic Surgery Nihon University Oyaguchi Kamicho, Itabashi-ku, Tokyo, Japan
Complication Avoidance	Minimally invasive approach, proper anatomical structure identification to avoid injury	Bipolar cautery dissection only over anterior spine, make sure to identify midline, ensure posterior disc space distraction to provide indirect foraminal decompression, pay attention to great vessels during cage and screw placement	Position to promote flexing at L5-S1, left-sided exposure with preservation of facets, foraminotomy on left side	L4-5 positive: two-stage with percutaneous screws, pedicle screws under fluoroscopy, compress on screws L5-S1 positive: minimally invasive, endoscope, no bone removal
Postoperative				
Admission	Floor	Floor	Floor	Floor
Postoperative complications feared	Durotomy, Nerve root injury, CSF leak	Vascular injury	Weakness, nerve root injury, CSF leak, discitis	L4-5 positive: injury to intestines, ureter, or vasculature L5-S1 positive: CSF leak
Anticipated length of stay	Outpatient or 1 day	Outpatient or 1 day	1 day	L4-5 positive: 1–2 weeks L5-S1 positive: 2–3 days
Follow up testing	Spine XRs in 6 weeks, 6 months, 12 months, 24 months	L-spine x-rays 6 weeks, 3 months, 6 months, 1 year after surgery	None	L4-5 positive: CT 7 days, 3 months after surgery L5-S1 positive: lumbar x-rays after surgery MRI: 1–3 months after surgery
Bracing	None	None	None	L4-5 positive: soft brace for 3–6 months L5-S1 positive: no bracing or possible 1 month soft brace
Follow up visits	2 weeks, 6 weeks, then as needed	2 weeks, 6 weeks, 3 months, 6 months, 1 year after surgery	7 days, 4 weeks after surgery	4 weeks after discharge

ALIF, Anterior lumbar interbody fusion; IOM, intraoperative monitoring; MIS, minimally invasive surgery; MRI, magnetic resonance imaging; OLIF, oblique lateral interbody fusion; PLL, posterior longitudinal ligament; SSEP, somatosensory evoked potential.

Differential diagnosis

- Disc degeneration
- Discitis
- Osteomyelitis

Important anatomical considerations

Axial back pain can be very difficult to manage as the workup can often be extended, leading to patient dissatisfaction. The cause of back pain can be both anatomical and nonanatomical. While a majority of the pain may be due to musculoskeletal pain, there is no way to definitively diagnose this. The goal of the preoperative workup is to try to identify the specific pain generator that may be the cause of the pain when possible. A number of elements in the lumbar spine can result in low back pain, which is driven by a degenerative process. Back pain may result from facet degeneration that may lead to pain over time. Degeneration joint of the facet, facet fracture due to degeneration causing spondylolisthesis, or instability may lead to back pain. As the facet degenerates, the facet joint may become filled with fluid, which can be identified on the MRI. Facet joint laxity or fracture can also lead to instability, which can be identified on flexion-extension x-rays.

Axial back pain can also result from disc degeneration. The identity of a single level of disc degeneration in an individual with overall healthy disc has been referred to as "black disc disease."[1–3] This is thought to be due to dehydration of the disc space leading to degeneration and acting as the pain generator in this patient. Although its accuracy for diagnosis is concerning, discography may sometimes serve as a tool for diagnosing the pain generator in these patients.[5] It should be noted that other causes of back pain such as acute fracture, infection, and neoplasm need to be ruled out.

Approaches to this lesion

The treatment for discogenic back pain for the most part is conservative in nature. Although some have advocated for radiofrequency ablation, there has not been consistent evidence showing improvement with this intervention.[6] However, it should be noted that there is evidence suggesting it is not superior to conservative management for improvement of pain and disability.[7] In very select cases, pain relief may be achieved via an anterior or posterior approach. These include potential interbody fusion through either a transforaminal lumbar interbody fusion (TLIF) or an anterior lumbar interbody fusion (ALIF). Both can be accomplished through a minimally invasive approach. The ultimate goal is to remove the offending disc and obtain fusion in hopes of relieving the back pain. In an anterior approach, an access surgeon is used to access the desired disc space, which is then prepped with an interbody placement and screw placement. Stand-alone anterior approach can be successful for these cases in the right patient population. Likewise, minimally invasive surgery or open TLIF can also be performed.

What was actually done

This patient was significantly debilitated with her pain and had exhausted all conservative management. She underwent a discogram that showed an annular tear at the diseased level with increased pain at the same level. After thorough discussion with the patient, she was offered a minimally invasive TLIF. The patient was placed on a Wilson frame on an OSI table. A stealth pin was placed in the posterior superior iliac spine (PSIS) and O-arm images were obtained. Intraoperative stealth was used to place pedicle screws through paraspinal incision 4 cm off midline. A pedicle-based retractor system was used. A TLIF was then performed. The patient tolerated the procedure well with significant pain relief postoperatively. She was discharged on postoperative day 2 with a lumbar corset while ambulating. Postoperative images show good location of the hardware (Fig. 15.4).

Commonalities among the experts

As expected, there was wide variation in the recommendations from our experts. These ranged from ongoing conservative management to anterior-posterior fusion. The experts required comprehensive evaluation prior to surgical intervention such as a discogram, disc injection, and even psychological evaluation. Of the experts who recommended surgical intervention, the least invasive approach offered was a left L5-S1 discectomy and foraminotomy. Another surgeon offered an ALIF with the goal of stabilization of the spine. The final expert offered a L4-5 OLIF with percutaneous screw placement if this was positive on the discogram. There was a consensus that the patient should be admitted to the floor postoperatively with planned hospitalization ranging from 1 to 3 days. Postoperative imaging was only recommended by our experts half the time.

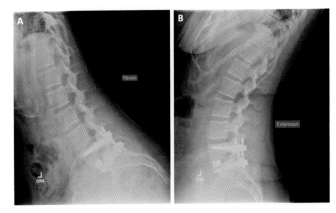

Fig. 15.4 Postoperative x-rays. (A) Lateral and (B) anteroposterior x-rays after surgery demonstrating instrumentation at L5-S1 with interbody fusion at L5-S1.

SUMMARY OF QUALITY OF EVIDENCE TO GUIDE SPECIFIC INTERVENTIONS FOR THIS CASE

- Evidence against radiofrequency ablation for discogenic back pain: level I
- Evidence against fusion for discogenic back pain: level I
- ALIF versus TLIF for interbody fusion: level II.2

REFERENCES

1. Buirski G, Silberstein M. The symptomatic lumbar disc in patients with low-back pain. Magnetic resonance imaging appearances in both a symptomatic and control population. *Spine (Phila Pa 1976)*. 1993;18(13):1808–1811.
2. Butler D, Trafimow JH, Andersson GB, McNeill TW, Huckman MS. Discs degenerate before facets. *Spine (Phila Pa 1976)*. 1990;15(2):111–113.
3. Schwarzer AC, Aprill CN, Derby R, Fortin J, Kine G, Bogduk N. The prevalence and clinical features of internal disc disruption in patients with chronic low back pain. *Spine (Phila Pa 1976)*. 1995;20(17):1878–1883.
4. Donelson R, Aprill C, Medcalf R, Grant W. A prospective study of centralization of lumbar and referred pain. A predictor of symptomatic discs and anular competence. *Spine (Phila Pa 1976)*. 1997;22(10):1115–1122.
5. Carragee EJ, Tanner CM, Yang B, Brito JL, Truong T. False-positive findings on lumbar discography. Reliability of subjective concordance assessment during provocative disc injection. *Spine (Phila Pa 1976)*. 1999;24(23):2542–2547.
6. Barendse GA, van Den Berg SG, Kessels AH, Weber WE, van Kleef M. Randomized controlled trial of percutaneous intradiscal radiofrequency thermocoagulation for chronic discogenic back pain: lack of effect from a 90-second 70 C lesion. *Spine (Phila Pa 1976)*. 2001;26(3):287–292.
7. Wang X, Wanyan P, Tian JH, Hu L. Meta-analysis of randomized trials comparing fusion surgery to non-surgical treatment for discogenic chronic low back pain. *J Back Musculoskelet Rehabil*. 2015;28(4):621–627.

16

Radiculopathy from foraminal stenosis

Fidel Valero-Moreno, MD

Introduction

Radiculopathy is one of the most common symptoms derived from degenerative changes in the cervical spine.[1] Radiculopathy is a disorder of the nerve roots and usually manifests as axial pain (neck/low back) radiating to the distribution of the affected nerve root.[2,3] The estimated prevalence of this condition is 3.5 cases per 1000 in the cervical spine.[3] This condition seems to peak around the fourth and fifth decades of life.[4,5] In the younger population, compromise of the neural foramen is often attributed to an acute injury.[6] Narrowing of the neural foramina with nerve root compromise occurs more frequently at the C7 level.[5,6] Patients may present with pain, paresthesia, sensory loss, progressive weakness, or a combination of these.[1] The development of specific symptoms and their magnitude vary according to the severity of foraminal narrowing and its impact on the neurovascular contents.[7] However, accurate correlations between the severity of stenosis and that of symptoms are not consistent among studies.[8] Magnetic resonance image (MRI) is generally the preferred imaging modality for the evaluation of degenerative changes of the spine, including the degree of foraminal stenosis.[1,7] In the absence of concerning signs or symptoms, conservative management with multimodal approaches is usually advocated for cervical radiculopathy as initial treatment.[4,7,9] Despite this, there is no high-level evidence available to predict which patients will fail conservative management.[9] In cases of severe or refractory pain, progressive neurological dysfunction, myelopathy, and failure of conservative treatment, surgical intervention is often required.[4,7,10]

Example Case

Chief complaint: left arm pain

History of present illness: This is a 59-year-old man with a history of 5 months of left arm pain in a C6 and C7 distribution. He has minimal neck pain. He has tried physical therapy, steroid injections, and pain injections without relief. The patient underwent an MRI of the cervical spine demonstrating the presence of chronic degenerative changes, with significant bilateral (left greater than right) foraminal stenosis at C5-C6 and C6-C7 levels mainly due to disc space collapse (Fig. 16.1).

Medications: aspirin

Allergies: no known drug allergies

Past medical and surgical history: none

Family history: noncontributory

Social history: smoker

Physical examination: awake, alert, and oriented to person, place, and time; cranial nerves II–XII intact; bilateral deltoids/ triceps/biceps 5/5; interossei 5/5; iliopsoas/knee flexion/ knee extension/dorsi, and plantar flexion 5/5

Reflexes: 2+ in bilateral biceps/triceps/brachioradialis with negative Hoffman; 2+ in bilateral patella/ankle; no clonus or Babinski; paresthesia in the distribution of left C6 and C7

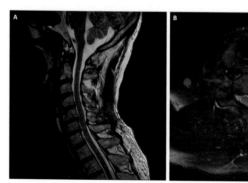

Fig. 16.1 Preoperative magnetic resonance image (MRI) of the cervical spine. (A) Sagittal T2 and **(B)** axial T2 images demonstrating multilevel cervical spondylosis, most marked at the C5-C6 and C6-C7 levels. Circumferential disc bulging with hypertrophic changes is noted at C5-C7 levels. Changes are more evident on the left side at both levels, including prominent left posterolateral disc osteophyte complex. Obliteration of the central canal and left anterior aspects of the cervical thecal sac at C5-C6 are also noted, including the lateral recess. Mild central spinal stenosis at C6-C7. There is also multilevel bilateral cervical facet arthropathy.

	Selby Chen, MD Neurosurgery Mayo Clinic Jacksonville, Florida, United States	Jason Cheung, MD Orthopaedic Surgery The University of Hong Kong, Queen Mary Hospital, Pokfulam, Hong Kong SAR, China	Brett A. Freedman, MD Sandra Hobson, MD Orthopaedic Surgery Mayo Clinic Rochester, Minnesota, United States	Rodrigo Navarro-Ramirez, MD Neurosurgery McGill University Montreal, Quebec, Canada
Preoperative				
Additional tests requested	EMG of left upper extremity	If i stated previously then fine. Otherwise i would do x-rays C-spine AP, flexion and extension instead of CT CT C-spine EMG/NCS	C-spine AP/lateral/flexion/ extension x-rays CT C-spine BMD Smoking cessation program	C-spine AP/flexion-extension x-rays CT C-spine
Surgical approach selected	C5-7 anterior cervical discectomy and fusion	If no improvement with conservative treatment, C5-7 anterior cervical discectomy and fusion	If stops smoking and no improvement with conservative treatment, C5-7 anterior cervical discectomy and fusion	Left C5-7 MIS tubular foraminotomy
Goal of surgery	Decompress left C6 and C7 nerve roots	Decompress left C6 and C7 nerve roots	Decompress left C6 and C7 nerve roots	Decompress left C6 and C7 nerve roots
Perioperative				
Positioning	Supine on a pillow	Supine	Supine on Jackson table, with Gardner-Wells tongs	Prone on Jackson table, with Mayfield pins
Surgical equipment	Fluoroscopy Surgical microscope	IOM (MEP/SSEP) Fluoroscopy Surgical microscope	Fluoroscopy IOM (MEP/SSEP/EMG) Surgical microscope	Fluoroscopy Tubular retractor system Surgical microscope
Medications	Steroids	Steroids	Tranexamic acid	None
Anatomical considerations	Carotid sheath, trachea, esophagus	Recurrent laryngeal nerve, vertebral artery, esophagus, uncovertebral joint location, and osteophytes	Anterior neck structures, vertebral artery	Lamina-facet landmark, ligamentum flavum, dura, nerve root
Complications feared with approach chosen	Nerve root palsy/injury, CSF leak	Inadequate decompression, dysphagia	Pseudoarthrosis, hematoma, dysphagia, esophageal injury, hoarseness	Pain, muscle spasms
Intraoperative				
Anesthesia	General	General	General	General
Exposure	C5-7	C5-7	C5-7	C5-7
Levels decompressed	C5-7	C5-7	C5-7	C5-7
Levels fused	C5-7	C5-7	C5-7	None

	Selby Chen, MD Neurosurgery Mayo Clinic Jacksonville, Florida, United States	Jason Cheung, MD Orthopaedic Surgery The University of Hong Kong, Queen Mary Hospital, Pokfulam, Hong Kong SAR, China	Brett A. Freedman, MD Sandra Hobson, MD Orthopaedic Surgery Mayo Clinic Rochester, Minnesota, United States	Rodrigo Navarro-Ramirez, MD Neurosurgery McGill University Montreal, Quebec, Canada
Surgical narrative	Position supine with pillow, right-sided paramedian incision is made after confirming level with x-ray, dissect down beyond platysma and identify carotid sheath, retract carotid sheath laterally and strap muscles/trachea/esophagus medially, prevertebral fascia is incised with Metzenbaum scissors, spinal needle is placed for localization, disc space is exenterated and PLL is resected, decompression extended out to bilateral neural foramina, palpate with nerve hook to confirm decompression, end plates prepared using high-speed bur, structural allograft placed under fluoroscopy, other disc prepared in similar fashion, cervical plate affixed anteriorly and secured in place with variable screws at C5-C6 and fixed screws at C7, AP and lateral fluoroscopic images are obtained, wound closed in anatomical layers with possible drain	Position supine, bolster placed behind scapula, right iliac crest also exposed if tricortical iliac crest autograft required, x-ray to check C5-7 and mark skin incision level, right-sided Robinson-Southwick approach, mark expected level with needle and confirm with x-ray, release longus colli to have enough lateral exposure, surgical microscope brought in, annulotomy of C5-7 and discectomy with complete disc and cartilaginous endplate removal, removal of PLL and any posterior osteophytes to expose dura, continue discectomy laterally and remove osteophytes at uncovertebral joint, cage filled with demineralized bone matrix and inserted in space with screw fixation, care to make sure screws are flush without prominence, Gelfoam between cage and esophagus, one deep fenestrated drain is placed, close in layers	Position supine, x-ray to plan incision centered over surgical level, place Gardner-Wells tongs with 15 lb of traction, incise skin down through subcutaneous fat, monopolar cautery to dissect through platysma, develop subplatysmal flaps, work through plane medial to sternocleidomastoid bluntly to create a plane lateral to strap muscles and medial to carotid sheath, confirm level with x-ray, dissect longus colli muscles off anterior surface of the spine in subperiosteal fashion, place appropriate sized self-retaining retractors, deflate and reinflate endotracheal cuff, bur anterior surface of disc space, large annulectomy at C5-6, remove annular pieces with pituitary, curettes to clean disc space, resect inferior lip of cephalad vertebral body with Kerrison, drill down bilateral uncus and posterior bars, release posterior annulus, remove PLL using nerve hooks to dissect and Kerrison to resect, resect posterolateral aspects of the uncus and entry zone of the foramen, confirm no residual compression in foramen with nerve hook, place lordotically tapered cage with demineralized bone matrix in the center of the cage, repeat at C6-7, place anterior C5-7 plate, final lateral x-ray, vancomycin in wound, layered closure	Position prone, identify levels using fluoroscopy or intraoperative navigation with reference array, two 2-cm skin incision and one or two fascial incisions, dock tube onto cervical facet, confirm location with x-ray, remove remnant muscle over spinal process/lamina/joint interface, find horizontal Y formed by upper/lower/interlaminar space under microscope, drill lamina until flavum is identified, dissect with curette and remove with Kerrison rongeur, remove bone until nerve can be seen from the top without removing more than 50% of the joint laterally, explore the nerve using a nerve hook, look for disc fragments or material compressing the nerve above and below the nerve, tube is removed under microscopic visualization, standard closure
Complication avoidance	Confirm foraminal opening with nerve hook, allograft placed under fluoroscopic guidance, intraoperative fluoroscopy to confirm position of hardware	Complete PLL removal, remove osteophyte laterally until foramina decompressed, insert cage with screws that are flush, gelfoam between cage and esophagus	Deflate and reinflate endotracheal cuff, open PLL, confirm no residual compression in foramen	MIS, tubular retractor, avoid anterior because of current smoking, preserve 50% of joint

	Selby Chen, MD Neurosurgery Mayo Clinic Jacksonville, Florida, United States	Jason Cheung, MD Orthopaedic Surgery The University of Hong Kong, Queen Mary Hospital, Pokfulam, Hong Kong SAR, China	Brett A. Freedman, MD Sandra Hobson, MD Orthopaedic Surgery Mayo Clinic Rochester, Minnesota, United States	Rodrigo Navarro-Ramirez, MD Neurosurgery McGill University Montreal, Quebec, Canada
Postoperative				
Admission	Floor	High dependency unit	Floor	Outpatient
Postoperative complications feared	Recurrent laryngeal nerve palsy, dysphagia, esophageal injury, neurological injury	Hematoma, acute tracheal compression	Pseudoarthrosis, hematoma, dysphagia, esophageal injury, hoarseness	Muscle spasms, neuropraxia
Anticipated length of stay	Overnight	2–3 days	1 day	Same day
Follow-up testing	AP and lateral cervical spine x-rays 6 weeks, 3 months, 6 months, 12 months, 24 months after surgery	Cervical x-rays at 6 weeks, 3 months, 6 months after surgery	C-spine AP and lateral x-rays C-spine flexion-extension x-rays 3 months, 6 months, 12 months after surgery CT C-spine 6 months after surgery ESR and CRP as inpatient	AP/lateral C-spine x-ray 2 weeks after surgery
Bracing	None	Rigid collar for 6 weeks	Miami J collar for 6 weeks	None
Follow-up visits	6 weeks after surgery	2 weeks, 6 weeks, 3 months, 6 months after surgery	2 weeks, 3 months, 6 months, 12 months after surgery	2 weeks, 1 month, 3 months after surgery

AP, Anteroposterior; BMD, bone mineral density; CRP, C-reactive protein; CT, computed tomography; EMG, electromyography; ESR, erythrocyte sedimentation rate; IOM, intraoperative monitoring; MEP, motor evoked potentials; MIS, minimally invasive surgery; NCS, nerve conduction study; PLL, posterior longitudinal ligament; SSEP, somatosensory evoked potentials.

Differential diagnosis

- Acute disc herniation
- Neoplasms within the spinal canal
- Primary nerve root tumors
- Epidural or vertebral metastases
- Polyradiculopathy of AIDS
- Peripheral nerve entrapment

Important anatomical and preoperative considerations

The neural foramen is created by the vertebral bodies, pedicles, discs, superior and inferior articular processes, and zygapophyseal joints. It is superiorly and inferiorly bounded by the pedicles of the adjacent vertebrae. The posterior aspect of the intervertebral disc forms a large area of its ventral boundary, whereas the joint capsule of the articular facets and the ligamentum flavum delimit most of its posterior edge.[7] The foramen is composed of three anatomical zones: entrance (internal), mid (intraforaminal), and exit (extraforaminal). The nerve root, dorsal root ganglion, radicular artery and vein, and lymphatics occupy the foramen. These structures are stabilized by transforaminal ligaments, especially in the lumbar segment.[7, 11] After passing through the foramen, the spinal nerves divide into anterior and posterior rami. The anterior division provides innervation to the extremities and truncal muscles, while the posterior rami distribute into the paraspinal muscles and the overlying skin.[11] In the cervical spine, the nerve roots pass through the foramina shortly after they are formed, but the lumbosacral nerve roots travel a considerable distance caudally to exit their corresponding vertebral level.[11] Foraminal stenosis can occur either as an acquired anatomical alteration (degenerative changes) or secondary to a congenital condition (achondroplasia).[7] Abnormal weight patterns generated over a functional unit of the spine (bone, joints, ligaments, discs) play a fundamental role in the development of instability, which in turn originates degeneration of these critical elements, causing foraminal stenosis.[7] The progressive narrowing of the intervertebral foramen may result in nerve root impingement, inflammation, or both, which eventually will cause radiculopathy.[12] Although the onset of symptoms is insidious, foraminal neuropathy will produce radicular symptoms and/or neurogenic claudication. Radicular symptoms can be influenced by spinal position. Usually, nerve root pain is exacerbated with spinal extension due to reduction of foraminal volume.[7]

Anteroposterior and lateral radiographs of the cervical and lumbar spine should be part of the initial evaluation of radiculopathy. These diagnostic modalities are helpful for the detection of disc space narrowing, facet hypertrophy, osteophytes, and spondylolisthesis.[4,7,9,13] MRI is the imaging modality of choice when evaluating cervical or lumbosacral radiculopathy.[4-6, 9] MRI can display important anatomical features including bony elements, spinal cord, soft tissue (sources of impingement), and nerve roots.[4, 12] Despite this, currently there is no consensus on the best moment to obtain this study.[9] A computed tomography (CT) scan can be employed as an addition to MRI for a better understanding of the osseous contribution to the foraminal encroachment, spur formation, or/and calcification of ligaments.[6, 9] Electromyography can assist to diagnose compressive and noncompressive radiculopathies and to differentiate the possible etiologies of radicular symptoms,[5, 6] but its interpretation is associated to false-positive and false-negative results if not corroborated with specific imaging findings.[4]

Currently, there are no established guidelines regarding indications for surgical treatment. Despite this, patients with persistent pain, progressive neurological symptoms, signs of instability, and failure of conservative treatment should be treated surgically.[4, 7, 9, 10] Conventional surgical strategies for cervical radiculopathy include open anterior and posterior approaches.[14] The most common procedure to address cervical radiculopathy is anterior cervical decompression and fusion (ACDF).[4, 9] Prospective and retrospective studies have demonstrated the efficacy of ACDF in treating cervical radiculopathy.[9] These analyses showed a significant and stable improvement in clinical status in around 90% of the patients.[4, 9, 15] The procedure implies a discectomy, which may be accompanied by an anterior foraminotomy. Following removal of disc material, an interbody graft is placed to restore intervertebral height. Thus this technique allows the achievement of direct and indirect decompression.[4, 9] Conscientious preoperative evaluation of vascular structures is mandatory.[9] Despite its high effectiveness rate, adjacent level pathology and pseudoarthrosis remain a concern following ACDF. The overall pseudoarthrosis rate is 2.6% but increases with the number of levels treated.[4] A posterior cervical foraminotomy can attain cervical decompression at multiple levels without the need for a fusion, thus eliminating the risk of pseudoarthrosis.[4, 9] Moreover, a posterior approach is a safer alternative for avoiding the vascular elements, such as the carotid and vertebral arteries, and can preserve motion in the spine. Up to 90% of the patients with radiculopathy experience symptom relief after posterior foraminotomy.[4, 9, 16]

What was actually done

The patient was diagnosed with left foraminal stenosis at the level of C5-C7 and this was confirmed on imaging. The patient was offered a 5 to 7 ACDF. After induction of general anesthesia, the patient was placed supine on the operating room table. Intraoperative C-arm confirmed the levels. Dissection of soft tissue and muscle was done. Operative microscope was then brought into the surgical field. A combination of curettes and a high-speed bur were used to remove the disk at C5-C6 and C6-C7. Once the spinal canal was identified, a left-sided total uncinatectomy was performed to decompress the C6 and C7 nerve roots. Additionally, posterior osteophytes were also removed using the high-speed bur and the posterior longitudinal ligament (PLL) was removed in these areas. Allograft spacers were introduced into the interspace. An anterior cervical plate was positioned, and six 16-mm constrained screws were placed. Locking mechanism was advanced and intraoperative fluoroscopy confirmed good positioning. The patient awoke in the operating room and was transferred to the floor and discharged on postoperative day 1. At follow-up visit, the patient remained stable, the pain was controlled, and there was no dysphagia. The patient underwent a postoperative radiographic evaluation that showed intact hardware from C5 to C7 (Fig. 16.2).

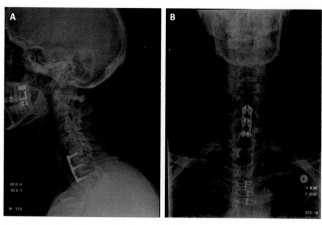

Fig. 16.2 Postoperative cervical x-rays. (A) Lateral and **(B)** anteroposterior x-rays of the cervical column demonstrating a C5-C7 anterior plate with paired body screws, with intact instrumentation and normal alignment and position. No fractures are seen.

Commonalities among the experts

Most advocated for a cervical spine CT scan as part of their preoperative additional testing. Half requested an electromyography evaluation and cervical column dynamic radiographs. The majority would perform discectomy and fusion through an anterior approach. Half recommended conservative treatment before attempting surgery. Most were cognizant of the vascular structures, esophagus, and crucial neck elements such as the recurrent laryngeal nerve. The most feared complications varied and included neurological dysfunction, inadequate decompression, and pseudoarthrosis, among others. Surgery was assisted by fluoroscopy and the surgical microscope. Half of the experts used perioperative steroids. Surgical nuances varied, but all coincided with adequate decompression of the C5-C7 levels. Most of the surgeons request cervical radiographs within 2 to 6 weeks after the surgery. Half advised the use of rigid collar for 6 weeks.

SUMMARY OF QUALITY OF EVIDENCE TO GUIDE SPECIFIC INTERVENTIONS FOR THIS CASE

- Surgical intervention for patients suffering from persistent severe pain, progressive neurological impairment, instability, and/or failure of conservative treatment: level II.2
- ACDF is effective to treat cervical radiculopathy with satisfactory long-term outcomes: level II.1
- Microsurgical decompression and posterior lumbar interbody fusion (PLIF) for lumbar foraminal stenosis have equivalent postoperative results: level II.1

REFERENCES

1. Engel G, Bender YY, Adams LC, et al. Evaluation of osseous cervical foraminal stenosis in spinal radiculopathy using susceptibility-weighted magnetic resonance imaging. *Eur Radiol.* 2019;29(4):1855–1862.
2. Rhee JM, Yoon T, Riew KD. Cervical radiculopathy. *J Am Acad Orthop Surg.* 2007;15(8):486–494.

3. Casey E. Natural history of radiculopathy. *Phys Med Rehabil Clin N Am*. 2011;22(1):1–5.
4. Iyer S, Kim HJ. Cervical radiculopathy. *Curr Rev Musculoskelet Med*. 2016;9(3):272–280.
5. Tarulli AW, Raynor EM. Lumbosacral radiculopathy. *Neurol Clin*. 2007;25(2):387–405.
6. Yoon SH. Cervical radiculopathy. *Phys Med Rehabil Clin N Am*. 2011;22(3):439–446. viii.
7. Choi YK. Lumbar foraminal neuropathy: an update on non-surgical management. *Korean J Pain*. 2019;32(3):147–159.
8. Ko S, Choi W, Lee J. The Prevalence of Cervical Foraminal Stenosis on Computed Tomography of a Selected Community-Based Korean Population. *Clin Orthop Surg*. 2018;10(4):433–438.
9. Woods BI, Hilibrand AS. Cervical radiculopathy: epidemiology, etiology, diagnosis, and treatment. *J Spinal Disord Tech*. 2015;28(5):E251–E259.
10. Schell A, Rhee JM, Holbrook J, Lenehan E, Park KY. Assessing Foraminal Stenosis in the Cervical Spine: A Comparison of Three-Dimensional Computed Tomographic Surface Reconstruction to Two-Dimensional Modalities. *Global Spine J*. 2017;7(3):266–271.
11. Li JM, Tavee J. Electrodiagnosis of radiculopathy. *Handb Clin Neurol*. 2019;161:305–316.
12. Kim S, Lee JW, Chai JW, et al. A New MRI Grading System for Cervical Foraminal Stenosis Based on Axial T2-Weighted Images. *Korean J Radiol*. 2015;16(6):1294–1302.
13. Ohba T, Ebata S, Fujita K, Sato H, Devin CJ, Haro H. Characterization of symptomatic lumbar foraminal stenosis by conventional imaging. *Eur Spine J*. 2015;24(10):2269–2275.
14. Oertel JM, Philipps M, Burkhardt BW. Endoscopic Posterior Cervical Foraminotomy as a Treatment for Osseous Foraminal Stenosis. *World Neurosurg*. 2016;91:50–57.
15. Bohlman HH, Emery SE, Goodfellow DB, Jones PK. Robinson anterior cervical discectomy and arthrodesis for cervical radiculopathy. Long-term follow-up of one hundred and twenty-two patients. *J Bone Joint Surg Am*. 1993;75(9):1298–1307.
16. Church EW, Halpern CH, Faught RW, et al. Cervical laminoforaminotomy for radiculopathy: Symptomatic and functional outcomes in a large cohort with long-term follow-up. *Surg Neurol Int*. 2014;5(Suppl 15):S536–S543.

17

Thoracic ligamentous hypertrophy causing stenosis

Kingsley Abode-Iyamah, MD

Introduction

Thoracic stenosis can lead to compression of the spinal cord as a result of spinal degeneration, hypertrophy of the facet and ligamentum flavum, ossification of the ligamentum flavum, and diffuse idiopathic skeletal hyperostosis, among others.[1–5] These changes may be the result of degenerative changes or microinstability at the location of the stenosis.[6] This can be especially true for stenosis due to adjacent segment disease from a prior surgical fusion.[7] Like cervical myelopathy, thoracic myelopathy can often present without diagnosis for years, leading to severe disability by the time a diagnosis is finally made. Symptoms may include gait imbalance, weakness, sensation loss, and even incontinence.

The management consideration becomes more complex when the stenosis is in the thoracolumbar junction. Surgical intervention may lead to destabilization when the stenosis is in thoracolumbar junction as the combination of decompression with the high mobility in this location can also lead to destabilization.[8]

Example Case

Chief complaint: leg weakness

History of present illness: A 28-year-old female with a history of low back pain as well as some pain going down the backs of her legs. She says this resolved on its own. More recently, she reports having had a fall and then a couple of weeks later started having leg weakness. She also describes numbness in her feet. Since that time, she has only been able to walk 10 to 15 yards without having to sit down. She uses a single-point cane for short distances and a wheelchair for longer distances. She does not report any new bowel or bladder issues. She underwent imaging and this was concerning for thoracic stenosis (Figs. 17.1 and 17.2).

Medications: metformin

Allergies: no known drug allergies

Past medical and surgical history: diabetes, morbid obesity

Family history: noncontributory

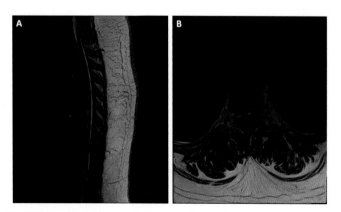

Fig. 17.1 Preoperative magnetic resonance images. (A) T2 sagittal and **(B)** T2 axial images demonstrating severe T9-T10 spinal canal stenosis and cord compression with cord edema/myelomalacia.

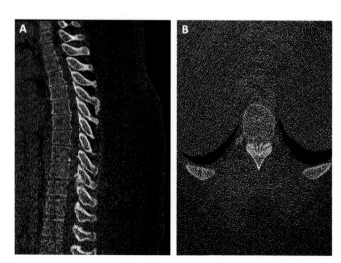

Fig. 17.2 Preoperative computed tomography scans. (A) Sagittal and **(B)** axial images demonstrating severe T9-T10 spinal canal stenosis with calcification of the ligamentum flavum.

Social history: retail, no smoking history, occasional alcohol

Physical examination: awake, alert, and oriented to person, place, and time; cranial nerves II–XII intact; bilateral deltoids/biceps/triceps 5/5; interossei 5/5; iliopsoas/knee flexion/knee extension 4+/5; dorsi and plantar flexion 4/5

Reflexes: 2+ in bilateral biceps/triceps/brachioradialis; 2+ in bilateral patella/ankle with positive clonus; right Babinski; negative Hoffman; sensation decreased in bilateral lower extremities

	Richard J. Bransford, MD Orthopaedic Surgery University of Washington Seattle, Washington, United States	Brett A. Freedman, MD Sandra Hobson, MD Orthopaedic Surgery Mayo Clinic Rochester, Minnesota, United States	Susana Núñez-Pereira, MD, PhD Orthopaedic Surgery Hospital Universitario Vall d'Hebron, Barcelona, Spain	Michael Y. Wang, MD Yingda Li, MBBS Neurosurgery University of Miami Miami, Florida, United States
Preoperative				
Additional tests requested	Upright scoliosis films	T-spine upright AP and lateral x-rays MRI L-spine MRI C-spine potentially BMD scans Hemoglobin A1C	T-spine x-rays High resolution T-spine CT Recheck MRI for edema or ligamentous injury	Pain drawing Postvoid residual Standing thoracic x-rays Check lateral scout MRI to ensure correct level counting upwards from lumbosacral spine, and x-rays to ensure 12 ribs in total Anesthesia evaluation
Surgical approach selected	T8-10 laminectomy and T8-10 posterior fusion	T9-10 laminectomy and fusion	T9-10 laminectomy	T9-10 laminectomy
Goal of surgery	Spinal cord decompression, stabilization of spine	Spinal cord decompression, stabilization of spine	Spinal cord decompression	Spinal cord decompression, prevent further neurological deterioration
Perioperative				
Positioning	Prone on Jackson table	Prone on Jackson table, with Gardner-Wells tongs and 15 lb of traction	Prone on Jackson table	Prone on Jackson table
Surgical equipment	IOM (MEP/SSEP) Fluoroscopy	IOM (MEP/SSEP/EMG) O-arm Surgical navigation Surgical microscope	IOM Fluoroscopy	IOM (MEP/ SSEP) Fluoroscopy Surgical microscope
Medications	Maintain MAPs >85	Tranexamic acid, MAP >80	None	Maintain MAPs >80, steroids
Anatomical considerations	Dura, spinal cord	Dura, spinal cord	Ligamentum flavum	Dura
Complications feared with approach chosen	Durotomy, spinal cord injury, incorrect level	Instability	Persistent compression Durotomy	Incorrect level, durotomy, cord injury, instability
Intraoperative				
Anesthesia	General	General	General	General
Exposure	T8-10	T9-10	T9-10	T9-10
Levels decompressed	T8-10	T9-10	T9-10	T9-10
Levels fused	T8-10	T9-10	None	None

	Richard J. Bransford, MD Orthopaedic Surgery University of Washington Seattle, Washington, United States	Brett A. Freedman, MD Sandra Hobson, MD Orthopaedic Surgery Mayo Clinic Rochester, Minnesota, United States	Susana Núñez-Pereira, MD, PhD Orthopaedic Surgery Hospital Universitario Vall d'Hebron, Barcelona, Spain	Michael Y. Wang, MD Yingda Li, MBBS Neurosurgery University of Miami Miami, Florida, United States
Surgical narrative	Position prone on Jackson table with face pillow, fluoroscopy to assess level, midline posterior incision, subperiosteal dissection to expose T8-10 posterior elements to transverse processes, place mono-axial pedicle screws using anatomy from T8-10 bilaterally, x-ray to confirm location, drill to create laminectomy troughs from inferior T8 to top of T10, remove lamina and spinous process with care of dura, clean edges with Kerrison punches while protecting dura, place rods and secure, decorticate and place autograft from lamina from T8-10, layered closure with subfascial drain	Preflip IOM, place Gardner-Wells tongs, position prone, incision planned with x-ray, dissect down through subcutaneous fat to level of deep dorsal fascia, fascia opened in line with incision, subperiosteal dissection preserving facet capsules, x-ray to confirm level, remove T9-10 facet capsule, expose associated lateral gutters for planned fusion bed, decorticate posterolateral gutter/lateral facet/lateral lamina, place T9-10 pedicle screws with anatomical landmarks and O-arm and surgical navigation, pedicle stimulation testing and intraoperative imaging, pack posterolateral gutters and facet joints with bone graft and demineralized bone matrix, T9-10 laminectomy with microscope using burs and Kerrison rongeurs, resect ligamentum flavum and medial facet capsules, confirm adequacy of decompression with a ball probe, place appropriately sized rods, place set screws and final tighten, layered closure with drain and incisional wound VAC	Position prone, IONM, confirm level with fluoroscopy (count ribs preoperatively and check with fluoroscopy, if any doubt, count from sacrum), midline posterior incision, split muscles to visualize affected lamina and spinous process, x-ray to confirm level, remove spinous process, facetectomy with small chisel, high-speed drill to remove lamina to identify where lamina merges with facet, identify and remove ligamentum flavum and bone with Kerrison, protecting dura. If there are some adherences, small fragments not compressing might be left in situ decompress both sides to minimize spinal cord manipulation, further decompression to make sure cord is decompressed, layered closure with drain	Position prone on Jackson with arms forward, level localization by counting up from sacrum or from AP fluoroscopic identification of 12th rib, midline incision, bilateral subperiosteal dissection, level confirmation with marker on pedicle, laminectomy to lamina-facet junction, Woodson elevator to free calcified ligamentum from dura, can leave portions adherent to dura floating if detached laterally, avoid downward pressure on thecal sac and have continuous monitoring, antibiotic irrigation, subfascial drain, layered closure
Complication avoidance	Anatomical pedicle screws, leave superior T8 and inferior T10 lamina, when dissecting care of ossification of ligamentum flavum	Preflip IOM, surgical navigation for pedicle screws, pedicle stimulation testing and intraoperative imaging, incisional wound VAC	Decompress widely to provide better visualization and minimize spinal cord manipulation	Level localization based on sacrum or 12th rib, dissect calcified ligament from dura, leave ligament in areas adherent, dural sealant if CSF leak sufficiently wide i.e. pedicle-to-pedicle decompression
Postoperative				
Admission	Floor	Floor	Floor	Floor
Postoperative complications feared	Epidural hematoma, medical complications	Infection, adjacent-level disease	CSF leak	CSF leak, spinal cord injury, iatrogenic instability, failure to improve
Anticipated length of stay	3 days	2–3 days	2–3 days	2–3 days
Follow-up testing	CT T-spine prior to discharge Upright T-spine x-rays prior to discharge, 3 months, 6 months, 1 year after surgery	T-spine upright AP and lateral x-rays prior to discharge, 3 months, 6 months after surgery ESR/CRP while inpatient CT T-spine 6 months after surgery	None	Physical therapy
Bracing	None	None	None	None
Follow-up visits	3–4 weeks, 3 months, 6 months, 1 year after surgery	2 weeks, 3 months, 6 months after surgery	2 and 6 weeks and 6 and 12 months	2 and 8 weeks after surgery

AP, Anteroposterior; BMD, bone mineral density; BMP, bone morphogenic protein; CRP, C-reactive protein; CSF, cerebrospinal fluid; CT, computed tomography; EMG, electromyogram; ESR, erythrocyte sedimentation rate; IOM, intraoperative monitoring; MAP, mean arterial pressure; MEP, motor evoked potentials; MIS, minimally invasive surgery; MRI, magnetic resonance imaging; SSEP, somatosensory evoked potentials; VAC, vacuum assisted closure.

Differential diagnosis

- Thoracic myelopathy
- Transverse myelitis
- Multiple sclerosis

Important anatomical considerations

The thoracic rib cage and its attachment to the sternum increases the stiffness of the thoracic spine and has been referred to as the fourth column. The thoracolumbar junction consists of T11 to L1 and represents a transition zone of the more stiff thoracic spine and more mobile lumbar spine containing two floating ribs. This transition from a more stiff spinal segment to a more mobile segment predisposes the thoracolumbar junction to increased mechanical movement, which can predispose this location not only to injury but also to destabilization.[9,10] While gross destabilization may not be apparent on dynamic x-rays, pneumatization of the disc space on flexion-extension films may also represent micro instability.[11]

Stenosis the thoracic spine results from hypertrophy of the facet and ligamentum flavum, ossification of the ligamentum flavum, diffuse idiopathic skeletal hyperostosis, disc herniation, or the combination of the above in an individual with congenital stenosis.[1-5] The thoracic spinal cord, unlike the cervical and lumbar spine, has reduced canal space and is the only segment of the spine that contains kyphosis. This combination of a reduced canal space and kyphosis predisposes patients to damage with additional compressive lesions in this location. Additionally, ventrally placed lesions may cause ongoing damage to the spinal cord as a result of draping of the cord over the mass.

Approaches to this lesion

Lesions in the thoracic spine can be approached via a posterior or anterior approach. The area of contention lies in whether decompression alone is sufficient in patients with hypertrophy of the facet and ligamentum flavum, ossification of the ligamentum flavum or diffuse idiopathic skeletal hyperostosis. Some believe that ligamentum hypertrophy represents the body's attempt to stabilize an already unstable segment. Therefore, a laminectomy alone may further destabilize these patients. Some authors have advocated for instrumentation when decompressing in the thoracolumbar spine.[11,18-19] Additionally, some authors have suggested a better outcome in those individuals who have undergone decompressive fusion compared with a laminectomy alone.[14-19]

What was actually done

The patient was brought to the operating room and positioned on an Allen bed and padded properly. Fluoroscopic imaging was used to count the ribs to confirm the proper level for laminectomy. The incision was marked and dissection was performed. The levels were confirmed again using intraoperative fluoroscopy. Mean arterial pressure of greater than 85 was maintained. The patient received 10 mg of dexamethasone prior to incision. A T9-10 laminectomy was performed. A drain was placed and each layer was closed. The incision was closed with 3 to 0 nylon with interrupted sutures given the patient's body habitus. The patient did well with improvement of her myelopathic symptoms. No additional imaging was done.

Commonalities among the experts

While all our experts agreed on a posterior approach for addressing this patient's pathology, there were differences in surgical management. Some surgeons recommended additional imaging such as scoliosis x-rays and thoracic x-rays, while another recommended magnetic resonance images of the lumbar and cervical spine. Additionally, some advocated for other tests including post void residual, bone mineral density scans, and hemoglobin A1C. Half recommended a laminectomy alone while the other half recommend a laminectomy and fusion. All had the same goal of decompressing the spinal cord; however, some recommended a fusion also to stabilize the spine at this location. Fluoroscopy and intraoperative monitoring were used by all experts. Additionally, the majority suggested mean arterial pressure goals intraoperatively. All would admit the patient to the floor postoperatively with an anticipated hospitalization being 2 to 3 days.

SUMMARY OF QUALITY OF EVIDENCE TO GUIDE SPECIFIC INTERVENTIONS FOR THIS CASE

- Intraoperative monitoring for myelopathy surgery: level II.1
- Fusion versus laminectomy alone for thoracic stenosis: level II.2

REFERENCES

1. Aizawa T, Sato T, Sasaki H, Kusakabe T, Morozumi N, Kokubun S. Thoracic myelopathy caused by ossification of the ligamentum flavum: clinical features and surgical results in the Japanese population. *J Neurosurg Spine.* 2006;5(6):514–519.
2. Aizawa T, Sato T, Sasaki H, Matsumoto F, Morozumi N, Kusakabe T, et al. Results of surgical treatment for thoracic myelopathy: minimum 2-year follow-up study in 132 patients. *J Neurosurg Spine.* 2007;7(1):13–20.
3. Kang KC, Lee CS, Shin SK, Park SJ, Chung CH, Chung SS. Ossification of the ligamentum flavum of the thoracic spine in the Korean population. *J Neurosurg Spine.* 2011;14(4):513–519.
4. Yang Z, Xue Y, Dai Q, Zhang C, Zhou HF, Pan JF, et al. Upper facet joint en bloc resection for the treatment of thoracic myelopathy caused by ossification of the ligamentum flavum. *J Neurosurg Spine.* 2013;19(1):81–89.
5. Zhang HQ, Chen LQ, Liu SH, Zhao D, Guo CF. Posterior decompression with kyphosis correction for thoracic myelopathy due to ossification of the ligamentum flavum and ossification of the posterior longitudinal ligament at the same level. *J Neurosurg Spine.* 2010;13(1):116–122.
6. Panjabi MM, Goel VK, Takata K. Physiologic strains in the lumbar spinal ligaments. An in vitro biomechanical study 1981 Volvo Award in Biomechanics. *Spine (Phila Pa 1976).* 1982;7(3):192–203.
7. Bastian L, Lange U, Knop C, Tusch G, Blauth M. Evaluation of the mobility of adjacent segments after posterior thoracolumbar fixation: a biomechanical study. *Eur Spine J.* 2001;10(4):295–300.
8. Yoganandan N, Maiman DJ, Pintar FA, Bennett GJ, Larson SJ. Biomechanical effects of laminectomy on thoracic spine stability. *Neurosurgery.* 1993;32(4):604–610.
9. Flouty O, Abode-Iyamah K, Ahmed R, Wilson S, Menezes AH. Junctional susceptibility of the pediatric spine: a case report. *Childs Nerv Syst.* 2015;31(5):797–800.
10. Jacobs RR, Asher MA, Snider RK. Thoracolumbar spinal injuries. A comparative study of recumbent and operative treatment in 100 patients. *Spine (Phila Pa 1976).* 1980;5(5):463–477.

11. Hitchon PW, Abode-Iyamah K, Dahdaleh NS, Grossbach AJ, El Tecle NE, Noeller J, et al. Risk factors and outcomes in thoracic stenosis with myelopathy: A single center experience. *Clin Neurol Neurosurg*. 2016;147:84–89.

12. Onishi E, Yasuda T, Yamamoto H, Iwaki K, Ota S. Outcomes of Surgical Treatment for Thoracic Myelopathy: A Single-institutional Study of 73 Patients. *Spine (Phila Pa 1976)*. 2016;41(22):E1356–E1363.

13. Osman NS, Cheung ZB, Hussain AK, Phan K, Arvind V, Vig KS, et al. Outcomes and Complications Following Laminectomy Alone for Thoracic Myelopathy due to Ossified Ligamentum Flavum: A Systematic Review and Meta-Analysis. *Spine (Phila Pa 1976)*. 2018;43(14):E842–E848.

14. Lesoin F, Rousseaux M, Autricque A, Reesaul Y, Villette L, Clarisse J, et al. Thoracic disc herniations: evolution in the approach and indications. *Acta Neurochir (Wien)*. 1986;80(1-2):30–34.

15. Patterson Jr. RH, Arbit E. A surgical approach through the pedicle to protruded thoracic discs. *J Neurosurg*. 1978;48(5):768–772.

16. Hurley ET, Maye AB, Timlin M, Lyons FG. Anterior Versus Posterior Thoracic Discectomy: A Systematic Review. *Spine (Phila Pa 1976)*. 2017;42(24):E1437–E1445.

17. Fessler RG, Sturgill M. Review: complications of surgery for thoracic disc disease. *Surg Neurol*. 1998;49(6):609–618.

18. Mixter WJBJ. Rupture of the intervertebral disc with involvement of the spinal canal. *New Engl Surg Soc*. 1934;211:210–215.

19. Hawk WA Spinal compression caused by ecchondrosis of the intervertebral fibrocartilage: with a review of the recent literature. *Brain*. 1936;59(2): 204–224.

18

C1–C2 facet arthropathy

Fidel Valero-Moreno, MD and Henry Ruiz-Garcia, MD

Introduction

Atlanto-axial (C1-C2) facet joint arthropathy is an underdiagnosed condition closely associated with the development of refractory occipital pain.[1,2] Prevalence increases with age, ranging from 5% in the sixth decade to 18% in the ninth decade of life.[1] Moreover, the atlanto-axial (CI-C2) facet joints are a common site of involvement in patients with inflammatory arthropathies, such as rheumatoid arthritis.[3,4] Older adult women are the most commonly affected.[4] Secondary occipital neuralgia in the setting of C1-C2 facet joint arthropathy is a well-known phenomenon; however, there are numerous possible causes of nonspecific chronic suboccipital pain (infections, trauma, neoplasms, congenital malformations), and therefore, the diagnosis is challenging and often neglected.[1,2,5] Headache, occipital pain, retro-auricular pain, and neck pain (usually unilateral) account for the most common symptoms associated with atlanto-axial facet arthropathy.[1] Additionally, rotation restriction toward the affected side is noted in most patients.[1,6] Cervicogenic headache has been implicated in 15% to 20% of chronic headaches cases.[7,8] Atlanto-axial arthropathy is rarely asymptomatic.[6] The pathophysiology of pain associated to C1-C2 arthropathy may be explained by the origination of aberrant axonal discharges (neuralgia) or nerve compression (radiculopathy).[9,10] Radiological diagnosis requires the confirmation of arthritis and vertical collapse of the facet joint on the side of neuralgia.[2] Alleviation of pain is the mainstay of treatment, and therefore pain reduction is the core determinant of a positive long outcome.[1,11] The primary indication for surgical intervention is C1-C2 osteoarthritis with unremitting pain after failed nonsurgical management.[1,2,5,9,12] Currently, posterior transarticular atlanto-axial fusion has proved to be an effective treatment to relieve intractable pain with a low rate of complications.[1,6,9,12] In this chapter, we present the case of a patient with persistent cervical pain localized on her left side.

Example Case

Chief complaint: neck pain

History of present illness: This is a 62-year-old female patient with a history of persistent neck pain localized on the left side. The pain is exacerbated with head turning. The patient does not report additional symptoms or arm pain. She has a history of previous surgical intervention of the cervical spine (Fig. 18.1).

Medications: aspirin

Allergies: no known drug allergies

Past medical and surgical history: anterior cervical discectomy and fusion

Family history: none

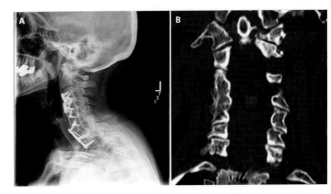

Fig. 18.1 Preoperative imaging of the cervical spine. (A) Preoperative lateral x-rays demonstrating previous anterior cervical discectomy and fusion, multilevel osseous foraminal narrowing secondary to facet, and uncovertebral joint hypertrophy. **(B)** Coronal reconstruction of computed tomography demonstrating severe arthrosis of the left C1-C2 facet joint, with vertical collapse of the joint on the side of pain (left), and no fusion is noted.

Social history: smoker
Physical examination: awake, alert, and oriented to person, place, and time; cranial nerves II–XII intact; bilateral deltoids/triceps/biceps 5/5; interossei 5/5; iliopsoas/knee flexion/knee extension/dorsi, and plantar flexion 5/5

Reflexes: 2+ in bilateral biceps/triceps/brachioradialis with negative Hoffman; 2+ in bilateral patella/ankle; no clonus or Babinski; sensation intact to light touch

	Sigurd Berven, MD Department of Orthopaedic Surgery UC San Francisco San Francisco, California, United States	Alvaro Camparo, MD Ramiro Barrera, MD Neurosurgery Hospital Padilla at Tucuman Universidad Nacional de Tucuman Tucuman, Argentina	Praveen Mummaneni, MD Brenton Pennicooke, MD Neurosurgery University of California at San Francisco San Francisco, California, United States	Baron Zarate Kalfopulos, MD Orthopaedic Surgery Instituto Nacional de Rehabilitacion Medica Sur Mexico City, Mexico
Preoperative				
Additional tests requested	SPECT C1-2 facet injection Neuromodulation trial MRI C-spine	Dynamic cervical x-ray CT Cervical angiography MRI C-spine	CT C-spine angiography MRI C-spine CT-guided C2 nerve block and ESI	SPECT/CT C-spine MRI C-spine EMG upper extremities
Surgical approach selected	If persistent pain despite nonoperative optimal care including neuromodulation, posterior C1-2 fusion	C1-3 posterior fusion	Avoid surgery because of smoker, but if responded to nerve block and had to, left C1-2 hemi-laminotomy for left C2 neurectomy	Avoid surgery because of smoker, but if responded to nerve block and had to, posterior C1-2 fusion with Gallie fusion
Goal of surgery	Stabilization of C1-2 segment	Deformity reduction, fusion	Relieve occipital pain	Relieve occipital pain
Perioperative				
Positioning	Prone, in Mayfield pins	Prone, in Mayfield pins	Prone on Jackson table, in Mayfield pins	Prone on a mask
Surgical equipment	O-arm Surgical navigation	Fluoroscopy	IOM (MEP/SSEP/EMG) Surgical navigation Intraoperative CT	IOM Fluoroscopy
Medications	None	NSAIDs	None	Tranexamic acid
Anatomical considerations	Vertebral artery, internal carotid artery, greater occipital nerve, spinal cord	Vertebral artery, C1-2 venous plexus, C2 nerves	Vertebral artery, spinal cord	C2 nerve roots, vertebral artery, thecal sac, C1-2 spinous process, C1 lateral mass, C2 pedicle
Complications feared with approach chosen	Instability, vertebral artery injury, spinal cord injury	Vertebral artery injury, C2 neuropathy	Spinal cord injury	Vertebral artery injury, durotomy, C1 lateral mass fracture, injury to C2 nerve root, venous plexus bleeding
Intraoperative				
Anesthesia	General	General	General	General
Exposure	C1-2	C1-3	C1-3	C1-3
Levels decompressed	None	None	C1-2	None
Levels fused	C1-2	C1-3	None	C1-2

	Sigurd Berven, MD Department of Orthopaedic Surgery UC San Francisco San Francisco, California, United States	Alvaro Camparo, MD Ramiro Barrera, MD Neurosurgery Hospital Padilla at Tucuman Universidad Nacional de Tucuman Tucuman, Argentina	Praveen Mummaneni, MD Brenton Pennicooke, MD Neurosurgery University of California at San Francisco San Francisco, California, United States	Baron Zarate Kalfopulos, MD Orthopaedic Surgery Instituto Nacional de Rehabilitacion Medica Sur Mexico City, Mexico
Surgical narrative	Position prone with Mayfield pins, visualize C1-2 with fluoroscopy, posterior midline C1-2 incision, subperiosteal exposure of C1-C2, cauterization of venous plexus behind C1 with bipolar, ligation of greater occipital nerve, Harms technique for posterior fixation at C1-2 with polyaxial C1 lateral mass screws and C2 pedicle screws, obtain local bone from underside of C1 ring/spinous process and lamina of C2, fusion using local bone and demineralized bone matrix, layered closure	Position prone with Mayfield pins, verify level with fluoroscopy, vertical midline skin incision from 2 cm superior to C1 to C4, subcutaneous tissue and muscle dissection, subperiosteal dissection of C1-3, place short thread screws in the lateral mass of C1 using high-speed drill and fluoroscopy, place C2 pars and C3 lateral mass screws using high-speed drill and fluoroscopy, placement of rods and close the system, placement of autologous bone graft, closure with drain	Position prone with Mayfield pins, lateral x-ray to plan incision, midline posterior incision, expose C1-3, attach navigation array, intraoperative CT and register with navigation system, left C1 inferior laminotomy and left C2 superior laminotomy to access left C1-2 foramen, identify and ligate and section C2 nerve root proximal to ganglion bilaterally, irrigate, layered closure	Position prone. 12–12 cm midline incision from C1-3, expose posterior arch of C1 (only 10 mm on each side)/C2 lamina until lateral mass, respect muscular insertions on C1 and C2 spinous processes, place C2 pedicle screws (25–30 degree cephalic and 30–35 degree medial angle) and C1 lateral mass (15 degree cephalic and 5–10 degree medial) screws, connect screws with rods and transverse connector, pass sublaminar wire beneath arch of C1 and around spinous process of C2 with cadaveric allograft between C2 spinous process and C1 posterior arch, decorticate C2 lamina/lateral mass/inferior edge of C1 posterior arch and apply demineralized bone matrix, layered closure
Complication avoidance	Ligation of greater occipital nerve, Harms technique for C1-2 screws	Screws under fluoroscopy, limiting levels of fusion	Surgical navigation, neurectomy	Limit exposure of C1 arch to 10 mm on each side, respect muscular insertions on C1 and C2 spinous processes, use transverse connector, avoid sublaminar C2 wire to avoid neural or dural injury
Postoperative				
Admission	Floor	ICU	Floor	Floor
Postoperative complications feared	Pseudoarthrosis, persistent pain, infection	Pseudarthrosis, neck pain, implant malposition, screw back out	Occipital neuralgia, C1-2 instability	Vertebral artery injury, wound infection, CSF leak, adjacent segment degeneration
Anticipated length of stay	2 days	3 days	3 days	3 days
Follow-up testing	C-spine AP/lateral x-ray prior to discharge, 4 weeks, 8–10 weeks, 6 months, 1 year, 2 years after surgery	C-spine x-ray after surgery, 1 month after surgery CT C-spine 3 months after surgery	C-spine AP and lateral x-ray, 6 weeks, 3 months, 6 months, 1 year, 2 years after surgery	C-spine x-ray 6 weeks, every 3 months for first year after surgery CT C-spine 12 months after surgery
Bracing	Cervical hard collar for 4 weeks	Philadelphia collar for 4 weeks	Miami J for 6 weeks	None
Follow-up visits	4 weeks, 8–10 weeks, 6 months, 1 year, 2 years after surgery	7 days, 1 month, 3 months after surgery	3 weeks, 6 weeks, 3 months, 6 months, 1 year, 2 years after surgery	2 weeks, 6 weeks, every 3 months for first year after surgery

AP, Anteroposterior; CSF, cerebrospinal fluid; CT, computed tomography; EMG, electromyography; ESI, epidural spinal injections; ICU, intensive care unit; IOM, intraoperative monitoring; MEP, motor evoked potential; MIS, minimally invasive surgery; NSAIDs, nonsteroidal antiinflammatory drugs; SPECT, single-photon emission computed tomography; SSEP, somatosensory evoked potential.

Differential diagnosis

- Cervical muscle strain
- Adjacent segment disease
- Junctional instability
- Occipital neuralgia
- Facet arthropathy

Important anatomical and preoperative considerations

The atlanto-axial facet joint is a synovial-lined joint that links the first two vertebral bodies. The primary movement of the atlanto-axial joint (AAJ) complex is rotation.[8] The largest degree of rotation in the neck occurs at the AAJ.[13] These vertebrae connect by two laterally and one centrally placed synovial joints.[8] Compressive forces, tears, and inflammatory processes can cause these joints to become painful. There is no vertebral disc between the occiput-atlas joint (OAJ) and the AAJ. The OAJ and the AAJ are innervated by the ventral rami of the first and second spinal nerves.[8] Behind the lateral articular masses, the first and second cervical nerves appear, and their respective ganglia rest on the vertebral arches of the axis and atlas. The greater occipital nerve (GON) originates from the lateral branch of the posterior ramus of C2.[8,14,15] This nerve emerges between bony surfaces and can be subject to stress by any movement of the head that tends to approximate these bony elements.[5,8,14,15] Unusual force applied to the neck or an aberrant nerve course can potentially predispose to the development of compression at the point the atlantal facet contacts the lamina of the axis.[14] The GON crosses the suboccipital triangle obliquely and then ascends rostrally along the rectus capitis posterior major. At this point, it receives a branch from the third occipital nerve.[14] The nerve pierces the tendon of the trapezius muscle and the deep cervical fascia below the superior nuchal line. Eventually, the GON divides into several terminal branches that join the lesser occipital nerve to supply the skin of the scalp as rostral as the coronal suture.[14]

Although less common, compression or irritation of the lesser occipital nerve (LON) may also lead to symptoms of occipital neuralgia. The ventral ramus of the second cervical nerve is the main origin of the LON, while the third cervical nerve contributes sporadically.[14] As the nerve crosses the lateral atlanto-axial articulation, specifically at the level of the posterosuperior articular process of the axis, compression can occur, especially when associated with degenerative changes.[14]

For patients with strong clinical and radiographic evidence of occipital neuralgia secondary to atlanto-axial arthropathy, the rationale for surgery is based on the presence of severe pain resistant to conservative treatment in concordance to the radiographic findings of the C1-C2 joint.[1,2,5,6,9,11] Posterior atlanto-axial fusion is widely accepted as the treatment of choice.[1,6] Although several techniques have been described (sublaminar or interspinous wires, transarticular screw fixation, C1-C2 screw-rod constructs),[16] atlanto-axial arthrodesis attained by placement of articular screws seems to be favored.[1,6,11] The risk of vertebral artery injury is around 4.1% for this procedure, and therefore a painstaking knowledge and evaluation of bony and vascular structures is essential before intervention to assure safer screw placement.[1] Despite the overall restriction in head rotation, C1-C2 fusion seems to offer a good long-term outcome for patients, especially in terms of pain relief.[1]

What was actually done

This patient with painful left C1-C2 facet arthropathy showed intense uptake at C1-C2 bone single-photon emission computed tomography (SPECT) scan. As she had a previous extensive anterior subaxial fusion, a C1-C4 posterior fusion was recommended to avoid a mobile interspace at C2-C3. After general anesthesia was provided, baseline somatosensory and motor evoked potentials studies were obtained. The responses were normal at baseline and unchanged throughout the operative procedure. Thereafter, the patient was turned into the prone position on the Jackson table. Head and neck were placed in neutral position using a Mayfield head holder, with a slightly head-up position throughout the operative procedure. A posterior upper cervical incision was made, and the subperiosteal dissection took place from C1 to C4. The C2 nerve roots were then divided bilaterally in order to provide access for C1 screw placement. After C1-C2 facet joints were entered and decorticated bilaterally, screws were placed into the lateral mass of C1 bilaterally under navigational image guidance with the assistance of an intraoperative O-arm. C2 pars screws were then placed, and a laminar screw was placed from left to right at C2 as the left C2 pars was quite small. Thereafter, lateral mass screws were placed at C3 and C4 bilaterally. Prebent rods measuring 55 mm in length were then attached to the polyaxial screw heads. A previously harvested block of tricortical iliac crest was secured in place at C1-C2 and the Songer cables were tightened and cut appropriately. A second spin with the O-arm showed good position of all screws and the sublaminar wires. Strips of bone morphogenic protein (BMP) sponge and iliac crest bone graft were placed into the facet joints at C1-C2 bilaterally. Additional BMP was placed in the C2-C3 and C3-C4 facet joints. Additional loose bone graft was placed over the posterior elements from C1 to C4 in order to create a robust fusion mass. Hemostasis was achieved, and the wound was closed in layers after vancomycin was applied into the wound. A hard cervical collar was applied to the patient's neck. Postoperative imaging revealed the position of the instrumentation (Fig. 18.2).

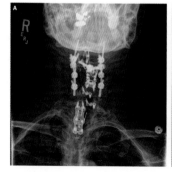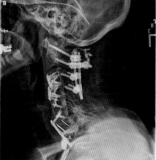

Fig. 18.2 Postoperative x-rays. (A) Lateral and **(B)** anteroposterior x-rays demonstrating C1-C4 fusion with bilateral pedicle screws and vertical rods as well as sublaminar wire construct C1-C2. Previous C3-T1 anterior cervical discectomy and fusion is noted similar to prior exam

Commonalities among the experts

All of the surgeons opted for a magnetic resonance imaging (MRI) of the cervical spine as part of the preoperative evaluation. Half requested a cervical computed tomography (CT) angiography for the study and evaluation of the vertebral artery relationships. Most of the experts advocated for conservative treatment as their initial management. Half recommended a posterior C1-C2 fixation if the patient failed conservative therapy. The main goal of surgery was occipital pain relief for half of the physicians, while the rest focused on stabilization and deformity reduction. All were aware of the vertebral arteries, and most considered the C2 neural elements and the spinal cord as important structures of which to be cognizant. The most feared complications were injury to the vertebral arteries, spinal cord, and C2 nerve roots. Surgery was generally attained with fluoroscopy, intraoperative monitoring, and surgical navigation. No special medications were recommended perioperatively. Although management approaches greatly varied, most coincided with posterior upper cervical fusion as the ideal strategy in case of surgical treatment. Following surgery, most admitted their patient to the floor. Half requested a cervical spine radiographs prior to discharge. All advocated for radiographical follow-up 4 to 6 months after surgery. Most recommended the use of a rigid collar for a minimum of 4 weeks after surgery.

SUMMARY OF QUALITY OF EVIDENCE TO GUIDE SPECIFIC INTERVENTIONS FOR THIS CASE

- Posterior fixation of the C1-C2 joint for patients suffering from unremitting pain despite conservative management is associated with long-term pain relief: level II.2

REFERENCES

1. Grob D, Bremerich FH, Dvorak J, Mannion AF. Transarticular screw fixation for osteoarthritis of the atlanto axial segment. *Eur Spine J.* 2006;15(3):283–291.
2. Yeom JS, Riew KD, Kang SS, et al. Distraction Arthrodesis of the C1-C2 Facet Joint with Preservation of the C2 Root for the Management of Intractable Occipital Neuralgia Caused by C2 Root Compression. *Spine (Phila Pa 1976).* 2015;40(20):E1093–E1102.
3. Halla JT, Hardin Jr. JG. The spectrum of atlantoaxial facet joint involvement in rheumatoid arthritis. *Arthritis Rheum.* 1990;33(3):325–329.
4. Halla JT, Hardin Jr. JG. Atlantoaxial (C1-C2) facet joint osteoarthritis: a distinctive clinical syndrome. *Arthritis Rheum.* 1987;30(5):577–582.
5. Janjua MB, Reddy S, El Ahmadieh TY, et al. Occipital neuralgia: A neurosurgical perspective. *J Clin Neurosci.* 2020;71:263–270.
6. Holly LT, Batzdorf U, Foley KT. Treatment of severe retromastoid pain secondary to C1-2 arthrosis by using cervical fusion. *J Neurosurg.* 2000;92(2 Suppl):162–168.
7. Taher F, Bokums K, Aichmair A, Hughes AP. C1-C2 instability with severe occipital headache in the setting of vertebral artery facet complex erosion. *Eur Spine J.* 2014;23(Suppl 2):145–149.
8. Hoppenfeld JD. Cervical facet arthropathy and occipital neuralgia: headache culprits. *Curr Pain Headache Rep.* 2010;14(6):418–423.
9. Pakzaban P. Transarticular screw fixation of C1-2 for the treatment of arthropathy-associated occipital neuralgia. *J Neurosurg Spine.* 2011;14(2):209–214.
10. Ehni G, Benner B. Occipital neuralgia and the C1-2 arthrosis syndrome. *J Neurosurg.* 1984;61(5):961–965.
11. Grob D. Surgery in the degenerative cervical spine. *Spine (Phila Pa 1976).* 1998;23(24):2674–2683.
12. Stemmler N, Solaroglu I, Aydin AL, et al. Unusual pain due to unilateral facet degeneration at the C1-2 level. *Turk Neurosurg.* 2014;24(3):430–433.
13. Menezes AH, Traynelis VC. Anatomy and biomechanics of normal craniovertebral junction (a) and biomechanics of stabilization (b). *Childs Nerv Syst.* 2008;24(10):1091–1100.
14. Cesmebasi A, Muhleman MA, Hulsberg P, et al. Occipital neuralgia: anatomic considerations. *Clin Anat.* 2015;28(1):101–108.
15. Hunter CR, Mayfield FH. Role of the upper cervical roots in the production of pain in the head. *Am J Surg.* 1949;78(5):743–751.
16. Lee JY, Im SB, Jeong JH. Use of a C1-C2 Facet Spacer to Treat Atlantoaxial Instability and Basilar Invagination Associated with Rheumatoid Arthritis. *World Neurosurg.* 2017;98:874.e813–874.e816.

19

Migrated interbody

Kingsley Abode-Iyamah, MD

Introduction

Transforaminal lumbar interbody interbody fusion (TLIF) and posterior lumbar interbody fusion (PLIF) have become common procedures for the treatment of degenerative lumbar disease such as spondylolisthesis, scoliosis, and spondylosis leading to foraminal stenosis.[1-5] Interbody cage placement is often used to increase fusion rate and stabilization of the instrumented segments. While this has shown to be advantageous to patient outcomes and fusion rates, migration of the interbody can occur following interbody cage placement.[6-10] While the interbody cage can migrate both anteriorly and posteriorly, the concerns differ depending on the direction of migration. For anterior migration, the main concerns are injury of the great vessels and bowel perforation, especially in grafts with ongoing migration or placed too far anteriorly. For posterior migration, the main concerns are nerve root compression, cauda equina syndrome, and spinal deformity. Although many small cohort studies exist looking at the risk of migration, a recent meta-analysis by Liu et al. found that pear-shaped disks and straight cages were the main risk factors for cage migration. Here, we discuss the approach to a posteriorly displaced cage migration causing deformity.

Example Case

Chief complaint: leg and back pain

History of present illness: A 52-year-old female with a history of L3-5 TLIF 2 years prior presents with back pain and leg pain. Immediately after surgery 2 years prior, the patient had worsening back pain and inability to stand up straight. She continued to have worsening back pain. She eventually had a magnetic resonance image (MRI) and was found to have kyphoscoliosis with migration of her L4-5 interbody cage posteriorly into the canal (Fig. 19.1). She was also noted to have hardware loosening on computed tomography (CT) (Fig. 19.2) and a kyphotic deformity on x-rays (Fig. 19.3).

Medications: sumatriptan

Allergies: no known drug allergies

Past medical and surgical history: back pain, L3-L5 TLIF

Family history: noncontributory

Social history: nurse, no smoking history, occasional alcohol

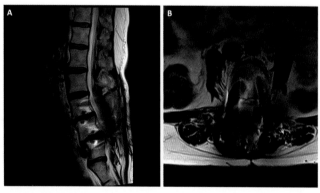

Fig. 19.1 Preoperative magnetic resonance images. (A) T2 sagittal and **(B)** T2 axial images demonstrating L4-5 kyphosis with interbody graft migration.

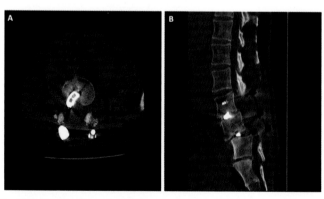

Fig. 19.2 Preoperative computed tomography scans. (A) Sagittal and **(B)** L4-5 kyphosis with interbody graft migration and resulting grade I spondylolisthesis of L4-5 with hardware at L4-5.

Physical examination: awake, alert, and oriented to person, place, and time; cranial nerves II–XII intact; bilateral deltoids/triceps/biceps 5/5; interossei 5/5; iliopsoas/knee flexion/knee extension/dorsi, and plantar flexion 5/5

Reflexes: 2+ in bilateral biceps/triceps/brachioradialis with negative Hoffman; 2+ in bilateral patella/ankle; no clonus or Babinski; sensation intact to light touch

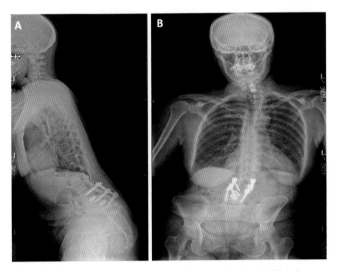

Fig. 19.3 Preoperative x-rays. (A) Anteroposterior (AP) and **(B)** lateral x-rays demonstrating coronal and sagittal imbalance.

	Todd J. Albert, MD Orthopaedic Surgery Hospital for Special Surgery Weill Cornell Medical College New York, New York, United States	Dean Chou, MD Rory Mayer, MD Neurosurgery University of California at San Francisco San Francisco, California, United States	Fabio Cofano, MD Neurosurgery University of Turin Spine Surgery Unit Humanitas Gradenigo Hospital Turin, Italy	Luis Rodrigo Diaz Iniguez, MD Orthopaedic Surgery Hospital Angeles Lindavista Mexico City, Mexico
Preoperative				
Additional tests requested	DEXA	DEXA (3–6 months of teriparatide if osteopenic or osteoporotic) L-spine flexion-extension x-rays Medicine evaluation	DEXA Previous x-rays	L-spine flexion-extension x-rays DEXA Parathyroid hormone level Calcium metabolism evaluation
Surgical approach selected	Stage 1: posterior exploration Stage 2: revision and removal of anterior L4-S1 cages Stage 3: posterior fusion	Stage 1: L4-5 ALIF with cage retrieval, L5-S1 ALIF; Stage 2: T10-pelvis posterior fusion with posterior column osteotomies and possible L4 PSO	Step 1: L3-L5 intersomatic arthrodesis after cage removal Stage 2: L5-S1 ALIF Stage 3: L3-S1 posterior reinstrumentation and fusion	L4-5 interbody removal, L2-S1 posterior fusion and L4-5 interbody replacement
Goal of surgery	Decompression, and restore sagittal and coronal alignment	Cage retrieval, correction of sagittal and coronal alignment, fusion across pseudoarthrosis	Restore sagittal and coronal alignment with resolution of pain, achievement of stable fusion	Decompression, stabilize spine, improve sagittal balance

	Todd J. Albert, MD Orthopaedic Surgery Hospital for Special Surgery Weill Cornell Medical College New York, New York, United States	Dean Chou, MD Rory Mayer, MD Neurosurgery University of California at San Francisco San Francisco, California, United States	Fabio Cofano, MD Neurosurgery University of Turin Spine Surgery Unit Humanitas Gradenigo Hospital Turin, Italy	Luis Rodrigo Diaz Iniguez, MD Orthopaedic Surgery Hospital Angeles Lindavista Mexico City, Mexico
Perioperative				
Positioning	Stage 1: prone Stage 2: supine Stage 3: prone	Stage 1: supine on flat top Jackson table Stage 2: prone on proaxis table	Stage 1: right lateral Stage 2: supine with slight Trendelenburg Stage 3: prone with hip extension	Prone
Surgical equipment	IOM (MEP/SSEP/EMG) Fluoroscopy BMP	IOM (MEP/SSEP/EMG) Fluoroscopy Surgical navigation Cell saver	IOM Fluoroscopy	IOM Fluoroscopy Vertebroplasty set
Medications	Tranexamic acid, paraspinal blocks	Tranexamic acid	None	Steroids, Pregabalin
Anatomical considerations	Nerve roots, dura, anterior vasculature	Stage 1: iliac vessels, aortic bifurcation, ureter Stage 2: dura, right L4 and L5 nerve roots, scar tissue	Psoas, lumbar plexus and vessels, iliac vessels	Dura, nerve root, vertebral body, bone density
Complications feared with approach chosen	Instrument failure, CSF leak, vascular injury, pseudoarthrosis	CSF leak, nerve root injury, pseudoarthrosis	Vascular injury, lumbar plexus injuries, inability to remove cages, durotomy	Neurological injury, vertebral fracture
Intraoperative				
Anesthesia	General	General	General	General
Exposure	Stage 1: L4-S1 Stage 2: L3-S1 Stage 3: L4-S1	Stage 1: L4-S1 Stage 2: T10-pelvis	Stage 1: L3-L5 Stage 2: L5-S1 Stage 3: L3-S1	L2-S1
Levels decompressed	L4-S1	L4-S1	L3-L5	L4-5
Levels fused	L3-S1	T10-pelvis	L3-S1	L2-S1
Surgical narrative	Stage 1: position prone, open previous posterior midline incision, subperiosteal dissection, explore hardware, remove pedicle screws from L4-S1 and rods, place new instrumentation with upsized instrumentation from L4-S1 with possible iliac fixation depending on purchase and bone quality, prepare fusion bed, obtain local bone graft, temporary closure	Stage 1: position supine, vascular surgery access, abdominal incision, retroperitoneal approach to anterior spine, mobilization of great vessels, expose L4-5 and L5-S1 disc spaces, discectomy at L4-5 with use of Cobb to aggressively distract disc space and mobilize cage for retrieval, placement of interbody cage at L4-5, discectomy and ALIF at L5-S1, avoid placement of any screw through buttress plate or integrated screw/plate into L4 vertebral body because of planned L4 PSO	Stage 1: left lateral approach for L3-L4 and L4-L5, dissect abdominal wall to reach retroperitoneal space, transpsoas approach to the L3-L4 and L4-L5 disc with aid of IOM, remove transforaminal cages by distracting disc spaces with spreader devices, position trabecular titanium cage trying to reach anterior part of disc space to achieve proper lordosis Stage 2 (same day): position supine, anterior retroperitoneal approach to L5-S1 disc space, careful discectomy with proper preparation of bony end plates, position hyper lordotic cage based on spinopelvic parameters	Position prone, midline skin incision, plane dissection to transpedicular system, remove rods, remove L5 pedicle screws, remove interbody, reduce the listhesis, reposition interbody in L4-5 space, place pedicle screws at L2 and L5-S1, contour rod to restore lumbar lordosis to improve sagittal balance, x-ray to confirm alignment and hardware location, layered closure

	Todd J. Albert, MD Orthopaedic Surgery Hospital for Special Surgery Weill Cornell Medical College New York, New York, United States	Dean Chou, MD Rory Mayer, MD Neurosurgery University of California at San Francisco San Francisco, California, United States	Fabio Cofano, MD Neurosurgery University of Turin Spine Surgery Unit Humanitas Gradenigo Hospital Turin, Italy	Luis Rodrigo Diaz Iniguez, MD Orthopaedic Surgery Hospital Angeles Lindavista Mexico City, Mexico
	Stage 2 (same day): position supine, vascular surgery to expose L3-S1 by retroperitoneal approach, remove L4-5 cage, remove L3-4 case if not solid, distract L4-5/L5-S1/possible L3-4, place large footprint lordotic cases with BMP for lordosis from L3-S1, layered closure Stage 3 (same day): position prone, open incision from stage 1, place rods, lock down, layered closure with subfascial drain	Stage 2 (2–3 days after stage 1): position prone, thoracolumbar incision, explant prior implants at L3-5, O-arm spine and navigated pedicle screw placements from T10-pelvis except for L4, perform posterior column osteotomies at L3-S1 to see if enough lordosis can be achieved, PSO if need more lordosis by placing short L3 and L5 screws that are buried deeper into the pedicles relative to the other pedicles, place L3-5 accessory rods across PSO site and separate rod construct T10-pelvis excluding L3 and L5 screws, expose dura from the pedicle of L3 to pedicle of L5, isolate L4 pedicles, PSO, closure of osteotomy with proaxis table, final tighten L3-5 accessory rods, size and place primary rods from T10-pelvis, use coronal bender for correction of coronal deformity, final tighten set screws, layered closure with two subfascial drains	Stage 3 (same day): position prone, open old incision, remove screws and reposition at L3-S1 bilaterally, posterior osteotomy of L5, compression between screws after rod positioning	
Complication avoidance	Stage 1 to upsize instrumentation with potential iliac fixation depending on purchase and bone quality, stage 2 exposure done by vascular surgery, lordotic cases from L3-S1, three staged approach	Stage 1 approach by vascular surgery, avoid anterior screws into L4 vertebral body, start with posterior column osteotomies to increase lordosis, PSO if need more lordosis, four-rod construct, coronal plane bender for coronal plane deformity	Three-stage approach, IOM to guide transpsoas approach, place cage as anterior as possible to promote lordosis, place hyperlordotic cage based on spinopelvic parameters	Reduce the listhesis, extend construct, replace hardware, contour rods to be more lordotic
Postoperative				
Admission	ICU	ICU	ICU	Floor
Postoperative complications feared	Infection, hematoma, medical complication	CSF leak, nerve root injury, bony fracture when retrieving cage	CSF leak, lumbar plexus injuries, infections	Neurological injury, vertebral fracture, infection
Anticipated length of stay	4–6 days	7 days	4–5 days	7 days

	Todd J. Albert, MD Orthopaedic Surgery Hospital for Special Surgery Weill Cornell Medical College New York, New York, United States	Dean Chou, MD Rory Mayer, MD Neurosurgery University of California at San Francisco San Francisco, California, United States	Fabio Cofano, MD Neurosurgery University of Turin Spine Surgery Unit Humanitas Gradenigo Hospital Turin, Italy	Luis Rodrigo Diaz Iniguez, MD Orthopaedic Surgery Hospital Angeles Lindavista Mexico City, Mexico
Follow-up testing	AP/lateral lumbar x-rays prior to discharge AP/lateral/flexion/ extension lumbar x-rays 3 months after surgery EOS entire spine 3 months after surgery	Standing scoliosis x-rays prior to discharge, 6 weeks, 3 months, 6 months, 1 year, and 2 years after surgery	Standing x-rays within 24 hours after surgery, 1, 3, 6, and 12 months after surgery	L-spine x-rays prior to discharge MRI L-spine 2 months after surgery
Bracing	Light lumbar wrap when out of bed and ambulating for 3–4 weeks	None	Semirigid brace for 30 days	Jewett brace for 2 months
Follow-up visits	3–4 weeks	2 weeks, 6 weeks, 3 months, 6 months, 1 year, and 2 years after surgery	1, 3, 6, and 12 months after surgery	2 weeks after surgery

ALIF, Anterior lumbar interbody fusion; AP, anteroposterior; BMP, bone morphogenic protein; CSF, cerebrospinal fluid; DEXA, dual-energy x-ray absorptiometry; EMG, electromyography; ICU, intensive care unit; IOM, intraoperative monitoring; MEP, motor evoked potential; MRI, magnetic resonance imaging; PSO, pedicle subtraction osteotomy; SSEP, somatosensory evoked potentials.

Differential diagnosis

- Interbody migration
- Pseudoarthrosis
- Hardware failure
- Adjacent segment disease

Important anatomical considerations

The vertebral body is connected anteriorly and posteriorly by the anterior and posterior longitudinal ligaments, respectively. The vertebrae have the intervertebral disc space, which absorbs the axial load on the spine. Anterior to the spinal column are the great vessels in the retroperitoneal space. Both the aorta and vena cava run together, bifurcating at the L4 space. Posterior to the vertebrae is the spinal canal, which contains the thecal sac. The exiting nerve root exits through the vertebral foramen below the pedicle of that level. Kambin's triangle is a right triangle over the dorsolateral space allowing safe placement of interbody cage while avoiding complications. Anteriorly migrated interbody cage can lead to compression or injury to the great vessels. This is best identified by computed tomography (CT) angiogram to better assess the integrity of the vessels. When there are concerns for vascular injury due to graft migration anteriorly, multidisciplinary care in coordination with a vascular surgeon is essential. Posteriorly migrated graft can lead to compression of the exiting or traversing nerve root. For posteriorly migrated graft, a CT myelogram is a useful diagnostic test as hardware artifact may make it difficult to identify the involved neural structures on a magnetic resonance image (MRI). Posterior migration can cause compression of the cauda equina, which can result in cauda equina syndrome. Both anterior and posterior interbody migration can result in kyphotic deformity, resulting in back pain and weakness.

Approaches to this lesion

The treatment of a migrated interbody graft is best achieved by addressing it from the direction of its migration. An anteriorly displaced graft, which requires retrieval, is best addressed from an anterior approach. This may require additional intervention such as an anterior lumbar interbody fusion (ALIF) or additional posterior instrumentation depending on the status of the previously placed pedicle screws. A posteriorly displaced graft causing neurological deficit or deformity should be approach posteriorly. This allows identification of important structures and careful dissection of these structures prior to removal of the graft. Additionally, a posterior approach allows the surgeon to address any complications directly such as a cerebrospinal fluid (CSF) leak. Furthermore, this approach allows addressing any deformity that may also result from the graft migration. Additional graft placement can be performed from a posterior approach. While an anterior approach can be attempted for a posteriorly displaced graft, it poses a risk of inability for direct repair of potential complications such as a CSF leak. As previously mentioned, any anterior approach will most likely also require additional posterior approach, especially when a deformity in involved.

What was actually done

The presented case shows a posteriorly displaced graft at L4-5 with focal kyphosis, spondylolisthesis, and deformity. The patient was taken to the operating room and positioned on an Orthopedic system Inc (OSI) table. A midline incision was made and the previous instrumentation identified. The previous instrumentation was removed and replaced and new instrumentation was placed from T11 to the pelvis. Following the instrumentation placement, dissection was carried out to identify the thecal sac. The thecal sac was found to be under severe tension. The interbody graft was identified and was

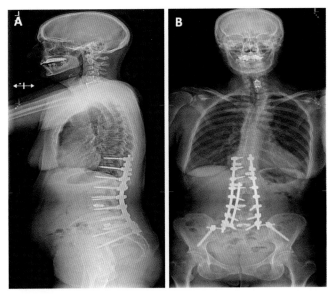

Fig. 19.4 Postoperative x-rays. (A) Lateral and **(B)** AP x-rays after instrumentation from T11 to pelvis with removal of the prior L4-5 interbody cage and correction of deformity.

and stability, including bone morphogenic protein and a vertebroplasty set. Half elected using tranexamic acid intraoperatively to minimize blood loss. While the majority were concerned about CSF leak and nerve injury, those who recommended an anterior approach were also concerned about vascular injury. The majority recommended postoperative admission to the intensive care unit with planned hospitalization for 4 to 7 days.

SUMMARY OF QUALITY OF EVIDENCE TO GUIDE SPECIFIC INTERVENTIONS FOR THIS CASE

- Intraoperative monitoring for deformity surgery: level II.1
- Anterior versus posterior approach for migration of cage: level II.2

scarred in place. The graft could not be easily mobilized, so the end plates of L4 and L5 were drilled to create some space to free the graft. Given the amount of tension on the thecal sac, this could not be mobilized medially. Dissection continued medially under the thecal sac to free the bony ingrowth into the graft until it could be easily mobilized. The graft was then removed, allowing relaxation of the thecal sac. Additionally, the intervertebral disc space was prepped and autograft was placed in the disc space for bony fusion. The instrumentation was rodded, correcting the deformity, and compression at the L4-5 disc space was performed to allow correction of the focal kyphosis. Intraoperative neuromonitoring was used throughout the case. Two hemovac drains were placed and each layer closed. The patient was mobilized on postoperative day 1 and discharged on postoperative day 5 with good pain control. Follow-up x-rays showed good placement of the hardware and correction of the kyphotic deformity (Fig. 19.4).

Commonalities among the experts

The plans for surgical intervention for this patient varied with most recommending an anterior approach for cage removal. Additionally, the majority recommended a staged procedure involving anterior and posterior approaches. While all the experts recommend extension of the fusion, this varied from one level above to multiple levels with one expert recommending the possibility of a three column osteotomy for correction of the sagittal imbalance. Only one expert recommended a posterior approach alone, similar to what was done for this patient. All our experts recommended the use of intraoperative monitoring and fluoroscopy. Half recommended agents to augment fusion

REFERENCES

1. Arnold PM, Robbins S, Paullus W, Faust S, Holt R, McGuire R. Clinical outcomes of lumbar degenerative disc disease treated with posterior lumbar interbody fusion allograft spacer: a prospective, multicenter trial with 2-year follow-up. *Am J Orthop (Belle Mead NJ)*. 2009;38(7):E115–E122.
2. Hayashi K, Matsumura A, Konishi S, Kato M, Namikawa T, Nakamura H. Clinical Outcomes of Posterior Lumbar Interbody Fusion for Patients 80 Years of Age and Older with Lumbar Degenerative Disease: Minimum 2 Years' Follow-Up. *Global Spine J*. 2016;6(7):665–672.
3. Liang Y, Shi W, Jiang C, Chen Z, Liu F, Feng Z, et al. Clinical outcomes and sagittal alignment of single-level unilateral instrumented transforaminal lumbar interbody fusion with a 4 to 5-year follow-up. *Eur Spine J*. 2015;24(11):2560–2566.
4. Takahashi T, Hanakita J, Minami M, Kitahama Y, Kuraishi K, Watanabe M, et al. Clinical outcomes and adverse events following transforaminal interbody fusion for lumbar degenerative spondylolisthesis in elderly patients. *Neurol Med Chir (Tokyo)*. 2011;51(12):829–835.
5. Watanabe K, Yamazaki A, Morita O, Sano A, Katsumi K, Ohashi M. Clinical outcomes of posterior lumbar interbody fusion for lumbar foraminal stenosis: preoperative diagnosis and surgical strategy. *J Spinal Disord Tech*. 2011;24(3):137–141.
6. Baeesa SS, Medrano BG, Noriega DC. Long-Term Outcomes of Posterior Lumbar Interbody Fusion Using Stand-Alone Ray Threaded Cage for Degenerative Disk Disease: A 20-Year Follow-Up. *Asian Spine J*. 2016;10(6):1100–1105.
7. Houten JK, Post NH, Dryer JW, Errico TJ. Clinical and radiographically/neuroimaging documented outcome in transforaminal lumbar interbody fusion. *Neurosurg Focus*. 2006;20(3):E8.
8. Park MK, Kim KT, Bang WS, Cho DC, Sung JK, Lee YS, et al. Risk factors for cage migration and cage retropulsion following transforaminal lumbar interbody fusion. *Spine J*. 2019;19(3):437–447.
9. Proubasta IR, Vallve EQ, Aguilar LF, Villanueva CL, Iglesias JJ. Intraoperative antepulsion of a fusion cage in posterior lumbar interbody fusion: a case report and review of the literature. *Spine (Phila Pa 1976)*. 2002;27(17):E399–E402.
10. Zhao FD, Yang W, Shan Z, Wang J, Chen HX, Hong ZH, et al. Cage migration after transforaminal lumbar interbody fusion and factors related to it. *Orthop Surg*. 2012;4(4):227–232.

20

Cervical myelopathy

Fidel Valero-Moreno, MD

Introduction

Myelopathy denotes any neurological deficit related to a pathology of the spinal cord. A spinal cord injury (SCI) can be produced by diverse etiologies such as trauma, ischemia, neoplasms, inflammatory processes, and infection. However, degenerative cervical myelopathy (DCM) is the most common cause of spinal cord dysfunction.[1-4] Degenerative myelopathy may result from spondylosis, disc herniation, or facet arthropathy, as well as ligamentous hypertrophy, calcification, or ossification.[3,5] DCM accounts for 54% of all the nontraumatic SCI in the United States.[3] This condition mainly affects aging people and is usually diagnosed during the fifth decade of life.[4,6] C5-C6 is the most commonly involved level regardless of gender and age.[7,8] The pathogenesis of neurological impairment hinges on the direct injury to neurons and glial cells, either from static or dynamic mechanical insults.[2] The spinocerebellar and corticospinal tracts are usually affected first.[1] Onset of symptoms is usually insidious, and initial complaints are frequently gait disturbances and fine motor deficits.[1] To establish a reliable correlation between the severity of symptomatology and the degree of radiographic compression is challenging.[1,2] Most of the abnormalities that contribute to the development of DCM can be demonstrated with a magnetic resonance image (MRI), and therefore an MRI should be routinely performed if cervical myelopathy is suspected.[1-4] Surgery is the standard treatment for DCM.[1,3,6,7,9] Cervical decompression halts disease progression and improves neurological outcomes, functional status, and quality of life.[1,4,9] Besides decompression of spinal cord, surgery should restore cervical alignment and address instability if present.[1] The ideal approach to attain the aforementioned is still a matter of debate. Several factors impact the surgical strategy, such as the localization of the compression (anterior or posterior), levels affected, and the need to preserve cervical lordosis.[6,8] Anterior approaches include discectomy and fusion and/or corpectomy, whereas common posterior techniques include laminectomy/laminoplasty and fusion.[1,3,6,7]

In this chapter, we present the case of a 68-year-old man presenting with gait disturbances/instability and hand atrophy with suspected cervical myleopathy.

Example Case

Chief complaint: instability

History of present illness: This is a 68-year-old man with a history of hand atrophy and gait instability for several weeks. He initially attributed these symptoms to his lumbar spine. He does have a history of prior lumbar laminectomy. The patient stated that he did have some difficulty with dexterity and balance and even suffered recurrent falls. He had some difficulty with urinary urgency, but he attributed this to his history of prostate cancer. Magnetic resonance image (MRI) and computed tomography (CT) of the cervical spine showed significant degenerative spinal canal stenosis with severe ventral compression of the spinal cord (Figs. 20.1 and 20.2).

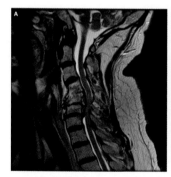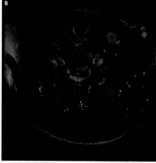

Fig. 20.1 Preoperative magnetic resonance image (MRI) of the cervical spine. **(A)** T2 sagittal and **(B)** axial images of the cervical spine demonstrating a severe cervical degenerative spinal stenosis. Severe anterior spinal cord compression is evident from C4 to C6 levels, where compression is markedly worse at the C6 level. There is thickening of the anterior and posterior longitudinal ligaments and ossification of the anterior longitudinal ligament from C3 to C6. A decrease of the intervertebral space between C5 and C6 is noted, and there is anterior fusion between the fourth and fifth cervical vertebrae. Cervical kyphosis of the cervical spine is apparent.

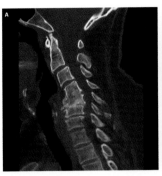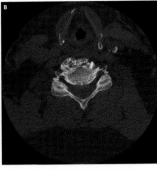

Fig. 20.2 Preoperative computed tomography (CT) of the cervical spine.
(A) Sagittal and **(B)** axial images demonstrating a kyphotic deformity of the
cervical spine and severe degenerative changes, including the fusion of C4 and C5
vertebrae, complete collapse of the anterior intervertebral space between C5 and C6,
ossification of the anterior longitudinal ligament, and osteophyte formation.

Medications: ramipril
Allergies: no known drug allergies.
Past medical and surgical history: prostatic cancer, hypertension
Family history: noncontributory
Social history: engineer, no smoking, no alcohol
Physical examination: awake, alert, and oriented to person, place,
and time; cranial nerves II–XII intact; unsteady gait. Bilateral
deltoids/triceps/biceps 5/5; interossei 4/5; iliopsoas/knee
flexion/knee extension/dorsi, and plantar flexion 5/5
Reflexes: 2+ in bilateral biceps/triceps/brachioradialis with
negative Hoffman; 2+ in bilateral patella/ankle; no clonus or
Babinski; sensation intact to light touch

	Richard Allen, MD, PhD Jakub Sikora, MD Orthopaedic Surgery University of California at San Diego San Diego, California, United States	Richard J. Bransford, MD Orthopaedic Surgery University of Washington Seattle, Washington, United States	Juan Fernando Ramon, MD Neurosurgery University Hospital Fundacion Santa Fe de Bogata Bogota, Columbia	Timothy F. Witham, MD Neurosurgery Johns Hopkins Baltimore, Maryland, United States
Preoperative				
Additional tests requested	Confirm no other source of pathology Swallow evaluation C-spine Flex/Ext X-rays	AP/lateral/flexion/extension C-spine x-rays Medicine evaluation C-spine Flex/Ext X-rays	AP/lateral/flexion/extension C-spine x-rays Medicine evaluation C-spine Flex/Ext X-rays	DEXA Standing scoliosis x-rays/EOS imaging Calcium, vitamin D, PTH, testosterone serum levels Medicine evaluation C-spine Flex/Ext X-rays
Surgical approach selected	Stage 1: C4-5 anterior cervical corpectomy, C6-7 ACDF, C3-6 plating fusion Stage 2: C5-C7 laminectomy and C2-T2 posterior fusion	Stage 1: C4-5 corpectomy and C6-7 ACDF Stage 2: C2-T2 posterior fusion and C3-6 laminectomy	C3-4 corpectomy	Stage 1: C4-5 corpectomy, C3-6 reconstruction, C3-6 plating Stage 2: C2-T2 fixation and fusion, possible C6-7 laminectomy
Goal of surgery	Decompress spinal cord, restore alignment, stabilize spine	Decompress spinal cord, restore lordosis and physiological alignment, stabilize spine	Decompress spinal cord, restore lordosis, stabilize spine	Decompress spinal cord, restoration of anatomical alignment, stabilization
Perioperative				
Positioning	Stage 1: supine with Gardner-Wells tongs Stage 2: prone, with Gardner-Wells tongs	Stage 1: supine on Jackson flat top with Gardner-Wells tongs Stage 2: prone on Jackson flip frame with Mayfield pins	Supine, no pins	Stage 1: supine with 10 pounds traction Stage 2: prone with pins
Surgical equipment	Fluoroscopy	IOM (MEP/SSEP/EMG) Fluoroscopy Surgical microscope	Fluoroscopy O-arm	Stage 1: IOM, fluoroscopy Stage 2: IOM, fluoroscopy, bone scalpel
Medications	Tranexamic acid	MAPs >85	None	Vitamin D/calcium supplements if needed, PTH analog if needed, MAP >85
Anatomical considerations	Vertebral arteries, PLL, thecal sac	Esophagus, sympathetic plexus, trachea, carotid artery, recurrent laryngeal nerve, vertebral arteries	Esophagus, larynx, vascular structures, uncincate process, PLL	Vertebral arteries, spinal cord, cervical nerve roots

	Richard Allen, MD, PhD Jakub Sikora, MD Orthopaedic Surgery University of California at San Diego San Diego, California, United States	Richard J. Bransford, MD Orthopaedic Surgery University of Washington Seattle, Washington, United States	Juan Fernando Ramon, MD Neurosurgery University Hospital Fundacion Santa Fe de Bogata Bogota, Columbia	Timothy F. Witham, MD Neurosurgery Johns Hopkins Baltimore, Maryland, United States
Complications feared with approach chosen	Dysphagia	Inadequate decompression, misalignment	Vascular injury, esophageal injury, recurrent laryngeal nerve injury	Spinal instability, inadequate decompression
Intraoperative				
Anesthesia	General	General	General	General
Exposure	Stage 1: C3-7 Stage 2: C2-T2	Stage 1: C3-7 Stage 2: C2-T2	C3-6	Stage 1: C3-7 Stage 2: C2-T2
Levels decompressed	Stage 1: C3-6 Stage 2: C5-7	Stage 1: C3-6 Stage 2: C3-6	C3-4	Stage 1: C3-6 Stage 2: C6-7
Levels fused	Stage 1: C3-7 Stage 2: C2-T2	Stage 1: C3-7 Stage 2: C2-T2	C3-6	Stage 1: C3-6 Stage 2: C2-T2
Surgical narrative	Stage 1: Position supine with Gardner-Wells tongs, modified left oblique neck incision through skin and platysma, modified Smith-Robinson approach releasing hyoid, develop subplatysmal flaps down through superficial and deep cervical fascia, subperiosteally dissect anterior cervical spine, confirm location with spinal needle, remove anterior osteophytes and flatten, C6-7 ACDF with microscope, place Caspar pins and retractor, annuolotomy and removal of disc, parallel the endplates with matchstick bur and avoid taking structural end plate, bur back to uncovertebral joints and posteriorly down to PLL, foraminotomies at C6-7, trial graft sizes and place structural allograft, move Caspar pins proximally, take annulotomy to C3 and perform C5-6 and C4-5 discectomy, begin corpectomy using matchstick and bur down to PLL on right then on left, resect freed vertebral body with Leksell, remove underlying PLL, identify entire dural sac, insert cage with allograft/autograft/demineralized bone matrix, place anterior cervical plate from C3-7, final AP and lateral x-rays, layered closure	Stage 1: position supine with 10–15 lb of traction in lordotic position, left-sided transverse incision in Langer's line centered about C5 body, dissection to longus colli with wide exposure and gentle pressure, place retractor and Caspar pins with one in C3 and one into C6 vertebral body, bring in microscope, C3-4 and C5-6 discectomy, create trough with drill at uncovertebral joints along C4 and C5 body on left and right, remove as much of the vertebral bodies as possible and save bone, remove posterior bone with up-angled curettes/Kerrison/pituitary rongeurs, dissect through PLL to see dura and ensure decompression, place cage from C3 to C6 with optimized lordosis and cage filled with autograft, remove Caspar pins, C6-7 discectomy through PLL, place lordotic corticocancellous allograft after decompression, place plate spanning from C3-7, close incision over drain	Position supine, head slightly extended, neutral, lateral x-ray to check level, right lateral horizontal incision, platysma dissection, identify border of sternocleidomastoid, open anterior cervical fascia, blunt finger dissection, palpate carotid artery, identify and retract larynx/thyroid/esophagus, put retractor on longus colli base, dissect levels as needed, place pins at C3 and C6, distract, C3-4 corpectomy, C4-5 discectomy, identify PLL and uncinate process, prepare end plates for implant, put PEEK implant with bone chips, x-ray to check position, screw fixation with plate, x-ray to confirm location and hardware, layered closure with drain	Stage 1: position supine on Mayfield horseshoe, position supine with 10 lb traction, postposition IOM, right-sided vertical incision along anterior border of sternocleidomastoid, localizing x-ray, Caspar pins at C3 and C6 for distraction, place self-retaining retractors, C3-4 and C5-6 discectomies, C4-5 corpectomies with drill to PLL, open and resect PLL to decompress cord and C4-6 nerve roots bilaterally, size and fill cage, place cage, remove weight from traction, remove distraction pins, place plate, layered closure with drain, x-ray

	Richard Allen, MD, PhD Jakub Sikora, MD Orthopaedic Surgery University of California at San Diego San Diego, California, United States	Richard J. Bransford, MD Orthopaedic Surgery University of Washington Seattle, Washington, United States	Juan Fernando Ramon, MD Neurosurgery University Hospital Fundacion Santa Fe de Bogata Bogota, Columbia	Timothy F. Witham, MD Neurosurgery Johns Hopkins Baltimore, Maryland, United States
	Stage 2 (same day): position prone with Gardner-Wells tongs, midline incision C2-T2, subperiosteal dissection, C5-7 laminectomy, C2 pedicle screws, C4-6 lateral mass crews aiming up and out approximately 15 degrees, place pedicle screws at C7-T2, instrument from C3-T2, decorticate, final tighten, set screws, place autograft and allograft, layered closure with Marcaine in subcutaneous space	Stage 2 (same day): replace tongs with Mayfield pins, flip into prone position, optimize lordosis of spine, subperiosteal exposure from C2 lateral mass to T2 transverse processes, place C2 pars/C3-6 lateral mass (Magerl technique)/T1-2 pedicle screws, laminectomy troughs from C3-6 at junction of lamina and lateral mass, remove lamina and ensure decompression, place lordotic rods from C2 pars to T2 pedicle screws and secure, decorticate from C2-T2 and place autograft from laminectomy mixed with demineralized bone matrix for fusion, layered closure with subfascial drain, take to ICU intubated		Stage 2 (next day): position prone with Mayfield pins, postposition IOM, expose C2-T2, C6-7 en bloc laminectomy with ultrasonic bone scalpel, drill pilot holes, drill screw holes, decorticate bone, place instrumentation and rods, x-ray, layered closure with drain
Complication avoidance	Two-staged approach, flatten anterior cervical spine to prevent dysphagia, perform discectomy prior to corpectomy to get appropriate interbody, do not remove structural end plate during discectomy, C7 pedicle screws	Traction during anterior approach, troughs along uncovertebral joints, dissect through PLL, optimize lordosis with anterior cage, two-staged approach, Magerl technique for cervical lateral mass screws	Anterior cervical approach with distraction, maintain PLL	Two-staged approach dependent on degree of decompression between stages, traction to help with alignment, open PLL, MRI between stages
Postoperative				
Admission	ICU	ICU	ICU	Intermediate care
Postoperative complications feared	Dysphagia, pseudoarthrosis, wound complications, instrument failure	Dysphagia, airway issues	Dysphagia, cervical hematoma, vascular injury, esophageal injury	Dysphagia, C5 palsy, CSF leak, instrument failure, pseudoarthrosis, esophageal injury
Anticipated length of stay	3–4 days	4–5 days	3–4 days	
Follow-up testing	C-spine x-rays 6 weeks, 3 months, 6 months, 1 year after surgery	CT C-T spine within 24 hours of surgery C-spine x-rays prior to discharge, 3 months, 6 months, 12 months after surgery	C-spine x-ray 1 month after surgery	MRI C-spine after stage 1 CT C-spine within 48 hours after stage 2 C-spine x-rays 6 weeks, 3 months, 6 months, 12 months after surgery
Bracing	Aspen brace for 10 weeks, soft collar all day for 2 weeks, soft collar at night only for 2 weeks	Miami J for 10–12 weeks	Hard collar for 4 weeks	Collar dependent on bone quality
Follow-up visits	2 weeks, 6 weeks, 3 months, 6 months, 1 year after surgery	4 weeks, 3 months, 6 months, 12 months after surgery	1 month after surgery	2 weeks, 6 weeks, 3 months, 6 months, 12 months after surgery

ACDF, Anterior cervical decompression and fusion; CT, computed tomography; DEXA, dual-energy x-ray absorptiometry; EMG, electromyography; ICU, intensive care unit; IOM, intraoperative monitoring; MAP, mean arterial pressure; MEP, motor evoked potentials; MRI, magnetic resonance imaging; PEEK, polyetheretherketone; PLL, posterior longitudinal ligament; PTH, parathyroid hormone level; SSEP, somatosensory evoked potentials.

Differential diagnosis

- Cervical stenosis
- Intramedullary spinal cord tumor
- Transverse myelitis
- Syringomyelia
- Peripheral nerve entrapment
- Normal pressure hydrocephalus

Important anatomical and preoperative considerations

The pathogenesis of DCM starts with the development of spondylosis. When patients with cervical spondylotic changes progress to spinal cord compression and clinical myelopathy, the condition is established.[1] Nevertheless, spondylosis alone does not account for the generation of symptoms, as static and dynamic factors are both involved in the development of DCM.[5,8] Static factors are related to congenital stenosis, or acquired stenosis, secondary to degenerative processes. Narrowing of the cervical spinal canal is an important predisposing factor for cervical myelopathy. The etiopathogenesis of canal stenosis is markedly diverse. Congenital anomalies such as achondroplasia may be associated to a reduced capacity of the spinal canal to sufficiently protect the spinal cord from ordinary age-related degenerative encroachments. Similarly, fusion of any two cervical vertebrae, as seen in Klippel-Feil syndrome, can lead to accelerated spondylosis.[8,10] Exaggerated spondylotic changes in adjacent segments may also be encountered in patients who underwent surgical fusion of cervical vertebrae.[8,10] Dynamic factors also significantly contribute to the pathological mechanisms producing myelopathy. Cord compression and irritation are exacerbated by neck motion. Stretching of the spinal cord occurs with neck flexion, which causes osteophytic spurs and intervertebral protruding discs to exert compression on the neural tissue. Compression of the spinal cord may also occur between the posterior margin of the vertebral body anteriorly and the laminae or ligamentum flavum posteriorly, principally during hyperextension of the neck.[8,10,11]

The intrinsic properties of the spinal cord seem to influence the development and degree of symptoms in the setting of DSM. The spinal cord is believed to reach its functional tolerance to pressure when the transverse area is reduced to less than 50% to 75% of the normal value. In other words, the degree of spinal cord compression necessary to induce clinical manifestations was determined to be between 50 and 60 mm^2 of its cross-sectional transverse area. These findings, reported by Kadanka et al., were significant when associated with MRI T2 hyperintensities on the spinal cord.[10,12,13] However, the different elements of the spinal cord vary in their susceptibility to external stress. The anterior white columns are relatively resistant to ischemia compared with the rest of the cord, whereas the gray matter is more fragile than the white matter.[13] Also, it has been reported that the spinal cord is more vulnerable to tensile forces than compressive ones.[13] Eventually, chronic compression or stretching of the spinal cord will trigger axonal demyelination, gliosis, scarring, degeneration of the tracts, and atrophy of the anterior horn cells.[3]

In patients with symptomatic DCM, surgical decompression is associated with significant and sustainable improvements in neurological outcomes, functional status, and health-related quality of life.[1,3,4,9] Although no consensus is available regarding the rationale for anterior and posterior approaches, certain characteristics such as the location of the compression, extent of the disease, and clinical features guide the surgical planning.[1,3,5,14] Anterior cervical decompression and fusion (ACDF) is considered the best treatment modality for anterior pathology, especially in the setting of kyphosis or hypolordosis, anterior osteophytes, and disc herniations.[14] ACDF is aimed for direct decompression of the spinal cord from a predominantly ventral pathology and restoration of cervical lordosis. ACDF is usually indicated for single-level to two-level disease.[1,5,6,14] Anterior decompression is relatively contraindicated in cases of stenosis from posterior pathology, compression originated behind the vertebral body, and ossification of the posterior longitudinal ligament (OPLL).[1] Despite this, anterior corpectomy may be a suitable option for patients suffering from severe anterior disease with significant OPLL (>60%).[14] Common complications associated with anterior approaches are dysphagia (incidence ranging from 0% to 24%) especially when treating C4-C6 levels, recurrent laryngeal nerve lesion (8%), and adjacent level disease (38%).[1,14]

In the presence of posterior pathology, a greater number of stenotic segments (>3), ligamentum flavum hypertrophy, and myelopathy on a neutral to lordotic cervical spine favor posterior approaches.[1,3,5,14,15] Posterior techniques include laminectomy alone, laminectomy and fusion, and laminoplasty.[9,14] Despite being an effective treatment for cervical spondylotic myelopathy and OPLL, laminectomy is less advocated in the current literature due to the high rate of postlaminectomy kyphosis and postoperative instability (15%–20%).[5,15] On the other hand, both laminectomy and fusion, as well as laminoplasty, represent effective and safe methods to treat DCM. Moreover, there are no significant differences in postoperative functional status between these procedures.[1,3,5,16] In patients with local kyphosis (>13 degrees), some authors recommend anterior decompression or posterior correction of kyphosis as an adjunct to laminoplasty.[14,15] The main complication associated with posterior approaches is iatrogenic kyphosis, which can occur even with preservation of the posterior elements as in laminoplasty.[1,14,15] Iatrogenic kyphosis is thought to be associated with the removal of the midline tension band when fusion is not performed and has been connected to progressive myelopathy, postural deformity, and intractable pain. The incidence of postlaminectomy kyphosis is around 20%.[1,14] A circumferential approach (combined) is less commonly indicated and is usually recommended for patients with fixed kyphosis, instability, and poor bone quality. An anterior-posterior approach may also be contemplated in the setting of patients with severe kyphotic angulation necessitating decompression of three or more levels.[1]

What was actually done

A C4-C6 anterior cervical corpectomy with anterior C3-C7 and posterior C2-T2 fusion was planned. The patient was brought to the operating room. Following intubation and induction of general anesthesia, the patient was placed in the supine position. All pressure points were padded. The patient's neck was slightly extended. Skin incision was made and dissection was carried out until the platysma was identified. The muscle was opened and the dissection was continued medial to the sternocleidomastoid muscle. Then, the carotid was identified and the dissection was performed medial to it. After opening of the prevertebral fascia, the vertebral body was identified. Fluoroscopy was brought into the procedure and the disc space C3-C4 was confirmed. Exposure was extended to the C6-C7 level. A discectomy was done at C3-C4 and C6-C7 until the posterior longitudinal ligament was identified. A corpectomy was then done from C4 down to C6. The posterior longitudinal ligament was identified and opened. The thecal sac was decompressed. A corpectomy cage was placed and filled with allograft. The cage was expanded to 55 mm. Optimal placement was confirmed with fluoroscopy. Then, a 60-mm four-level anterior plate was secured at C3 and C7. The instrumentation was secured. Platysma was approximated and dermal and wound were closed. The patient was kept intubated and placed in Mayfield pins. The patient was flipped to the prone position. The patient's head was held in a three-pin head holder and secured to the operating table. The planned incision was marked out, and the patient was prepped and draped. Posterior skin incision was done. Dissection was made with Bovie cautery and the spinous processes and laminae were identified. Dissection continued laterally to the lateral masses. In the thoracic spine, the transverse processes was identified. Rostrally, C2 was recognized. Intraoperative fluoroscopy confirmed the axis level. C2 pars screws were placed, followed by lateral mass screws from C3 to C6 except bilaterally at C5, where only screws on the left side were placed. The C7 level was skipped and pedicle screws were placed at T1 and T2. With a high-speed bur, a laminectomy was created from C6 to C7. Bone was elevated and saved for autograft, and the spinal cord was decompressed. A titanium rod was brought into place and cut to fit the instrumentation. The rod was placed, secured in place, and final tightened. Fluoroscopy confirmed good placement of the instrumentation. The wound was irrigated and allograft was placed along the lateral and medial grooves. Intraoperative neuromonitoring was performed during the full case and was maintained throughout the entire case. A drain was placed and the muscle and dermal layer were approximated. The skin was closed. The patient was flipped back to the supine position and kept intubated and transferred to the intensive care unit for observation. The patient tolerated the procedure well without any immediate postoperative complications. The patient was extubated on postoperative day 1, and no dysphagia was noted. At follow-up, the patient reported significant improvement of balance, and x-rays of the cervical spine showed an intact hardware with stable alignment (Fig. 20.3).

Commonalities among the experts

Most of the surgeons requested a medicine evaluation as part of their preoperative assessment. Half opted for dynamic radiographs of the cervical spine. The majority would pursue surgery through a combined (circumferential) approach, and just one surgeon chose a pure anterior decompression. All aimed for decompression of the spinal cord, restoration of cervical alignment, and stabilization of the spine. Most were aware of the vascular structures, esophagus, and critical neural elements. Feared complications varied and included vascular injury, dysphagia, postoperative instability, and damage to the recurrent laryngeal nerve. Surgery was generally attained with fluoroscopy and intraoperative monitoring, with no special perioperative medications. Although surgical schemes were different, most shared the concept of anterior cervical corpectomy and decompression during the first stage, followed by posterior laminectomy and fusion in the second stage. Most admitted their patients to the intensive care unit following surgery. Half requested a cervical CT scan within the first 48 perioperative hours. Most preferred cervical radiographs within the first 6 postoperative weeks. Most recommended follow-up for at least 1 year after surgery. All surgeons advocated for the use of collar after the intervention.

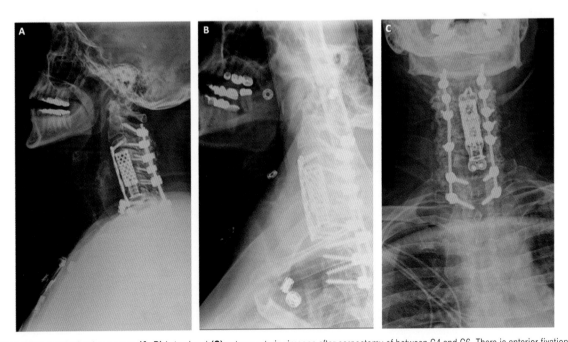

Fig. 20.3 Postoperative cervical spine x-rays. (A–B) Lateral and **(C)** anteroposterior images after corpectomy of between C4 and C6. There is anterior fixation with an anterior plate and screw fixation from C3 to C7. The posterior instrumented fusion extends from C2 to T2. The hardware is intact with stable alignment.

SUMMARY OF QUALITY OF EVIDENCE TO GUIDE SPECIFIC INTERVENTIONS FOR THIS CASE

- Anterior or posterior surgical decompression in cervical myelopathy related to sustainable improved functional outcomes, neurological status, and quality of life: level II.1
- Anterior cervical decompression and fusion for ventral pathology with single-level to two-level disease, kyphosis, and disc herniation: level III
- Posterior decompression for posterior pathology involving more than three segments and ligamentum flavum hypertrophy in a neutral or lordotic cervical spine: level III

REFERENCES

1. Iyer A, Azad TD, Tharin S. Cervical Spondylotic Myelopathy. *Clin Spine Surg*. 2016;29(10):408–414.
2. Karadimas SK, Gatzounis G, Fehlings MG. Pathobiology of cervical spondylotic myelopathy. *Eur Spine J*. 2015;24(Suppl 2): 132–138.
3. Tetreault L, Goldstein CL, Arnold P, et al. Degenerative Cervical Myelopathy: A Spectrum of Related Disorders Affecting the Aging Spine. *Neurosurgery*. 2015;77(Suppl 4):S51–S67.
4. Davies BM, Mowforth OD, Smith EK, Kotter MR. Degenerative cervical myelopathy. *BMJ*. 2018;360:k186.
5. Wilson JR, Tetreault LA, Kim J, et al. State of the Art in Degenerative Cervical Myelopathy: An Update on Current Clinical Evidence. *Neurosurgery*. 2017;80(3s):S33–S45.
6. Montano N, Ricciardi L, Olivi A. Comparison of Anterior Cervical Decompression and Fusion versus Laminoplasty in the Treatment of Multilevel Cervical Spondylotic Myelopathy: A Meta-Analysis of Clinical and Radiological Outcomes. *World Neurosurg*. 2019; 130(530–536):e532.
7. Tracy JA, Bartleson JD. Cervical spondylotic myelopathy. *Neurologist*. 2010;16(3):176–187.
8. Toledano M, Bartleson JD. Cervical spondylotic myelopathy. *Neurol Clin*. 2013;31(1):287–305.
9. Fehlings MG, Ibrahim A, Tetreault L, et al. A global perspective on the outcomes of surgical decompression in patients with cervical spondylotic myelopathy: results from the prospective multicenter AO Spine international study on 479 patients. *Spine (Phila Pa 1976)*. 2015;40(17):1322–1328.
10. Matsunaga S, Komiya S, Toyama Y. Risk factors for development of myelopathy in patients with cervical spondylotic cord compression. *Eur Spine J*. 2015;24(Suppl 2):142–149.
11. Milligan J, Ryan K, Fehlings M, Bauman C. Degenerative cervical myelopathy: Diagnosis and management in primary care. *Can Fam Physician*. 2019;65(9):619–624.
12. Badhiwala JH, Ahuja CS, Akbar MA, et al. Degenerative cervical myelopathy - update and future directions. *Nat Rev Neurol*. 2020;16(2):108–124.
13. Kadanka Z, Kerkovsky M, Bednarik J, Jarkovsky J. Cross-sectional transverse area and hyperintensities on magnetic resonance imaging in relation to the clinical picture in cervical spondylotic myelopathy. *Spine (Phila Pa 1976)*. 2007;32(23):2573–2577.
14. Klineberg E. Cervical spondylotic myelopathy: a review of the evidence. *Orthop Clin North Am*. 2010;41(2):193–202.
15. Cho SK, Kim JS, Overley SC, Merrill RK. Cervical Laminoplasty: Indications, Surgical Considerations, and Clinical Outcomes. *J Am Acad Orthop Surg*. 2018;26(7):e142–e152.
16. Heller JG, Edwards CC, 2nd, Murakami H, Rodts GE. Laminoplasty versus laminectomy and fusion for multilevel cervical myelopathy: an independent matched cohort analysis. *Spine (Phila Pa 1976)*. 2001;26(12):1330–1336.

21

Failed back surgery syndrome

Fidel Valero-Moreno, MD

Introduction

Although the term involves controversy, failed back surgery syndrome (FBSS) is defined as lumbar pain with or without radicular symptom that persists or appears after one or several surgical interventions.[1–3] FBSS is not necessarily the consequence of a failed surgical procedure but rather a mismatch between the outcome and the patient's and surgeon's presurgical expectations.[1,3,4] Specific reasons for pain, including infection, pseudomeningocele, and/or hematoma, should be ruled out before establishing FBSS as a diagnosis.[5,6] The incidence of FBSS ranges between 10% and 40%.[2,7–10] Moreover, low back pain lifetime prevalence is estimated to range between 60% and 85%,[1,3,6,7] with an estimated global incidence of 9.4%.[3] Therefore, low back pain represents a critical health problem and entails significant social, financial, and psychological consequences for the patients.[3] Preoperative patient-related conditions such as anxiety, hypochondriasis, and cognitive impairment may negatively influence surgical outcomes. Similarly, poor patient selection and inadequate surgical planning are well known predisposing factors for the development of this syndrome.[1,7] Insufficient decompression of the lateral recess or the neural foramen is the most common cause of failed surgical technique leading to FBSS, accounting for 25% to 29% of the cases.[6,7] Postoperative issues may also contribute and include recurrent disc herniations (in up to 15% of the patients), epidural fibrosis (20%–36%), and postsurgical instability.[4,6] Diagnosis of this condition must include a careful matching of the clinical presentation with the suspected anatomical anomaly, as well as a psychosocial assessment that includes behavioral elements such as anxiety disorder and secondary gain.[11] Treating patients with chronic pain persisting after spine surgery is extremely challenging and requires multidisciplinary medical approaches.[10] Currently, there are no high-level studies supporting specific management strategies for FBSS.[10,11] However, after excluding clear indications for decompression or restoration of physiological spine balance, treatment of FBSS should begin with conservative management (including cognitive behavioral therapies), followed by minimally invasive procedures, and finally surgical interventions.[1,3,7,11,12] Surgical treatment for FBSS is controversial and is sometimes associated with worsening of the clinical symptoms.[4] Studies report that no more than 30% of the patients have a successful outcome after a second surgery and that the percentage of patients experiencing resolution of their symptoms diminishes with each subsequent surgical procedure.[1,5,7] Therefore, surgical treatment for FBSS is reserved for patients with clear anatomical or pathological cause for their pain, typically after failure of nonsurgical treatment.[7] We present a case of a 63-year-old male presenting with chronic pain and radicular symptoms after multiple spine surgeries and diagnosis concerning for FBSS.

Example case

Chief complaint: lower limb pain

History of present illness: This is a 63-year-old male with a history of multiple lumbar surgeries, including instrumented fusion and three revision laminectomies. The patient presented with persistent bilateral lower extremity pain, with the pain markedly worse in his left leg. His pain has been constant for many years with a recent worsening. His last surgery was 1 year prior and latest imaging showed solid fusion of his lumbar construct. Additionally, a lumbosacral magnetic resonance imaging (MRI) was performed, demonstrating findings compatible with arachnoiditis (Fig. 21.1).

Medications: oxycodone, fentanyl patch

Allergies: no known drug allergies

Past medical and surgical history: chronic pain, previous L2-sacrum fusion and decompression with three revisions and last surgery was complicated by cerebrospinal fluid leakage

Family history: none

Social history: smoker

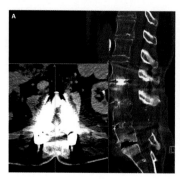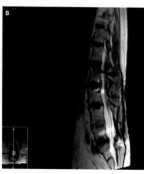

Fig. 21.1 Preoperative images. (A) Computed tomography axial and sagittal views of the lumbosacral spine demonstrating prior solid fusion at L2-S1 levels. There is diffuse osteopenia as well as degenerative changes including irregularities involving the end plates and osteophytes. The patient is markedly hypolordotic at L3 to S1 levels and no compensatory changes are noted. **(B)** T2-sagittal lumbar magnetic resonance images demonstrating the previous fusion at L2 to S1 levels, degenerative changes including osteochondrosis and osteophytes from L2 to L5. There is decreased intervertebral space at L4-L5 and significant disc protrusion at L3-L4 and L5-S1. As mentioned above, loss of lumbar lordosis is evident. There is an image suggestive of lumbosacral arachnoiditis (empty theca sign).

Physical examination: awake, alert, and oriented to person, place, and time; cranial nerves II–XII intact; bilateral deltoids/triceps/biceps 5/5; interossei 5/5; iliopsoas/knee flexion/knee extension/dorsi, and plantar flexion 5/5

Reflexes: 2+ in bilateral biceps/triceps/brachioradialis with negative Hoffman; 2+ in bilateral patella/ankle; no clonus or Babinski; sensation diminished in his lower left limb with an L4, L5 distribution.

	Richard Allen, MD, PhD Jakub Sikora, MD Orthopaedic Surgery University of California at San Diego San Diego, California, United States	Rafid Al-Mahfoudh, MBChB Neurosurgery Brighton and Sussex University Hospitals Brighton, United Kingdom	Aron Lazary, MD, PhD Orthopaedic Surgery Buda Health Center Semmelweis University Budapest, Hungary	Allan D. Levi, MD, PhD Meng Huang, MD Neurosurgery University of Miami Miami, Florida, United States
Preoperative				
Additional tests requested	Full-length standing 36-inch scoliosis x-rays CT T-L spine myelogram DEXA	SPECT CT NCS/EMG L-spine standing x-rays Pain management evaluation	Full spines standing x-rays L-spine flexion-extension x-rays	L-spine upright AP/lateral/flexion-extension x-rays DEXA
Surgical approach selected	Stage 1: posterior removal of instrumentation, L4-S1 revision decompression with laminectomy, L2-4 exploration of fusion Stage 2: L5-S1 ALIF Stage 3: L2-pelvis fusion including pelvic bolts	T9-10 thoracic laminectomy and insertion of spinal cord stimulator lead for trial	Stage 1: removal of S1 implant Stage 2: L5-S1 ALIF	Revision L5-S1 fusion with lateral MIS L5-S1 ALIF (XALIF), prone L5-S1 MIS revision fusion
Goal of surgery	Spinal canal decompression, solid fusion	Pain management	Stabilization, lordosis correction, L5-S1 fusion	Restore intervertebral height, indirect decompression of L5-S1 foramina, achieve solid arthrodesis at L5-S1 with improvement of lordosis to improve spinal-pelvic parameters
Perioperative				
Positioning	Stage 1: prone on Jackson table Stage 2: supine Stage 3: prone on Jackson table	Prone on Montreal mattress	Stage 1: prone Stage 2: supine	Stage 1: right lateral decubitus on radiolucent table Stage 2: prone on Jackson table

	Richard Allen, MD, PhD Jakub Sikora, MD Orthopaedic Surgery University of California at San Diego San Diego, California, United States	Rafid Al-Mahfoudh, MBChB Neurosurgery Brighton and Sussex University Hospitals Brighton, United Kingdom	Aron Lazary, MD, PhD Orthopaedic Surgery Buda Health Center Semmelweis University Budapest, Hungary	Allan D. Levi, MD, PhD Meng Huang, MD Neurosurgery University of Miami Miami, Florida, United States
Surgical equipment	Fluoroscopy Osteotomes Vertebroplasty set	Fluoroscopy Surgical microscope	Fluoroscopy	IOM (MEP, SSEP) Instrument removal set Anterior and posterior instrumentation Pulse oximetry for left leg Fluoroscopy Surgical navigation Isocentric C-arm for cone beam CT Cobalt drill
Medications	Tranexamic acid	None	None	Gabapentin, Celebrex, steroids, bupivacaine liposome injection suspension with bupivacaine 1:1, Toradol
Anatomical considerations	Thecal sac, middle sacral arteries, sympathetic plexus	Thecal sac, lamina	Stage 1: thecal sac Stage 2: peritoneum, iliac artery and veins	Common iliac vessels and branches, peritoneum, ureter, sympathetic plexus
Complications feared with approach chosen	Pseudoarthrosis, vascular complications	Epidural fibrosis	Stage 1: dural tear Stage 2: peritoneal and iliac vessel injury, hypogastric plexus injury	CSF leak
Intraoperative				
Anesthesia	General	General	General	General
Exposure	Stage 1: L2-S1 Stage 2: L5-S1 Stage 3: L2-sacrum	T9-10	Stage 1: L5-S1 Stage 2: L5-S1	Stage 1: L5-S1 anteriorly Stage 2: L5-S1
Levels decompressed	Stage 1: L4-S1 Stage 2: L5-S1 Stage 3: None	T9-10	Stage 1: None Stage 2: L5-S1	L5-S1
Levels fused	Stage 1: L2-S1 Stage 2: L5-S1 Stage 3: L2-pelvis	None	Stage 1: None Stage 2: L5-S1	L5-S1

	Richard Allen, MD, PhD Jakub Sikora, MD Orthopaedic Surgery University of California at San Diego San Diego, California, United States	Rafid Al-Mahfoudh, MBChB Neurosurgery Brighton and Sussex University Hospitals Brighton, United Kingdom	Aron Lazary, MD, PhD Orthopaedic Surgery Buda Health Center Semmelweis University Budapest, Hungary	Allan D. Levi, MD, PhD Meng Huang, MD Neurosurgery University of Miami Miami, Florida, United States
Surgical narrative	Stage 1: position prone, incision over previous midline scar at L2-sacrum, expose previous instrumentation and fusion site, remove all set screws and rods, evaluate L2-4 fusion site and screw stability, leave screws in if no concern of pseudoarthroses, remove screws and upsize and/or redirect if concern of loosening, assess decompression and perform revision laminectomy and decompression L4-S1, place S2 anterior iliac screws, preliminary closure Stage 2 (same day): position supine, vascular surgery performs anterior retroperitoneal approach, L5-S1 annulotomy, release disc space with Cobb retractors, remove disc, expand space further with trials and serially dilate space carefully, decompress entire disc material and take cartilage end plates off, ensure nice punctate bleeding in bone bed before rasping, impact 18/20 degree PEEK cage with BMP-2 and cellular bone matrix, place two stabilizing screws through interbody into L5 and S1, vascular surgery closure Stage 3 (same day): position prone, contour two rods appropriately, place rods with set screws, copiously irrigate, decorticate, place autograft and BMP-2/demineralized bone matrix/cancellous chips, take final AP and lateral image, verify placement of instrumentation, powder vancomycin into wound, layered closure with drain and Marcaine in subcutaneous tissue	Position prone, paramedian needle to localize operative level, midline incision, bilateral muscle dissection, placement of McCulloch retractor, check x-ray to confirm T9-10 level, microscope brought in, laminectomy with high-speed drill, remainder of lamina removed with flavectomy once bone thinned, paddle tunneller and placement of spinal cord stimulator, tunnel out separate incision and connected to further lead that is tunneled percutaneously to the skin, closure in layers	Stage 1: position prone, open caudal 5–6 cm of the posterior scar, dissection down to L5-S1 segment, cut rods under L5 screws and remove S1 screws, layered closure with drain Stage 2: position supine, 6 cm horizontal skin incision half-way between navel and pubic symphysis, explore rectus sheath and cut linea alba, mobilize rectus muscle fibers to left from medial to lateral, explore posterior rectus sheet and use arcuate line to approach retroperitoneal fat, peritoneum bluntly mobilized and retracted cranially, identify left iliac artery by palpation, identify medially the promontorium and bluntly dissect retroperitoneal tissue in front of L5-S1 disc, clean disc surface by blunt dissection with bipolar cautery, cut anterior anulus fibrosus and disc space, place a large hyperlordotic 20–30 degree ALIF cage based on preoperative x-ray filled with synthetic bone substitute or allograft, fix cage with screws or plates, standard closure without drain	Stage 1 (lateral XALIF): right lateral decubitus with left side up on radiolucent table with bed rail mounted retractor holders placed rostral on ipsilateral side and caudal on contralateral side, spine needles and fluoroscopy to localize and guide Wiltse approach to S1 screw heads, inject 5 mL of bupivacaine mixture into tracts prior to opening, incision and monopolar cautery to identify S1 tulip heads, remove set screw, pack off incisions, check cross table AP and mark midline with proper Ferguson angle, true lateral imaging to identify anterior/posterior boundaries of disc space and lordotic angle, extend line anteriorly to midline and split difference with AP mark and ASIS, approach surgeon performs retroperitoneal opening and access to disc space, set retractor blades, confirm disc level and medial-lateral positioning with fluoroscopy, ALIF with sequential distraction/dilation of disc space, achieve 20 degree hyperlordotic implant with proper interference fit, keep trial in place for 5 minutes to ensure no IOM changes from baseline, place implant with extrasmall BMP and cellular allograft, place anterior plate/screws with appropriate size to avoid collision with posterior transpedicular instrumentation, close anterior incision with closure of abdominal wall fascia, staple posterior incision closed. Stage 2 (revision posterior instrumentation): transfer patient prone on Jackson table, right PSIS pin placement with frame, cone beam CT for navigation, reopen incision with navigation guidance to remove L5 set screws, cobalt drill to cut rods proximal to L5 screw head, remove rods and L5-S1 screws, replace with 1 mm larger screws under navigation, retap at S1 with under navigation with powered undersized tap to breach anterior cortical wall to facilitate bicortical fixation, replace roads and screws, final cone beam CT to evaluate hardware, inject remainder of bupivacaine solution into paraspinal muscles, no drain

	Richard Allen, MD, PhD Jakub Sikora, MD Orthopaedic Surgery University of California at San Diego San Diego, California, United States	Rafid Al-Mahfoudh, MBChB Neurosurgery Brighton and Sussex University Hospitals Brighton, United Kingdom	Aron Lazary, MD, PhD Orthopaedic Surgery Buda Health Center Semmelweis University Budapest, Hungary	Allan D. Levi, MD, PhD Meng Huang, MD Neurosurgery University of Miami Miami, Florida, United States
Complication avoidance	Multistaged approach, examine fusion construct, upsize screws if needed, vascular surgery to help with approach, ensure nice punctate bleeding in bone bed before rasping, BMP to help fusion	Spinal cord stimulator trial	Two stage approach, remove implant posteriorly to allow more lordosis anteriorly, anatomical retroperitoneal approach to L5-S1 disc space, dissect with bipolar cautery near disc space, place hyperlordotic ALIF cage	Identify S1 tulips first, retroperitoneal approach, restore lordosis with hyper lordotic implant, keep trial in for 5 minutes to ensure no IOM changes, surgical navigation, bicortical S1 pedicle screws, postinstrumentation cone beam CT
Postoperative				
Admission	Floor	Floor	Floor	Floor/step down unit
Postoperative complications feared	Vascular injury, ileus, FI complications, infections, dural tear	Malposition of stimulator, epidural hematoma	Stage 1: dural tear, infection Stage 2: peritoneal and iliac vessel injury, hypogastric plexus injury	Ileus, L5 nerve root traction injury, ischemic leg, sympathetic plexus injury
Anticipated length of stay	3 days	2–3 days	3 days	2–4 days
Follow-up testing	L-spine x-rays 1 month, 3 months, 6 months, 1 year, 2 years after surgery	Trial stimulation	L-spine x-ray after drain removal	Upright AP/lateral lumbar x-rays
Bracing	TLSO for 12 weeks	None	None	Soft lumbo-sacral orthotic
Follow-up visits	2 weeks, 1 month, 3 months, 6 months, 1 year, 2 years after surgery	1–2 days for implantation of generator if trial stimulation successful	3 months, 6 months, 12 months after surgery	2 weeks after surgery with nurse visit, 6 and 12 weeks with x-rays, 9 months with lumbar CT and 36 in AP and lateral upright x-rays

ALIF, Anterior lumbar interbody fusion; AP, anteroposterior; BMP, bone morphogenic protein; CSF, cerebrospinal fluid; CT, computed tomography; DEXA, dual-energy x-ray absorptiometry; EMG, electromyography; IOM, intraoperative monitoring; MAP, mean arterial pressure; MEP, motor evoked potentials; MIS, minimally invasive surgery; NCS, nerve conduction study; PEEK, polyetheretherketone; PSIS, posterior superior iliac spine; SPECT, single-photon emission computerized tomography; SSEP, somatosensory evoked potentials; TLSO, thoracic lumbar sacral orthosis.

Differential diagnosis

- Recurrent disc herniation
- Hardware malfunction/malposition
- Nerve root compression/foraminal stenosis
- Epidural abscess/hematoma
- Malingering/psychological disorders
- Failed back syndrome

Important anatomical and preoperative considerations

Knowledge of the potential sources of pain in patients with FBSS is critical to accurately diagnosing and treating these conditions.[1,13] Imaging represents the simplest initial approach to this condition; however, a thorough neurological examination and pain evaluation must complement radiological assessment in order to avoid false positive findings. Additional surgical interventions based on incomplete or inaccurate diagnosis carry a high risk of further morbidity.[1,11,13] Therefore, the choice of imaging modality hinges on the underlying suspected diagnosis.[1] Meticulous pain assessment is required and should be aimed at determining its precise location and origin.[3,11,13] Pain patterns vary and may display an axial (low back) or radicular distribution (one or both lower limbs).[4,13] Poorly located pain in a nondermatomal configuration is often associated with psychosocial conditions and sometimes even malingering.[4,13] Lower extremity pain, especially when radiating below the knee, is generally linked to nerve compression. A neglected pathology should be considered as the origin of pain, when the symptoms are similar to the preoperative status.[13] The most common causes include an incorrect site of surgery and insufficient surgery such as missed extruded disc fragment or suboptimal foraminal decompression.[3,13] On the other hand, new onset radicular pain immediately after surgery should raise concern about hardware malposition including pedicle screws and interbody implants.[3,11,13] Hematoma and abscess usually present as a new radicular pain during the early postoperative period (1–5 days).[3] In cases with predominant back pain, symptomatology could be the result of spinal instability, disrupted discs, or facet joint abnormalities.[13]

Image evaluation should start with basic standard radiographs with full standing flexion and extension x-rays. Plain radiographs are useful for assessing spinal deformities, changes in lordosis, and sagittal balance, and may demonstrate spondylolisthesis even with normal magnetic resonance imaging (MRI) results.[1,3,12] However, MRI represents the gold standard for visualization of the spine in FBSS.[1,3,12] MRI allows the differentiation of disc herniation from postsurgical fibrosis, identification of perineural scar tissue, and recurrent disc herniation as the origin of pain.[1] In some cases, visualization of the presence and severity of fibrosis is not possible or not accurate. Therefore more specific diagnostic procedures may be indicated such as epiduroscopy, which identifies severe fibrosis in 91% of the patients.[14,15] Computed tomography (CT) provides a superior image of osseous changes within the spine, including facet arthropathy, dimensions of the canals, and pseudoarthrosis.[3,12] In cases of severe image distortion due to surgical instrumentation, a CT myelography with contrast is indicated.[12]

In patients with FBSS and no indication for urgent surgery, conservative treatment including medication and physical therapy should be the first-line management.[1,3] Additionally, psychotherapy may be effective in certain cases in which stress reduction and cognitive behavioral therapy may translate into pain reduction.[3] Pharmacological treatment is multimodal and sometimes debated (especially opioids).[3] Medications include antiepileptics, nonsteroidal antiinflammatory drugs (NSAIDs), steroids, antidepressants, and opioids. NSAIDs have shown to be superior to placebo for reducing low back pain.[1] Gabapentin and pregabalin (anticonvulsants) are commonly used to treat neuropathic pain and may play a role in preventing postoperative pain.[1,3,7] Moreover, pregabalin is also associated to preoperative pain relief.[1] In most of FBSS cases, opioids or derivatives are required.[7] The use of opioids is currently recommended for only short-term therapy.[7] The combination of naloxone and oxycodone is associated with a lower risk of constipation and a better analgesic effect in comparison to oxycodone or morphine alone.[1,7] However, opioids do not improve long-term pain or functional outcomes.[12] Muscle relaxants such as thiocolchicoside are a reliable treatment option for patients with muscle spasm–associated low back pain.[7]

Spinal cord stimulation (SCS) is often quoted as the most effective modality of semi-invasive treatment in patients with neuropathic limb pain.[1,3] The exact mechanism is not completely understood.[7] The PROCESS study demonstrated improved outcomes with SCS compared with conventional medical medicine (CMM) alone in the treatment of neuropathic pain from FBSS. The percentage of patients experimenting reduction in pain after 6 months of treatment was 9% in the CMM-alone group versus 48% in the CMM + SCS group.[1,3,7,16] Epidural injections are the most commonly used semi-invasive procedure to treat radicular pain.[3,12] Epidural steroids provide limited short-term pain relief and activity improvement through inflammation inhibition.[7,12,17] The main approaches to epidural injection are interlaminar and transforaminal for the lumbar spine and caudal approach for sacral nerve involvement.[3,12] Despite this, due to procedural complexity, the high risk of infection, serious potential neurological complications, and the lack of strong evidence in favor of epidural injections, infiltration should be considered

as a last resort modality.[7,12] As mentioned earlier, surgical management of FBSS can be offered to patients with a clear documented anatomical or pathological cause for their pain who have failed medical or minimal-invasive treatment.[1,3,7,12] Surgery for FBSS is associated with high morbidity and corresponding low rates of success.[3] Moreover, the success rate of surgical intervention decreases with every reoperation.[7,12] Nonetheless, certain irrefutable indications for surgery remain such as bowel or bladder dysfunction, significant myelopathy with obvious neurological impairment, spinal cord injury by screws or rods, instability, and pseudoarthrosis.[7,12]

What was actually done

The patient was admitted to the hospital and thoroughly examined by our team. A judicious neurological and radiographic evaluation was done. Due to the absence of hematoma, abscess, and critical anatomical and hardware-related abnormalities, it was decided that surgical intervention was not the best treatment modality for the patient. Instead, due to the presence of arachnoiditis at the lumbosacral level and the predominant radicular unremitting pain, a thoracic SCS was performed (Fig. 21.2). After the procedure, the patient experienced significant pain relief in both lower extremities.

Commonalities among the experts

All opted for spine x-rays to assess the preoperative status, with half recommending full-length standing x-rays and half dynamic x-rays of the lumbar spine. Also, half requested bone density scans. The majority would perform a posterior revision of the previous fusion, followed by an anterior lumbar interbody fusion (ALIF) at the L5-S1 level. The main goals of the surgery for half of the surgeons were spinal decompression, lordosis correction, and obtaining a solid arthrodesis. Most were cognizant of the thecal sac and local vascular structures. Feared complications greatly varied among surgeons and included pseudoarthrosis, vascular injury, epidural fibrosis, dural tears, and cerebrospinal fluid leak. Surgery was generally pursued with fluoroscopy, microscope, and intraoperative monitoring. There were no commonalities regarding perioperative medications. All admitted their patients to the floor following surgery. Half requested lumbar x-rays before discharge. Half advocated for the use

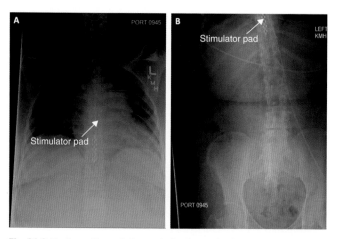

Fig. 21.2 Postoperative anterior-posterior thoracolumbar x-rays. (A) Thoracic and **(B)** lumbar images demonstrating spinal cord stimulator pad at T8-T10 levels. No abnormal displacement is noted.

of thoracic lumbar sacral orthosis. Half advocated for initial follow-up 2 weeks after surgery and periodic radiographic evaluation within at least the first postoperative year.

SUMMARY OF QUALITY OF EVIDENCE TO GUIDE SPECIFIC INTERVENTIONS FOR THIS CASE

- SCS is an effective treatment for neuropathic limb pain with improved outcomes in comparison with conventional medical medicine: level I.
- Epidural steroid injections provide short-term pain relief for radicular symptoms: level II.2.

REFERENCES

1. Daniell JR, Osti OL. Failed Back Surgery Syndrome: A Review Article. *Asian Spine J.* 2018;12(2):372–379.
2. Rigoard P, Gatzinsky K, Deneuville JP, et al. Optimizing the Management and Outcomes of Failed Back Surgery Syndrome: A Consensus Statement on Definition and Outlines for Patient Assessment. *Pain Res Manag.*. 2019;2019:3126464.
3. Baber Z, Erdek MA. Failed back surgery syndrome: current perspectives. *J Pain Res.* 2016;9:979–987.
4. Onesti ST. Failed back syndrome. *Neurologist.* 2004;10(5):259–264.
5. Cho JH, Lee JH, Song KS, et al. Treatment Outcomes for Patients with Failed Back Surgery. *Pain Physician.* 2017;20(1):E29–e43.
6. Chan CW, Peng P. Failed back surgery syndrome. *Pain Med.* 2011;12(4):577–606.
7. Sebaaly A, Lahoud MJ, Rizkallah M, Kreichati G, Kharrat K. Etiology, Evaluation, and Treatment of Failed Back Surgery Syndrome. *Asian Spine J.* 2018;12(3):574–585.
8. Weir S, Samnaliev M, Kuo TC, et al. The incidence and healthcare costs of persistent postoperative pain following lumbar spine surgery in the UK: a cohort study using the Clinical Practice Research Datalink (CPRD) and Hospital Episode Statistics (HES). *BMJ Open.* 2017;7(9):e017585.
9. Shapiro CM. The failed back surgery syndrome: pitfalls surrounding evaluation and treatment. *Phys Med Rehabil Clin N Am.* 2014;25(2):319–340.
10. Chen YC, Lee CY, Chen SJ. Narcotic Addiction in Failed Back Surgery Syndrome. *Cell Transplant.* 2019;28(3):239–247.
11. Hazard RG. Failed back surgery syndrome: surgical and nonsurgical approaches. *Clin Orthop Relat Res.* 2006;443:228–232.
12. Hussain A, Erdek M. Interventional pain management for failed back surgery syndrome. *Pain Pract.* 2014;14(1):64–78.
13. Guyer RD, Patterson M, Ohnmeiss DD. Failed back surgery syndrome: diagnostic evaluation. *J Am Acad Orthop Surg.* 2006;14(9):534–543.
14. Amirdelfan K, Webster L, Poree L, Sukul V, McRoberts P. Treatment Options for Failed Back Surgery Syndrome Patients With Refractory Chronic Pain: An Evidence Based Approach. *Spine (Phila Pa 1976).* 2017;42(Suppl 14):S41–s52.
15. Avellanal M. [Epiduroscopy]. *Rev Esp Anestesiol Reanim.* 2011;58(7):426–433.
16. Kumar K, Taylor RS, Jacques L, et al. Spinal cord stimulation versus conventional medical management for neuropathic pain: a multicentre randomised controlled trial in patients with failed back surgery syndrome. *Pain.* 2007;132(1-2):179–188.
17. Parr AT, Diwan S, Abdi S. Lumbar interlaminar epidural injections in managing chronic low back and lower extremity pain: a systematic review. *Pain Physician.* 2009;12(1):163–188.

22

Osteoporotic compression fracture

Fidel Valero-Moreno, MD

Introduction

Vertebral compression fracture (VCF) is the most common complication of osteoporosis.[1,2] Osteoporotic VCFs can lead to pain, functional disability, and decreased quality of life.[1] These types of fractures are related to significant rates of morbidity and mortality and, with their overall high prevalence, lead to serious health and economic problems.[1,3] VCFs occur in 25% of postmenopausal women over 50 years of age. This increases to 40% in those older than 80 years.[4,5] Furthermore, it is estimated that VCFs affect 700,000 patients in the United States annually.[2,5] These fractures are associated with a 16% reduction in an expected 5-year survival.[1] More than two-thirds of the patients with compression fractures are asymptomatic. When symptoms are present, abrupt onset of axial pain is the most common complaint. Most of the fractures are diagnosed between the T8 and L4 levels.[2] Osteoporotic fractures are associated with anterior loss of vertebral height, kyphosis, and a higher risk for secondary fractures.[2,6] Moreover, spinal deformity is linked to decreased pulmonary function, impaired gait, reduced mobility, and psychosocial stress.[1,4] Lateral radiographs with or without anteroposterior views are usually sufficient for the diagnosis. An anterior wedge fracture is the classical radiographic finding.[2,7] Further imaging is indicated in the setting of neurological deficit or instability assessment.[7] Goals of treatment include pain relief, restoration of function, and prevention of future fractures.[2,4,7] Pain relief is the priority when treating VCFs, especially in the older adult population.[1] Standard nonsurgical management includes bed rest, analgesics, and bracing.[1] Percutaneous vertebral augmentation in the form of vertebroplasty or kyphoplasty is recommended for patients with inadequate pain relief after conservative management.[2,5,8,9] In the uncommon cases with neurological deterioration or instability, surgical intervention should be considered.[8] In this chapter, we present a case of a young patient with a history of metastatic brain cancer and multiple compression fractures in the thoracic and lumbar spine.

Example case

Chief complaint: low back pain

History of present illness:
This is a 46-year-old female patient with a history of metastatic breast cancer who presented with new onset lower back pain and decreased mobility in the setting of osteoporosis. She had a previous spinal radiation and multiple thoracolumbar vertebral fractures treated with kyphoplasty. New spine radiographs demonstrated superior end plate fractures of L2 and L4 (Fig. 22.1).

Medications: fentanyl patch

Allergies: no known drug allergies

Past medical and surgical history: stage IV breast cancer, chronic pain, previous kyphoplasties for pathological vertebral fractures

Family history: none

Social history: former smoker

Physical examination: awake, alert, and oriented to person, place, and time; cranial nerves II–XII intact; bilateral deltoids/triceps/biceps 5/5; interossei 5/5; iliopsoas/knee flexion/knee extension/dorsi, and plantar flexion 5/5

Reflexes: 2+ in bilateral biceps/triceps/brachioradialis with negative Hoffman; 2+ in bilateral patella/ankle; no clonus or Babinski; sensation intact to light touch

	Todd J. Albert, MD Orthopaedic Surgery Hospital for Special Surgery Weill Cornell Medical College New York, New York, United States	Richard J. Bransford, MD Orthopaedic Surgery University of Washington Seattle, Washington, United States	Adrian Casey, MD Neurosurgery National Hospital for Neurosurgery and Neurosurgery Queen Square, Holborn, London, United Kingdom	Nicholas Theodore, MD Dr. A. Karim Ahmed Ann Liu, MD Neurosurgery Johns Hopkins University Baltimore, Maryland, United States
Preoperative				
Additional tests requested	CT T- and L-spine MRI T- and L-spine	DEXA Oncology evaluation	MRI complete spine CT chest/abdomen/pelvis DEXA Oncology evaluation Endocrinology/osteoporosis evaluation	CT T- and L-spine MRI T- and L-spine Standing scoliosis x-rays Oncology evaluation Pain management
Surgical approach selected	L4 vertebroplasty	Pain control	L2 and L4 kyphoplasty	Pain control and TLSO
Goal of surgery	Pain control		Pain control, prevent further collapse and instability	
Perioperative				
Positioning	Prone on Jackson table		Prone on Montreal mattress	
Surgical equipment	Surgical navigation		Surgical navigation Fluoroscopy	
Medications	None		None	
Anatomical considerations	Nerves, vascular structures		Thecal sac, nerve roots	
Complications feared with approach chosen	Cement extrusion, misdirected trocars		Progressive vertebral collapse	
Intraoperative				
Anesthesia	General		General	
Exposure	L4		L2, L4	
Levels decompressed	None		None	
Levels fused	None		None	
Surgical narrative	Position prone, surgical navigation registration, cannulate pedicles, insert cement, standard closure		Position prone, preoperative level check, AP and lateral x-ray for insertion of Jamshidi needles in L2 and L4 pedicles, AP check until posterior wall passed, lateral x-ray check for needle depth, inject cement, check for absence of cement leak, remove needles, standard closure	
Complication avoidance	Surgical navigation		Surgical navigation, x-rays to determine medial-lateral and anterior-posterior needle placement	
Postoperative				
Admission	Floor	Floor	Floor	
Postoperative complications feared	Neurological deterioration, ongoing pain	Neurological deterioration, ongoing pain	Infection, cement leakage, vascular complication	
Anticipated length of stay	Overnight	Overnight	Overnight	
Follow-up testing	AP/lateral T- and L-spine x-rays prior to discharge and 3 months after surgery	AP/lateral T- and L-spine x-rays 3 weeks after discharge	L-spine x-rays 3–6 weeks after surgery MRI or CT L-spine 6 weeks after surgery if needed	Standing scoliosis x-rays within 72 hours and 6 weeks after discharge
Bracing	None	TLSO for comfort	None	TLSO when out of bed for 8 weeks
Follow-up visits	2–3 weeks	3 weeks after discharge	6 weeks after surgery	2 weeks and 6 weeks after discharge

AP, Anteroposterior; *CT*, computed tomography; *DEXA*, dual-energy x-ray absorptiometry; *MRI*, magnetic resonance imaging; *TLSO*, thoracic lumbar sacral orthosis.

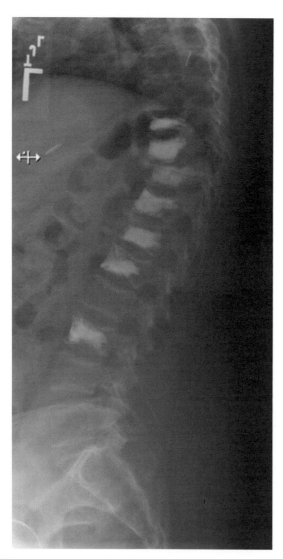

Fig. 22.1 Preoperative radiographs of the thoracolumbar spine. Lateral x-rays showing previous T8-T12 deformities and kyphoplasties. There is marked thoracic kyphosis, more evident at a previously treated compression fracture at T9. There is multilevel disc space narrowing and the presence of superior end plates fractures of the L2 and L4 vertebrae with mild compression deformity. L1 and L3 compression fractures with prior augmentations.

Differential diagnosis

- Osteoarthritis
- Musculoskeletal pain
- Spinal stenosis
- Multiple myeloma
- Bone neoplasms
- Metastatic tumors
- Osteomyelitis
- Scheuermann disease

Important anatomical and preoperative considerations

Osteoporotic fractures of the vertebral column are commonly associated with anatomical and mechanical changes such as diminished ventral height of vertebrae, increased kyphosis, and predisposition to secondary fractures.[1] The frequency of

secondary fractures increases with the number of deformities.[1,6] Once a patient develops a compression fracture, the risk of another fracture, independent of bone density status, increases fivefold.[10] Most of the VCFs occur at the thoracolumbar junction (T12-L2) and the midthoracic region (T6-T8).[7,10] VCFs involve a particular mechanism that is characterized by collapsed trabecular bone rather than a break.[10] These fractures can be classified in three types and based on the portion of the body affected.[10] Half of all compression fractures are wedge-type, involving compression of the anterior segment of the vertebral body. Wedge variant fractures usually occurs at the midthoracic region.[10] Biconcave type fractures represent approximately 17% of the compression fractures. The central part of the vertebral body is compressed while the anterior and posterior remain unaffected.[10] The third type is the crush fracture, accounting for about 13% of VCFs. This involves either compression of the entire anterior or posterior portions of the vertebral body.[10] Some vertebral fractures may be considered unstable. Fractures with more than 50% loss of vertebral height, significant fragment retropulsion, more than 25 to 35 degrees of kyphosis, and fractures with significant involvement of the posterior ligamentous elements should be considered unstable.[7] Compression fractures in the lumbar spine may cause greater disability than those in the throacic region.[10]

Initial imaging studies include anteroposterior and lateral radiographs of the spine. Well demarcated fracture lines may suggest an acute condition, whereas sclerotic margins and osteophytes would point to a chronic fracture.[7] Characteristic radiographic findings of VCFs include a decrease in vertebral body height of at least 20% or a 4 mm reduction from the original height.[2] Intravertebral clefts can be a radiographic sign of avascular necrosis in the vertebral body.[10] Magnetic resonance imaging (MRI) and computed tomography (CT) are indicated for fractures extending to the posterior column or when there is suspected retropulsion or spinal cord/nerve roots involvement.[2,7] In patients with no symptom relief after conservative treatment, or progressive neurological signs, CT or MRI should be considered.[2] Dual-energy x-ray absorptiometry (DEXA) should be considered in patients harboring VCFs to evaluate for osteoporosis and determine disease severity.[2]

The main goals of the treatment for VCFs are pain relief, mobility restoration, and risk reduction for deformity and further vertebral fractures.[10] The initial strategy to treat VCFs has been conservative management including bed rest, analgesics, and bracing.[1,3,4,7,10,11] Initial therapy usually includes narcotic analgesics, use of an external orthosis, and the administration of calcitonin.[4] However, conservative treatment often fails. Medical management is frequently ineffective to reduce pain, improve mobility, and restore vertebral height or realignment.[1,2,4,10,12] Just 50% of the patients receiving conservative management will achieve pain reduction, and most of them fail within the first 3 months of treatment.[2] Moreover, although narcotics attain good rates of pain control, they are poorly tolerated by the older adult population due to significant side effects such as constipation, confusion, and respiratory depression.[4] Bed rest as part of the management for VCFs should be carried out cautiously as prolonged inactivity is linked to further loss of bone mass and deep venous thrombosis (DVT).[2,13] External orthosis is most commonly used to prevent kyphotic deformity; however, there is a lack of evidence to support its efficacy.[4,7]

Percutaneous vertebral augmentation should be offered when conservative methods have not provided pain relief or in the setting of unremitting pain affecting the patient's quality of life.[1-3,5,9] Surgically treated patients have a 43% reduced risk in mortality compared with nonsurgically treated patients.[1] Vertebral augmentation procedures include percutaneous vertebroplasty (PVP) and balloon kyphoplasty (BKP). Both methods focus on preventing further loss of vertebral height, correcting kyphotic deformity, and decreasing pain.[2,10,12] Immediate pain relief is experienced by 85% to 95% of the patients after undergoing one of these procedures[10] and is associated with significantly greater pain relief, decreased kyphosis, functional recuperation, and improvement in quality of life compared with nonsurgical treatments.[3,5,11,12] PVP is attained through a percutaneous transpedicular injection of liquid cement, medical cement, or polymethylmethacrylate (PMMA) into a collapsed vertebral body without previous balloon inflation.[2,4,7] PVP can reduce pain in up to 75% to 100% of the patients shortly after the procedure. The mean volume of cement injected is 2.2 mL.[10] In BKP, a balloon is used in the first stage to create a cavity in the broken vertebra, which allows for compaction of the spongy bone pushing the end plates in the cranial and caudal directions, thus increasing the vertebral body height.[10] The second stage, after removal of the inflatable tamps, is followed by the injection of PMMA.[1,10,12] The mean volume of cement injected is 3.9 mL.[10] Kyphoplasty is able to restore vertebral height by 50% to 70% and reduce kyphosis by 6 to 10 degrees.[10] BKP and PVP outcomes in terms of pain reduction are similar, whereas the degree of increase of vertebral body height and reduction of the kyphotic angle is superior after BKP.[1,3] Cement leakage and new adjacent or nonadjacent vertebral fractures are the most common complications associated with these procedures.[1] Cement leakage is usually asymptomatic and its overall rate is 14.6%. This complication is generally more pronounced after PVP.[1] New fractures of vertebrae occur after PVP and BKP at approximately equivalent rates.[1]

What was actually done

The patient was consented for a balloon kyphoplasty of L2 and L4. The patient was brought to the operating room and induced under general anesthesia. The patient was positioned prone on a Jackson table and all the pressure points were carefully padded. Fluoroscopy was brought into position. The L2 fracture was treated first, followed by the L4 level. The pedicles were marked out on the skin with the assistance of AP fluoroscopy. A dissector canula was passed down the left L2 pedicle into the vertebral body. The trocar was removed, leaving the working canula in place. The tract was drilled and the balloon was placed. Similar procedure was performed on the right side. The balloons were inflated to a total volume of 2.5 mL and maximum pound force per square inch (psi) of 190 on each side. After this, the balloons were deflated and removed. Under live lateral fluoroscopy, PMMA was injected into each side of the vertebral body to a total fill of 2.4 mL bilaterally. On the L4 level, the balloons were inflated to a total volume of 1.5 mL on the right side and 2.5 mL on the left, with a maximum psi of 185 bilaterally. Under live lateral fluoroscopy, PMMA was slowly injected to a total fill of 1.5 mL on the right and 2.5 mL on the left. All cannulas were removed, and anteroposterior

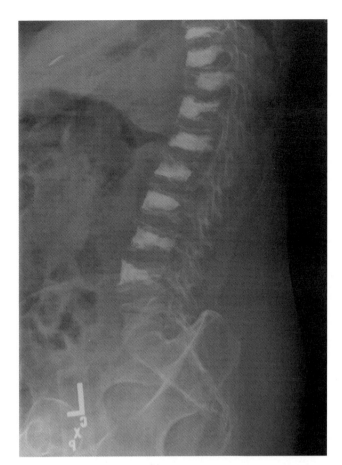

Fig. 22.2 Postoperative plain lateral radiographs of the lumbar spine showing good deposition of cement within the L2 and L4 vertebrae. There is no evidence of new compression fractures, and the lumbar lordosis is maintained. No listhesis is noted.

and lateral fluoroscopy showed good location and volume of the cement. The patient was taken to the recovery room in stable condition. The patient was discharged home the same day. At the first follow-up, the patient showed excellent progress and was pain-free. Plain radiographs showed cement deposition in both vertebrae and no evidence of new fractures (Fig. 22.2).

Commonalities among the experts

The majority of the surgeons opted for an MRI of the thoracic and lumbar spine as additional preoperative assessment. Half would complement their evaluation with a CT scan of the thoracolumbar spine and a DEXA. Treatment strategies greatly varied among experts, where half would pursue conservative modalities including pain control and thoracolumbar orthosis, one would perform vertebroplasty, and one surgeon recommended kyphoplasty. All aimed for pain control as the main goal of management. Although therapeutic approaches varied, most were concerned about the likelihood of neurological deterioration. Physicians performing vertebral augmentation were cognizant of the nerve roots and vascular structures. The most feared complication related to the procedure was cement extrusion. Vertebral augmentation was attained with surgical navigation and fluoroscopy. Following treatment, all admitted their patients to the floor. Anteroposterior and lateral radiographs before discharge were recommended by one surgeon, and after discharge by the rest. All advocated for follow-up between 3 and 6 weeks after discharge.

SUMMARY OF QUALITY OF EVIDENCE TO GUIDE SPECIFIC INTERVENTIONS FOR THIS CASE

- Vertebral augmentation with vertebroplasty or balloon kyphoplasty, reduce pain associated to VCFs, and improve function compared with conservative management: level I
- BKP and PVP show similar efficiency in terms of pain reduction and restoration of function: level I
- BKP increases vertebral body height and reduces kyphotic wedge angle more than PVP: level I

REFERENCES

1. Boonen S, Wahl DA, Nauroy L, et al. Balloon kyphoplasty and vertebroplasty in the management of vertebral compression fractures. *Osteoporos Int*. 2011;22(12):2915–2934.
2. McCarthy J, Davis A. Diagnosis and Management of Vertebral Compression Fractures. *Am Fam Physician*. 2016;94(1):44–50.
3. Svedbom A, Alvares L, Cooper C, Marsh D, Ström O. Balloon kyphoplasty compared to vertebroplasty and nonsurgical management in patients hospitalised with acute osteoporotic vertebral compression fracture: a UK cost-effectiveness analysis. *Osteoporos Int*. 2013;24(1):355–367.
4. Goldstein CL, Chutkan NB, Choma TJ, Orr RD. Management of the Elderly With Vertebral Compression Fractures. *Neurosurgery*. 2015;77(Suppl 4). S33-45.
5. Savage JW, Schroeder GD, Anderson PA. Vertebroplasty and kyphoplasty for the treatment of osteoporotic vertebral compression fractures. *J Am Acad Orthop Surg*. 2014;22(10):653–664.
6. Lee JH, Lee DO, Lee JH, Lee HS. Comparison of radiological and clinical results of balloon kyphoplasty according to anterior height loss in the osteoporotic vertebral fracture. *Spine J*. 2014;14(10): 2281–2289.
7. Musbahi O, Ali AM, Hassany H, Mobasheri R. Vertebral compression fractures. *Br J Hosp Med (Lond)*. 2018;79(1):36–40.
8. Bernardo WM, Anhesini M, Buzzini R. Osteoporotic vertebral compression fracture - Treatment with kyphoplasty and vertebroplasty. *Rev Assoc Med Bras (1992)*. 2018;64(3):204–207.
9. Courtney SW, Radcliffe E, Cress L, West B. What are the best treatments for reducing osteoporotic compression fracture pain? *J Fam Pract*. 2019;68(1):E28–e29.
10. Dewar C. Diagnosis and treatment of vertebral compression fractures. *Radiol Technol*. 2015;86(3):301–320. quiz 321-303.
11. Voormolen MH, Mali WP, Lohle PN, et al. Percutaneous vertebroplasty compared with optimal pain medication treatment: short-term clinical outcome of patients with subacute or chronic painful osteoporotic vertebral compression fractures. The VERTOS study. *AJNR Am J Neuroradiol*. 2007;28(3):555–560.
12. Yuan WH, Hsu HC, Lai KL. Vertebroplasty and balloon kyphoplasty versus conservative treatment for osteoporotic vertebral compression fractures: A meta-analysis. *Medicine (Baltimore)*. 2016;95(31):e4491.
13. Esses SI, McGuire R, Jenkins J, et al. The treatment of symptomatic osteoporotic spinal compression fractures. *J Am Acad Orthop Surg*. 2011;19(3):176–182.

23

Hangman's fracture

Oluwaseun O. Akinduro, MD

Introduction

Traumatic fractures of the second cervical vertebra account for nearly 20% of all acute cervical spinal fractures with approximately 8.5% of surviving patients having neurological deficits after the injury.[1] The low rate of neurological deficits with these injuries has been attributed to the relatively wide canal at the level of the axis.[2] C2 fractures can be classified as odontoid fractures, hangman's fractures, or fractures of the body of C2. Bilateral fractures of the par interarticularis are termed *hangman's fractures*. They were first described in 1866 by Samuel Haughton after noting this fracture pattern in people who had been subjected to execution by hanging.[3] This was termed traumatic spondylolisthesis of the axis when it was noted that this same fracture pattern was seen in many individuals after motor vehicle collisions. The mechanism of injury that was originally described for hangman's fractures was hyperextension and distraction, but modern-day hangman's fractures seen after motor vehicle collisions are typically caused by hyperextension and compression.[4] The most commonly used classification scheme for axis fracture is a modification of the Effendi classification, which classifies fractures based on their morphology (Table 23.1).[5,6] Most patients with stable traumatic spondylolisthesis of the axis can be managed with traction and external orthosis.[7] Surgery is generally preferred for type III fractures and those who fail to achieve proper alignment with traction and immobilization. In this chapter, we will review the case of a patient with a C2 hangman fracture and review the pertinent anatomy, treatment options, and final treatment strategy for this specific case.

Example case

Chief complaint: neck pain after motor vehicle collision
History of present illness: This is a 52-year-old female who presented to the emergency room with neck pain after a motor vehicle collision. She has midline neck tenderness to palpation. She does not have any neurological symptoms in her extremities. Computed tomography scans of the cervical spine were obtained, which revealed evidence of a fracture through bilateral pars interarticularis (Fig. 23.1).
Medications: antidepressants
Allergies: no known drug allergies
Past medical history: depression, anxiety
Past surgical history: noncontributory
Family history: none
Social history: none
Physical examination: awake, alert, and oriented to person, place, and time; cranial nerves II–XII intact; bilateral deltoids/triceps/biceps 5/5; interossei 5/5; iliopsoas/knee flexion/knee extension/dorsi, and plantar flexion 5/5
Reflexes: 2+ in bilateral biceps/triceps/brachioradialis with negative Hoffman; 2+ in bilateral patella/ankle; no clonus or Babinski; sensation intact to light touch
Laboratories: all within normal limits

Table 23.1 Effendi and Levine Classification for Traumatic Spondylolisthesis of C2

	Description	Stability	Management
Type I	Fracture lines vertical and posterior to vertebral body	Stable	Cervical collar or halo
Type II	>3mm of subluxation, disruption of C2–3 disk	May lead to early instability	Halo traction and then immobilization in a halo vest; may require stabilization for instability
Type IIA	Oblique fracture with >11 degrees angulation	Unstable	No traction with increased angulation; may need stabilization
Type III	Disruption of the bilateral C2–3 joint	Unstable	Surgical stabilization

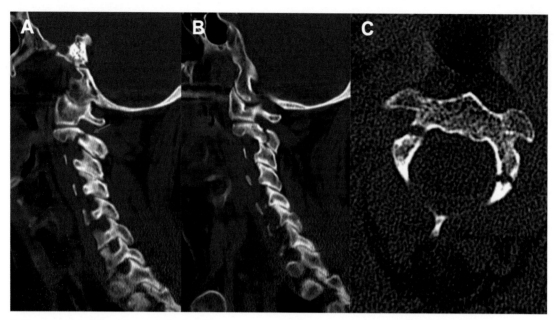

Fig. 23.1 Computed tomography imaging of the cervical spine. (A) Sagittal image through the left pars interarticularis. **(B)** Sagittal image through the right pars interarticularis. **(C)** Axial image at the level of C2 revealing bilateral obliquely oriented fractures through the C2 pars interarticularis. Red arrow highlights fracture line.

	Ali A Baaj, MD Neurosurgery Weill Cornell New York, New York, United States	Ahmed S. Barakat, MD Orthopaedic Surgery University of Cairo Cairo, Egypt	Michael G. Fehlings, MD, PhD Neurosurgery University of Toronto Western Toronto, Canada	Alexander R. Vaccaro, MD, PhD, MBA Orthopaedic Surgery Thomas Jefferson University Philadelphia, Pennsylvania, United States
Preoperative				
Additional tests requested	MRI C-spine to assess ligaments and spinal cord CTA to assess vertebral artery	Flexion-extension cervical x-rays under supervision MRI C-spine CTA C-spine	MRI C-spine CTA to assess vertebral artery CT complete spine AP/lateral cervical x-rays	MRA or CTA to evaluate vertebral arteries
Surgical approach selected	Posterior C1-C3 fusion	Conservative management	Hard collar initially, if there is nonunion or displacement then posterior C1-3 fusion	Hard collar for 6 weeks
If young patient	Potential collar	Same approach	Same approach	Same approach
If older adult patient	Fusion	Same approach	Fusion	Same approach
Goal of surgery	Prevent subluxation and spinal cord injury		Achieve fusion, long-term stability, maintain neurological status	
Perioperative				
Positioning	Prone with Mayfield pins		Prone with Mayfield pins	
Surgical equipment	IOM Surgical navigation or fluoroscopy		IOM (MEP/SSEP) Surgical microscope O-arm Surgical navigation BMP	
Medications	+/- Steroids, maintain MAPs		None	
Anatomical considerations	Vertebral artery, avoid spinal manipulation		Vertebral artery, C2 pedicle anatomy, spinal cord, dura, C2 nerve roots	

	Ali A Baaj, MD Neurosurgery Weill Cornell New York, New York, United States	Ahmed S. Barakat, MD Orthopaedic Surgery University of Cairo Cairo, Egypt	Michael G. Fehlings, MD, PhD Neurosurgery University of Toronto Western Toronto, Canada	Alexander R. Vaccaro, MD, PhD, MBA Orthopaedic Surgery Thomas Jefferson University Philadelphia, Pennsylvania, United States
Complications feared with approach chosen	Pseudoarthrosis, spinal cord injury		Pseudoarthrosis, spinal cord injury, vertebral artery injury, C2 neuralgia, epidural bleeding, malpositioned instrumentation	
Intraoperative				
Anesthesia	General		General	
Exposure	C1-3		C1-3	
Levels decompressed	None		None	
Levels fusion	C1-3		C1-3	
Surgical narrative	Head is pinned, placed prone with care, fluoroscopy to confirm cervical alignment, subperiosteal dissection from C1-3, bilateral lateral mass screws at C1 and C3, secure with rods, decortication of joins and auto/allograft used for fusion		Asleep fiberoptic intubation, head is pinned, sandwich flip using Allen table, position prone with pins, posterior midline incision, expose C1-3, attach reference frame, O-arm spin, expose C1 lateral mass with control of epidural venous plexus, section C2 nerve roots in preganglionic fashion if needed, drill and tap C1 lateral masses/left C2 pedicle/C3 lateral masses, place polyaxial screws and connect with rods, remove C2-3 spinous process, combine autograft with small unit of BMP for bone grafting, decorticate posterior elements of C1-3, place local bone graft and BMP, layered closure with subfascial drain, local wound anesthetic and vancomycin powder	
Complication avoidance	Surgical navigation, limit to C1-3		Fiberoptic intubation, sandwich flip, surgical navigation, limit to C1-3, preganglionic section C2 if needed to assess C1 lateral mass, avoid right C2 pedicle, BMP	
Postoperative				
Admission	Stepdown unit	Floor	Stepdown unit	Floor
Postoperative complications feared	Infection, vertebral artery injury		Infection, non/union, hardware failure, epidural hematoma, C2 neuralgia	
Anticipated length of stay	2-3 days	1 day	3 days	1 day
Follow-up testing	CT C-spine or x-rays	AP and lateral cervical x-rays 2 weeks after discharge CT cervical spine 8 weeks after discharge Cervical x-rays flexion-extension 8 weeks, 6 months, 24 months after discharge	Cervical x-rays 6 weeks, 3 months, 6 months, 12 months, 24 months after surgery CT C-spine 6 months after surgery	Cervical x-rays 6 weeks, 3 months, 6 months after discharge

	Ali A Baaj, MD Neurosurgery Weill Cornell New York, New York, United States	Ahmed S. Barakat, MD Orthopaedic Surgery University of Cairo Cairo, Egypt	Michael G. Fehlings, MD, PhD Neurosurgery University of Toronto Western Toronto, Canada	Alexander R. Vaccaro, MD, PhD, MBA Orthopaedic Surgery Thomas Jefferson University Philadelphia, Pennsylvania, United States
Bracing	Cervical collar when out of bed	Aspen collar for 8 weeks	Hard collar for 6 weeks	Hard collar for 6 weeks
Follow-up visits	2 weeks for wound check; 3, 12, and 24 months with x-rays	2 weeks	6 weeks, 3 months, 6 months, 12 months, 24 months after surgery	6 weeks, 3 months, 6 months after discharge

AP, Anteroposterior; *CT*, computed tomography; *CTA*, computed tomography angiography; *BMP*, bone morphogenic protein; *IOM*, intraoperative monitoring; *MAP*, mean arterial pressure; *MEP*, motor evoked potentials; *MRA*, magnetic resonance angiography; *MRI*, magnetic resonance imaging; *SSEP*, somatosensory evoked potentials.

Differential diagnosis

- Axis fracture
- Atlas fracture
- Cervical muscle strain
- Spinal cord injury

Important anatomical considerations

The second cervical vertebra has multiple neurovascular associations that must be considered when planning either anterior or posterior approach to the region. The C1-2 joint also allows for a significant portion of the flexion, extension, and axial rotation of the cervical spine, so preservation of this motion should be a priority for fractures that are deemed stable. The third segment of the vertebral artery may be encountered during lateral dissection of the C2 lateral mass in the foramen transversarium. The artery then courses medially behind the lateral mass of C1 prior to entering a groove along the rostral surface of the lateral portion of the posterior arch of C1 prior to extending superiorly into the foramen magnum.[8] The vertebral artery can be found in the suboccipital triangle, bordered by the rectus capitis posterior major and the superior and inferior oblique muscles. The location of the C2 nerve roots nerve roots may obstruct placement of C1 lateral mass screws, as the screw may be in contact with the nerve root causing pain and discomfort for patients. The C2 nerve root may be sacrificed without clinically significant sequelae other than numbness in the posterior aspect of the head. The C2 pedicle must be reviewed preoperatively to determine the feasibility of C2 pedicle screws. It is important to review the pedicle anatomy with thin cut multiplanar CT images, as the pedicle size will vary according the plane of the axial images.[9,10] When approaching the upper cervical spine from an anterior approach, one must review the relationship of the carotid artery, esophagus, trachea, vagus nerve, and the hypoglossal nerve. The hypoglossal nerve may be encountered behind the posterior belly of the digastric muscle during dissection in the upper cervical spine, thus care must be taken to avoid a postoperative deficit.

Approaches to this lesion

Management approaches for hangman's fractures include traction with halo immobilization, anterior cervical decompression and fusion (ACDF) of C2-C3, and posterior cervical instrumentation from C1 to C3. There is a wide range of posterior instrumentation techniques, with the Gallie fusion being one of the earliest to be described, being the Gallie fusion, which involves use of a bone graft that is secured with a wire under the C1 lamina and the C2 spinous process.[11] Posterior instrumentation techniques have evolved over time, and now the most commonly used method for fixation is C1 lateral mass screws with C2 pars or pedicle screws. Posterior instrumentation techniques result in excellent fusion rates, but the range of motion of the atlanto-axial joint is eliminated, restricting head on neck rotation. For this reason, many surgeons opt for an ACDF in order to partially preserve this motion across the C1-2 joint. An ACDF of C1-2 is challenging due to the rotral location and corresponding neurovascular structures. This should only be performed by experienced spine surgeons with possible inclusion of an experienced head and neck surgeon.

What was actually done

This patient presented with pain in her neck due to a hangman's fracture and also had pain secondary to a fractured left forearm, a fractured sternum, and an L1 compression fracture. She was managed conservatively and has progressively improved in her pain, although it did not get completely back to normal. She was placed into a rigid cervical collar and had a follow-up computed tomography (CT) scan of the cervical spine at 1-month intervals. She was seen in clinic at 4 months after her accident and had incomplete healing of her fracture line at that time, but she was doing well clinically. At 6 months after her accident, she was seen in the clinic and had complete absence of neck pain. Flexion-extension imaging, as well as repeat CT scan of the cervical spine, revealed no motion and partial healing of the fracture (Figs. 23.2 and 23.3). At this time, she was weaned from her cervical collar.

Commonalities among the experts

There was a general consensus among the experts as to the necessity of further advanced imaging. All four experts planned for magnetic resonance imaging (MRI) and a CT angiogram to evaluate the ligamentous structures and the vertebral artery. Three experts planned for conservative management, with one of them opting to proceed with surgery if management in a cervical collar resulted in nonunion or fracture displacement. One surgeon planned for posterior C1-3 fusion to prevent fracture subluxation and subsequent spinal cord injury. The surgeon that planned for surgical management with failed conservative management also planned for a posterior C1-3 fusion with lateral mass screws at C1 and C3. All surgeons planned for follow-up imaging, but there was variation in the time points, with only two surgeons obtaining imaging up to 24 months after the injury.

SUMMARY OF QUALITY OF EVIDENCE TO GUIDE SPECIFIC INTERVENTIONS FOR THIS CASE

■ Hangman's fractures may initially be managed with external immobilization in most cases using either a halo or cervical collar: level III
■ Surgical stabilization should be considered in cases of severe angulation of C2 on C3 and when the C2-3 facet joint is disrupted: level III
■ Fractures with <11 degrees of angulation may be initially reduced using cervical traction: level III

REFERENCES

1. Greene KA, Dickman CA, Marciano FF, Drabier JB, Hadley MN, Sonntag VK. Acute axis fractures. Analysis of management and outcome in 340 consecutive cases. *Spine (Phila Pa 1976)*. 1997;22:1843–1852.
2. Mollan RA, Watt PC. Hangman's fracture. *Injury*. 1982;14:265–267.
3. Haughton, S. (1866). IV. On hanging, considered from a mechanical and physiological point of view. The London Edinburgh and Dublin Philosophical Magazine and Journal of Science, 32(213), 23–34.
4. Pryputniewicz DM, Hadley MN. Axis fractures. *Neurosurgery*. 2010;66:68–82.
5. Effendi B, Roy D, Cornish B, Dussault RG, Laurin CA. Fractures of the ring of the axis. A classification based on the analysis of 131 cases. *J Bone Joint Surg Br*. 1981;63-B:319–327.
6. Levine AM, Edwards CC. The management of traumatic spondylolisthesis of the axis. *J Bone Joint Surg Am*. 1985;67:217–226.
7. Francis WR, Fielding JW, Hawkins RJ, Pepin J, Hensinger R. Traumatic spondylolisthesis of the axis. *J Bone Joint Surg Br*. 1981;63-B:313–318.
8. Tubbs RS, Shah NA, Sullivan BP, Marchase ND, Cohen-Gadol AA. Surgical anatomy and quantitation of the branches of the V2 and V3 segments of the vertebral artery. Laboratory investigation. *J Neurosurg Spine*. 2009;11:84–87.
9. Davidson CT, Bergin PF, Varney ET, Jones LC, Ward MS. Planning C2 pedicle screw placement with multiplanar reformatted cervical spine computed tomography. *J Craniovertebr Junction Spine*. 2019;10:46–50.
10. Yin D, Oh G, Neckrysh S. Axial and oblique C2 pedicle diameters and feasibility of C2 pedicle screw placement: Technical note. *Surg Neurol Int*. 2018;9:40.
11. Gallie WE. Skeletal Traction in the Treatment of Fractures and Dislocations of the Cervical Spine. *Ann Surg*. 1937;106:770–776.

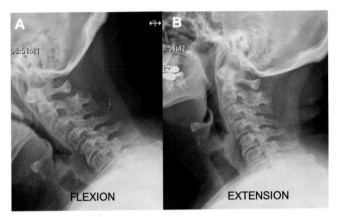

Fig. 23.2 Lateral x-rays of the cervical spine. (A) Flexion and **(B)** extension images reveal no evidence of dynamic instability.

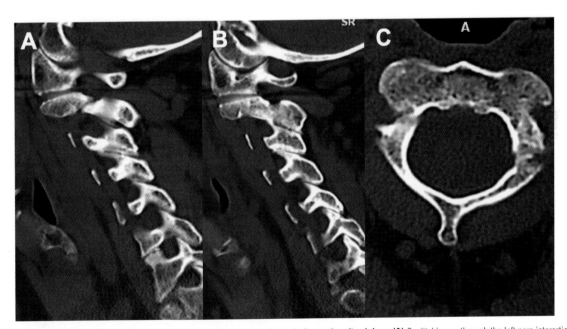

Fig. 23.3 Computed tomography imaging of the cervical spine obtained approximately 6 months after injury. (A) Sagittal image through the left pars interarticularis. **(B)** Sagittal image through the right pars interarticularis. **(C)** Axial image at the level of C2 redemonstrates obliquely oriented fractures through bilateral pars interarticularis. There is evidence of formation of bone into the fracture lines, indicating partial healing.

24

Compression fracture with back pain

Kingsley Abode-Iyamah, MD

Introduction

Osteoporotic vertebral fracture is increasing in prevalence with our aging population. It has a reported incidence of 30% to 50% in those over the age of 50.[1] This condition often affects postmenopausal women and can result spontaneously or following minor trauma. Osteoporotic fractures are suspected to total more than 3 million by 2025, which is an increase of 48%, surpassing a national burden of $25 billion dollars in 2025 with a cumulative 10-year burden of $228 billion.[2,3] Vertebral compression fractures result in frequent neurosurgical consultation particularly in older adult and postmenopausal women.[4,5] The most common presenting symptom is back pain. Occasionally, patients may complain of subjective weakness secondary to limited mobility and pain but without objective findings. Rarely, neurological deficit can occur from compression of the nerve root or compression of the spinal cord. The treatment is typically nonsurgical, although in rare causes surgical intervention may be warranted. The Thoracolumbar Injury Classification and Severity score has been developed and widely accepted as a scoring system to identify those requiring surgical intervention by scoring based on fracture type, neurological deficit, and integrity of posterior ligament complex (Table 24.1).[5]

Example case

Chief complaint: back pain
History of present illness: A 62-year-old female with a history of seizures suffered a fall and presented with back pain. She was admitted for ongoing back pain, which was poorly controlled. The pain improved in the recumbent position and worsened with ambulation. She denies weakness or bowel/bladder dysfunction. She underwent imaging which revealed a compression fracture (Figs. 24.1–24.3).
Medications: none
Allergies: no known drug allergies
Past medical and surgical history: hypertension, osteoporosis, reflux
Family history: noncontributory

Table 24.1 Thoracolumbar Injury Classification and Severity score used to guide management of thoracolumbar fractures

Morphology	Compression	1
	Burst	2
	Translation/rotation	3
	Distraction	4
Neurological status	Intact	0
	Nerve root	2
	Complete cord	2
	Incomplete cord	3
	Cauda equina	3
Integrity of posterior ligamentous complex	Intact	0
	Suspected	2
	Injured	3
Total points		0–3 nonsurgical
		4 +/– surgery
		>4 surgery

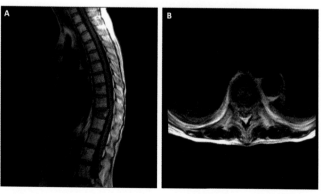

Fig. 24.1 Preoperative magnetic resonance imaging. (A) T2 sagittal and **(B)** T2 axial images demonstrating T10 compression fracture with focal kyphosis.

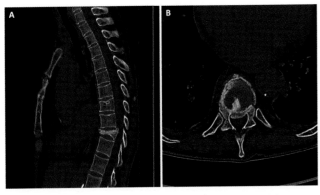

Fig. 24.2 Preoperative computed tomography scans. (A) Sagittal and **(B)** axial images demonstrating a T10 compression fracture with focal kyphosis.

Social history: office worker, no smoking history, occasional alcohol

Physical examination: awake, alert, and oriented to person, place, and time; cranial nerves II–XII intact; bilateral deltoids/triceps/biceps 5/5; interossei 5/5; iliopsoas/knee flexion/knee extension/dorsi, and plantar flexion 5/5

Reflexes: 2+ in bilateral biceps/triceps/brachioradialis with negative Hoffman; 2+ in bilateral patella/ankle; no clonus or Babinski; sensation intact to light touch

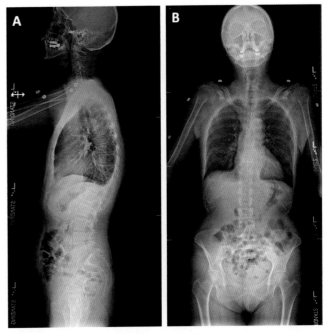

Fig. 24.3 Preoperative x-rays. (A) Anteroposterior (AP) and **(B)** lateral x-rays demonstrating a T10 compression fracture with focal kyphosis but no global imbalance present.

	Carlo Bellabarba, MD Orthopaedic Surgery University of Washington Harborview Medical Center Seattle, Washington, United States	Sutipat Pairojboriboon, MD Orthopaedic Surgery Vichaiyut Hospital Phyathai, Thailand	Nicholas Theodore, MD Ann Liu, MD, A. Karim Ahmed, MD Neurosurgery Johns Hopkins University Baltimore, Maryland, United States	Clemens Weber, MD, PhD Neurosurgery Stavanger University Hospital Stavanger, Norway
Preoperative				
Additional tests requested	DEXA Neurology evaluation	MRI T-spine STIR DEXA Anesthesia evaluation Rheumatology evaluation Hip x-rays	PMR consultation for physical therapy and conservative pain management DEXA Osteoporosis labs 1. TLSO fitting if pain unable to be controlled 2. Repeat XR in 6 weeks	DEXA
Surgical approach selected	T10 corpectomy vis costotransversectomy, T8-L1 fusion with possible cement augmentation	T8-L1 fusion with indirect reduction of T10	If fails pain control and TLSO brace, T9–10 laminectomy with robot-assisted T8–12 fusion	Surgery only for instability
Approach if 21 years of age	Posterior instrumented fusion alone	T10 corpectomy and T8-L1 fusion	Shorter fusion T9–11 fusion	Same approach
Approach if 80 years of age	Same approach	Conservative management	Conservative management	Same approach
Goal of surgery	Stabilization, fusion, long-term relief of pain	Reduce risk of neurological deterioration, stabilize spine and prevent progressive deformity, correct sagittal alignment	Decrease back pain	Stabilize spine
Perioperative				
Positioning	Prone	Prone, no pins, on Wilson frame	Prone, no pins, on Jackson table	Prone, no pins

	Carlo Bellabarba, MD Orthopaedic Surgery University of Washington Harborview Medical Center Seattle, Washington, United States	Sutipat Pairojboriboon, MD Orthopaedic Surgery Vichaiyut Hospital Phyathai, Thailand	Nicholas Theodore, MD Ann Liu, MD, A. Karim Ahmed, MD Neurosurgery Johns Hopkins University Baltimore, Maryland, United States	Clemens Weber, MD, PhD Neurosurgery Stavanger University Hospital Stavanger, Norway
Surgical equipment	IOM (MEP/SSEP) Fluoroscopy PMMA	Fluoroscopy Surgical navigation PMMA	IOM (MEP/SSEP) Fluoroscopy Robotic navigation system	Fluoroscopy Surgical navigation
Medications	Tranexamic acid	Antiosteoporotic medication	Steroids	None
Anatomical considerations	Spinal column and pedicles, rib cage, pleura, spinal cord and nerve roots, neurovascular bundle, great vessels	Ribs for counting, pedicles, spinal cord	Spinal canal, nerve roots	Spinous process, facet joints
Complications feared with approach chosen	Pneumothorax, infection, medical complications, nonunion	Retropulsed fragment while positioning, cortical pedicle breach, spinal cord injury	Neurological injury, adjacent segment disease, failure of construct	Bleeding
Intraoperative				
Anesthesia	General	General	General	General
Exposure	T8-L1	T8-L1	T9–12	T9-T11
Levels decompressed	T9–11	T10	T9–10	T10
Levels fused	T8-L1	T8-L1	T9–12	T9–11
Surgical narrative	Preflip IOM signals, position prone, midline longitudinal incision centered over fractured vertebrae, subperiosteal exposure to transverse process two to three levels above and below depending on the length of the construct, expose right of fractured vertebrae on right side along its dorsal surface 4–5 cm lateral to transverse process, place pedicle fenestrated screws under fluoroscopic guidance, laminectomy from pedicle above to pedicle below fracture level, two-level bilateral facetectomy above and below pedicle of fractured level, remove right T10 transverse process, left-side temporary rod, expose rib circumferentially, section rib approximately 5 cm from costovertebral joint, dissect costovertebral attachments and remove rib fragments, ligate nerve within neurovascular bundle medial to dorsal root ganglion, dissect bluntly around right lateral aspect of vertebral body, slide malleable ribbon retractor anterior to vertebral body, incise annulus at T9–10 and T0–11 on right, resect bulk of T10, drill pedicle down on left side, use osteotome along left side of posterior cortex to osteotomize between disc above and below, fold posterior cortex into corpectomy defect on right to complete corpectomy, resect cartilaginous end plates above and below, place expandable cage filled with corpectomy bone with x-ray and pack bone graft around it, cement screw augmentation and vertebroplasties above and below if osteoporotic, place right-sided contour rod, replace left temporary rod with full length rod, x-rays to confirm alignment and hardware position, decorticate remaining posterior elements and add morcellized bone graft, BMP if considered for nonunion, vancomycin powder in wound, layered closure over drain	Preflip IOM signals, log roll into prone position on Wilson frame, x-rays to identify surgical level, mark T10 vertebral lesion, longitudinal midline incision over spinous process, dissect down along spinous process and along lamina to facets, tip of spinous process used to confirm T10 level, place pedicle screws from T8–L1 based on anatomical landmarks and screw size based on preoperative CT, fluoroscopic images to help assess placement, assess screw placement with O-arm, inject PMMA under pressure through fenestrated titanium screws except T10, connect rods to screws, indirect reduction of injured vertebra, reposition retropulsed fragment with ligamentotaxis, final fluoroscopic image, closure with local anesthetic and subfascial drains	Position prone, attach tracker and reference array, intraoperative x-ray to register to preoperative CT, incision from T8–12, subperiosteal dissection, trajectories are planned for instrumentation, instrumentation with robot including possibility of percutaneous screws, T9–10 laminectomy with or without facetectomies to decompress spinal canal if needed, decorticate facet joints and place demineralized bone matrix, place top loading rods and caps, final x-ray to confirm placement of hardware, wound irrigated with antibiotic solution, place vancomycin powder, drain placement as needed, layered closure	Midline incision, dissection of paraspinous muscles, confirm level with fluoroscopy, surgical navigation, pedicle screws at T9 and T11, laminectomy at T10, no drain

	Carlo Bellabarba, MD Orthopaedic Surgery University of Washington Harborview Medical Center Seattle, Washington, United States	Sutipat Pairojboriboon, MD Orthopaedic Surgery Vichaiyut Hospital Phyathai, Thailand	Nicholas Theodore, MD Ann Liu, MD, A. Karim Ahmed, MD Neurosurgery Johns Hopkins University Baltimore, Maryland, United States	Clemens Weber, MD, PhD Neurosurgery Stavanger University Hospital Stavanger, Norway
Complication avoidance	Preflip signals, laminectomy and facetectomy from pedicle to pedicle, ligate nerve in neurovascular bundle, malleable ribbon to protect surrounding structures, cement screw augmentation and vertebroplasties above and below if osteoporotic, BMP if concerned for nonunion	Preflip signals, anatomical landmarks for screws, fluoroscopy to help assess screw placement, O-arm to assess screws, placement of fenestrated screws for PMMA, ligamentotaxis to fix retropulsed fragment	Robotic navigation, facetectomies as needed	Minimize levels involved, avoid surgery if possible
Postoperative				
Admission	ICU	ICU	Floor	Floor
Postoperative complications feared	Pneumothorax, infection, medical complications, nonunion	Spinal cord injury, PMMA extravasation	Neurological injury, adjacent segment disease, failure of construct	Screw misplacement
Anticipated length of stay	3–5 days	3–4 days	3–4 days	2–3 days
Follow-up testing	CT T-L spine prior to discharge T-L spine upright x-rays in recovery and prior to discharge, 3 months 6 months, 12 months after surgery	BMD Thoracic x-rays 3 months and each visit after surgery CT thoracolumbar spine 6 months after surgery	Standing scoliosis x-rays within 72 hours of surgery, 6 weeks after surgery	CT scans after surgery and 12 months later
Bracing	None	None	TLSO when out of bed for 8–12 weeks	None
Follow-up visits	3 weeks, 3 months, 6 months, 12 months after surgery	2 weeks, 3 months intervals until 1 year after surgery	2 weeks and 6 weeks after surgery	3 months and 1 year after surgery

BMD, Bone mineral density; *BMP*, bone morphogenic protein; *CT*, computed tomography; *DEXA*, dual-energy x-ray absorptiometry; *ICU*, intensive care unit; *IOM*, intraoperative monitoring; *MEP*, motor evoked potentials; *MIS*, minimally invasive surgery; *MRI*, magnetic resonance imaging; *PMMA*, polymethylmethacrylate; *SSEP*, somatosensory evoked potentials; *STIR*, short tau inversion recovery; *TLSO*, thoracic lumbar sacral orthosis.

Differential diagnosis

- Compression fracture
- Burst fracture
- Osteomyelitis

Important anatomical considerations

A compression fracture is the result of anterior loading on the vertebrae with failure of the anterior column. These fractures are defined by injury to one end plate without involvement of the posterior wall of the vertebrae. By definition, these fractures do not involve the posterior ligamentous complex and are therefore not considered unstable. The most common cause of these fractures is osteoporosis and most commonly seen in older adult and postmenopausal woman. Other risk factors of osteoporosis and resulting compression fracture include low body weight, sedentary lifestyle, smoking, and chronic use of steroids. The fractures most commonly occur in the thoracic spine but can be found throughout the entire spinal column. The ongoing compression from the initial fracture and angulation can progress over time especially if the underlying cause is not addressed. Furthermore, additional compression fractures can develop over time, as a person is four times more likely to develop additional compression fractures after one occurs.[6–9] Progressive kyphosis leading to focal kyphotic deformity can cause increasing back pain and may ultimately lead to instability.[10, 11] This occurs when the focal kyphosis leads to splaying of the facet and loss of posterior ligamentous complex integrity.

Approaches to this lesion

The main treatment for compression fracture is conservative in nature. This typically involves bed rest in the acute setting. Treatment with pain medication, muscle relaxants, and bracing are also essential in early treatment for pain control and early mobilization. Healing of the fractured vertebrae typically results in improvement of symptoms and is followed by physical therapy. Initial treatment should also take into consideration the underlying cause of the compression fracture when it is due to osteoporosis. When conservative management fails and there is intractable back pain, surgical intervention can be considered. The timing for treatment with vertebroplasty/kyphoplasty is of debate and is most frequently considered for acute and subacute fractures and have been shown to improve pain up to 24 months.[12] Although there have been studies showing rapid pain relief and functional recovery with augmentation, recent randomized studies have not shown a benefit.[13–16] When there is deformity associated with the compression fracture, a more definitive surgical intervention should be considered. This becomes tricky in patients with poor bone quality. Treatment options for deformity includes instrumentation with or without screw augmentation to improve screw pullout strength.[17, 18] In some cases, a corpectomy may be considered if there is retropulsion of the fracture causing spinal cord compression. Bracing is typically advocated in the postoperative period to reduce risk of screw pullout. Additionally, the use of a bone stimulator should also be considered as well as bone morphogenetic protein intraoperatively. The postoperative treatment of the underlying bone quality is also extremely important to prevent further compression fractures, which includes anabolic mediation to promote bone quality and density.[19]

What was actually done

This patient was first attempted on conservative management with bracing and mobilization, but this was unsuccessful. She continued to have ongoing back pain preventing mobilization. Vertebroplasty/kyphoplasty was not considered for this patient given the chronicity of the fracture as identified on magnetic resonance imaging (MRI) and computed tomography (CT) scan (Figs. 24.1–24.2), focal angulation, and retropulsed fragment of the fracture. Given that the patient had failed conservative management, she was offered open instrumented fixation. The patient was taken to the operating room where she was positioned on an Orthopedic system Inc (OSI) table. A midline incision was performed and exposure of the thoracic spine from T8 to T12 was performed. Instrumentation was placed two levels above and below the fracture. Screw augmentation was not performed on this case as the bone quality was adequate. Postoperatively the patient was braced with a Jewett brace and imaging showed good location of the hardware (Fig. 24.4). The patient was evaluated by Endocrinology and started on teriparatide for treatment of her osteoporosis.

Commonalities among the experts

The majority of our experts agreed surgical intervention was necessary after the nonsurgical approach had failed. One expert only offered surgery if the patient's fracture was

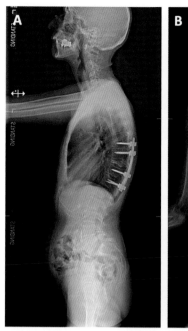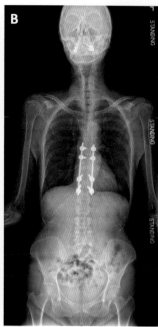

Fig. 24.4 Postoperative x-rays. (A) Lateral and **(B)** AP x-rays demonstrating instrumentation from T8-T12 and correction of the kyphotic deformity.

demonstrated to be unstable. Of those that offered surgical intervention, all offered a posterior approach with two experts offering construct extending from T8 to L1 and one expert offering construct from T8 to T12. One expert recommended corpectomy at T10, and the other offered laminectomy of T9–10. Half planned on cement screw augmentation, with two others expressing the need for intraoperative monitoring. There was a consensus that fluoroscopy was needed if surgical intervention was pursued. All our experts expressed the need for additional imaging postoperatively.

SUMMARY OF QUALITY OF EVIDENCE TO GUIDE SPECIFIC INTERVENTIONS FOR THIS CASE

- Cement augmentation of pedicle screws in osteoporosis: level II.2
- Intraoperative monitoring for deformity surgery: level II.1

REFERENCES

1. Ballane G, Cauley JA, Luckey MM, El-Hajj Fuleihan G. Worldwide prevalence and incidence of osteoporotic vertebral fractures. *Osteoporos Int.* 2017;28(5):1531–1542.
2. Ebot J, Bohnen AM, Abode-Iyamah K. Bilateral Acute Osteoporotic Lumbar Pedicle Fracture Presenting with Associated Neurological Deficit: A Case Report and Review of Literature. *Cureus.* 2020;12(3):e7273.
3. Lewiecki EM, Leader D, Weiss R, Williams SA. Challenges in osteoporosis awareness and management: results from a survey of US postmenopausal women. *J Drug Assess.* 2019;8(1):25–31.
4. Luthman S, Widen J, Borgstrom F. Appropriateness criteria for treatment of osteoporotic vertebral compression fractures. *Osteoporos Int.* 2018;29(4):793–804.

5. McCarthy J, Davis A. Diagnosis and Management of Vertebral Compression Fractures. *Am Fam Physician*. 2016;94(1):44–50.

6. Cauley JA, Hochberg MC, Lui LY, et al. Long-term risk of incident vertebral fractures. *JAMA*. 2007;298(23):2761–2767.

7. Klotzbuecher CM, Ross PD, Landsman PB, Abbott 3rd TA, Berger M. Patients with prior fractures have an increased risk of future fractures: a summary of the literature and statistical synthesis. *J Bone Miner Res*. 2000;15(4):721–739.

8. Melton 3rd LJ, Atkinson EJ, Cooper C, O'Fallon WM, Riggs BL. Vertebral fractures predict subsequent fractures. *Osteoporos Int*. 1999;10(3):214–221.

9. van der Klift M, de Laet CE, McCloskey EV, et al. Risk factors for incident vertebral fractures in men and women: the Rotterdam Study. *J Bone Miner Res*. 2004;19(7):1172–1180.

10. Adams MA, Dolan P. Biomechanics of vertebral compression fractures and clinical application. *Arch Orthop Trauma Surg*. 2011;131(12):1703–1710.

11. Pollintine P, Luo J, Offa-Jones B, Dolan P, Adams MA. Bone creep can cause progressive vertebral deformity. *Bone*. 2009;45(3):466–472.

12. Kaufmann TJ, Jensen ME, Schweickert PA, Marx WF, Kallmes DF. Age of fracture and clinical outcomes of percutaneous vertebroplasty. *AJNR Am J Neuroradiol*. 2001;22(10):1860–1863.

13. Alvarez L, Alcaraz M, Perez-Higueras A, et al. Percutaneous vertebroplasty: functional improvement in patients with osteoporotic compression fractures. *Spine (Phila Pa 1976)*. 2006;31(10):1113–1118.

14. Buchbinder R, Osborne RH, Ebeling PR, et al. A randomized trial of vertebroplasty for painful osteoporotic vertebral fractures. *N Engl J Med*. 2009;361(6):557–568.

15. Ploeg WT, Veldhuizen AG, The B, Sietsma MS. Percutaneous vertebroplasty as a treatment for osteoporotic vertebral compression fractures: a systematic review. *Eur Spine J*. 2006;15(12):1749–1758.

16. Wardlaw D, Cummings SR, Van Meirhaeghe J, et al. Efficacy and safety of balloon kyphoplasty compared with non-surgical care for vertebral compression fracture (FREE): a randomised controlled trial. *Lancet*. 2009;373(9668):1016–1024.

17. Elder BD, Lo SF, Holmes C, et al. The biomechanics of pedicle screw augmentation with cement. *Spine J*. 2015;15(6):1432–1445.

18. Liu MY, Tsai TT, Lai PL, Hsieh MK, Chen LH, Tai CL. Biomechanical comparison of pedicle screw fixation strength in synthetic bones: Effects of screw shape, core/thread profile and cement augmentation. *PLoS One*. 2020;15(2):e0229328.

19. Kendler DL, Marin F, Zerbini CAF, et al. Effects of teriparatide and risedronate on new fractures in post-menopausal women with severe osteoporosis (VERO): a multicentre, double-blind, double-dummy, randomised controlled trial. *Lancet*. 2018;391(10117):230–240.

25

Burst fracture without PLC injury

Kingsley Abode-Iyamah, MD

Introduction

Thoracolumbar vertebral body fractures are a common cause of spinal injury, where burst fractures account for up to 58% of all thoracolumbar fractures.[1] These fractures can lead to pain and neurological deficit. In other cases, they may remain asymptomatic. The fracture itself may also lead to kyphotic deformity and spinal instability. When there is evidence of instability, kyphotic deformity, or even neurological deficit, surgical intervention is often recommended. These treatments can range from instrumentation alone to instrumentation and decompression via laminectomy or a combination of laminectomy and corpectomy. The management becomes difficult in those patients who are neurologically intact. In these patients, the most common presenting symptom is back pain. Occasionally, patients may complain of subjective weakness secondary to limited mobility and pain, but without objective findings. The management of patients who remain neurologically intact with thoracolumbar burst fracture becomes highly variable. This variability has led to the development of multiple scoring systems to help guide management. Of the available scoring system to determine which patient with thoracolumbar fracture will require surgical intervention, the Thoracolumbar Injury Classification and Severity (TLICS) score has been developed and widely accepted as a scoring system to identify those requiring surgical intervention by scoring based on fracture type, neurological deficit, and integrity of posterior ligamentous complex (see Chapter 24, Table 1).[2] Typically those with intact posterior ligamentous complex who are neurologically intact would not meet criteria for surgical intervention. The management of this subgroup of patients can become somewhat difficult as they are typically limited by their back pain. There have been numerous articles reporting excellent outcomes with conservative management, while others report advantage of surgical intervention in these patients.[3–15] Management in these patients should be therefore individualized when these patients fail conservative management, which includes pain control, bracing, and physical therapy for early mobilization.

Example case

Chief complaint: back pain

History of present illness: A 64-year-old female suffered a fall with ongoing back pain. She was seen in the emergency room for this ongoing back pain. She noted that the pain improved in the recumbent position and worsened with ambulation. She denied any weakness or bowel/bladder dysfunction. She underwent imagines that revealed a T11–12 burst fracture with retropulsed bone fragments (Figs. 25.1–25.3).

Medications: none

Allergies: no known drug allergies

Past medical and surgical history: hypertension, osteoporosis

Family history: noncontributory

Social history: secretary, no smoking history, occasional alcohol

Physical examination: awake, alert, and oriented to person, place, and time; cranial nerves II–XII intact; bilateral deltoids/triceps/biceps 5/5; interossei 5/5; iliopsoas/knee flexion/knee extension/dorsi, and plantar flexion 5/5

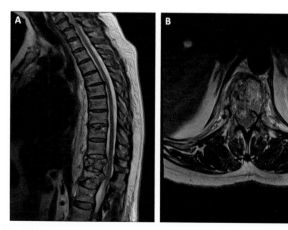

Fig. 25.1 Preoperative magnetic resonance images. (A) T2 sagittal and **(B)** T2 axial images demonstrating T11 and 12 burst fracture and a T8 compression fracture with retropulsed bone fragments.

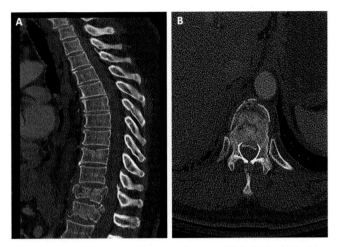

Fig. 25.2 Preoperative computed tomography scans. (A) Sagittal and **(B)** axial images demonstrating T11 and T12 burst fracture and a T8 compression fracture with retropulsed bone fragments.

Reflexes: 2+ in bilateral biceps/triceps/brachioradialis with negative Hoffman; 2+ in bilateral patella/ankle; no clonus or Babinski; sensation intact to light touch

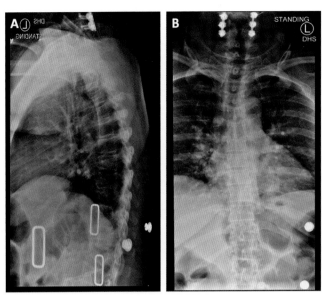

Fig. 25.3 Preoperative x-rays. (A) Anteroposterior (AP) and **(B)** lateral x-rays demonstrating T11 and T12 burst fracture and a T8 compression fracture; no kyphotic deformity.

	Pedro Luis Bazán, MD Spine Surgeon HIGA San Martín La Plata (Chief Orthopaedic) Hospital Italiano La Plata Instituto de Diagnóstico La Plata La Plata, Buenos Aires, Argentina	Sigurd Berven, MD Orthopaedic Surgery University of California at San Francisco San Francisco, California, United States	Michelle J. Clarke, MD Neurosurgery Mayo Clinic Rochester, Minnesota, United States	Mohamed A.R. Soliman, MD, MSc, PhD Neurosurgery Cairo University Cairo, Egypt
Preoperative				
Additional tests requested	DEXA	DEXA	DEXA	MRI cervical spine
	Scoliosis standing x-rays		Osteoporosis labs	DEXA
Hounsfield Units in CT				Medicine, endocrine, anesthesia evaluation
Surgical approach selected	T10-L1 percutaneous fusion	If fails to mobilize with brace, T10-L1 percutaneous posterior fusion with T9 kyphoplasty	If develops progress deformity or pain, T12-L1 laminectomy and T9-L3 posterior fusion	T11-12 laminectomy and T10-L1 posterior fusion
Approach if 21 years of age	Same approach	Nonoperative	Same approach +/– 1 level	Same approach
Approach if 80 years of age	Same approach with augmentation	Same approach	Same approach	MIS approach
Goal of surgery	Stabilize spine	Stabilize spine with early mobilization, pain improvement, avoid progressive deformity	Decompress neural elements, stabilize spine/restore biomechanics	Stabilize spine with early mobilization, pain improvement, decompress thecal sac, avoid progressive deformity
Perioperative				
Positioning	Prone	Prone on Jackson table	Pone on Jackson table	Prone on Jackson table, no pins
Surgical equipment	Fluoroscopy	Fluoroscopy	Fluoroscopy	Fluoroscopy
		Kyphoplasty set	O-arm	IOM
		PMMA	Ultrasound	Surgical navigation
				Ultrasound
				Surgical microscope

	Pedro Luis Bazán, MD Spine Surgeon HIGA San Martín La Plata (Chief Orthopaedic) Hospital Italiano La Plata Instituto de Diagnóstico La Plata La Plata, Buenos Aires, Argentina	Sigurd Berven, MD Orthopaedic Surgery University of California at San Francisco San Francisco, California, United States	Michelle J. Clarke, MD Neurosurgery Mayo Clinic Rochester, Minnesota, United States	Mohamed A.R. Soliman, MD, MSc, PhD Neurosurgery Cairo University Cairo, Egypt
Medications	Maintain MAP	Acetaminophen, gabapentin	None	Steroids, maintain MAP, possible osteoporotic medication
Anatomical considerations	Transverse process, pedicles, vertebral body	Spinal cord, descending aorta	Spinal cord, pedicle orientation	Spinal cord, pedicle orientation
Complications feared with approach chosen	Cortical violation	Progressive kyphosis, prolonged immobilization, junctional pathology	Spinal instability, spinal cord injury, ongoing neural compression	Spinal cord injury, dural tear and CSF leak, screw malposition, delayed instability and progressive kyphosis, delayed mobilization with medical complications
Intraoperative				
Anesthesia	General	General	General	General
Exposure	T10-L1	T10-L1	T9-L3	T10-L1
Levels decompressed	None	None	T12-L1	T11-12
Levels fused	T10-L1	T10-L1	T9-L3	T10-L1
Surgical narrative	Position prone, x-ray to confirm alignment and level, percutaneous screw placement using biplanar localization of T10-L1 pedicles bilaterally, percutaneous titanium rod, standard closure	Preflip MEP, position prone, postflip MEP, biplanar localization of T10-L1 pedicles, percutaneous placement of T10-L1 pedicle screws bilaterally, augment T10 and L1 screws with PMMA, T9 kyphoplasty, percutaneous titanium rod, standard closure	Position prone, fluoroscopy to mark levels and plan incision, midline incision, dissect to transverse processes bilaterally, laminectomy over both fractures levels if there is neural compression, place all pedicle screws using Lenke technique, O-arm spine to confirm screw placement, contour rods, use ligamentotaxis if there is concern for a fragment in the canal by locking in screws above and below fracture and distracting, confirm decompression with ultrasound or O-arm, footed tamp if ongoing compression on fragment, final tighten screws, decorticate, arthrodesis using autograft and allograft, close in layers over a drain	Position prone, IOM setup and checked, intraoperative fluoroscopy to mark levels and visualize fracture, midline skin incision and dissection down to fascia, subperiosteal dissection to expose posterior elements including facet capsule and transverse processes one level above higher fracture and two levels below lower fracture, registration of surgical navigation, entry points based on navigation and intraoperative fluoroscopy, drill entry point with high-speed drill, size and length of screws estimated with preoperative images and navigation, place pedicle screws one level above higher fracture and two levels below lower fracture, intraoperative spin to confirm screw position, decortication of spinous process/laminae/facet joints, laminectomy of fracture levels with high-speed drill and Kerrison rongeurs, adequate decompression confirmed with ultrasound, if still compression can push fractured fragments forward with Epstein curette, place slightly kyphotic rod, lay autograft on decorticated bone, closure in layers with subfascial drain
Complication avoidance	Percutaneous placement of pedicle screws	Pre- and postflip MEP, percutaneous placement of pedicle screws, augment screws with PMMA	Pedicle screws using Lenke technique, O-arm spin to confirm position of screws, ligamentotaxis if necessary, ultrasound or O-arm to confirm decompression	Surgical navigation, ultrasound to determine adequacy of decompression, push fractured fragments forward if necessary for better decompression

	Pedro Luis Bazán, MD Spine Surgeon HIGA San Martín La Plata (Chief Orthopaedic) Hospital Italiano La Plata Instituto de Diagnóstico La Plata La Plata, Buenos Aires, Argentina	Sigurd Berven, MD Orthopaedic Surgery University of California at San Francisco San Francisco, California, United States	Michelle J. Clarke, MD Neurosurgery Mayo Clinic Rochester, Minnesota, United States	Mohamed A.R. Soliman, MD, MSc, PhD Neurosurgery Cairo University Cairo, Egypt
Postoperative				
Admission	Floor	Floor	Floor	Floor
Postoperative complications feared	Infection, hardware failure	Kyphosis, pulmonary complications	Kyphosis, pseudoarthrosis	Screw malposition, instrumentation failure, worsening neurological function, CSF leak
Anticipated length of stay	1 day	2 days	3–4 days	1–2 days
Follow-up testing	T-L spine x-rays within 24 hours of surgery T-L flexion/extension x-rays 1 month after surgery CT T-L spine 3 months after surgery	36-inch standing films prior to discharge, 4 weeks, 3 months, 6 months, 1 year, 2 years after surgery Likely removal of implants 1 year after surgery	Possible endocrinology evaluation Standing x-rays at 6 weeks, 6 months, 1 year after surgery CT T-L spine 1 year after surgery	CT T-L spine within 24 hours of surgery and 6 months after surgery
Bracing	None	TLSO for comfort	None	None
Follow-up visits	2 weeks, 1 month, 2 months, 3 months, 6 months, 1 year after surgery	4 weeks, 3 months, 6 months, 1 year, 2 years after surgery	6 weeks, 6 months, 1 year after surgery	10–14 days, 4 weeks, 3 months, 6 months, 1 year after surgery

CSF, cerebrospinal fluid; *CT*, computed tomography; *DEXA*, dual-energy x-ray absorptiometry; *IOM*, intraoperative monitoring; *MAP*, mean arterial pressure; *MEP*, motor evoked potentials; *MIS*, minimally invasive surgery; *MRI*, magnetic resonance imaging; *PMMA*, polymethylmethacrylate; *SSEP*, somatosensory evoked potentials; *TLSO*, thoracic lumbar sacral orthosis.

Differential diagnosis

- Burst fracture
- Compression fracture
- Osteomyelitis

Important anatomical considerations

A burst fracture is the result of axial loading on the vertebrae with failure of the superior and inferior end plates. These fractures routinely involve fracture of the lamina and its involvement does not make the fracture unstable. An important component of the assessment of a patient with a burst fracture is whether or not there is the existence of retropulsion of bone fragments. Retropulsed vertebral fragments can cause neurological deficit or radiculopathy depending on its location. Additionally, assessment of the posterior ligamentous complex is a key component in the decision making for management strategy. The posterior ligamentous complex is composed of the ligamentum flavum, facet capsule, and interspinous and supraspinous ligaments. The integrity of these ligaments can be assessed looking at the short tau inversion recovery (STIR) magnetic resonance images, where hyperintensity of these ligaments may suggest an unstable fracture. Furthermore, the integrity of the posterior longitudinal ligament can also play a key role in guiding treatment options. Lastly, another key component is the fracture type using the load sharing classification (degree of comminution and apposition of the fracture fragments, and the kyphotic deformity) can also help determine those patients with an intact or disrupted posterior ligamentous complex.[3,16–18]

Approaches to this lesion

The main treatment for thoracolumbar burst fractures with intact posterior ligamentous complex is bracing and early mobilization. The patient initially presented with back pain, which may require bed rest in the immediate setting. Treatment with pain medication, muscle relaxants, and bracing is also essential in the early treatment for pain control and early mobilization. Healing of the fractured vertebrae typically results in improvement of symptoms and is followed by physical therapy. When the patient fails conservative management with bracing and is unable to mobilize, fixation is considered. While open fracture fixation was commonly used, minimally invasive approaches with percutaneous fixation have recently gained popularity.[19,20] Recent publications comparing open instrumentation and fusion with percutaneous instrumentation alone show no difference in hardware failure. With percutaneous instrumentation, there is also an opportunity to remove the instrumentation in the future once bony healing is confirmed on imaging. Whether performing open instrumentation or percutaneous instrumentation, advancement in instrumentation now allows ligamentous taxis in patients with retropulsed bone fragments that may need reduction.[21,22] This can only be performed when the posterior longitudinal ligament is intact and allows tension on this ligament to reduce the fracture fragment from the spinal canal. Very rarely those with burst fractures causing focal kyphosis may require repair of the anterior column. Depending on the location of the fracture, this can be performed from a lateral or a posterior approach. Posterior fixation with short versus long segment fixation (instrumentation one level above and below versus two levels above and below the fracture) has long been debated.[23] While both have shown good outcomes, there is evidence that short segment fixation may not have equal fixation compared with long segment fixations.[23-27] However, most recently Wei et al. conducted a randomized trial that demonstrated that short and monosegmental fixation is equally effective and reliable with shorter operative time and less blood loss.[26] Importantly, instrumentation of the fracture sight may increase the rate of fixation when short segment is used.[24] The use of vertebroplasty at the fracture sight has also been explored and may increase the chances of fusion.[28,29]

What was actually done

This patient was first attempted to be managed conservatively with bracing and mobilization, but this was unsuccessful. She continued to have ongoing back pain preventing mobilization. Vertebroplasty/kyphoplasty was not considered for this patient given the chronicity of the fracture as identified on magnetic resonance imagine and computed tomography scans (Figs. 25.1 and 25.2), as well as the presence of focal angulation and retropulsed fragments into the canal. Given that the patient had failed conservative management, she was offered open instrumented fixation. The patient was taken to the operating room and positioned on an Orthopedic system Inc (OSI) table. A midline incision was performed and exposure of the thoracolumbar spine from T7 to L2 was performed. Instrumentation was placed two levels above and below the fracture site, and ligamentous taxi was used to reduce the retropulsed bony fragments. Screw augmentation was not performed on this case because of the adequate bone quality. Postoperatively the patient was braced with a Jewett brace. Postoperative imaging showed good position of the hardware and resolution of the retropulsed bony fragments (Fig. 25.4).

Commonalities among the experts

Most of our experts recommended initial conservative management and surgical intervention if the patient failed conservative management. All also recommended that the patient undergo workup for osteoporosis with a dual-energy x-ray absorptiometry scan. If conservative management failed, all experts recommended surgical intervention. Half recommended percutaneous T10-L1 instrumentation, with one suggesting use of kyphoplasty. The other half recommended open laminectomy and fusion from T12 to L1, although the level of fusion varied from T9-L3 to T11-L3. All experts uniformly agreed on the need for intraoperative fluoroscopy, while two experts recommend intraoperative ultrasound to assess canal decompression. Half recommended maintaining elevated mean arterial pressure goals throughout the case. There was consensus that the patient should be admitted to the floor postoperatively with expected hospitalization stay ranging from 1 to 4 days. Bracing was only recommended by one expert. All recommended additional postoperative imaging.

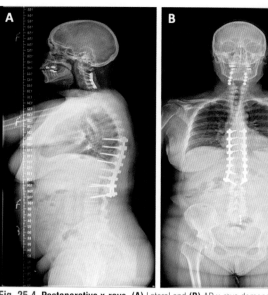

Fig. 25.4 Postoperative x-rays. (A) Lateral and **(B)** AP x-rays demonstrating instrumentation from T7 to L2.

SUMMARY OF QUALITY OF EVIDENCE TO GUIDE SPECIFIC INTERVENTIONS FOR THIS CASE

- Short versus monosegmental fixation segment fixation for burst fracture: level I
- Screw augmentation for burst fracture: level II.1

REFERENCES

1. Alanay A, Acaroglu E, Yazici M, Oznur A, Surat A. Short-segment pedicle instrumentation of thoracolumbar burst fractures: does transpedicular intracorporeal grafting prevent early failure? *Spine (Phila Pa 1976)*. 2001;26(2):213–217.
2. Vaccaro AR, Lehman Jr. RA, Hurlbert RJ, et al. A new classification of thoracolumbar injuries: the importance of injury morphology, the integrity of the posterior ligamentous complex, and neurologic status. *Spine (Phila Pa 1976)*. 2005;30(20):2325–2333.
3. Dai LY, Jiang LS, Jiang SD. Conservative treatment of thoracolumbar burst fractures: a long-term follow-up results with special reference to the load sharing classification. *Spine (Phila Pa 1976)*. 2008;33(23): 2536–2544.
4. Danisa OA, Shaffrey CI, Jane JA, et al. Surgical approaches for the correction of unstable thoracolumbar burst fractures: a retrospective analysis of treatment outcomes. *J Neurosurg*. 1995;83(6):977–983.
5. Hitchon PW, Abode-Iyamah K, Dahdaleh NS, et al. Nonoperative Management in Neurologically Intact Thoracolumbar Burst Fractures: Clinical and Radiographic Outcomes. *Spine (Phila Pa 1976)*. 2016; 41(6):483–489.
6. Hitchon PW, He W, Dahdaleh NS, Moritani T. Risk factors for supplementary posterior instrumentation after anterolateral decompression and instrumentation in thoracolumbar burst fractures. *Clin Neurol Neurosurg*. 2014;126:171–176.
7. Hitchon PW, He W, Viljoen S, et al. Predictors of outcome in the non-operative management of thoracolumbar and lumbar burst fractures. *Br J Neurosurg*. 2014;28(5):653–657.
8. Hitchon PW, Torner J, Eichholz KM, Beeler SN. Comparison of anterolateral and posterior approaches in the management of thoracolumbar burst fractures. *J Neurosurg Spine*. 2006;5(2):117–125.
9. Hitchon PW, Torner JC, Haddad SF, Follett KA. Management options in thoracolumbar burst fractures. *Surg Neurol*. 1998;49(6):619–626. discussion 26-7.

10. Mumford J, Weinstein JN, Spratt KF, Goel VK. Thoracolumbar burst fractures. The clinical efficacy and outcome of nonoperative management. *Spine (Phila Pa 1976)*. 1993;18(8):955–970.

11. Siebenga J, Leferink VJ, Segers MJ, et al. Treatment of traumatic thoracolumbar spine fractures: a multicenter prospective randomized study of operative versus nonsurgical treatment. *Spine (Phila Pa 1976)*. 2006;31(25):2881–2890.

12. Thomas KC, Bailey CS, Dvorak MF, Kwon B, Fisher C. Comparison of operative and nonoperative treatment for thoracolumbar burst fractures in patients without neurological deficit: a systematic review. *J Neurosurg Spine*. 2006;4(5):351–358.

13. Tropiano P, Huang RC, Louis CA, Poitout DG, Louis RP. Functional and radiographic outcome of thoracolumbar and lumbar burst fractures managed by closed orthopaedic reduction and casting. *Spine (Phila Pa 1976)*. 2003;28(21):2459–2465.

14. Verlaan JJ, Diekerhof CH, Buskens E, et al. Surgical treatment of traumatic fractures of the thoracic and lumbar spine: a systematic review of the literature on techniques, complications, and outcome. *Spine (Phila Pa 1976)*. 2004;29(7):803–814.

15. Wood K, Buttermann G, Mehbod A, Garvey T, Jhanjee R, Sechriest V. Operative compared with nonoperative treatment of a thoracolumbar burst fracture without neurological deficit. A prospective, randomized study. *J Bone Joint Surg Am*. 2003;85(5):773–781.

16. McCormack T, Karaikovic E, Gaines RW. The load sharing classification of spine fractures. *Spine (Phila Pa 1976)*. 1994;19(15):1741–1744.

17. Parker JW, Lane JR, Karaikovic EE, Gaines RW. Successful short-segment instrumentation and fusion for thoracolumbar spine fractures: a consecutive 41/2-year series. *Spine (Phila Pa 1976)*. 2000;25(9):1157–1170.

18. Radcliff K, Kepler CK, Rubin TA, et al. Does the load-sharing classification predict ligamentous injury, neurological injury, and the need for surgery in patients with thoracolumbar burst fractures?: Clinical article. *J Neurosurg Spine*. 2012;16(6):534–538.

19. Chu JK, Rindler RS, Pradilla G, Rodts Jr. GE, Ahmad FU. Percutaneous Instrumentation Without Arthrodesis for Thoracolumbar Flexion-Distraction Injuries: A Review of the Literature. *Neurosurgery*. 2017;80(2):171–179.

20. Ntilikina Y, Bahlau D, Garnon J, et al. Open versus percutaneous instrumentation in thoracolumbar fractures: magnetic resonance imaging comparison of paravertebral muscles after implant removal. *J Neurosurg Spine*. 2017;27(2):235–241.

21. Charles YP, Walter A, Schuller S, Aldakheel D, Steib JP. Thoracolumbar fracture reduction by percutaneous in situ contouring. *Eur Spine J*. 2012;21(11):2214–2221.

22. Steib JP, Charles YP, Aoui M. In situ contouring technique in the treatment of thoracolumbar fractures. *Eur Spine J*. 2010;19(Suppl 1). S66-8.

23. Dobran M, Nasi D, Brunozzi D, et al. Treatment of unstable thoracolumbar junction fractures: short-segment pedicle fixation with inclusion of the fracture level versus long-segment instrumentation. *Acta Neurochir (Wien)*. 2016;158(10):1883–1889.

24. Kapoen C, Liu Y, Bloemers FW, Deunk J. Pedicle screw fixation of thoracolumbar fractures: conventional short segment versus short segment with intermediate screws at the fracture level-a systematic review and meta-analysis. *Eur Spine J*. 2020;29(10):2491–2504.

25. Tezeren G, Kuru I. Posterior fixation of thoracolumbar burst fracture: short-segment pedicle fixation versus long-segment instrumentation. *J Spinal Disord Tech*. 2005;18(6):485–488.

26. Wei FX, Liu SY, Liang CX, et al. Transpedicular fixation in management of thoracolumbar burst fractures: monosegmental fixation versus short-segment instrumentation. *Spine (Phila Pa 1976)*. 2010;35(15). E714-20.

27. Wu Y, Chen CH, Tsuang FY, Lin YC, Chiang CJ, Kuo YJ. The stability of long-segment and short-segment fixation for treating severe burst fractures at the thoracolumbar junction in osteoporotic bone: A finite element analysis. *PLoS One*. 2019;14(2):e0211676.

28. Liao JC, Chen WJ. Short-Segment Instrumentation with Fractured Vertebrae Augmentation by Screws and Bone Substitute for Thoracolumbar Unstable Burst Fractures. *Biomed Res Int*. 2019;2019:4780426.

29. Liao JC, Chen WP, Wang H. Treatment of thoracolumbar burst fractures by short-segment pedicle screw fixation using a combination of two additional pedicle screws and vertebroplasty at the level of the fracture: a finite element analysis. *BMC Musculoskelet Disord*. 2017;18(1):262.

26

Fracture after kyphoplasty

Fidel Valero-Moreno, MD, Henry Ruiz-Garcia, MD and William Clifton, MD

Introduction

Kyphoplasty is a minimally invasive technique for the treatment of pathological compression fractures and osteoporotic compression fractures of the spine. This procedure represents a valuable treatment option for patients and their families, especially in terms of pain relief and improvement of the quality of life.[1] Kyphoplasty successfully relieves acute pain in the vast majority of patients with pathological and osteoporotic fractures[2] and increases the biomechanical stability by partially restoring vertebral height.[3] Several complications can occur including extrusion of cement into the spinal canal, hematoma, osteomyelitis, and adjacent vertebral fractures.[4] However, refracture after cemented vertebral augmentation by kyphoplasty is relatively rare. Refracture occurs at 3.4 months after kyphoplasty on average and has an incidence rate of 12.5%.[5–7] The pathogenesis of this condition is linked to technical factors and patient-related conditions, such as advanced osteoporosis, high body mass index, and low bone mineral density (BMD).[5–7] Conservative treatment, such as antiosteoporosis medication and back brace, are effective for the treatment of refracture. Nevertheless, surgical decompression and stabilization can be required in the setting of a new neurological deficit.[5] Herein, we present the case of a 69-year-old woman with acute back pain 1 day after a kyphoplasty.

Example case

Chief complaint: back pain

History of present illness: This is a 69-year-old female who has acute worsening of back pain after an L1 kyphoplasty 1 day prior. She has no leg symptoms and no genitourinary symptoms. Because of the worsening back pain, she underwent x-rays (Fig. 26.1) and magnetic resonance imaging (Fig. 26.2) that demonstrated refracture at the previous kyphoplasty site. Computed tomography scans (not shown) showed bilateral L1 pedicle and posterior element fractures.

Medications: bisphosphonates

Allergies: no known drug allergies

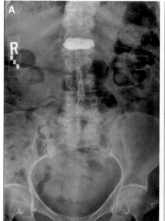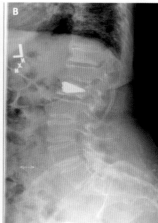

Fig. 26.1 Preoperative x-rays. (A) Anteroposterior (AP) and **(B)** sagittal x-rays demonstrating interval vertebral augmentation at L1 with partial restoration of vertebral body height. Mild inferior end plate compression deformity at T12 that was new since prior examination.

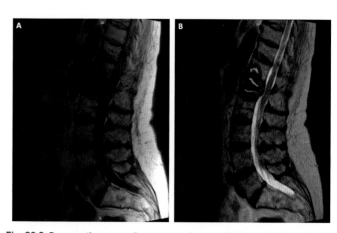

Fig. 26.2 Preoperative magnetic resonance images. (A) T1 and **(B)** T2 sagittal images demonstrating interval vertebral augmentation of the L1 compression fracture with mild central spinal stenosis at the L1 level. In addition, there is a prominent Schmorl's node in the anterior inferior aspect of the T12 end plate, with mild loss of vertebral body height and marrow edema.

Past medical and surgical history: mastectomy for stage 1 BRCA neg cancer 10 years previous

Family history: none

Social history: no smoking, no alcohol

Physical examination: awake, alert, and oriented to person, place, and time; cranial nerves II–XII intact; bilateral deltoids/ biceps/triceps 5/5; interossei 5/5; iliopsoas/knee flexion/ knee extension/dorsi, and plantar flexion 5/5

Reflexes: 2+ in bilateral biceps/triceps/brachioradialis; 2+ in bilateral patella/ankle; no clonus or Babinski; negative Hoffman; sensation intact to light touch; FABER negative; hip motion testing negative; straight leg raise negative

	Michelle J. Clarke, MD Neurosurgery Mayo Clinic Rochester, Minnesota, United States	Christopher J. Dewald, MD Orthopaedic Surgery Rush University Medical Center Chicago, Illinois, United States	Jeff D. Golan, MD Neurosurgery McGill University Montreal, Quebec, Canada	Luiz Robert Vialle, MD Orthopaedic Surgery Pontifical Catholic University of Parana Curitiba, Brazil
Preoperative				
Additional tests requested	DEXA Endocrinology evaluation Standing x-rays in brace	Standing x-rays ESR/CRP	None	Axial MRI CT T-spine T12 needle biopsy if lesion seen
Adjuvant therapy	Osteoporotic treatment TLSO brace	None	Osteoporotic treatment Jewett brace	None
Surgical approach selected	Conservative management	If convinced this is the source of pain and depending on standing balance and SVA, Stage 1: T10-L3 fusion with posterior column osteotomies as needed Stage 2 (if needed based on SVA): T12-L2 discectomy with interbody fusion and possible L1 corpectomy	Conservative management	If convinced this is the source of pain, L1 corpectomy and T10-L2 fusion
Surgical approach if 21 years old	Same approach	Same approach	Same approach	Anterior or posterior
Surgical approach if 80 years old	Same approach	Same approach	Same approach	Same
Goal of surgery		Stabilization, improve sagittal balance		Decompression, stabilization
Perioperative				
Positioning		Stage 1: prone on Jackson table Stage 2: right lateral decubitus		Lateral
Surgical equipment		Fluoroscopy Bone cement		Fluoroscopy MIS retractors
Medications		None		None
Anatomical considerations		Never roots, spinal canal, great vessels, bowel, kidneys		Vascular anatomy, diaphragm insertion
Complications feared with approach chosen		Bow injury, injury to great vessels, nerve root injury, pseudoarthrosis, spinal instrumentation failure, adjacent level kyphosis		Inferior vena cava injury
Intraoperative				
Anesthesia		General		General
Exposure		Stage 1: T10-L3 Stage 2: T12-L2		T12-L2
Levels decompressed		Stage 1: None Stage 2: T12-L2		L1–2
Levels fused		Stage 1: T10-L3 Stage 2: T12-L2		T12-L2

	Michelle J. Clarke, MD Neurosurgery Mayo Clinic Rochester, Minnesota, United States	Christopher J. Dewald, MD Orthopaedic Surgery Rush University Medical Center Chicago, Illinois, United States	Jeff D. Golan, MD Neurosurgery McGill University Montreal, Quebec, Canada	Luiz Robert Vialle, MD Orthopaedic Surgery Pontifical Catholic University of Parana Curitiba, Brazil
Surgical narrative		Position prone, midline posterior incision, expose bone, place pedicle screws from T10-L3 using anatomy, place cement through pedicles at T10 and T11 using x-rays, determine whether alignment proper, determine Smith-Peterson osteotomies as needed, remove inferior facets with osteotome and ligamentum flavum with Leksell rongeur, remove superior facets to complete osteotomy, place rods with appropriate lordosis, place locking caps, layered closure with drains Possible stage 2 (2–3 days later) standing x-rays show more anterior support is needed, position right lateral decubitus, identify 12th rib, incise skin and dissect to rib tip, bluntly dissect through lateral abdominal musculature, enter into retroperitoneal space, sweep retroperitoneal tissue anteriorly and identify psoas muscle with fingertip, palpate bulging discs beneath psoas, retract psoas muscle posterior and incise T12-L1 and L1–2 discs back to posterior annulus, place two PEEK cages or L1 corpectomy with expandable cage with 1/3 ilium to fit defect, layered closure		Lateral position similar to an OLIF, psoas muscle identification after peritoneum retraction, corridor between peritoneum and psoas enlarged with dissection and vascular retraction until L1 vertebral body well defined, sometimes diaphragm pillar needs to be cut for the T12-L1 disc to be exposed, ligate lumbar artery at L1 level, place MIS retractor, L1 corpectomy and removal of cement, care with thecal sac, preparation of the T12 and L2 end plates for mesh, lace mesh filled with allograft bone, bone material send for pathological analysis, closure of muscle layers without drain, percutaneous posterior T10-L2 fusion
Complication avoidance		Support top of construct with cement, determine Smith-Peterson osteotomies as needed based on positioning in Jackson table, staged procedure if more anterior support needed based on standing x-rays, palpate bulging discs beneath psoas		Lateral approach, care with thecal sac, percutaneous posterior fusion to supplement, concern for breast cancer metastasis
Postoperative				
Admission		Floor		ICU
Postoperative complications feared		Adjacent vertebral fracture, loss of fixation, proximal or distal junction kyphosis		Deep vein thrombosis, hardware pull out, adjacent fracture
Anticipated length of stay				3 days
Follow-up testing	Thoracolumbar x-rays in 4 weeks in brace CT thoracolumbar spine 3 and 6 months	Standing x-rays 3 weeks after surgery	Thoracolumbar x-rays in 2–4 weeks	Physical therapy Thoracolumbar x-rays after surgery, 2 weeks, monthly for 6 months after surgery
Bracing	TLSO brace for 6 months	TLSO brace for 6 weeks	Jewett brace for 4 weeks	None
Follow-up visits	4 weeks, 3 months, 6 months	3 weeks after surgery	2–4 weeks	2 weeks, monthly for 6 months after surgery

BMP, Bone morphogenic protein; *CRP*, C-reactive protein; *CT*, computed tomography; *DEXA*, dual-energy x-ray absorptiometry; *ESR*, erythrocyte sedimentation rates; *ICU*, intensive care unit; *IOM*, intraoperative monitoring; *MAP*, mean arterial pressure; *MEP*, motor evoked potentials; *MIS*, minimally invasive surgery; *MRI*, magnetic resonance imaging; *PEEK*, polyether ether ketone; *SSEP*, somatosensory evoked potentials; *SVA*, sagittal vertical axis; *TLSO*, thoracic lumbar sacral orthosis.

Differential diagnosis

- Osteoporotic fracture
- Metastatic lesion

Important anatomical and preoperative considerations

The spine is the most common location for osteoporotic fractures[8] and is the primary osseous target of metastatic cancer.[2] Osteoporotic fractures of the vertebral column constitute at least 50% of all the osteoporotic fractures in the United States.[8] Compression fractures are a common complication of these conditions and around 30% of patients may suffer from adverse sequelae, including chronic pain, fatigue, kyphosis, and neurological impairment.[2, 8] Kyphoplasty was designed to restore vertebral height by expanding a balloon to elevate the end plate and create a cavity for cementation.[9] Balloon kyphoplasty differentiates from percutaneous vertebroplasty (PVP) as it includes the insertion of an inflatable tamp, in order to reduce deformity and allow the injection of polymethylmethacrylate (PMMA) at a low pressure to prevent leakage.[10]

Kyphoplasty is a relatively safe and minimally invasive procedure and has shown its effectiveness in providing quick pain relief and improving quality of life. Despite this, recollapse of the augmented vertebra can occur, causing severe back pain and dysfunction.[7] Severe osteoporosis, fracture level in the thoracolumbar region, and the presence of an intravertebral cleft are vertebral-related factors that might contribute to the development of cemented vertebrae refracture.[2, 3, 5, 7, 11, 12] Interestingly, patients with intravertebral clefts have nearly a twofold increased risk of subsequent fracture after vertebroplasty.[12] Technical issues believed to be associated with refracture are usually related to the amount of cement and its distribution within the vertebral body.[5, 7, 12] Although the ideal volume of cement is controversial and there is no consensus,[6] a high dose of cement (> 3.5 cc) in a reasonable range can reduce the possibility of postsurgical refracture.[7] Interestingly, a higher restoration of the vertebral height is related to increased paravertebral soft tissue tension, leading to increased mechanical loading and refracture.[3]

Patients with compression fractures and intravertebral clefts experiencing worsening pain consistent with the site of prior kyphoplasty should be followed up closely. Refracture and neurological compromise must be ruled out.[5, 12, 13] Before any additional surgical intervention, magnetic resonance imaging must rule out the presence of other conditions that may be causing recurrent pain, such as adjacent fracture or cement leakage.[13, 14] Retreatment with vertebroplasty is an accepted management modality for subsequent refracture of previously treated vertebra. Repeat percutaneous vertebroplasty successfully treats unresolved symptoms and provides pain relief in most cases.[13–15]

What was actually done

A positron emission tomography (PET) scan was performed to stage the patient's previous history of breast cancer, and this did not reveal any malignant lesion. Computed tomography and magnetic resonance scans of the lumbar spine confirmed the diagnosis of L1 compression fracture status post vertebroplasty and bilateral pedicle fractures at L1,

with spinal instability and conus compression. The patient was taken to the operating room for a T10-L4 instrumented fusion with intraoperative somatosensory and motor evoked potential monitoring. After general anesthesia took place, the patient was positioned prone on the Jackson table, and the head was fixed in neutral position with Gardner-Wells tongs and 15 lb of axial traction. A midline incision from T10 to L4 was done, followed by subperiosteal dissection. Beginning at L4, the pedicles were probed using a gearshift probe. Screws were placed after a ball-tip probe confirmed the intraosseous position. The pedicles were not tapped due to the osteoporotic nature of her spine. Pedicle screws were placed from L4 up to T10 level bilaterally with the exception of L1, which had fractured pedicles and posterior elements. After placing all the screws, a C-arm helped to confirm their correct position. Two contoured titanium rods were secured bilaterally. Thereafter, the facets and lamina were decorticated bilaterally, bone morphogenic protein (BMP) was then placed within the facet joints at each level from T10 to L4, and corticocancellous chips were distributed over the dorsal aspect of the spine bilaterally. Two Hemovac drains were placed, and the wound was closed in anatomical layers after vancomycin powder was distributed. There were no intraoperative complications and postoperative x-ray showed successful instrumentation (Fig. 26.3). The patient was discharged to rehabilitation with ankle foot orthosis (AFO) braces on postoperative day 4.

Commonalities among the experts

The majority of the surgeons performed an image study of the thoracic spine for a better understanding of the preoperative status. Preoperative adjuvant therapy was not employed when a surgical approach was preferred. However, brace placement and osteoporotic treatment was recommended by the surgeons opting for a conservative management. Surgical strategy involved stabilization through thoracolumbar fusion and L1 corpectomy. Surgery was accomplished with the aid of fluoroscopy, and no particular perioperative medications were requested. The surgeons considered the identification and preservation of blood vessels as the key anatomical feature during the approach. The most feared complications

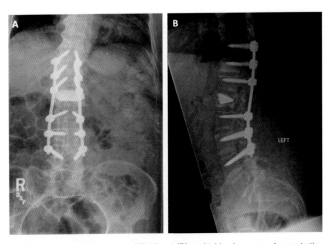

Fig. 26.3 Postoperative x-rays. (A) AP and **(B)** sagittal lumbar x-rays demonstrating interval posterior spinal fixation rod and pedicle screw placement from T10 through L4. Hardware was intact. Previous augmentation at L1 appeared unchanged and no new compression deformities are appreciated.

were adjacent vertebral fracture and hardware dysfunction. Postoperative admission varied between intensive care unit and regular ward. All advocated for thoracolumbar x-rays 2 to 4 weeks after either conservative or surgical management. Most of the surgeons recommended bracing for a period that varied considerably from 4 weeks to 6 months.

SUMMARY OF QUALITY OF EVIDENCE TO GUIDE SPECIFIC INTERVENTIONS FOR THIS CASE

- Spinal column stabilization after adequate surgical intervention: level III
- Bracing as part of conservative management: level III

REFERENCES

1. Cho JH, Ha JK, Hwang CJ, Lee DH, Lee CS. Patterns of Treatment for Metastatic Pathological Fractures of the Spine: The Efficacy of Each Treatment Modality. *Clin Orthop Surg.* 2015;7(4):476–482.
2. Rajah G, Altshuler D, Sadiq O, Nyame VK, Eltahawy H, Szerlip N. Predictors of delayed failure of structural kyphoplasty for pathological compression fractures in cancer patients. *J Neurosurg Spine.* 2015;23(2):228–232.
3. Yu W, Xu W, Jiang X, Liang D, Jian W. Risk Factors for Recollapse of the Augmented Vertebrae After Percutaneous Vertebral Augmentation: A Systematic Review and Meta-Analysis. *World Neurosurg.* 2018;111:119–129.
4. Takahashi S, Hoshino M, Yasuda H, et al. Characteristic radiological findings for revision surgery after balloon kyphoplasty. *Sci Rep.* 2019;9(1):18513.
5. Li X, Lu Y, Lin X. Refracture of osteoporotic vertebral body after treatment by balloon kyphoplasty: Three cases report. *Medicine (Baltimore).* 2017;96(49):e8961.
6. Kim DJ, Kim TW, Park KH, Chi MP, Kim JO. The proper volume and distribution of cement augmentation on percutaneous vertebroplasty. *J Korean Neurosurg Soc.* 2010;48(2):125–128.
7. Li YX, Guo DQ, Zhang SC, et al. Risk factor analysis for re-collapse of cemented vertebrae after percutaneous vertebroplasty (PVP) or percutaneous kyphoplasty (PKP). *Int Orthop.* 2018;42(9):2131–2139.
8. Rajasekaran S, Kanna RM, Schnake KJ, et al. Osteoporotic Thoracolumbar Fractures-How Are They Different? Classification and Treatment Algorithm. *J Orthop Trauma.* 2017;31(Suppl 4):S49–s56.
9. Alamin T, Kleimeyer JP, Woodall JR, Agarwal V, Don A, Lindsey D. Improved biomechanics of two alternative kyphoplasty cementation methods limit vertebral recollapse. *J Orthop Res.* 2018;36(12):3225–3230.
10. Song D, Meng B, Chen G, et al. Secondary balloon kyphoplasty for new vertebral compression fracture after initial single-level balloon kyphoplasty for osteoporotic vertebral compression fracture. *Eur Spine J.* 2017;26(7):1842–1851.
11. Feng L, Feng C, Chen J, Wu Y, Shen JM. The risk factors of vertebral refracture after kyphoplasty in patients with osteoporotic vertebral compression fractures: a study protocol for a prospective cohort study. *BMC Musculoskelet Disord.* 2018;19(1):195.
12. Trout AT, Kallmes DF, Lane JI, Layton KF, Marx WF. Subsequent vertebral fractures after vertebroplasty: association with intraosseous clefts. *AJNR Am J Neuroradiol.* 2006;27(7):1586–1591.
13. Choi SS, Hur WS, Lee JJ, Oh SK, Lee MK. Repeat vertebroplasty for the subsequent refracture of procedured vertebra. *Korean J Pain.* 2013;26(1):94–97.
14. Chen LH, Hsieh MK, Liao JC, et al. Repeated percutaneous vertebroplasty for refracture of cemented vertebrae. *Arch Orthop Trauma Surg.* 2011;131(7):927–933.
15. Yang SC, Chen WJ, Yu SW, Tu YK, Kao YH, Chung KC. Revision strategies for complications and failure of vertebroplasties. *Eur Spine J.* 2008;17(7):982–988.

27

Pure bone thoracolumbar chance fracture

Oluwaseun O. Akinduro, MD

Introduction

The thoracolumbar junction is a region of biomechanical transition from the relatively stiff thoracic spine to the more flexible lumbar spine, which makes it susceptible to injury from high-velocity trauma. Fractures of the thoracolumbar junction are associated with an approximately 25% risk of spinal cord injury.[1] Historically, there has been a general lack of consensus regarding the surgical management of thoracolumbar fractures, primarily driven by presence of level I evidence supporting the use of orthosis for patients with stable burst fractures and no neurological deficits.[2] Many clinicians have developed strategies to better classify thoracolumbar fractures and determine which fractures would be considered unstable and require instrumentation. In this chapter, we will discuss the most frequently employed classification

systems while we discuss the presentation and management of a patient with a thoracolumbar fracture.

Example case

Chief complaint: mid back pain

History of present illness: This is an 81-year-old female who was seen in the emergency room after a car accident. She has mid back pain with midline palpation and no leg symptoms. The patient underwent a computed tomography (CT) and magnetic resonance imaging (MRI) of the lower thoracic and lumbar spine concerning for a pure bone Chance fracture of T12 (Fig. 27.1).

Medications: Eliquis, hydrochlorothiazide, tramadol

Allergies: no known drug allergies

Past medical history: atrial fibrillation, previous stroke

Past surgical history: L4–5 and L3–4 anterior lumbar interbody fusion

Family history: no history of malignancies

Social history: no smoking, no alcohol use

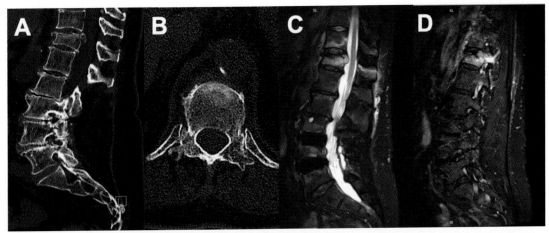

Fig. 27.1 Preoperative computed tomography (CT) and magnetic resonance imaging (MRI) of the thoracolumbar spine. (A) Mid sagittal and **(B)** axial CT centered at the level of T12 images demonstrating a fracture extending from the T12 vertebral body into the posterior elements of the spine. A small fragment of retropulsed bone can also be visualized. The axial image demonstrates fracture lines extending through bilateral pedicles. **(C)** Mid sagittal T2 and **(D)** sagittal short tau inversion recovery (STIR) MRI demonstrating mild retropulsion of a bone fragment, with no significant impingement on the spinal cord. The STIR image demonstrates a significant amount of edema in the T12 vertebral body as well as soft tissue edema posteriorly.

Physical examination: awake, alert, and oriented to person, place, and time; cranial nerves II–XII intact; bilateral deltoids/triceps/biceps 5/5; interossei 5/5; iliopsoas/knee flexion/knee extension/dorsi, and plantar flexion 5/5

Reflexes: 2+ in bilateral biceps/triceps/brachioradialis with negative Hoffman; 2+ in bilateral patella/ankle and no clonus or Babinski, sensation intact to light touch
Laboratories: all within normal limits

	Jason Cheung, MD Orthopaedic Surgery The University of Hong Kong Queen Mary Hospital Pokfulam, Hong Kong SAR, China	Scott Daffner, MD Orthopaedic Surgery West Virginia University Morgantown, West Virginia, United States	Gordon Deen, MD Neurosurgery Mayo Clinic Jacksonville, Florida, United States	Michael G. Fehlings, MD, PhD Neurosurgery University of Toronto Toronto, Canada
Preoperative				
Additional tests requested	Serum tumor markers Hematology evaluation Cardiology consultation Osteoporosis medication Blood tests including bone profile Osteoporosis investigation	Upright AP and lateral T- and L-spine x-rays Vitamin D level Endocrinology evaluation	None	CT complete spine T- and L-spine x-rays CT chest and abdomen Hematology evaluation Medicine evaluation
Surgical approach selected	TLSO brace, osteoporosis medication	If kyphotic deformity, intractable pain, and/or neurological deficit, posterior T10-L2 cement-augmented fusion	TLSO brace, no surgery offered	T11-L1 posterior percutaneous fusion
Surgical approach if 21 years old	Same approach	Percutaneous fixation	Same approach	TLSO brace
Surgical approach if 80 years old	Same approach	Open fusion	Same approach	Same approach
Goal of surgery	Depends on the findings above but if tumor related we will require biopsy, staging and stabilization and adjuvant treatment as necessary	Stabilization of spine, early mobilization		Stabilization of fracture, pain control, maintain neurological function
Perioperative				
Positioning		Prone on Jackson table		Prone
Surgical equipment		IOM (MEP/SSEP) Fluoroscopy Bone cement		IOM (MEP/SSEP) Fluoroscopy O-arm Surgical navigation
Medications		Maintain MAP >80		None
Anatomical considerations		Pedicles, nerve roots, spinal cord, T9-10 and L2-3 facet capsules		Pedicles
Complications feared with approach chosen		Pseudoarthrosis, instrumentation failure		Epidural hematoma, malpositioned screws, loss of fixation, medical complications
Intraoperative				
Anesthesia		General		General
Exposure		T10-L2		T11-L1
Levels decompressed		None		None
Levels fused		T10-L2		T11-L1

	Jason Cheung, MD Orthopaedic Surgery The University of Hong Kong Queen Mary Hospital Pokfulam, Hong Kong SAR, China	Scott Daffner, MD Orthopaedic Surgery West Virginia University Morgantown, West Virginia, United States	Gordon Deen, MD Neurosurgery Mayo Clinic Jacksonville, Florida, United States	Michael G. Fehlings, MD, PhD Neurosurgery University of Toronto Toronto, Canada
Surgical narrative		Preflip IOM, position prone, recheck IOM, midline posterior incision, standard exposure of T10-L2, take care to not disrupt T9-10 or L2-3 facet capsules, expose just enough over transverse processes to be able to identify landmarks, place fenestrated screws bilaterally from T10-L2 avoiding T12, confirm position of screws with x-ray, inject 1–1.5 cc of cement through each screw under fluoroscopy, contour titanium rods and seat within screw heads, apply end caps and tighten, irrigate wound, decorticate exposed lamina and T10-L2 facet joints, place bone graft and/or extender, layered closure with possible drain		Delay surgery by 72 hours because of anticoagulant, sandwich flip on Allen table, position prone, check alignment with fluoroscopy, mark T10-L1 levels, small incision over T10 spinous process and clamp reference frame to T10 spinous process, O-arm spin and register navigation, stab incisions to cannulate T11-L1 bilateral pedicles with K-wires, place percutaneous dilators and cannulate pedicles bilaterally, place rod percutaneously, tighten all connections, confirm hardware location with fluoroscopy, infiltrate each incision with anesthetic
Complication avoidance		Preflip IOM, take care to not disrupt T9-10 or L2-3 facet capsules, cement augmented screws, avoid cement in T12 (fracture level), use less rigid rods		Delay surgery due to anticoagulant, surgical navigation, percutaneous fusion
Postoperative				
Admission	Floor	Stepdown unit	Floor	Floor
Postoperative complications feared		Anemia, infection, instrumentation failure, adjacent segment degeneration		Epidural hematoma, malpositioned screws, loss of fixation, medical complications
Anticipated length of stay	2–3 days	2 days	2–3 days	2–3 days
Follow-up testing	Thoracic spine x-rays 3 months and 6 months after discharge	CT T-L spine prior to discharge Upright T- and L-spine x-ray prior to discharge, 6 weeks, 3 months Outpatient physical therapy 3 months after surgery Flexion/extension x-rays 6 months, 12 months, 24 months after surgery	Thoracic spine x-rays 2 and 4 weeks after discharge	T-L spine x-rays prior to discharge, 6 weeks, 3 months, 6 months, 12 months, 24 months after surgery CT 6 months after surgery Resume anticoagulation after 2 weeks Osteoporosis evaluation
Bracing	TLSO brace for 3 months	None	Aspen TLSO brace for 6 weeks	None
Follow-up visits	3 months and 6 months after discharge	2 weeks, 6 weeks, 3 months, 6 months, 12 months, 24 months after surgery	6 weeks after discharge	6 weeks, 3 months, 6 months, 12 months, 24 months after surgery

AP, Anteroposterior; *CT*, computed tomography; *IOM*, intraoperative monitoring; *MAP*, mean arterial pressure; *MEP*, motor evoked potentials; *SSEP*, somatosensory evoked potentials; *TLSO*, thoracic lumbar spine orthosis.

Differential diagnosis

- Pure bone Chance fracture
- Burst fracture
- Acute disc herniation
- Muscle strain

Important anatomical considerations

Denis originally classified the thoracolumbar spine into an anterior middle and posterior column.[3] The anterior column includes the anterior longitudinal ligament and the anterior two-thirds of the vertebral body and disc. The middle column includes the posterior one-third of the vertebral body and disc and the posterior longitudinal ligament. The posterior column includes the facet joints and capsules, pedicles, ligamentum flavum, supraspinous, and interspinous ligaments. The three-column model has mostly been replaced by more modern classification schemes such as the AO classification and the Thoracolumbar Spine Injury Classification and Severity (TLICS) score (Table 27.1).[4, 5] TLICS is a numerical grading scale that has the added benefit of its ability to guide decision making for clinicians, with a score >4 indicating the need for surgical intervention.

Transition zones of the spine such as the cervicothoracic and thoracolumbar spine have unique biomechanical properties that must be considered when planning surgery in these locations. The facet joints of the thoracic spine are oriented in a coronal plane and the lumbar spine is oriented in a sagittal plane. The coronal orientation allows for added lateral bending in the thoracic region, while the sagittal orientation allows for increased flexion and extension in the lumbar spine. Also, the articulation of the thoracic spine with the rib cage and

anterior articulation of the ribs with the sternum allows for added stability of the thoracic spine.[6] The lower thoracic ribs (T11 and 12) do not articulate with the sternum, making these levels more susceptible to injury than the thoracic levels above. The most important anatomical consideration when planning for surgical fusion of the thoracolumbar spine is the posterior ligamentous complex (PLC). The PLC includes the facet joints, posterior longitudinal ligament, ligamentum flavum, interspinous ligaments, and supraspinous ligaments. The PLC is a major determinant of stability in the thoracolumbar spine and a primary component of the TLICS score. Another important consideration is the location of the conus medullaris, which typically terminates in the middle third of the L1 vertebral body.[7] Compression of the conus medullaris will lead to upper motor neuron weakness, while compression of the nerve roots immediately caudal to the conus will lead to lower motor neuron weakness.

Approaches to this lesion

The first consideration when determining how to approach and manage this lesion is to determine whether to offer surgical stabilization of this fracture. If the decision is made to proceed with surgical stabilization of this fracture, the primary options to consider are open and percutaneous stabilization of the spine. Minimally invasive procedures have become more prevalent in spinal stabilization, with multiple studies showing that minimally invasive procedures allow for minimized pain, muscle disruption, blood loss, and noninferior outcomes compared with conventional open procedures.[8, 9] Although there has been an increase in minimally invasive procedures, many surgeons prefer open procedures due to the added visualization and robust arthrodesis that can be obtained from drilling the posterolateral gutters and laying bone graft. Stabilization is often augmented with cement for patients with diminished bone mineral density. Open approaches to the thoracolumbar spine include posterior, lateral, and anterior. The use of one approach over another is typically determined by the need for decompression and the location of the compression. When the compression can only be adequately addressed via an anteriorly approach, one should consider having a vascular surgeon assist with the exposure. The primary risk during an anterior approach is injury to the great vessels such as the aorta and the vena cava. The artery of Adamkiewicz is also most commonly located on the left between T8 and L1, thus a preoperative angiogram should be considered if lateral dissection is required, placing this artery at risk.[10]

What was actually done

This patient was noted to have evidence of a pure bony Chance fracture, with extension into the posterior column. The treatment options were discussed with the patient and the decision was made to proceed with surgical stabilization of the fracture. The patient had prior anterior instrumentation from L3 to L5, so instrumentation was planned from T10 to L5 rather than stopping short of her prior instrumentation. The patient was brought into the operating room and was placed under general anesthesia. Neuromonitoring was used with motor and somatosensory evoked potentials. Mayfield pins were placed prior to the patient being flipped into the prone position onto a Jackson table. An incision was made and monopolar cautery was used to perform a subperiosteal dissection proceeded down the spinous processes and lamina bilaterally. Upon

Table 27.1 The Thoracolumbar Spine Injury Classification and Severity (TLICS) score	
Characteristics	**Points**
Fracture Morphology	
No abnormality	0
Compression	1
Burst	2
Rotation/translation	3
Distraction	4
Posterior Ligamentous Complex (PLC)	
Intact	0
Indeterminate	2
Disrupted	3
Neurological Status	
Intact	0
Root injury	2
Complete injury	2
Incomplete injury	3
Cauda equina syndrome	3
0–3: nonsurgical management; 4: indeterminate, surgeons' preference, >4 surgical management	

completion of the exposure, the stealth frame was clamped to the most rostral spinous process and the O-arm brought in to register the navigation. Pedicle screws were placed from T10 to the L5 in the normal fashion using navigation, and placement was confirmed with another O-arm spin. Rods were then placed from T10 to L5 and secured with set screws. The wound was copiously irrigated with bacitracin irrigation prior to arthrodesis. An arthrodesis was performed from T10 to L5 followed by placement of allograft. The patient was taken to the recovery unit followed by the floor and was found to have no new neurological deficits. Postoperative imaging confirmed good placement of the instrumentation (Fig. 27.2).

Commonalities among the experts

There was a split among the surgeons regarding the treatment that would be offered for the patient. Half planned to offer surgical stabilization, and half of the surgeons planned for conservative management with bracing. The two surgeons that planned for instrumented fusion planned for a minimally invasive percutaneous approach, from either T11 to L2 or T10 to L1. There was agreement regarding the care of the patient during admission, with all surgeons recommending the floor or a stepdown unit for the patient's care. The surgeons also planned for a 2- to 3-day hospital stay, and all planned for imaging to be completed after discharge.

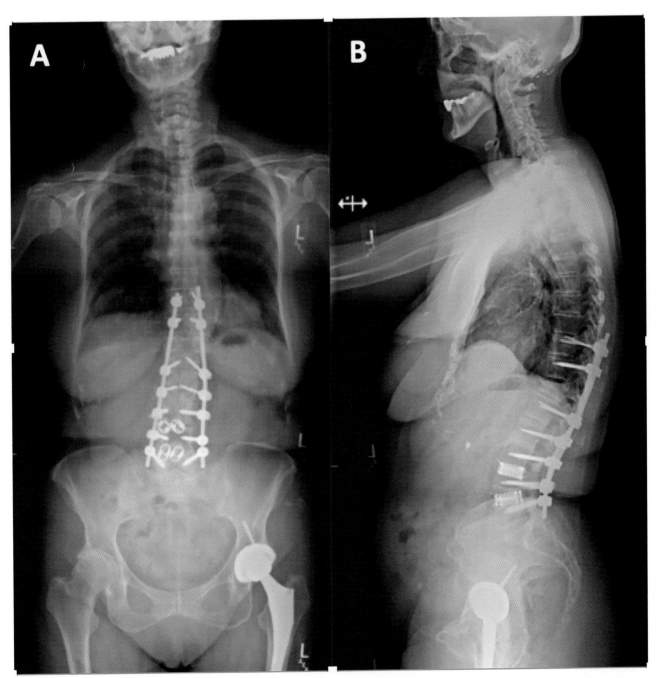

Fig. 27.2 Postoperative standing scoliosis x-rays. (A) Anteroposterior and **(B)** lateral images demonstrating hardware from T10 to L5 with good placement of the pedicle screws.

SUMMARY OF QUALITY OF EVIDENCE TO GUIDE SPECIFIC INTERVENTIONS FOR THIS CASE

- Minimally invasive percutaneous pedicle screw fixation results in noninferior outcomes compared with traditional open fixation for thoracolumbar fractures and is associated with decreased blood loss and shorter operative time but more intraoperative radiation usage: level IIA
- Operative treatment of patients with stable thoracolumbar burst fractures is not associated with improved long-term outcomes compared with nonoperative treatment: level IA

REFERENCES

1. Chapman JR, et al. Thoracolumbar flexion-distraction injuries: associated morbidity and neurological outcomes. *Spine (Phila Pa 1976)*. 2008;33(6):648–657.
2. Wood K, et al. Operative compared with nonoperative treatment of a thoracolumbar burst fracture without neurological deficit. A prospective, randomized study. *J Bone Joint Surg Am*. 2003;85(5):773–781.
3. Denis F. The three column spine and its significance in the classification of acute thoracolumbar spinal injuries. *Spine (Phila Pa 1976)*. 1983;8(8):817–831.
4. Vaccaro AR, et al. AO Spine thoracolumbar spine injury classification system: fracture description, neurological status, and key modifiers. *Spine (Phila Pa 1976)*. 2013;38(23):2028–2037.
5. Rihn JA, et al. A review of the TLICS system: a novel, user-friendly thoracolumbar trauma classification system. *Acta Orthop*. 2008;79(4):461–466.
6. Andriacchi T, et al. A model for studies of mechanical interactions between the human spine and rib cage. *J Biomech*. 1974;7(6):497–507.
7. Soleiman J, et al. Magnetic resonance imaging study of the level of termination of the conus medullaris and the thecal sac: influence of age and gender. *Spine (Phila Pa 1976)*. 2005;30(16):1875–1880.
8. Yang M, et al. Comparison of clinical results between novel percutaneous pedicle screw and traditional open pedicle screw fixation for thoracolumbar fractures without neurological deficit. *Int Orthop*. 2019;43(7):1749–1754.
9. Koreckij T, Park DK, Fischgrund J. Minimally invasive spine surgery in the treatment of thoracolumbar and lumbar spine trauma. *Neurosurg Focus*. 2014;37(1):E11.
10. Taterra D, et al. Artery of Adamkiewicz: a meta-analysis of anatomical characteristics. *Neuroradiology*. 2019;61(8):869–880.

28

Central cord syndrome without instability

Kingsley Abode-Iyamah, MD

Introduction

Central cord syndrome was first described by Schneider et al. in 1954 as a syndrome of disproportionate motor weakness of the upper limbs compared with the lower limbs, bladder dysfunction (urinary retention), and variable sensory changes.[1] It is the result of injury to the spinal cord and falls within the spectrum of acute spinal cord injuries. It is the most common form of incomplete spinal cord injury in adults and results in a characteristic neurological deficit where there is worse deficit in the upper extremities compared with the lower extremities, variable sensory changes, and urinary retention. It is typically seen in patients with either known or undiagnosed spinal canal stenosis of the cervical spine who suffer a traumatic event leading to the deficit. Due to the underlying cervical spondylosis typically associated with central cord syndrome, it is most commonly found in the older adult population.[2,3] It is most commonly seen following hyperextension injury as a result of a fall in which the neck is extended. This results in contusion at the site of the injury, causing edema of the spinal cord and resulting symptoms. While there is typically no acute fracture associated with the injury on imaging, in some cases there can be a fracture or even an acute disc herniation associated with the injury.[1,4,5] The initial diagnosis of central cord syndrome may be difficult given that a patient's imaging only shows degenerative changes without acute spinal column injury. Additionally, there may be comorbidities or associated injuries that may require optimization prior to addressing the central cord syndrome. While early treatment options of posterior decompression and myelotomy showed poor outcome, recent surgical techniques have shown improved outcomes.[6,7] Although some still advocate for nonoperative management, the timing of treatment for patients who present with central cord syndrome is highly debated, with some advocating for early intervention and others for delayed surgical intervention.[8–12]

Example case

Chief complaint: arm and leg weakness

History of present illness: A 51-year-old male presented after a syncopal fall following a coughing fit. Immediately upon regaining consciousness, he was unable to move his arms or legs for approximately 1 to 2 hours. He slowly regained some strength and was able to call emergency services. He continued to have significant weakness, in upper greater than lower extremities, upon arrival. Imaging was done and showed compression at the C3-4 region with an osteophyte complex on magnetic resonance imaging and computed tomography (Figs. 28.1 and 28.2).

Medications: amlodipine, cetirizine, flonase, lisinopril

Allergies: no known drug allergies

Past medical and surgical history: hypertension

Family history: noncontributory

Social history: construction worker, no smoking history, occasional alcohol

Physical examination: awake, alert, and oriented to person, place, and time; cranial nerves II–XII intact

Motor: LUE: 4/5 deltoid, 5/5 biceps, 5/5 triceps, 5/5 wrist extension, 4/5 grip, 4/5 finger abduction

Right upper extremity: 2/5 deltoid, 2/5 biceps, 2/5 triceps, 2/5 wrist extension, 1/5 grip, 1/5 finger abduction

Left lower extremity: 5/5 strength psoas, quad, hamstring, tibialis anterior, extensor hallicus longus, gastrocnemius

Right lower extremity: 5/5 psoas, 5/5 quad, 5/5 hamstring, 4/5 tibialis anterior, 4/5 extensor hallicus longus, 4/5 gastrocnemius

Sensation intact; decreased to pinprick on left from T3 down; normal patellar and brachioradialis reflexes bilaterally

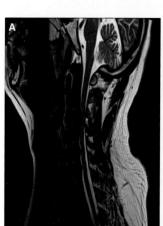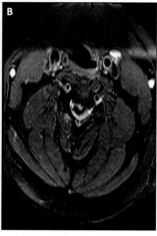

Fig. 28.1 Preoperative magnetic resonance images. (A) T2 sagittal and **(B)** T2 axial images demonstrating C3-4 osteophyte with cord compression and cord signal change.

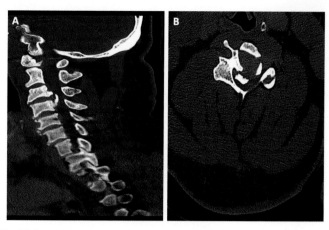

Fig. 28.2 Preoperative computed tomography images. (A) Sagittal and **(B)** axial images demonstrating a C3-4 calcified bridging osteophyte with canal stenosis.

	Carlo Bellabarba, MD Orthopaedic Surgery University of Washington Harborview Medical Center Seattle, Washington, United States	Bhavuk Garg, MD Orthopaedic Surgery All India Institute of Medical Sciences New Delhi, India	Allan D. Levi, MD, PhD Meng Huang, MD Neurosurgery University of Miami Miami, Florida, United States	Davide Nasi, MD Neurosurgery Polytechnic University of Marche, Umberto Ancona, Italy
Preoperative				
Additional tests requested	Medicine evaluation	Complete spine MRI	None	None
Adjuvant therapy	None	Monitor and if no improvement, then surgery	Monitor in ICU with MAP >85 for total of 48 hours	Monitor, pursue surgery within 15 days
Surgical approach selected	C3-4 laminoplasty	C4 corpectomy and C3-4 ACDF	C3-4, C4-5 ACDF with partial C3 and total C4 corpectomy after neurological status plateaus	C3-4 ACDF
Surgical approach if 21 years old	Same approach	Same approach	Same approach	Same approach
Surgical approach if 80 years old	C3-4 laminectomy, C2-5 posterior instrumented fusion	Same approach	C3-5 laminectomy and fusion	Same approach
Goal of surgery	Spinal cord decompression, preserving spinal stability and motion	Spinal cord decompression, anterior fixation	Spinal cord decompression from ventral osteophyte-disc complex	Spinal cord decompression, anterior fixation
Perioperative				
Positioning	Prone with Mayfield pins on Jackson table	Supine, no pins	Supine neutral with minimal extension with Mayfield pins	Supine with slight neck extension with Mayfield pins
Surgical equipment	IOM (MEP/SSEP) Fluoroscopy	Fluoroscopy IOM Surgical microscope Ultrasonic bone scalpel	IOM (MEP/SSEP) Isocentric C-arm for cone beam CT Fluoroscopy Surgical navigation Navigated drills Anterior cervical retractors Anterior instrumentation with expandable corpectomy cage Dural substitute and fibrin glue	Fluoroscopy Surgical microscope

	Carlo Bellabarba, MD Orthopaedic Surgery University of Washington Harborview Medical Center Seattle, Washington, United States	Bhavuk Garg, MD Orthopaedic Surgery All India Institute of Medical Sciences New Delhi, India	Allan D. Levi, MD, PhD Meng Huang, MD Neurosurgery University of Miami Miami, Florida, United States	Davide Nasi, MD Neurosurgery Polytechnic University of Marche, Umberto Ancona, Italy
Medications	Maintain MAP	Tranexamic acid	MAP goal >85	Steroids
Anatomical considerations	Paraspinal muscular attachments to C2, spinal cord and nerve roots	Vertebral artery, internal carotid artery, esophagus	Esophagus/pharynx, trachea, carotid sheath, vertebral arteries	Carotid sheath, cervical spinal column, intervertebral disc, PLL, osteophyte, spinal cord
Complications feared with approach chosen	C5 palsy, loss of cervical spine motion, progressive kyphotic malalignment, persistent neck pain	Dural tear, neurological worsening	Dysphagia, dysphonia, airway compromise	Dysphonia, spinal cord injury, implant failure, esophageal injury, vascular injury
Intraoperative				
Anesthesia	General	General	General	General
Exposure	C3-4	Anterior C3-4	Anterior C3-5	Anterior C3-4
Levels decompressed	C3-4	C3-4	C3-5	C3-4
Levels fused	None	C3-4	C3-5	C3-4
Surgical narrative	Fiberoptic intubation, preflip IOM, midline incision centered over C3-4 levels, preserve paraspinal attachments to C2, expose junction of lamina with lateral masses on left hinge side and preserving facet capsules on opening side, confirm levels with x-ray, gently rotate posterior arches of C3 and 4 toward hinge side while using curette to release ligament along opening side, instrument across laminoplasty defect using 6mm bicortical screws through the lamina medially and 8mm screws into the lateral mass laterally, x-rays to confirm alignment and hardware position, vancomycin powder in wound, layered closure over drain	Intubation with fiberoptic intubation and avoid further neck extension, IOM, standard Smith-Robinson approach from left, C3-4 discectomy under microscope with C4 partial corpectomy, gradual burring of ossified posterior longitudinal ligament, avoid use of Kerrison, use nerve hook to lift ossified ligament fragments, leave ossified ligament floating to dura if adherent, large ACDF cage filled with calcium phosphate, cervical locking plate with screws in C3 and lower half of C4, complete C4 corpectomy if not possible to place screws in C4 and use corpectomy with plate fixation, from C3-5	Intubation with fiberoptic scopes, maintain MAPs >85, IOM with MEP/SSEP baselines, neutral head position with Mayfield pins, extend head after baseline IOM obtained, ENT approach, expose C3-5, Caspar pins on C3 and C5 for distraction, discectomy at C3-4 and C4-5 with resection of PLL and posterior osteophytes, intraoperative cone beam CT and navigation registration, C4 corpectomy with navigated drill, partial inferior C3 corpectomy to remove posterior osteophyte, place expandable interbody, remove Caspar pins, place anterior plate with bicortical purchase using lateral fluoroscopy, subplatysmal drain	Position supine, incision made parallel to disc spaced localized by x-ray, undermine platysma, plane medial to sternocleidomastoid identified and bluntly dissected, carotid palpated, plane medial to carotid developed with blunt dissection, spine palpated, prevertebral fascia entered, disc level confirmed with x-ray, Cloward retractors and distractors used, disc annuelctomy performed, cartilaginous end plate is removed from bony end plate with curettes, osteophyte drilled down to PLL, PLL entered with nerve hook and resected with Kerrison punches, visualize dural plane, PEEK/carbon cage filled with bone and placed in disc space, place anterior cervical plate aligned in midline and fixed with screws with x-ray, layered closure
Complication avoidance	Baseline IOM, preserve paraspinal attachments to C2, laminoplasty using 6mm bicortical screws through the lamina medially and 8mm screws into the lateral mass laterally	Baseline IOM, avoid Kerrison rongeurs if possible, leave ossified ligament floating to dura if adherent, complete corpectomy if needed	Baseline IOMs, ENT approach for high cervical region, intraoperative cone beam CT and navigation	Limit to one level, blunt dissection toward spine, prepare endplates

	Carlo Bellabarba, MD Orthopaedic Surgery University of Washington Harborview Medical Center Seattle, Washington, United States	Bhavuk Garg, MD Orthopaedic Surgery All India Institute of Medical Sciences New Delhi, India	Allan D. Levi, MD, PhD Meng Huang, MD Neurosurgery University of Miami Miami, Florida, United States	Davide Nasi, MD Neurosurgery Polytechnic University of Marche, Umberto Ancona, Italy
Postoperative				
Admission	ICU	ICU	ICU	Floor
Postoperative complications feared	C5 palsy, loss of cervical spine motion, progressive kyphotic malalignment, persistent neck pain	CSF leak, esophageal injury Recurrent laryngeal nerve injury, superior laryngeal nerve injury	Dysphagia, dysphonia, airway compromise from neck hematoma	Dysphonia, spinal cord injury, implant failure, esophageal injury, vascular injury
Anticipated length of stay	2–3 days	1–2 days	1–2 days	5 days
Follow-up testing	CT C-spine prior to discharge C-spine x-rays upright AP/lateral prior to discharge C-spine AP/lateral/flexion/extension x-rays 3 weeks, 3 months, 6 months, 12 months after surgery	CT C-spine prior to discharge	AP/lateral upright x-ray Inpatient rehab evaluation	MRI C-spine 3 months after surgery
Bracing	Soft collar for 2 weeks	Soft collar for 2–3 weeks	Rigid collars for 8 weeks	None
Follow-up visits	3 weeks, 3 months, 6 months, 12 months after surgery	1 week, 2 weeks after surgery	2 weeks after surgery with nurse visit, 6 weeks with AP/lateral x-rays, 12 weeks with AP/lateral flexion/extension cervical CT	2 weeks, 3 months after surgery

ACDF, Anterior cervical decompression and fusion; *AP,* anteroposterior; *BMP,* bone morphogenic protein; *CT,* computed tomography; *DEXA,* dual-energy x-ray absorptiometry; *ENT,* ear nose and throat; *ICU,* intensive care unit; *IOM,* intraoperative monitoring; *MAP,* mean arterial pressure; *MEP,* motor evoked potentials; *MIS,* minimally invasive surgery; *MRI,* magnetic resonance imaging; *PEEK,* polyetheretherketone; *PLL,* posterior longitudinal ligament; *SSEP,* somatosensory evoked potential.

Differential diagnosis

- Spinal cord injury
- Transverse myelitis
- Multiple sclerosis

Important anatomical considerations

Central cord syndrome is the result of contusion of the spinal cord due to hyperextension injury. This typically results from existing stenosis of the spinal canal from a disc-osteophyte complex or ligamentum hypertrophy and is therefore more commonly seen in the older adult population.[1–5] Although more common in older adults, there is a bimodal age distribution in patients presenting with central cord syndrome. While the older adult population typically present following a fall, younger patients present after a high-energy mechanism such as motor vehicle accident resulting in unstable fracture, acute disc herniation, or congenital stenosis.[13–15]

Contusion of the spinal cord as a result of the stenosis or fracture causes injury to axons in the medial portion of the spinal cord and spares those on the lateral portion of the spinal cord. This results in more severe injury to motor axon of the upper extremities with less damage to that of the lower extremities. Sensory dysfunction is typically present although variable, while urinary dysfunction in the form of retention is typically present. Patients may also present with bradycardia and hypotension due to unregulated vagal input from loss of the sympathetic input.[16] Most patients present with severe neurological deficit, which rapidly improves over the first 24 hours before plateauing. The timing for intervention has therefore been highly debated with some recommending early intervention within 24 hours and others allowing the patient to first recover and then perform surgical intervention in a delayed fashion after the neurological recovery plateaus.[9, 10, 17]

Approaches to this lesion

The initial management of central cord syndrome is stabilization of the cervical spine in a rigid collar and admission to the intensive care unit. Mean arterial pressure of 85 to 90 should be maintained to prevent secondary injury of the spinal cords with fluids, blood products, or pressors.[18] There is no role for high-dose steroids in the management of acute spinal cord injury and has been associated with worse outcomes.[19–21] Some authors advocate for nonsurgical management which may be appropriate for patients with medical comorbidities that make them poor surgical candidates, those with very mild neurological deficit, or those with rapidly improving symptoms. When surgical intervention is warranted, the timing of surgical intervention is highly debated. Early research on spinal cord injury suggests worse outcome with early internvention, and, as a result, some authors advocate delaying surgical intervention for several weeks.[1, 7, 22–24] More recent research with the use of modern neuroanesthesia shows benefits with early intervention.[18] While most surgeons agree that neurological examination should plateau prior to intervention, patients with ongoing neurological compression or worsening examination may benefit from early surgical intervention.[12, 25] When surgical intervention is warranted, the approach can vary from anterior to posterior. In patients with loss of cervical lordosis, anterior compression from a disc, or disc-osteophyte complex, an anterior approach to remove the offending agent is most appropriate. When there is maintenance of cervical lordosis, stenosis from hypertrophe of the ligamentum flavum, or congenital stenosis, posterior cervical laminectomy without or without fusion should typically be undertaken.

What was actually done

The patient was admitted to the neuroscience intensive care unit after evaluation in the emergency department and placed in a hard cervical collar. An arterial line was placed, and a mean arterial pressure (MAP) of 85 to 90 mm Hg was maintained. Given the initial improvement following the injury, the patient was maintained on elevated MAP management for 72 hours. After the patient's neurological exam plateaued, he was taken to the operating room for surgical intervention. The patient was brought to the operating room for planned C4 corpectomy and C3-5 anterior cervical fusion. Intraoperatively, the patient received a one-time dose of dexamethasone to minimize surgical edema. Intraoperative neuromonitoring was performed throughout the case. There was a cerebral spinal fluid leak noted intraoperatively, which was repaired with a dural sealant. A drain was placed and left to gravity only and removed on postoperative day 1. The patient was discharged to an inpatient rehabilitation facility on postoperative day 7 where he continued his remarkable recovery. Postoperative imaging showed good location of the instrumentation (Fig. 28.3).

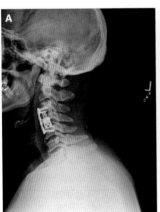
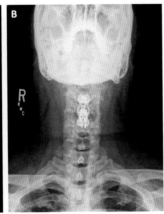

Fig. 28.3 Postoperative x-rays. (A) Lateral and **(B)** anteroposterior x-rays demonstrating a C4 corpectomy and C3-5 anterior cervical decompression and fusion.

Commonalities among the experts

Half of our experts requested further evaluation of the patient. While one expert recommended complete spinal magnetic resonance imaging, the other recommended Medicine consult for evaluation of the patient. The majority recommended a period of monitoring prior to surgical intervention, which ranged from 2 to 15 days, although only one recommended MAP goals greater than 85. While most surgeons recommended an anterior approach for this case, one surgeon did recommend a laminoplasty. Of those that recommended an anterior approach, two recommended a corpectomy at C4 and one recommended a C3-4 anterior cervical decompression and fusion. All were in agreement with the use of intraoperative fluoroscopy and the majority favored the used of intraoperative monitoring. Additionally, half recommended elevated intraoperative MAP goals. The majority recommended admission to the intensive care unit after surgery with hospital stays ranging from 1 to 5 days.

SUMMARY OF QUALITY OF EVIDENCE TO GUIDE SPECIFIC INTERVENTIONS FOR THIS CASE

- Timing of surgery for central cord syndrome: level II.1
- MAP goals for central cord syndrome: level II.1
- Avoidance of steroids for central cord syndrome: level II.1

REFERENCES

1. Schneider RC, Cherry G, Pantek H. The syndrome of acute central cervical spinal cord injury; with special reference to the mechanisms involved in hyperextension injuries of cervical spine. *J Neurosurg*. 1954;11(6):546–577.
2. Gupta R, Bathen ME, Smith JS, Levi AD, Bhatia NN, Steward O. Advances in the management of spinal cord injury. *J Am Acad Orthop Surg*. 2010;18(4):210–222.
3. Rowshan K BN. Central cord syndrome: acute decompression versus watch and wait. *The cervical spine*. 2012;5:1594.
4. Taylor AR. The mechanism of injury to the spinal cord in the neck without damage to vertebral column. *J Bone Joint Surg Br*. 1951;33-B(4):543–547.
5. Taylor AR, Blackwood W. Paraplegia in hyperextension cervical injuries with normal radiographic appearances. *J Bone Joint Surg Br*. 1948;30B(2):245–248.
6. Samuel AM, Grant RA, Bohl DD, Basques BA, Webb ML, Lukasiewicz AM, et al. Delayed surgery after acute traumatic central cord syndrome is associated with reduced mortality. *Spine (Phila Pa 1976)*. 2015;40(5):349–356.
7. Schneider RC, Thompson JM, Bebin J. The syndrome of acute central cervical spinal cord injury. *J Neurol Neurosurg Psychiatry*. 1958;21(3):216–227.
8. Aarabi B, Alexander M, Mirvis SE, Shanmuganathan K, Chesler D, Maulucci C, et al. Predictors of outcome in acute traumatic central cord syndrome due to spinal stenosis. *J Neurosurg Spine*. 2011;14(1):122–130.
9. Anderson KK, Tetreault L, Shamji MF, Singh A, Vukas RR, Harrop JS, et al. Optimal Timing of Surgical Decompression for Acute Traumatic Central Cord Syndrome: A Systematic Review of the Literature. *Neurosurgery*. 2015;77(Suppl 4):S15–S32.
10. Fehlings MG, Vaccaro A, Wilson JR, Singh A, D WC, Harrop JS, et al. Early versus delayed decompression for traumatic cervical spinal cord injury: results of the Surgical Timing in Acute Spinal Cord Injury Study (STASCIS). *PLoS One*. 2012;7(2):e32037.
11. Kepler CK, Kong C, Schroeder GD, Hjelm N, Sayadipour A, Vaccaro AR, et al. Early outcome and predictors of early outcome in patients treated surgically for central cord syndrome. *J Neurosurg Spine*. 2015;23(4):490–494.

12. Stevens EA, Marsh R, Wilson JA, Sweasey TA, Branch Jr. CL, Powers AK. A review of surgical intervention in the setting of traumatic central cord syndrome. *Spine J*. 2010;10(10):874–880.

13. Harrop JS, Sharan A, Ratliff J. Central cord injury: pathophysiology, management, and outcomes. *Spine J*. 2006;6(6 Suppl):198S–206S.

14. Jung SK, Shin HJ, Kang HD, Oh SH. Central cord syndrome in a 7-year-old boy secondary to standing high jump. *Pediatr Emerg Care*. 2014;30(9):640–642.

15. Ramirez NB, Arias-Berrios RE, Lopez-Acevedo C, Ramos E. Traumatic central cord syndrome after blunt cervical trauma: a pediatric case report. *Spinal Cord Ser Cases*. 2016;2:16014.

16. Evans LT, Lollis SS, Ball PA. Management of acute spinal cord injury in the neurocritical care unit. *Neurosurg Clin N Am*. 2013;24(3):339–347.

17. Lenehan B, Fisher CG, Vaccaro A, Fehlings M, Aarabi B, Dvorak MF. The urgency of surgical decompression in acute central cord injuries with spondylosis and without instability. *Spine (Phila Pa 1976)*. 2010;35(21 Suppl):S180–S186.

18. Bono C GS. Management of acute traumatic spinal cord injury. *Curr Treat Options Neurol*. 2004;17:334.

19. Bracken MB, Shepard MJ, Holford TR, Leo-Summers L, Aldrich EF, Fazl M, et al. Administration of methylprednisolone for 24 or 48 hours or tirilazad mesylate for 48 hours in the treatment of acute spinal cord injury. Results of the Third National Acute Spinal Cord Injury Randomized Controlled Trial. National Acute Spinal Cord Injury Study. *JAMA*. 1997;277(20):1597–1604.

20. Hugenholtz H. Methylprednisolone for acute spinal cord injury: not a standard of care. *CMAJ*. 2003;168(9):1145–1146.

21. Nesathurai S. Steroids and spinal cord injury: revisiting the NASCIS 2 and NASCIS 3 trials. *J Trauma*. 1998;45(6):1088–1093.

22. Divi SN, Schroeder GD, Mangan JJ, Tadley M, Ramey WL, Badhiwala JH, et al. Management of Acute Traumatic Central Cord Syndrome: A Narrative Review. *Global Spine J*. 2019;9(1 Suppl):89S–97S.

23. Farmer J, Vaccaro A, Albert TJ, Malone S, Balderston RA, Cotler JM. Neurologic deterioration after cervical spinal cord injury. *J Spinal Disord*. 1998;11(3):192–196.

24. Marshall LF, Knowlton S, Garfin SR, Klauber MR, Eisenberg HM, Kopaniky D, et al. Deterioration following spinal cord injury. A multicenter study. *J Neurosurg*. 1987;66(3):400–404.

25. Chen TY, Dickman CA, Eleraky M, Sonntag VK. The role of decompression for acute incomplete cervical spinal cord injury in cervical spondylosis. *Spine (Phila Pa 1976)*. 1998;23(22):2398–2403.

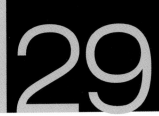

Penetrating spine trauma

Fidel Valero-Moreno, MD, Jaime L. Martinez Santos, MD and William Clifton, MD

Introduction

Penetrating injuries to the spine are often caused by gunshot wounds (GSWs).[1] Most of the literature supporting the management guidelines of GSWs to the spine stem from military and combat medicine.[2] The overall incidence of civilian GSWs has increased and causes 13% to 17% of all traumatic spine injuries, but this varies depending on the country.[3] Civilian GSWs typically occur with low-caliber weapons but still create devastating injuries. Civilian spinal GSWs are typically caused by low-velocity (<1000 ft/second) projectiles, and battle-related injuries by high-velocity firearms (2000–3000 ft/second) often involving multiple spinal levels.[4,5] This condition represents a long-term impairment and disability, especially in younger individuals.[4,6] Functional outcomes from penetrating injuries are worse than those from blunt trauma based on the likelihood of having a spinal cord injury.[6] The surgical intervention of patients with penetrating spine trauma is widely debated, and there is currently a paucity of high-level evidence supporting a standard of surgical care.[3,4] The heterogeneity of injury patterns in penetrating spine injuries makes the classification and treatment algorithm an extremely challenging task.[4] In this chapter, we present a case that demonstrates an example of surgical management of a penetrating GSW to the spine with resulting conus injury.

Example case

Chief complaint: gunshot wound to the spine

History of present illness: This is a 39-year-old man who was brought to the emergency department after sustaining a gunshot wound to the lower back. The patient was fully conscious and presented with a lower limb paraplegia. Imaging was concerning for a GSW to the spine (Fig. 29.1).

Medications: none

Allergies: no known drug allergies

Past medical and surgical history: none

Family history: noncontributory

Social history: multidrug use and ethanol abuse

Physical examination: awake, alert, oriented to person, place, and time; cranial nerves II–XII intact; bilateral deltoids/biceps/triceps 5/5; interossei 5/5; iliopsoas/knee flexion/knee extension/dorsi, and plantar flexion 0/5

Reflexes: 2+ in bilateral biceps/triceps/brachioradialis; 3+ in bilateral patella/ankle; positive Babinski; negative Hoffman; L3 sensory level; no rectal tone

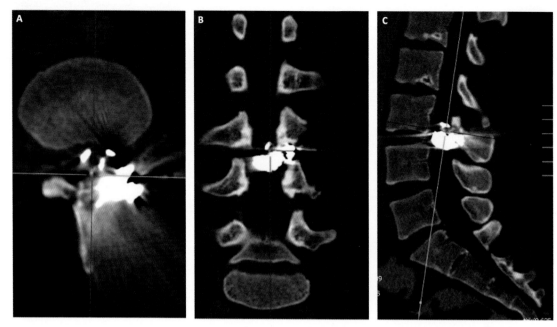

Fig. 29.1 Preoperative postcontrast computed tomography (CT) bone windows. (A) Axial, **(B)** coronal, and **(C)** Sagittal views images demonstrating a metallic artifact (bullet) within the posterolateral spinal canal at the L3-4 level. The bullet had fractured the left lamina and broke into the left L3-4 zygapophyseal joint. No spondylolisthesis is evident. In addition, there is disruption of the posterior ligament complex as the bullet went across the interlaminar ligament (ligamentum flavum), facet capsular ligament, and posterior longitudinal ligament (PLL). The bullet and its fragments occupy the whole anteroposterior diameter of the spinal canal on the left and displace the cauda equina nerve roots to the right.

	Ignacio Barrenechea, MD Neurosurgery Grupo Gamma Rosario, Santa Fe, Argentina	Luis Rodrigo Diaz Iniguez, MD Orthopaedic Surgery Hospital Angeles Lindavista Mexico City, Mexico	Patrick C. Hsieh, MD Neurosurgery University of Southern California Los Angeles, California, United States	Alexander R. Vaccaro, MD, PhD, MBA Orthopaedic Surgery Thomas Jefferson University Philadelphia, Pennsylvania, United States
Preoperative				
Additional tests requested	L-spine sitting x-rays Hepatitis B/C, HIV, syphilis testing Cardiology evaluation Trauma survey Infectious disease evaluation	L-spine x-ray	Toxicology panel CT abdomen/pelvis	Trauma survey
Surgical approach selected	L3 hemilaminectomy, removal of bullet fragments, duraplasty, possible L3-4 fusion	L3-4 laminectomy, removal of bullet and fragments, possible L3-4 posterior fusion if instability present	L3-4 laminectomy, removal of bullet with duraplasty, L3-4 posterior spinal fusion, possible lumbar drain placement	Delayed surgery 6–8 weeks, L3-4 laminectomy
Surgical approach if 55 years old Surgical approach if 80 years old	Same approach Conservative management	Same approach Same approach	Same approach Same approach	Same approach Conservative management
Goal of surgery	Cauda equina decompression, avoid infection/fragment migration/toxic metal	Remove fragments, decompress neural elements	Cauda equina decompression, removal of mass effect, dura repair	Cauda equina decompression, removal of mass effect, dura repair

	Ignacio Barrenechea, MD Neurosurgery Grupo Gamma Rosario, Santa Fe, Argentina	Luis Rodrigo Diaz Iniguez, MD Orthopaedic Surgery Hospital Angeles Lindavista Mexico City, Mexico	Patrick C. Hsieh, MD Neurosurgery University of Southern California Los Angeles, California, United States	Alexander R. Vaccaro, MD, PhD, MBA Orthopaedic Surgery Thomas Jefferson University Philadelphia, Pennsylvania, United States
Perioperative				
Positioning	Prone on Wilson frame	Prone	Prone on Jackson table	Prone
Surgical equipment	Fluoroscopy Surgical microscope	Fluoroscopy	IOM (MEP/SSEP/sphincter) Fluoroscopy Surgical microscope O-arm Lumbar drain	IOM Fluoroscopy Lumbar drain
Medications	Maintain MAP	Steroids	Steroids, liposomal bupivacaine	None
Anatomical considerations	Cauda equina, pars interarticularis, lumbar facets and pedicles, dura	Neurological tissue, pedicles, intervertebral disc	Thecal sac, cauda equina nerve roots	Thecal sac, cauda equina nerve roots
Complications feared with approach chosen	Spinal instability, CSF leak, neurological deterioration	Progressive neurological injury, fragment migration, infection	Cauda equina nerve injury, enlarging dural injury	Cauda equina nerve injury
Intraoperative				
Anesthesia	General	General	General	General
Exposure	L3	L3-4	L3-4	L3-4
Levels decompressed	L3	L3-4	L3-4	L3-4
Levels fused	L3-4	L3-4	L3-4	None
Surgical narrative	Position prone, x-ray to plan incision, midline incision, fascia incised and opened underneath skin edge with monopolar cautery, detach left lumbar muscles off L3 lamina, hemilaminotomy under microscopic visualization with high-speed bur, keep ligamentum flavum as dural protection during bone work, resect ligamentum flavum with angled Kerrison rongeurs, bluntly dissect dura to identify dural defect, carefully dissect bullet fragments off cauda equina roots, explore extent of L3-4 facet and L3 pedicle damage, L3-4 pedicle screw fusion if signs of instability are found, pack area with fat and fibrin flue if cannot primarily repair, layered closure with no drain, maintain bullet and bullet fragments for ballistic investigation	Position prone, midline skin incision, plane dissection, laminectomy over bullet, remove bullet and fragments, evaluate disc injury as well as pedicles and stability, L3-4 pedicle screws if there is instability, irrigate wound, layered closure	Position prone, baseline MEP/SSEP with anal sphincter, expose L3-4 level and confirm with x-rays, placement of L3-4 pedicle screw tracts, L3-4 laminectomy with left L3-4 facetectomy, removal of extradural bullet fragment, explore thecal sac, examine dura integrity, open dura and remove bullet fragments under microscopic visualization, close dura with water-tight closure and perform duraplasty if needed, arthrodesis and placement of bone graft and osteo biologics at L3-4, dural only and fibrin flue, drain placement in epidural space, topic vancomycin and tobramycin, wound closure in layers, lumbar drain placement if concerned about closure	Position prone, plan incision based on x-ray, minimally invasive approach, subperiosteal dissection, confirm correct levels, laminectomy by trying to identify edges of visible dura, tack dura back with sutures, remove encapsulated bullet fragments, close dura as bed as possible with patch if needed, place lumbar drain through separate stab incision, layered closure, place patient on bed rest for 3–5 days with <15 cc/hr drainage, observe for infection
Complication avoidance	Use ligamentum flavum to protect dura during bone work, fuse if instability is found, primary dural repair if possible, attempt primary repair of dura	Explore disc injury, posterior fusion if instability present	Remove extradural bullet first, explore dural integrity, duraplasty if needed, lumbar drain if CSF leak rate concern is high	Delay surgery 6–8 weeks to allow for assessment of neurological function and encapsulation of bullet, minimally invasive approach, lumbar drain placement

| | Ignacio Barrenechea, MD
Neurosurgery
Grupo Gamma
Rosario, Santa Fe, Argentina | Luis Rodrigo Diaz
Iniguez, MD
Orthopaedic
Surgery
Hospital Angeles
Lindavista
Mexico City, Mexico | Patrick C. Hsieh, MD
Neurosurgery
University of Southern
California
Los Angeles, California,
United States | Alexander R. Vaccaro,
MD, PhD, MBA
Orthopaedic Surgery
Thomas Jefferson
University
Philadelphia,
Pennsylvania,
United States |

Postoperative				
Admission	ICU	Floor vs. ICU	Floor	Floor
Postoperative complications feared	Spinal instability, CSF leak, neurological deterioration	Infection, progressive neurological injury	CSF leak, medical complications	CSF leak, infection, cauda equina nerve root injury
Anticipated length of stay	5 days	2 days	5–7 days	5–7 days
Follow-up testing	CT L-spine within 48 hours of surgery	L-spine x-ray after surgery CT L-spine within 48 hours EMG 2 months after surgery	L-spine x-rays before discharge, 3 months, 6 months, 12 months, annually after surgery	L-spine x-rays after surgery, 6 weeks, 3 months, 6 months, annually after surgery
Bracing	None	None	None	None
Follow-up visits	3 weeks, 6 weeks, 3 months, 1 year after surgery	2 weeks after surgery	2–3 weeks, 6 weeks, 3 months, 6 months, 12 months, annually after surgery	2 weeks, 6 weeks, 3 months, 6 months, annually after surgery

CSF, Cerebrospinal fluid; *CT*, computed tomography; *EMG*, electromyography; *ICU*, intensive care unit; *IOM*, intraoperative monitoring; *MEP*, motor evoked potential; *SSEP*, somatosensory evoked potential.

Differential diagnosis

- Spinal stab wounds
- Explosive-related injury
- Penetrating spinal cord injury
- Spinal shock
- Epidural hematoma

Important anatomical and preoperative considerations

Most of the penetrating spine injuries are caused by stab wounds and GSWs.[3] The vast majority of penetrating injuries caused by explosive mechanisms are combat-related lesions.[7] Functional impairment and prognosis is worse for patients with GSWs than those with stab wounds.[3] Several factors contribute to the increased severity of the lesion; however, projectile speed, design, and fragmentation play a fundamental role.[3,7–9] Three mechanisms of tissue damage can be identified: direct impact of the projectile, shock waves of bullet impaction, and the formation of a temporary cavitation.[3,4,9] Civilian spinal GSWs cause damage mainly by a direct mass effect.[4] Penetrating spinal injuries caused by gunshots can be classified in three groups,[3] based on the location of the bullet: Type I when fragments are located inside the canal, type II if the whole bullet is allocated in the canal, and type 3 when the bullet is found in the intervertebral space. Most cases present with a type I lesion.[3] The risk of paralysis is significantly higher in patients with bullet fragments in the spinal canal.[3]

The thoracic spine is overall the most common spinal level affected by GSWs and the cervical spine is involved in most of the cases presenting with a complete neurological deficit.[3,4] Injuries in the cervical spine are often related to loss of the airway and frequently require emergency intubation. Moreover, penetrating cervical injury represents a high risk for vascular disruption of the internal carotid and vertebral arteries,[3] and computed tomography angiography or magnetic resonance angiography should be considered before surgical planning. Hemopneumothorax and damage to vital organs are the most prevalent lesions in the thoracic spine penetrating injury.[3] Perforation of abdominal viscera must be recognized and promptly treated due to the high risk of infection. In cases of lumbosacral GSWs, the presence of significant bleeding must be anticipated and rapidly managed.[3] Despite the lack of consensus or guidelines for the appropriate administration and duration of antibiotics, it is traditionally accepted among orthopedic surgeons and neurosurgeons that antibiotic therapy must be started immediately in all cases for 48 to 72 hours, with emphasis on patients with perforation of the gastrointestinal tract.[3,6,10]

Surgical treatment for penetrating spine injury remains controversial. It is widely accepted that surgical intervention does not improve neurological deficits,[3,4] and some authors advocate to reserve surgery only to prevent worsening of the current neurological status.[6] Furthermore, several studies reported that patients undergoing surgery and those treated conservatively showed similar degrees of neurological improvement.[2,3] However, certain patients can benefit from surgical management, mainly when presenting with incomplete and progressive deficits and lower lesions, such as bullets located in the lumbar region.[4] Thus laminectomy should be considered in patients harboring incomplete neurological deficits, especially when a cauda equina syndrome is identified and in those whose imaging shows evidence of bone or metal fragments in the spinal canal.[3]

What was actually done

The patient was brought to the operating room for exploration of penetrating injury, decompression, and possible duraplasty. The patient underwent intubation and general anesthesia, was positioned prone on the operating table, and pressure points were adequately padded. Somatosensory and motor evoked potential monitoring was utilized during the intervention. Level was confirmed with intraoperative fluoroscopy. Skin incision was made. Dissection was carried out with Bovie cautery. The posterior elements of the affected level were exposed, and some foreign bodies were identified. Several bullet fragments were cautiously removed from the facet and lamina, which were compressing the thecal sac. A laminectomy was performed at L4, including lower L3 and upper L5 as well. There were no signs of dural violation. After several Valsalva maneuvers, no cerebrospinal fluid leak was seen. The pedicles of the spinal levels above and below the level of injury were able to be palpated, confirming adequate decompression of the spinal canal. The wound was copiously irrigated and no signs of active bleeding were noted. The muscles were approximated and the wound closed in a regular fashion. Extubation was done in the operating room. The patient awoke with improvement in his neurological status and was transferred to the intensive care unit. At 3-month follow-up, the patient completely recovered. Radiographs showed postoperative expected changes and no foreign bodies (Fig. 29.2).

Commonalities among the experts

Half of the surgeons chose spinal x-rays for the evaluation of bony anatomy and trauma survey to assess the presence of life-threatening injuries. The majority would perform a L3-L4 laminectomy in the prone position, with removal of bullet and fragments. Posterior lumbar two-level decompression and fusion was advocated by most of the surgeons to ensure neural relief and stability. In the setting of a patient older than 80 years old, half of the surgeons would prefer conservative management. All targeted for removal of fragments and neural elements decompression as the main goals of surgery. Half would perform a duraplasty. Most were aware of the cauda equina nerve roots, lumbar pedicles, and thecal sac. The most feared approach-related complication was damage to the caudal equina and the risk of neurological deterioration. All the surgeons would perform the surgical procedure under fluoroscopy, and half of them would utilize lumbar drainage. Half of the physicians advocated for steroids as a perioperative medication. Surgical nuances and strategies varied but coincided in the importance of adequate foreign body removal and neurological preservation. The most feared complication was a cerebrospinal fluid leak. Following surgery, the majority would admit their patients to the floor and order a lumbar x-ray. Half of the surgeons recommended a computed tomography scan within 48 hours after surgery.

SUMMARY OF QUALITY OF EVIDENCE TO GUIDE SPECIFIC INTERVENTIONS FOR THIS CASE

- Posterior decompression and fusion to provide neural release and stabilization: level III
- The main goals of surgery are bullet and fragment removal and neural decompression: level III

REFERENCES

1. Isiklar ZU, Lindsey RW. Low-velocity civilian gunshot wounds of the spine. *Orthopedics*. 1997;20(10):967–972.
2. Heiden JS, Weiss MH, Rosenberg AW, Kurze T, Apuzzo ML. Penetrating gunshot wounds of the cervical spine in civilians. Review of 38 cases. *J Neurosurg*. 1975;42(5):575–579.
3. de Barros Filho TE, Cristante AF, Marcon RM, Ono A, Bilhar R. Gunshot injuries in the spine. *Spinal Cord*. 2014;52(7):504–510.
4. Sidhu GS, Ghag A, Prokuski V, Vaccaro AR, Radcliff KE. Civilian gunshot injuries of the spinal cord: a systematic review of the current literature. *Clin Orthop Relat Res*. 2013;471(12):3945–3955.
5. Szuflita NS, Neal CJ, Rosner MK, Frankowski RF, Grossman RG. Spine Injuries Sustained by U.S. Military Personnel in Combat are Different From Non-Combat Spine Injuries. *Mil Med*. 2016;181(10):1314–1323.
6. Morrow KD, Podet AG, Spinelli CP, et al. A case series of penetrating spinal trauma: comparisons to blunt trauma, surgical indications, and outcomes. *Neurosurg Focus*. 2019;46(3):E4.
7. Blair JA, Possley DR, Petfield JL, Schoenfeld AJ, Lehman RA, Hsu JR. Military penetrating spine injuries compared with blunt. *Spine J*. 2012;12(9):762–768.
8. Kumar A, Wood 2nd GW, Whittle AP. Low-velocity gunshot injuries of the spine with abdominal viscus trauma. *J Orthop Trauma*. 1998;12(7):514–517.
9. Lin SS, Vaccaro AR, Reisch S, Devine M, Cotler JM. Low-velocity gunshot wounds to the spine with an associated transperitoneal injury. *J Spinal Disord*. 1995;8(2):136–144.
10. Pasupuleti LV, Sifri ZC, Mohr AM. Is extended antibiotic prophylaxis necessary after penetrating trauma to the thoracolumbar spine with concomitant intraperitoneal injuries? *Surg Infect (Larchmt)*. 2014;15(1):8–13.

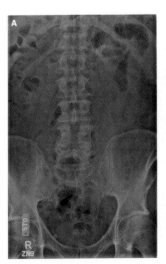
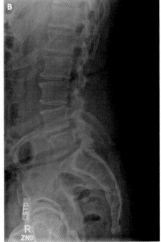

Fig. 29.2 Postoperative lumbar spine x-rays. (A) Anteroposterior and **(B)** lateral images demonstrating postoperative changes including a L4 laminectomy and partial laminectomy of lower L3 and upper L5 vertebrae. No evidence of foreign bodies.

30

C1 fracture

Oluwaseun O. Akinduro, MD

Introduction

Cervical spinal cord injury is a devastating complication most commonly caused by motor vehicle collisions and falls from heights. Upper cervical spinal cord injuries may result in neurogenic shock, respiratory failure, and loss of motor in the upper and lower extremities, often leaving patients bed bound and connected to a ventilator for life. For this reason, injuries of the upper cervical spine must be managed with extreme care and urgency. The craniocervical junction (CVJ) is the most mobile portion of the spine, with complex associations between numerous ligaments and joints. Isolated fractures of the axis are known as Jefferson fractures, named after Sir Geoffrey Jefferson who described them in 1920. These fractures are typically stable and rarely result in neurological injury, but the primary concern is whether the transverse ligament remains intact, as this will guide the treatment of these patients. The most commonly used classification system for Jefferson fractures was described by Landells and Van Peteghem.[1] In this system, type I fractures involve only a single arch of C1, type II fractures involve both the anterior and posterior arch, and type III fractures are fractures of the C1 lateral mass. Type I and III fractures are typically managed with external orthosis for 8 to 12 weeks with fusion rates nearing 100%.[2,3] Type II fractures can be managed conservatively as well with orthosis as long as the transverse ligament is intact.[4] One method for determining stability of the transverse ligament is with the rule of Spence, which states that the ligament is likely disrupted if an open mouth odontoid x-ray shows combined lateral displacement of C1 on C2 of 7 mm or greater.[5] Disruption of the transverse ligament should prompt consideration for surgical stabilization of the fracture. In this chapter, we will discuss the presentation and management of a patient with an isolated fracture of C1 and discuss the relevant anatomy and surgical approaches.

Example case

Chief complaint: neck pain after fall

History of present illness: A 56-year-old male who presents to the emergency room after a fall from a ladder, approximately 10 ft in height. He has arm paresthesias but no weakness. He has a spinal cord stimulator and cannot undergo magnetic resonance imaging (MRI). Computed tomography (CT) imaging revealed evidence of a C1 fracture (Fig. 30.1).

Medications: Dilaudid, Advil, acetaminophen

Allergies: no known drug allergies

Past medical history: chronic pain

Past surgical history: multiple lumbar laminectomies, spinal cord stimulator

Family history: noncontributory

Social history: daily alcohol consumption

Physical examination: awake, alert, and oriented to person, place, and time; cranial nerves II–XII intact; bilateral deltoids/biceps/triceps 5/5; interossei 5/5; iliopsoas/knee flexion/knee extension/dorsi, and plantar flexion 5/5

Reflexes: 2+ in bilateral biceps/triceps/brachioradialis; 3+ in bilateral patella/ankle; positive Babinski; positive Hoffman's bilaterally; diffuse allodynia present in bilateral upper extremities

Laboratories: all within normal limits

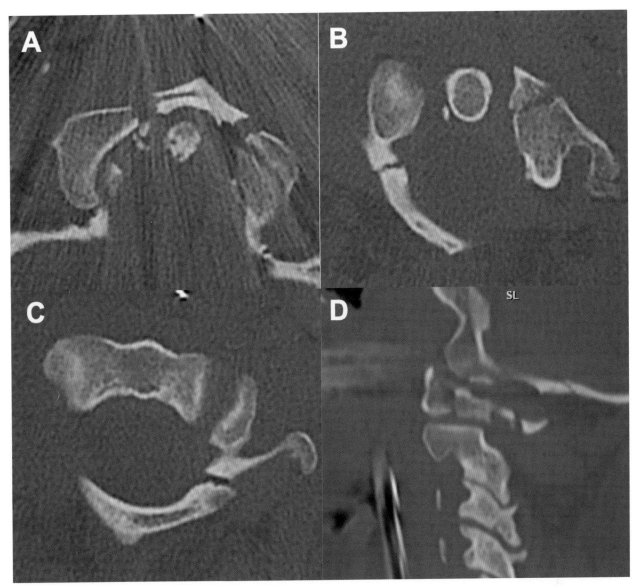

Fig. 30.1 Preoperative computed tomography (CT) image of the cervical spine. (A) Axial image at the rostral aspect of the dens. **(B)** Axial image at the level of the midbody of the dens. **(C)** Axial image at the level of the C2 vertebral body. **(D)** Sagittal image demonstrating multiple fractures of the C1 arch. The C1 neural arch is fractured in two places anteriorly and two places posterolaterally. A fracture also runs through the anterior aspect of the left C1 articular process. There is a small defect in the medial aspect of the right C1 articular pillar and a very small ossific fragment at the right lateral aspect of the dens, which likely represents an avulsion fracture of the right transverse ligament.

	Ciaran Bolger, MD Royal College of Surgeons Catherine Moran, MD Neurosurgery Tallaght University Hospital Dublin, Ireland	Gordon Deen, MD Neurosurgery Mayo Clinic Jacksonville, Florida, United States	K. Daniel Riew, MD Orthopaedic Surgery Columbia University New York, New York, United States	Baron Zarate Kalfopulos, MD Orthopaedic Surgery Instituto Nacional de Rehabilitacion Medica Sur Mexico City, Mexico
Preoperative				
Additional tests requested	CT myelogram	None	CT myelogram CTA	MRI C-spine C-spine AP/lateral x-ray Open-mouth x-ray
Surgical approach selected	Posterior C1-2 fusion	Miami J collar, no surgery offered	Halo vest and no surgery unless instability and lack of healing; if instability after immobilization, then posterior C1-2 fusion	Posterior C1-2 fusion

(continued on next page)

	Ciaran Bolger, MD Royal College of Surgeons Catherine Moran, MD Neurosurgery Tallaght University Hospital Dublin, Ireland	Gordon Deen, MD Neurosurgery Mayo Clinic Jacksonville, Florida, United States	K. Daniel Riew, MD Orthopaedic Surgery Columbia University New York, New York, United States	Baron Zarate Kalfopulos, MD Orthopaedic Surgery Instituto Nacional de Rehabilitacion Medica Sur Mexico City, Mexico
Surgical approach if 21 years old Surgical approach if 80 years old	Same approach Same approach	Same approach Same approach	C1 lateral mass screws and rods Hard collar	Same Minerva jacket
Goal of surgery	Stabilize spine, maintain joint integrity, promote healing, reduce pain, prevent neurological deterioration		Stabilize spine	Stabilize spine, early mobilization
Perioperative				
Positioning	Prone, with pins		Prone	Prone, no pins
Surgical equipment	Fluoroscopy Surgical navigation		Fluoroscopy Surgical microscope	Fluoroscopy IOM
Medications	MAP>80		Steroids	None
Anatomical considerations	Spinal cord, vertebral artery, C2-3 joint, C2 nerve root		Vertebral artery, C2 nerve, venous plexus, spinal cord	Vertebral artery, C2 nerve, thecal sac, spinous process
Complications feared with approach chosen	Instability		Hematoma, displacement of screws, medical complications	Vertebral artery injury, durotomy, C1 lateral mass fracture, C2 nerve root injury, venous plexus bleeding
Intraoperative				
Anesthesia	General		General	General
Exposure	Occiput-C2		Occiput-C2	C1-3
Levels decompressed	None		None	None
Levels fused	C1-2		C1-2	C1-2
Surgical narrative	Position prone with neck flexion, midline incision occiput to C2, expose C1 arch and posterior elements of C2, subperiosteal dissection medial border of C2 to expose pedicle and C1-2 joint bilaterally, dissect lateral to vertebral foramen, insert C2 pedicle screws with fluoroscopy/PediGuard/ surgical navigation if available, dissect C1 arch laterally and stay inferior to arch to expose C1 lateral mass, insert lag screw with preservation of C2 nerve root if possible, maintain venous hemostasis with bipolar/ hemostatic agents, secure screws to rods bilaterally, confirm with x-ray, closure in layers		If halo did not work, position prone in neutral head position, expose C1-2, leave muscles attach to caudal edge of C2, place C1 lateral mass screws and C2 pedicle screws, alternatively can use C1-2 transarticular screws, bone graft with allograft iliac crest wired in to directly compress it into C1 posterior arch and C2 lamina/spinous process, intraoperative CT to confirm position of hardware	Position prone, midline incision, expose C1-3 spinous process, expose posterior arch of C1 (<10 mm on each side) and lamina of C2 until lateral mass, make an entry point for C2 pedicle screw with polish drill that is 25–30 degrees cephalad and 30–35 degrees medial, drill C1 lateral mass with 15 degrees cephalad and 5–10 degrees medially, connect screws with longitudinal rods with transverse connector, decorticate C2 lamina and lateral mass and inferior edge of C1 posterior arch, use demineralized bone matrix, layered closure
Complication avoidance	Insert C2 pedicle screw with PediGuard or stealth navigation, preserve C2 root if possible, stay on the underside of the C1 arch		Leave muscles attach to caudal edge of C2, structural allograft at C1 posterior arch, intraoperative CT	Limit posterior arch of C1 exposure, respect muscular insertions on C1 and C2 spinous process, use transverse connector

	Ciaran Bolger, MD Royal College of Surgeons Catherine Moran, MD Neurosurgery Tallaght University Hospital Dublin, Ireland	Gordon Deen, MD Neurosurgery Mayo Clinic Jacksonville, Florida, United States	K. Daniel Riew, MD Orthopaedic Surgery Columbia University New York, New York, United States	Baron Zarate Kalfopulos, MD Orthopaedic Surgery Instituto Nacional de Rehabilitacion Medica Sur Mexico City, Mexico
Postoperative				
Admission	Floor	Floor	Floor	Floor
Postoperative complications feared	Malunion, infection		Hematoma, displacement of screws, medical complications	Vertebral artery injury, wound infection, CSF leak
Anticipated length of stay	3–5 days	2–3 days	1–2 days	2 days
Follow-up testing	C-spine x-ray prior to discharge CT C-spine 3 months and 6 months after surgery if necessary Possibly remove screws 6 months after surgery	C-spine x-rays 1 month after discharge CT C-spine 2 months after discharge	C-spine flexion-extension x-rays 4–6 weeks after halo vest placement if no surgery C-spine standing AP/lateral x-rays at 6 weeks, 6 months, 1 year after surgery	C-spine x-rays 6 weeks and every 3 months for first year after surgery CT C-spine 12 months after surgery
Bracing	None	Hard collar for 2 months	None	None
Follow-up visits	2 weeks, 3 months, 6 months after surgery	6 weeks after discharge	6 weeks, 6 months, 1 year after surgery	2 weeks, 6 weeks, every 3 months for first year after surgery

AP, Anteroposterior; *CSF*, cerebrospinal fluid; *CT*, computed tomography; *CTA*, computed tomography angiography; *IOM*, intraoperative monitoring; *MAP*, mean arterial pressure; *MRI*, magnetic resonance imaging.

Differential diagnosis

- C1 fracture
- Cervical muscle strain
- Normal synchondrosis (pediatrics)
- Spinal cord injury
- Chiari malformation
- Syringomyelia

Important anatomical considerations

The anatomy of the CVJ is complex as this junction allows for a significant amount of the mobility of the cervical spine and the ligamentous structures must allow for axial rotation and lateral bending while maintaining enough stability to protect the spinal cord. The vertebral arteries must be considered when performing surgeries within this area, as damage to the vertebral artery can result in significant morbidity.[6] The third segment of the vertebral artery typically courses lateral to the C2 lateral mass and then superolateral in a groove on the lateral border of C1. There can be variability in the location and course of this vessel, so preoperative vascular imaging is necessary to avoid complications related to vascular injury. Some patients may have a high riding vertebral artery or ponticulus posticus, a bony arch overlying the dorsal aspect of the atlas, which would make dorsolateral dissection dangerous.[7,8] This can typically be identified on preoperative lateral x-rays. The intrinsic ligaments of the CVJ include the cruciate ligament, tectorial membrane, alar ligament, apical ligament, and anterior atlanto-occipital membrane.[9] These ligaments provide a majority of the stability for this region. The cruciate ligament is a cross-shaped structure that is considered the most important ligament of the CVJ. Its transverse portion inserts into the medial portion of bilateral C1 lateral masses and prevents posterior translation of the odontoid process. The vertical part attaches the C2 body to the anterior portion of the foramen magnum, rostral to the tectorial membrane and caudal to the apical ligament. The paired alar ligaments connect the posterior portion of the odontoid process to the medial borders of the C1 lateral masses and occipital condyles. These ligaments help prevent overrotation of the upper cervical spine and also work with the tectorial membrane to prevent excessive flexion. The tectorial membrane is a continuation of the posterior longitudinal ligament and continues into the foramen magnum. The apical ligament attaches the tip of the odontoid to the anterior portion of the foramen magnum, helping to prevent distraction. The anterior atlanto-occipital membrane prevents hyperextension of the head. The C2 nerve root must be considered, as it typically traverses over the location that the C1 lateral mass screw will be placed and thus may lead to a postoperative pain syndrome in the distribution of the C2 nerve root. The two options are to place lag screws that avoid the C2 nerve root or to sacrifice the root and counsel the patient before surgery about the loss of sensation to the back of the head.

Approaches to this lesion

This patient presented with a C1 fracture with disruption of the transverse ligament as noted on imaging. Due to the transverse ligament disruption, this fracture is considered unstable, and the patient should be considered for surgical fixation of the fracture. The most commonly employed method of fixation for this fracture is a posterior C1-2 instrumented fusion. This can be done with a variety of fixation techniques. If the C1 lateral mass is intact, C1 lateral mass screws are an option for fixation. Fixation of C2 can be completed with C2 pedicle or pars screws. Surgeons must perform rigorous review of the preoperative imaging, as there is significant variation in the size of the C2 pedicle, making this unsafe when the pedicles are inadequately sized.[10] Biomechanical studies have shown that there is no significant difference in pullout strength between C2 pars and C2 pedicle screws.[11] Fixation can also be performed with transarticular screws, which have a more rostral trajectory than pars/pedicle screws.[12] Fluoroscopy should be used to aid the trajectory, which will be straight up across the C1 and C2 articular surfaces and into the lateral mass of C1.[13] Vascular injury of the vertebral arteries occurs relatively more frequently with placement of transarticular screws, so surgeons must closely analyze the preoperative imaging to fully assess the course of the artery prior to screw placement.[6] For patients with fractured or inadequate C1 lateral masses, other fixation options include laminar screws and wiring techniques. Studies have shown adequate pullout strength for these fixation techniques. For patients who are not managed with surgical stabilization, another treatment option is for halo fixation.

What was actually done

This is a patient that presented with C1 Jefferson burst fracture with fracturing of the anterior and posterior arches in two places. There was also radiographic evidence of transverse ligament rupture. Since the lateral mass was mostly intact, the decision was made to proceed with a posterior C1 lateral mass and C2 pedicle/pars screw construct. There was evidence of a fracture line through the anterior portion of the left C1 lateral mass, so a screw at this location would need to avoid pushing the fractured bone anteriorly. The patient was taken to the operating room and placed into the prone position with a Mayfield head clamp. An incision was marked and prepped from the occiput to below the level of C3 to have adequate exposure. A subperiosteal dissection was carried down to C1 and C2, being aware that the posterior arch of C1 was fractured. Careful attention was also paid to the lateral dissection around the superior margin of the C2 lateral mass in order to avoid inadvertent vertebral artery injury. The C2 nerve root was encountered during dissection of the C1 lateral mass, and its trajectory prevented optimal placement of C1 lateral mass screws. The nerve was then sacrificed prior to placement of the C1 lateral mass screw to prevent a postoperative neuropathy in the distribution of C2. The C2 pars screws were placed and the screws were connected with a rod. The incision was copiously irrigated and closed in anatomical layers. The patient was awoken in the operative room with no new neurological deficits. Postoperative x-rays revealed adequate placement of the screw/rod construct (Fig. 30.2).

Commonalities among the experts

Management of C1 fractures remains controversial, as there is evidence showing that even select patients with type II fractures and transverse ligament disruption may fuse without surgical fixation. There was a split among the surgical

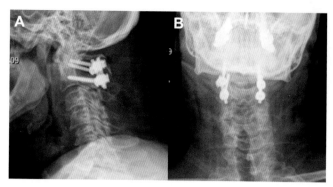

Fig. 30.2 Postoperative cervical spine x-rays. (A) Lateral and **(B)** anteroposterior images demonstrating adequate placement of C1 lateral mass and C2 pars screws.

experts, with half opting for instrumented fixation and the other half planning for conservative management with external orthosis. Half would not alter their management strategy for a 21-year-old or 80-year-old patient, with fusion being the option of choice for the younger patient and conservative management for an older patient. The majority of the surgeons planned for obtaining more imaging, including a computed tomography myelogram, magnetic resonance imaging, and/or x-rays. The surgical technique described was similar for the surgeons, with a consensus regarding the stabilization method of posterior C1-2 fixation. Although there are other options for instrumentation techniques, there was also consensus for use of C1 lateral mass and C2 pedicle screws, if feasible. The surgeons all agreed that the primary anatomical considerations would be the C2 nerve roots as well as the vertebral arteries. The surgeons all planned to transfer to patients to the floor after surgery, with discharge ranging from 1 to 2 days and up to 3 to 5 days after surgery.

SUMMARY OF QUALITY OF EVIDENCE TO GUIDE SPECIFIC INTERVENTIONS FOR THIS CASE

- If the transverse ligament is intact in isolated Jefferson's fractures, cervical immobilization alone will likely result in adequate healing of the fracture: level III
- Isolated Jefferson's fractures with a damaged transverse ligament should undergo evaluation for possible C1-C2 instrumentation, but these patients can also be treated with halo fixation with adequate outcomes: level III

REFERENCES

1. Landells CD, Van Peteghem PK. Fractures of the atlas: classification, treatment and morbidity. *Spine (Phila Pa 1976)*. 1988;13(5):450–452.
2. Kontautas E, et al. Management of acute traumatic atlas fractures. *J Spinal Disord Tech*. 2005;18(5):402–405.
3. Hadley MN, et al. Acute traumatic atlas fractures: management and long term outcome. *Neurosurgery*. 1988;23(1):31–35.
4. Dickman CA, et al. Neurosurgical management of acute atlas-axis combination fractures. A review of 25 cases. *J Neurosurg*. 1989;70(1):45–49.
5. Spence Jr KF, Decker S, Sell KW. Bursting atlantal fracture associated with rupture of the transverse ligament. *J Bone Joint Surg Am*. 1970;52(3):543–549.

6. Akinduro OO, et al. Neurological outcomes following iatrogenic vascular injury during posterior atlanto-axial instrumentation. *Clin Neurol Neurosurg*. 2016;150:110–116.

7. Arslan D, et al. The Ponticulus Posticus as Risk Factor for Screw Insertion into the First Cervical Lateral Mass. *World Neurosurg*. 2018;113:e579–e585.

8. Tambawala SS, et al. Prevalence of Ponticulus Posticus on Lateral Cephalometric Radiographs, its Association with Cervicogenic Headache and a Review of Literature. *World Neurosurg*. 2017;103:566–575.

9. Offiah CE, Day E. The craniocervical junction: embryology, anatomy, biomechanics and imaging in blunt trauma. *Insights Imaging*. 2017;8(1):29–47.

10. Hur JW, et al. Accuracy and Safety in Screw Placement in the High Cervical Spine: Retrospective Analysis of O-arm-based Navigation-assisted C1 Lateral Mass and C2 Pedicle Screws. *Clin Spine Surg*. 2019;32(4):E193–E199.

11. Koller H, et al. A biomechanical rationale for C1-ring osteosynthesis as treatment for displaced Jefferson burst fractures with incompetency of the transverse atlantal ligament. *Eur Spine J*. 2010;19(8):1288–1298.

12. Cyr J, et al. Fixation strength of unicortical versus bicortical C1-C2 transarticular screws. *Spine J*. 2008;8(4):661–665.

13. Paramore CG, Dickman CS, Sonntag VK. The anatomical suitability of the C1-2 complex for transarticular screw fixation. *J Neurosurg*. 1996;85(2):221–224.

31

Acute spinal cord injury

Kelly Gassie, MD and Oluwaseun O. Akinduro, MD

Introduction

The estimated global incidence of spinal cord injury (SCI) is difficult to specify as there is wide variation between regions and discrepancies in reporting.[1] It has been reported, however, that there are around 68 cases of SCI per million population and a prevalence as high as 116 per million in people ages 65 and older.[2] The economic burden of SCI is an estimated 4 billion dollars in the United States alone.[3] Likely due to more advanced medical treatments, increased safety and regulatory efforts and imaging modalities, the incidence of complete SCIs has decreased compared with incomplete injuries.[4] However, the incidence of high cervical SCI has nearly doubled since the 1970s.[5] Although the global incidence is difficult to estimate, SCI occurs three to four times more often in males than in females, with a bimodal age distribution occurring between 15 and 29 years and a second peak after 65 years of age.[5,6] Also, the average age of SCI has increased from 28 years old in the 1970s to around 37 years old, which may be explained by the increasing median age of the overall population.[5] The most common cause of SCI remains motor vehicle accidents, falls, recreation, and even violence.[1] Patients >65 years of age are at an increased risk of SCI due to age-related degeneration. Underlying cervical spinal stenosis is an increased risk to have neurological morbidity in any hyperflexion or hyperextension injury of the cervical spine, whether that be from a ground level fall or high velocity motor vehicle accident. Older patients with degenerative narrowing of the spinal canal are at a higher risk even in the context of a minor trauma just based on these aged-related changes.[7,8]

SCIs may be categorized as complete or incomplete based on patient presentation. Complete SCIs result in complete loss of motor and sensory function below the level of neurological injury, while incomplete injuries preserve some motor or sensation. The American Spinal Injury Association (ASIA) impairment scale was developed to classify the severity of SCIs and is important to use when diagnosing these patients. In older patients, central cord syndrome is the most common SCI.[9] Central cord syndrome typically presents in patients with upper extremity motor deficits greater than lower extremity and generally has a good prognosis. In this chapter, we discuss the presentation and management of a patient with an acute SCI, relevant surgical anatomy, and possible treatment options to consider.

Example case

Chief complaint: neck pain and weakness after fall

History of present illness: This is a 67-year-old male who presents to the emergency department after a ground level fall. He complains of upper and lower extremity paresthesias and that he cannot lift his arms. The patient had a magnetic resonance image (MRI) that revealed evidence of multilevel cervical stenosis and an area of increase T2 signal at C3-4, concerning for an acute spinal cord injury (Fig. 31.1).

Medications: acetaminophen, apixaban

Allergies: no known drug allergies

Past medical history: osteoarthritis, atrial fibrillation with rapid ventricular rate

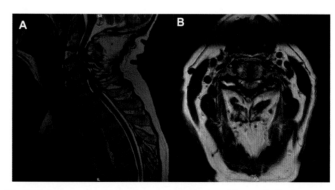

Fig. 31.1 Preoperative magnetic resonance images of the cervical spine.
(A) Sagittal and **(B)** axial T2 images demonstrating severe central canal stenosis with spinal cord compression and increased T2 signal within the spinal cord.

Past surgical history: transurethral resection of the prostate (TURP)
Family history: noncontributory
Social history: none
Physical examination: awake, alert, and oriented to person, place, and time; cranial nerves II–XII intact; Bilateral deltoids 1/5; bilateral biceps and triceps 2/5; bilateral lower extremities diffusely 3/5; rectal tone present; diffuse allodynia present in bilateral upper extremities; Hoffman's + in bilateral arms; upgoing toes bilaterally
Laboratories: all within normal limits

	Michelle J. Clarke, MD Neurosurgery Mayo Clinic Rochester, Minnesota, United States	Takeshi Hara, MD Neurosurgery Juntendo University Hongo, Bunkyo-ku, Tokyo, Japan	Peter Jarzem, MD Orthopaedic Surgery McGill University Montreal General Hospital Montreal, Canada	Frank M. Phillips, MD Orthopaedic Surgery Rush University Chicago, Illinois, United States
Preoperative				
Additional tests requested	Anesthesia evaluation	CT C-spine C-spine flexion-extension x-rays CTA C-spine	C-spine upright x-rays CT C-spine Medicine evaluation	C-spine x-rays CT C-spine
Surgical approach selected	C2-T1 laminectomy and C2-T2 posterior fusion	C3-4 laminectomy, C3-5 fusion	C2-6 laminoplasty	C3-4, C4-5, and possible C5-6 ACDF
Surgical approach if 21 years old Surgical approach if 80 years old	Same approach Same approach	Same approach Same approach	Same approach Same approach	Same approach Same approach
Goal of surgery	Decompress spinal cord, stabilize spine	Decompress spinal cord, stabilize spine	Decompress spinal cord, maintain spine mobility	Decompress neural elements
Perioperative				
Positioning	Prone with pins on Jackson table	Prone with pins	Prone with pins	Supine
Surgical equipment	IOM (MEP/SSEP) Fluoroscopy	IOM (MEP) Fluoroscopy	Fluoroscopy	IOM (MEP/SSEP) Fluoroscopy
Medications	Steroids	Steroids	Steroids, maintain MAPs	Maintain MAPs
Anatomical considerations	Spinal cord, vertebral artery	Spinal cord, vertebral artery, nerve roots	Spinal cord, C5 nerve root, muscle attachments at C2 and C7	Spinal cord, vertebral artery
Complications feared with approach chosen	Persistent compression	Spinal cord and/or nerve root injury, vertebral artery injury	Epidural hematoma, wound infection C5 palsy	Neural injury
Intraoperative				
Anesthesia	General	General	General	General
Exposure	C2-T2	C2-5	C2-7	C3-6
Levels decompressed	C2-T1	C3	C3-6	C3-6
Levels fused	C2-T2	C3-4	None	C3-6

	Michelle J. Clarke, MD Neurosurgery Mayo Clinic Rochester, Minnesota, United States	Takeshi Hara, MD Neurosurgery Juntendo University Hongo, Bunkyo-ku, Tokyo, Japan	Peter Jarzem, MD Orthopaedic Surgery McGill University Montreal General Hospital Montreal, Canada	Frank M. Phillips, MD Orthopaedic Surgery Rush University Chicago, Illinois, United States
Surgical narrative	Preflip baseline MEP, position prone, postflip MEP to confirm stable, x-ray to localize level and plan incision, midline incision, dissect to lateral mass and transverse processes bilaterally, laminectomy using Adson rongeur, lateral mass screws from C3-7 and possible C7 using Magrel technique, pedicle screws at T1 and T2 using Lenke technique, C2 pedicle screws freehand using Wolinsky technique, contour rods, adjust head if necessary, final tighten screws, x-rays to confirm location of hardware and contour of rods, arthrodesis using autograft and allograft, close in layers over a drain	Preflip IOM, position prone, neutral position, midline incision, subperiosteal dissection exposing caudal parts of C2-C5, C3 laminectomy and removal of ligamentum flavum, place C3-4 lateral mass screws with fluoroscopy to confirm direction of screws, place titanium rods, layered closure	Position prone, expose C2-C7 preserving muscle attachments to C2 and C7, remove spinous processes of C2-6, trim to make 12 mm laminoplasty spacers, attach spacers to arch plates, C2-3 and C6-7 laminotomies, remove ligamentum flavum, create longitudinal partial thickness laminotomy on right side and full thickness laminotomy down to ligamentum flavum on left using bur, pry open laminoplasty door from left side with hinge on right with use of Cobb, open to 12 mm and insert spacer starting at C6 going up to C3 with skipping C4, screw spacers onto remaining lamina and lateral masses, close with drain	Fiberoptic intubation, preposition IOM, position supine with neck in neutral position, postposition IOM, standard anterior cervical approach, transverse incision, dissect between carotid sheath and esophagus/trachea, perform anterior cervical discectomy with removal of portions of adjacent vertebral bodies depending on extent of retrovertebral compression, place interbody fusion cage/structural allograft, anterior instrumentation, layered closure
Complication avoidance	Pre- and postflip MEP, Magrel technique for lateral mass screws, Lenke technique for pedicle screws, C2 pedicle screws using Wolinksy technique, adjust head if necessary	Preflip IOM, limit construct to desired levels	Maintain muscle attachments to C2 and C7, laminoplasty with hinge door	Pre- and postposition IOM, remove of portions of adjacent vertebral bodies depending on extent of retrovertebral compression
Postoperative				
Admission	ICU	ICU	ICU	Floor
Postoperative complications feared	Progression spinal cord injury	Infection, instability, CSF leak, vertebral artery injury	Epidural hematoma, wound infection C5 palsy	Neural injury
Anticipated length of stay	3–4 days	10 days	3–5 days	2–3 days
Follow-up testing	Standing x-rays before discharge, 6 weeks, 6 months, 1 year after surgery CT cervical spine 1 year after surgery Physical therapy evaluation	CT C-spine within 24 hours, 3 months after surgery C-spine x-ray within 24 hours of surgery	None	C-spine x-rays 6 weeks, 3 months, 6 months, 1 year after surgery
Bracing	None	Soft collar for 3 months	Soft collar for 2 weeks	Philadelphia collar for 6 weeks
Follow-up visits	6 weeks, 6 months, 1 year after surgery	2–3 weeks, 3 months after surgery	6 weeks after surgery	2 weeks, 6 weeks, 3 months, 6 months, 1 year after surgery

ACDF, Anterior cervical decompression and fusion; *CT*, computed tomography; *CTA*, computed tomography angiography; *ICU*, intensive care unit; *IOM*, intraoperative monitoring; *MAP*, mean arterial pressure; *MEP*, motor evoked potential; *SSEP*, somatosensory evoked potential.

Differential diagnosis

- Acute SCI
- Central cord syndrome
- Severe cervical spondylosis
- Cervical spine fracture
- Transverse myelitis

Important anatomical considerations

Studies have shown that the most common level of spondylosis in the cervical spine has been C5-6, followed by C6-7, C4-5, C3-4, and finally C2-3.[10, 11] The cervical spine has seven vertebra and contributes to the mobility of the vertebral column in flexion, extension, lateral flexion, and rotation.[12] Anatomical factors of the cervical spine differ between the subaxial levels (C3-7) and the atlas (C1) and axis (C2). C3-C7 vertebra consist of a body, arch, and processes, with small but broad bodies.[12] Spinous processes of C3-C6 are bifid and C7 usually consists of the longest and most prominent spinous process. The C7 spinous process can often be palpated in most persons. Each cervical vertebral body has a transverse foramen in which the vertebral artery typically enters at C6.[12] Uncovertebral joints are unique to the cervical spine and are formed by the articular surface on each side of the posterolateral inferior part of one vertebral body, and the uncinate process projecting superiorly form the posterolateral vertebral body below.[13] These joints play an important role in the stability of the cervical spine and are involved with the facet joints as stabilizers with respect to the motion of the cervical spine.[14] The atlas (C1) and the atlas (C2) are distinct form the subaxial cervical spine levels. C1 does not have a spinous process nor a body and is the widest of the cervical vertebra; it is a ring-shaped bone with two lateral masses and an anterior and posterior arch.[12] C2 plays an intimate role with C1, as the dens projects upward from the body of C2 and serves as a pivot around which C1 rotates.[12] There are also significant ligaments that play critical parts in the steadiness of the cervical spine, in particular atlanto-axial stability. The most important ligament is the transverse ligament, which acts as a stabilizing band and constrains the posterior aspect of the dens to the anterior atlas arch.[15] Any compression on the spinal cord may lead to edema or hematoma formation.[16] Due to the anatomical layout of the tracts within the spinal cord, the edema affecting the central cord may cause injury to the lateral corticospinal tracts, affecting primarily the upper extremity due to the somatotopic organization of the upper extremity fibers being more medially located versus the more lateral lower extremity fibers. Whether the injury is due to traumatic, compressive forces, or vascular compromise within the spinal cord, degeneration of the axons at and near the level of the injury is the likely cause of persistent neurological findings.[17] Understanding the anatomy of the cervical spine will aid in the diagnosis and pathophysiology behind acute SCI, as many of these anatomical parts that contribute to underlying spinal stenosis also contribute to spinal cord dysfunction in traumatic conditions or even, as in our case, minor falls.

Approaches to this lesion

In any patient with a suspected spinal cord lesion, immediate immobilization should take place with the focus on initial stabilization and maintenance of airway, breathing, and circulation per trauma management guidelines. In a serious SCI, one must be aware that the spinal and neurogenic shock are very real threats and would need respiratory and hemodynamic stabilization. Once a patient has initially been assessed and stabilized, a full neurological examination is paramount. This can sometimes be challenging in a polytrauma situation, but obtaining a neurological exam in an efficient manner will aid in directing treatment and prognostication. The American Spinal Injury scale is important for prognostication and management and to determine whether the injury is complete or incomplete. The presence of any motor or sensation below the level of injury would determine an incomplete SCI and thus there is a known increased rate of improved function in these patients versus complete SCI patients.[18] Once the appropriate examination and stabilization for these patients has occurred, it is imperative to obtain imaging that will aid in diagnosis and treatment. In any concern for SCI, typical imaging modalities obtained are magnetic resonance imaging (MRI), computed tomography (CT), and plain films. CT scans, however, are more commonly used in an acute setting versus plain films. It is important to determine the mechanism of injury, any fractures, acute disc herniations, and any possible ligamentous injury. Once this has been determined, using other scales, such as the SLICS score (Table 31.1) in the subaxial cervical spine if any fractures are present, may guide treatment. In central cord syndrome, also termed "man in a barrel syndrome," patients present usually after a fall or trauma which has caused hyperextension of the spine with underlying cervical stenosis, resulting in weakness in the arms with relative preservation of lower extremity strength.[18,19] It often occurs in older adult patients with underlying cervical stenosis and can be associated with fractures or acute disc herniations.[16]

Table 31.1 The Subaxial Injury Classification and Severity (SLIC) score

Characteristics	Points
Fracture morphology	
No abnormality	0
Compression	1
Burst	2
Distraction (hyperextension, perched facet)	3
Rotation/translation (jumped facets, unstable teardrop)	4
Disoligamentous complex (DLC)	
Intact	0
Indeterminate	1
Disrupted	2
Neurological status	
Intact	0
Root injury	1
Complete injury	2
Incomplete injury	3
Continuous cord compression in setting of neurological deficit	+1

0–3: nonsurgical management; 4: indeterminate, surgeons' preference, >4 surgical management.

Management of SCIs, in particular central cord syndrome, are highly debated as there is no high-level evidence to guide treatment recommendations.[20,31] When one considers all factors at stake for acute SCIs, including associated disc herniations and/or fractures, decisions may be based on each individual's situation and surgeon preference. Anterior, posterior, and combined approaches have been widely discussed and debated in the literature for treating these patients. Training, personal experience, and patient individual circumstance play a role in the decision-making process; however, there are certain considerations in this disease process that are known in the treatment algorithm. There are factors that should always be taken into consideration including sagittal alignment, anatomical location of the compressive pathology, instability presence, neck anatomy, bone quality, and number of compressed levels.[5,12] Conservative treatment is usually a part of any treatment algorithm, and timing of surgery, if warranted, has been debated. Patients should have mean arterial pressure goals of 85 to 90 mm Hg, but duration is typically surgeon-dependent. Many studies have tried to define timing of surgery for patients, and there have been variable reports in the literature.[21–27] In patients with acute fractures needing stabilization or ongoing spinal cord compression with progressively worsening examination or neurological deterioration, surgery should be undertaken as soon as medically feasible, or within 24 to 48 hours.

There is also no high-level evidence for surgical intervention. Approaches are typically chosen based on individual presentation, morphology of injury, associated fractures, or disc herniations and surgeon preference. Anterior approaches offer many advantages including direct decompression of anterior spinal cord compression, muscle sparing dissection, lower infection rates, and correction of kyphosis, but they are less ideal when more than three levels of the spine are involved. When posterior pathology is present, anterior approaches are not ideal.[13] Posterior approaches allow for wider decompressions and spinal cord posterior drift unless there is significant preoperative kyphosis, but they have greater risks of wound infection, postoperative muscle pain, and C5 palsy.[13] Combined approaches may be considered with both anterior and posterior pathology present, focal kyphosis, and needs of multilevel decompression. Combined approaches, however, increase operative time and often requiring staging.[13] In terms of recovery, patients typically will double their ASIA motor scores (Table 31.2) at the 1-year follow-up, and multiple studies have shown that patients who present with mild or moderate impairment are more likely to have a good recovery.[28–30] Currently, the literature is not clear on which approach is ideal. Treatment algorithms rely on the patient individuality pending the pathology present as discussed earlier. Methods of anterior approaches include anterior cervical decompression and fusion (ACDF),

anterior cervical corpectomy and fusion, and cervical arthroplasty. Posterior approaches include laminoplasty or laminectomy with or without fusion.

What was actually done

An MRI was obtained which revealed severe central canal stenosis with spinal cord compression and increased T2 signal within the spinal cord (Fig. 31.1). The patient was taken to the operating room for a combined anterior and posterior approach in the same day. Part 1 consisted of a decompressive laminectomy between C2 and C6. The patient was placed in the sitting position with neuromonitoring, including somatosensory and motor-evoked potential. An incision was made from C2 to C6 and subperiosteal dissection was done to expose C2 to C6, which were subsequently removed for adequate decompression of the spinal cord. After obtaining hemostasis and closing in anatomical layers, the patient was placed supine on the operating table and a transverse incision was planned for our multilevel ACDF. A transverse incision was made and the anteromedial border of the sternocleidomastoid muscle was identified. The common carotid artery was palpated inferior and lateral and bluntly dissected until the prevertebral fascia and anterior cervical spine were identified. An ACDF was done at the C3-4, C4-5, and C5-6 levels, in that order. Postoperatively the patient was taken to the intensive care unit for monitoring. Postoperative figures showed stable hardware placement and adequate decompression (Fig. 31.2).

Table 31.2 **ASIA Impairment Scale**	
A	Complete: no motor or sensory below the level of injury
B	Incomplete: sensory but no motor below the level of injury
C	Incomplete: motor function <3/5 in more than half of muscles below the level of injury
D	Incomplete: motor function >3/5 in more than half of muscles below the level of injury
E	Normal

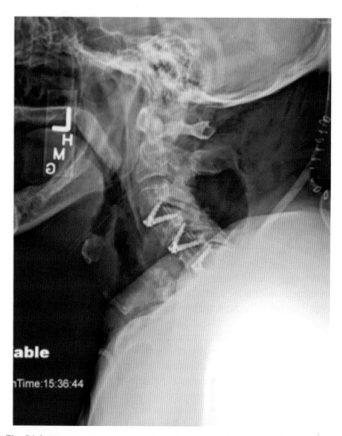

Fig. 31.2 Postoperative cervical spine lateral x-rays. Lateral x-rays demonstrating good alignment of cervical spine and anterior cervical discectomy and fusion hardware in place from C3-6.

Commonalities among the experts

Our panel of expert surgeons agreed with obtaining a more thorough assessment including anesthesia and medicine evaluations, flexion-extension x-rays, and a CT of the cervical spine before proceeding with operative intervention. Three surgeons planned a posterior approach. This included a C2-T1 laminectomy and fusion, a C3-4 laminectomy and fusion, and a C2-6 laminoplasty, all with prone positioning. Three surgeons would have used neuromonitoring during the procedure. Our expert panel agreed that the same approach would have been chosen if the patient had been young or old, with the main goals of decompressing the spinal cord. The majority would have given preincisional steroids, and two surgeons mentioned maintaining mean arterial pressure goals during the procedure. The majority would have placed the patient in the intensive care unit after surgery. Follow-up testing differed substantially between our panel of experts including timing of postoperative imaging, what type of imaging, and bracing. The majority would have kept the patient in a brace for 2 weeks to 3 months.

SUMMARY OF QUALITY OF EVIDENCE TO GUIDE SPECIFIC INTERVENTIONS FOR THIS CASE

- Spinal immobilization of all trauma patients with SCI is recommended: level II
- The ASIA international standards are recommended as the preferred neurological examination tool: level II
- Radiographic assessment of cervical spine is not recommended in awake, alert, not intoxicated patients without neck pain or other serious injuries: level I
- In the awake, symptomatic patient, high-quality CT imaging of the cervical spine is recommended: level II
- Administration of steroids for acute SCI is not recommended: level II
- Early administration of deep vein thrombosis prophylaxis (within 72 hours) is recommended: level II
- Aggressive multimodality management of patients with central cord syndrome is recommended: level III

REFERENCES

1. Lee BB, Cripps RA, Fitzharris M, et al. The global map for traumatic spinal cord injury epidemiology: update 2011, global incidence rate. *Spinal Cord.* 2014;52:110–116.
2. Smith S, Purzner T, Fehlings M. The Epidemiology of Geriatric Spinal Cord Injury. *Top Spinal Cord Inj Rehabil.* 2010;15:54–64.
3. Ma VY, Chan L, Carruthers KJ. Incidence, prevalence, costs, and impact on disability of common conditions requiring rehabilitation in the United States: stroke, spinal cord injury, traumatic brain injury, multiple sclerosis, osteoarthritis, rheumatoid arthritis, limb loss, and back pain. *Arch Phys Med Rehabil.* 2014;95(5):986–995.
4. Witiw CD, Fehlings MG. Acute Spinal Cord Injury. *J Spinal Disord Tech.* 2015 Jul;28(6):202–210.
5. Devivo MJ. Epidemiology of traumatic spinal cord injury: trends and future implications. *Spinal Cord.* 2012;50:365–372.
6. Van den Berg ME, Castellote JM, Mahillo-Fernandez I, et al. Incidence of spinal cord injury worldwide: a systemic review. *Neuroepidemiology.* 2010;34:184–192.
7. Karadmias SK, Gatzounis G, Fehlings MG. Pathobiology of cervical spondylotic myelopathy. *Eur Spine J.* 2015;24 Suppl 2:132–138.
8. Beattie MS, Manley GT. Tight squeeze, slow burn: inflammation of the aetiology of cervical myelopathy. *Brain.* 2011;134(Pt 5):1259–1261.
9. Chen S, Mohammed A, Auriat A, et al. Spinal Cord Injury and Central Cord Syndrome in *Spine Surgery in an Aging Population.* Brooks N, Strayer A, ed. 1st edition. *Thieme*; 2019.
10. Boden SD, Mcgown PR, Davis DO, et al. Abnormal magnetic-resonance scans of the cervical spine in asymptomatic subjects. A prospective investigation. *J Bone Joint Surg Am.* 1990;71:1178–1184.
11. Matsumoto M, Okada E, Ichihara D, et al. Modic changes in the cervical spine: prospective 10-year follow-up study in asymptomatic subjects. *J Bone Joint Surg Br.* 2012;94:678–683.
12. Bleys, RLAW. Anatomy of the Cervical Spine. AO Spine Masters Series. Vialle L, ed. 1st Edition. *Thieme*; 2015. doi:10.1055/b-003-122260.
13. Palmieri F, Cassar-Pullicino VN, Dell-Atti C, et al. Uncovertebral joint injury in cervical face dislocation: the headphones sign. *Euro Radiology.* 2006;16:1312–1315.
14. Clausen JD, Goel VK, Traynelis VC, et al. Uncinate processes and Luschka joints influence the biomechanics of the cervical spine: quantification using a finite element model of the C5-6 segment. *J Orthop Res.* 1997;3:342–347.
15. Bransford RJ, Alton TB, Patel AR, et al. Upper cervical spine trauma. *J Am Acad Orthop Surg.* 2014;22(11):718–729.
16. Brooks NP. Central Cord Syndrome. *Neurosurg Clin N Am.* 2017;28(1):41–47.
17. Jimenez O, Marcillo A, Levi ADO. A histopathological analysis of the human cervical spinal cord in patients with acute traumatic central cord syndrome. *Spinal Cord.* 2000;38(9):532–537.
18. Harrop JS, Sharan A, Ratliff J. Central cord injury: pathophysiology, management, and outcomes. *Spine J.* 2006;6(6) Suppl:198S–206S.
19. Butterfield MC, DeBlieux P, Palacios E. Man in a barrel: acute central cord syndrome after minor injury. *J Emerg Med.* 2015;48(3):333–334.
20. Aarabi B, Hadley BN, Dhall SS, et al. Management of acute traumatic central cord syndrome (ATCCS). *Neurosurgery.* 2013;72:195–204.
21. Guest J, Eleraky MA, Apostolides PJ, et al. Traumatic central cord syndrome: results of surgical management. *J Neurosurg.* 2002;1(Suppl):25–32.
22. Song J, Mizuno J, Nakagawa H, et al. Surgery for acute subaxial traumatic central cord syndrome without fracture or dislocation. *J Clin Neurosci.* 2005;12(4):438–443.
23. Chen L, Yang H, Yang T, et al. Effectiveness of surgical treatment for traumatic central cord syndrome clinical article. *J Neurosurg Spine.* 2009;10(1):3–8.
24. Lenehan B, Fisher CG, Vaccara A, et al. The urgency of surgical decompression in acute central cord injuries with spondylosis and without instability. *Spine.* 2010(21 Suppl):S180–S186.
25. Aarabi B, Alexander M, Mirvis SE, et al. Predictors of outcome in acute traumatic central cord syndrome due to spinal stenosis. *J Neurosurg Spine.* 2011;14(1):122–130.
26. Chen TY, Lee ST, Lui TN, et al. Efficacy of surgical treatment in traumatic central cord syndrome. *Surg Neurol.* 1997;48(5):435–440.
27. Andrew SE, Robert M, John AW, et al. A review of surgical intervention in the setting of traumatic central cord syndrome. *The Spine Journal.* 2010;10(10):874–880.
28. Waters RL, Adkins RH, Sie IH, et al. Motor recovery following spinal cord injury associated with cervical spondylosis: a collaborative study. *Spinal Cord.* 1996;34(12):711–715.
29. Shrosbree RD. Acute central cervical spinal cord syndrome-aetiology, age incidence and relationship to the orthopaedic injury. *Spinal Cord.* 1977;14(4):251–258.
30. Tow AM, Kong KH. Central cordy syndrome: functional outcome after rehabilitation. *Spinal Cord.* 1998;36(3):156–160.
31. Hadley MN, Walters BC. Introduction to the Guidelines for the Management of Acute Cervical Spine and Spinal Cord Injuries. *Neurosurgery.* 2013;72(3 Suppl):5–16.

32

Chronic L5 pars fractures with back pain and spondylolisthesis

Oluwaseun O. Akinduro, MD

Introduction

The pars interarticularis represents a small piece of bone that connects the facet to the pedicle. Given its small size and location, the pars is prone to fracture from multiple sources. Pars fractures can lead to back pain and leg pain with foraminal stenosis,[1] and it can also lead to lumbar spondylolisthesis, which is described as ventral subluxation of one vertebrae body on the other. It is classified as congenital/dysplastic, isthmic, degenerative, traumatic, or pathological based on the classification of Wiltse-Newman-MacNab, which has become the most widely accepted classification system (see Chapter 1, Table 2).[2] The degree of slippage is graded based on the Meyerding classification, scored from I to V (see Chapter 1, Table 1).[1] Grade I spondylolisthesis is defined as slippage less than 25%, grade II is displacement up to 50%, grade III is displacement up to 75%, grade IV is displacement of greater than 75%, and grade V is a complete subluxation of one body on another and is referred to as spondyloptosis.

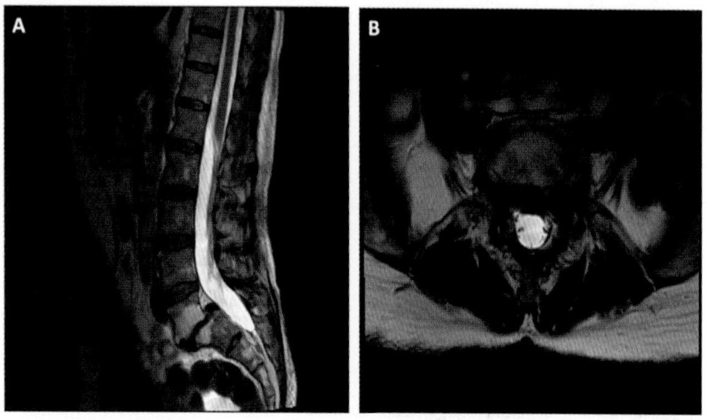

Fig. 32.1 Preoperative magnetic resonance imaging. (A) T2 sagittal and **(B)** T2 axial images demonstrating grade II spondylolisthesis with foraminal stenosis.

Example case

Chief complaint: left leg pain and weakness

History of present illness: A 58-year-old female who is very active presents with a several-year history of pain and numbness in her left leg. It has worsened over the past 6 months. She now notices a foot drop after walking for a prolonged period of time. This does improve with rest. She also has back pain that is improved with rest. She has tried physical therapy with minimal improvement. She underwent imaging and this revealed chronic pars fractures of L5 with spondylolisthesis (Figs. 32.1–32.3).

Medications: estradiol, hydroxychloroquine

Allergies: adhesive, aspirin

Past medical and surgical history: malignant melanoma, Sjogren syndrome

Family history: noncontributory

Social history: office work, no smoking history, occasional alcohol

Physical examination: awake, alert, and oriented to person, place, and time; cranial nerves II–XII intact; bilateral deltoids/triceps/biceps 5/5; interossei 5/5; iliopsoas/knee flexion/knee extension/dorsi, and plantar flexion 5/5

Reflexes: 2+ in bilateral biceps/triceps/brachioradialis with negative Hoffman; 2+ in bilateral patella/ankle; no clonus or Babinski; sensation intact to light touch

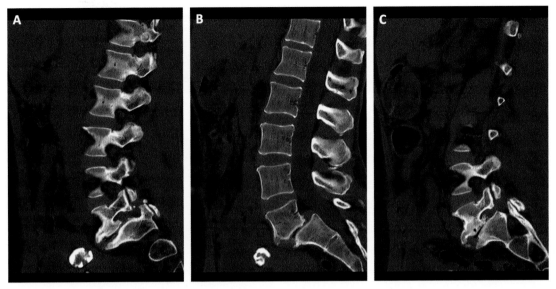

Fig. 32.2 Preoperative computed tomography (CT) scans. (A) right parasagittal, **(B)** Sagittal CT, and **(C)** left parasagittal images demonstrating bilateral chronic pars fracture with grade II spondylolisthesis and foraminal stenosis.

	Lorin M. Benneker, MD Orthopaedic Surgery Spine Unit, Sonnenhofspital Bern, Switzerland	Carlo Bellabarba, MD Orthopaedic Surgery University of Washington Harborview Medical Center Seattle, Washington, United States	Jeff D. Golan, MD Neurosurgery McGill University Montreal, Quebec, Canada	James S. Harrop, MD Neurosurgery Jefferson University Philadelphia, Pennsylvania, United States
Preoperative				
Additional tests requested	EOS® complete spine with spino-pelvic parameters DEXA Facet injections	None	None	None
Surgical approach selected	Stage 1: L5-S1 ALIF Stage 2: percutaneous posterior L5-S1 fusion	L5-S1 laminectomy, TLIF, posterior instrumented fusion	Left L5-S1 TLIF	Anterior L5-S1 graft with posterior L5-S1 instrumented fusion
Surgical approach if 21	ALIF	Same approach	Same approach	Same approach
Surgical approach if 80	Posterior decompression	Same approach	Same approach with caution	TLIF
Goal of surgery	Decompress left L5-S1 nerve roots, restoration of sagittal profile, fusion to improve back pain	Decompress left L5-S1 nerve roots, realignment, stabilization of spondylolisthesis	Decompress left L5-S1 nerve roots	Decompress spinal cord, stabilize lumbar spine
Perioperative				
Positioning	Stage 1: supine with maximum lordosis Stage 2: prone	Prone on Wilson table	Prone	Stage 1: supine Stage 2: prone with no pins on Jackson table
Surgical equipment	IOM Fluoroscopy	IOM (MEP/SSEP) Fluoroscopy BMP	Fluoroscopy	Fluoroscopy
Medications	None	None	None	None
Anatomical considerations	Iliac vessels, parasympathetic plexus, L5 nerve roots	L5 nerve roots, L5-S1 pedicles, L5 pars interarticularis	Exiting L5 nerve roots, bony end plates of L5 and S1	Aorta, iliac vessels, inferior vena cava, L5 pars

	Lorin M. Benneker, MD Orthopaedic Surgery Spine Unit, Sonnenhofspital Bern, Switzerland	Carlo Bellabarba, MD Orthopaedic Surgery University of Washington Harborview Medical Center Seattle, Washington, United States	Jeff D. Golan, MD Neurosurgery McGill University Montreal, Quebec, Canada	James S. Harrop, MD Neurosurgery Jefferson University Philadelphia, Pennsylvania, United States
Complications feared with approach chosen	L5 neuropraxia, persistent back pain	L5 nerve root palsy, failure of fixation, infection	Obtain adequate lordosis, instability	Pseudoarthrosis, kyphosis, intracanal fibrosis
Intraoperative				
Anesthesia	General	General	General	General
Exposure	Stage 1: L5-S1 Stage 2: L5-S1	L5-S1	L5-S1	L5-S1
Levels decompressed	Stage 1: L5-S1 Stage 2: None	L5-S1	L5-S1	L5-S1 foramina indirectly
Levels fused	Stage 1: L5-S1 Stage 2: L5-S1	L5-S1	L5-S1	L5-S1
Surgical narrative	Stage 1: position supine with maximum lordosis, horizontal skin incision, split rectus, retroperitoneal exposure of L5-S1, confirm disc space with x-ray, discectomy and decompression through disc space after sequential distraction and reposition of segment, insertion of trial cages under fluoroscopic control, lordotic angle should be around 20 degrees based on preoperative calculations, insertion of final cage filled with allo/autograft and angular-stable screw fixation, soft drain, closure Stage 2 (same day): position prone, stab incisions and transpedicular placement of k-wires under fluoroscopic control, thread and insert poly axial screws, insert rods, angular-stable fixation in S1, sequential reduction to L5, closure	Position prone, midline longitudinal incision, subperiosteal exposure of L5-S1 interlaminar space out to L5 transverse process and S1 ala, place L5-S1 bilateral pedicle screws under fluoroscopy, place L5 screw heads more anterior than S1 to facilitate reduction, wait of L5 screw placement if challenging, place S1 screws bicortically with fix angled screws, AP x-ray to confirm acceptable screw position, L5-S1 laminectomy, identify L5 nerve root and decompress along its course through the foramen, L5-S1 discectomy, place bilateral rods with securing to S1 first, use reduction forceps to engage L5 to the rod, distract slightly across screws but avoid tension on L5 nerve root, end plate preparation by resection of cartilaginous part of end plate, apply interbody spacer packed with bone graft and BMP from most symptomatic side while protecting L5 and S1 nerve roots, verify appropriate position, compress across L5 and S1 nerve roots to enhance lordosis and compress across interbody, x-rays to confirm alignment and hardware position, decorticate remaining L5 and S1 posterior elements and apply BMP and morcellized bone graft, vancomycin powder, layered closure over a drain	Position prone with encouraged lordosis, midline incision for L5-S1 laminectomy, procurement of local bone, bilateral exposure of Kambin triangle, restore disc height by alternating distractions on left/right side using graduate disc distractors, place banana cage at anterior aspect of interbody space, place percutaneous L5-S1 pedicle screws using fluoroscopy, compress for lordosis, fill extra autologous bone in interbody space	Stage 1: general surgery exposure, fluoroscopy to identify L5-S1 disc space, anterior discectomy, L5-S1 interbody, close Stage 2: prone on Jackson table, minimally invasive L5-S1 pedicle screws
Complication avoidance	2 staged approach, sequential distraction of disc space, calculate preop lordotic angle, percutaneous pedicle screws	Place L5 screw heads more anterior than S1 to facilitate reduction, wait of L5 screw placement if challenging, place S1 screws bicortically with fix angled screws, BMP, place interbody from most symptomatic side	Hybrid approach, alternating distraction, percutaneous screws	Two-stage, minimally invasive posterior fusion

	Lorin M. Benneker, MD Orthopaedic Surgery Spine Unit, Sonnenhofspital Bern, Switzerland	Carlo Bellabarba, MD Orthopaedic Surgery University of Washington Harborview Medical Center Seattle, Washington, United States	Jeff D. Golan, MD Neurosurgery McGill University Montreal, Quebec, Canada	James S. Harrop, MD Neurosurgery Jefferson University Philadelphia, Pennsylvania, United States
Postoperative				
Admission	Floor	Floor	Floor	Spine Unit
Postoperative complications feared	L5 neuropraxia, persistent back pain	L5 nerve root palsy, failure of fixation, infection	Radiculopathy, pseudoarthrosis, graft subsidence, pain	Continued pain, nerve root injury
Anticipated length of stay	4 days	2 days	2–3 days	3–5 days
Follow-up testing	L-spine standing x-rays within 2 days, 2 months, 12 months after surgery	CT L-spine prior to discharge L-spine upright AP/lateral x-rays prior to discharge L-spine upright AP/lateral/flexion/ extension x-rays 3 months, 6 months, 12 months after surgery	Standing x-rays and CT prior to discharge, physiotherapy	Lumbar x-rays 2 weeks after surgery
Bracing	None	None	None	6 weeks
Follow-up visits	2 months, 6 months, 12 months after surgery	3 weeks, 3 months, 6 months, 12 months after surgery	4–6 weeks and 6 months after surgery	2 weeks with APP, 3 months, 6 months, 1 year, 2 years after surgery

ALIF, Anterior lumbar interbody fusion; *AP*, anteroposterior, *APP*, advanced practice provider; *BMP*, bone morphogenic protein; *CT*, computed tomography; *DEXA*, dual-energy x-ray absorptiometry; *IOM*, intraoperative monitoring; *MEP*, motor evoked potential; *SSEP*, somatosensory evoked potential; *TLIF*, transforaminal lumbar interbody fusion.

Differential diagnosis

- Par fracture
- Isthmus spondylolisthesis
- Pedicle fracture

Important anatomical considerations

This is a case of spondylolisthesis due to pars fracture resulting in a grade II spondylolisthesis (see Chapter 1, Tables 1–2). While there is severe foraminal stenosis, there is no canal or lateral recess stenosis. There are a few important points to consider when determining the approach for a patient with spondylolisthesis. All patients undergoing surgical treatment should first exhaust conservative management. When considering the best surgical approach for this patient, it is important to take into consideration the patient's back pain. To rule out dynamic instability, it is generally recommended that flexion-extension x-rays be done (Fig. 32.3). Additionally, if considering an instrumented procedure, consideration should be given to obtaining a bone density scan to evaluate for osteoporosis. A CT scan is also helpful for evaluating bony details (Fig. 32.2). More recently, Chan et al. performed a prospective study that spinal fusion was superior to laminectomy alone for patients with spondylolisthesis.[3]

Approaches to this lesion

The treatment of spondylolisthesis can vary significantly and can be separated into open, minimally invasive, and anterior approaches.[3] In the open approach, one can consider a laminectomy alone versus a laminectomy and fusion. With an open laminectomy, the goal is decompression of the central

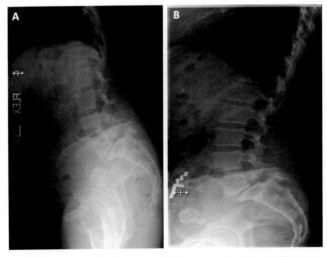

Fig. 32.3 Preoperative lumbar x-rays. (A) Anteroposterior (AP) and **(B)** lateral lumbar x-rays demonstrating bilateral pars fracture with grade II spondylolisthesis without dynamic instability.

and lateral recess stenosis. More recently, Chan et al. showed through a prospective study that spinal fusion was superior to laminectomy alone for patients with spondylolisthesis.[4] However, randomized controlled trials have failed to consistently show positive results for the use of fusion in patients with grade 1 spondylolisthesis. Inclusion of fusion with a laminectomy allows one to increase the degree of decompression with instrumented fusion to allow stabilization. Just as above, minimally invasive approach allows one to accomplish

similar results with less destruction of the paraspinal musculature. Both open and minimally invasive instrumentation can
be accomplished with interbody fusion. Anterior approaches
can be accomplished via an anterior lumbar interbody fusion
followed by laminectomy or a lateral approach followed by
percutaneous pedicle screw placement and decompression.
A recent meta-analysis found that although lumbar lordosis, segmental lordosis, and disc height are improved with
an anterior approach, there were no statistical differences in
postoperative back and leg pain and patient disability when
compared to posterior approaches.[3]

What was actually done

This patient, who has exhausted conservative management,
was offered a posterior approach. In addition to the magnetic
resonance imaging (MRI), which with the patient presented
(Fig. 32.1), a computed tomography scan (Fig. 32.2) and
flexion-extension x-rays of the lumbar spine were obtained
(Fig. 32.3). Although the flexion-extension x-ray did not reveal
a dynamic instability, given the grade II spondylolisthesis in
addition to the back pain, the decision was made to perform
a minimally invasive transforaminal interbody fusion with
bilateral facetectomy and decompression. Instrumentation
was accomplished via two paraspinal incision 4 cm off midline using intraoperative navigation system with O-Arm
(Medtronic, Minneapolis, Minnesota 55432). A transforaminal lumbar interbody fusion (TLIF) pedicle-based retraction
system (NuVasive, San Diego, CA, 92121) was used to allow
tissue retraction rostral-caudally as well as medial tissue
retraction. Bilateral facetectomy was performed and decompression was done. An interbody fusion was then accomplished via a transforaminal approach. No intraoperative
monitoring was performed during the case. Reduction of the
spondylolisthesis was accomplished via manual reduction.
The patient tolerated the procedure well with improvement
of all symptoms and discharged on postoperative day 1.
On subsequent follow-up, the patient continued to do well.
Postoperative imaging showed good location of the instrumentation (Fig. 32.4).

Commonalities among the experts

There was an even split among our surgeons on recommendations of anterior-posterior approach versus a posterior-only
approach for management of this patient's spondylolisthesis.
While half recommended an anterior lumbar interbody fusion
(ALIF) followed by posterior percutaneous instrumentation,
the other half recommended a L5-S1 TLIF. While there was
consensus on the use of intraoperative fluoroscopy, half recommended the use of intraoperative monitoring.[5] The complication most concerning was L5 nerve root injury followed

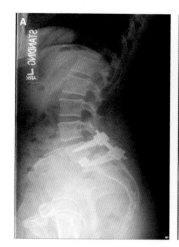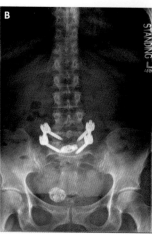

Fig. 32.4 Postoperative lumbar x-rays. (A) Lateral and **(B)** AP lumbar x-rays
demonstrating instrumentation at L5-S1 with L5-S1 interbody placement and
reduction of L5-S1 spondylolisthesis.

by pseudoarthrosis. Bracing was not typically recommended.
The expected hospitalization stay ranged from 2 to 7 days
with planned postoperative imaging recommended among
all surgeons.

**SUMMARY OF QUALITY OF EVIDENCE TO GUIDE SPECIFIC
INTERVENTIONS FOR THIS CASE**

- Bracing following lumbar fusion: level I
- Intraoperative monitoring for lumbar fusion: level II.1
- ALIF versus TLIF for spondylolisthesis: level I

REFERENCES

1. HW M. Spondylolisthesis. *Surg Gynecol Obstet*. 1932;54:371–377.
2. Wiltse NP LL, MacNab I. Classification of spondylosis and
   spondylolisthesis. *Clin Orthop*. 1976;117:23–29.
3. Chan AK, Bisson EF, Bydon M, Glassman SD, Foley KT, Potts EA,
   et al. Laminectomy alone versus fusion for grade 1 lumbar
   spondylolisthesis in 426 patients from the prospective Quality
   Outcomes Database. *J Neurosurg Spine*. 2018;30(2):234–241.
4. Cho JY, Goh TS, Son SM, Kim DS, Lee JS. Comparison of Anterior
   Approach and Posterior Approach to Instrumented Interbody
   Fusion for Spondylolisthesis: A Meta-analysis. *World Neurosurg*.
   2019;129:e286–e293.
5. Parker SL, Amin AG, Farber SH, McGirt MJ, Sciubba DM, Wolinsky
   JP, et al. Ability of electromyographic monitoring to determine the
   presence of malpositioned pedicle screws in the lumbosacral spine:
   analysis of 2450 consecutively placed screws. *J Neurosurg Spine*.
   2011;15(2):130–135.

33

Cervical jumped facets

Oluwaseun O. Akinduro, MD

Introduction

Fractures of the subaxial spine are typically caused by high-velocity injuries such as motor vehicle collisions, falls, and high-impact sports. The subaxial spine consists of the cervical vertebra numbered three to seven and is more mobile than the upper cervical and upper thoracic spine. The incidence of traumatic spinal cord injuries is about 40 per million persons per year with fractures of the subaxial spine accounting for approximately two-thirds of all cervical spinal cord fractures.[1,2] In this chapter, we discuss the presentation and management of a patient with bilateral jumped facets and then relevant surgical anatomy and possible treatment options.

Example case

Chief complaint: neck pain after fall
History of present illness: 81-year-old male who fell from a 5-foot ladder onto his back. He has neck pain and midline tenderness to palpation. He has a pacemaker and cannot undergo magnetic resonance imaging (MRI). He underwent a cervical spine computed tomography (CT) that was concerning for spinal fractures (Fig. 33.1).

Medications: warfarin, diuretics
Allergies: no known drug allergies
Past medical history: congestive heart failure, atrial fibrillation
Past surgical history: pacemaker, coronary bypass graft
Family history: none
Social history: former smoker
Physical examination: awake, alert, and oriented to person, place, and time; cranial nerves II–XII intact; bilateral deltoids/triceps/biceps 5/5; interossei 5/5; iliopsoas/knee flexion/knee extension/dorsi, and plantar flexion 5/5
Reflexes: Bilateral upper extremity 2+ in bilateral biceps/triceps/brachioradialis and Hoffman's present bilaterally; ataxic gait
Laboratories: all within normal limits

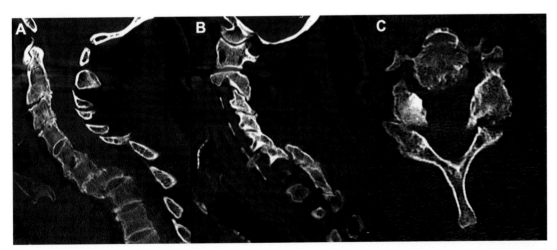

Fig. 33.1 Preoperative computed tomography scans of the cervical spine. (A), Midsagittal, **(B)**, sagittal off midline, and **(C)**, axial images demonstrating anterolisthesis of C6 on C7 and a focal kyphotic deformity, with evidence of dislocation of the C6-7 joint, with the inferior articulating process of C6 joint "jumped" in respect to the superior articulating processes of C7.

	Carlos A. Bagley, MD Neurosurgery University of Texas Southwestern Dallas, Texas, United States	Alvaro Camparo, MD Ramiro Barrera, MD Neurosurgery Hospital Padilla – Tucuman Universidad Nacional de Tucuman Tucuman, Argentina	Peter Jarzem, MD Orthopaedic Surgery McGill University Montreal General Hospital Montreal, Canada	Alexander R. Vaccaro, MD, PhD, MBA Orthopaedic Surgery Thomas Jefferson University Philadelphia, Pennsylvania, United States
Preoperative				
Additional tests requested	C-spine upright x-rays CT T-L spine Trauma evaluation Medicine evaluation Cardiology evaluation	Cervical traction with x-rays CT angiography	CT angiography Medicine evaluation Hematology evaluation	CT C-spine with contrast Potential CT myelogram
Surgical approach selected	C7 laminectomy, C4-T2 fusion	Posterior C6-7 fusion	Awake closed reduction with traction, C7 laminectomy C4-T2 fusion	C6-7 ACDF
Surgical approach if 25 Surgical approach if 60	Anterior approach Anterior approach	Same approach Same approach	Similar approach with less levels Similar approach with less levels	Same approach Same approach
Goal of surgery	Stabilize spine, decompress neural structures	Stabilize spine, fusion	Reduce dislocation, avoid spinal cord injury, stabilize spine	Stabilize spine
Perioperative				
Positioning	Prone, in pins	Prone, in Mayfield pins	Supine for traction with Gardner-Wells tongs, prone for fusion	Supine
Surgical equipment	IOM (MEP/SSEP) Fluoroscopy	Fluoroscopy	Fluoroscopy	IOM (MEP/SSEP) Fluoroscopy
Medications	Pregabalin	NSAIDs	Steroids, tranexamic acid, maintain MAP	Steroids, MAP >85
Anatomical considerations	C7 nerve root, thecal sac, spinal cord, vertebral artery	Vertebral artery, cervical lateral masses	Spinal cord, C5/C7/C8 nerve roots	Vertebral artery, anterior epidural space
Complications feared with approach chosen	C8 radiculopathy, spinal cord injury, dysphagia, cardiac event	Vertebral artery injury, cervical spine lateral mass rupture	Spinal cord injury, infection, hematoma, C5 palsy	Neurological injury
Intraoperative				
Anesthesia	General	General	General	General
Exposure	C4-T2	C5-T1	C4-T2	C6-7
Levels decompressed	C7	None	C7	None
Levels fused	C4-T2	C6-7	C4-T2	C6-7
Surgical narrative	Fiberoptic intubation in cervical collar, position prone, confirm neutral head position, obtain IOM, linear incision from C4-T2, subperiosteal dissection to expose spinous processes/lamina/lateral masses/facets/transverse processes, drill pilot holes for T1-2 bilateral pedicel screws using anatomical landmarks, cannulate and palpate	Position prone, cervical traction with fluoroscopy, vertical midline incision from C5-T1, subcutaneous tissue and muscle dissection, subperiosteal dissection of C6 and C7, place C6 and C7 lateral mass screws using high-speed drill and fluoroscopy, place bars and close system, placement of autologous bone graft from iliac crest, closure with drain	Stage 1: supine position, apply Gardner-Wells tongs on Jackson table, place bolster under shoulder, apply traction while monitoring neurological examination and frequent lateral or oblique x-rays, start with 10 lb and add 10 lb at 3–5 minute intervals until reduced, reduce weight to 20 lb once reduced	Position supine, anterior approach if unable to adequately visualize anterior epidural space, x-ray to identify level, transverse incision, dissection between carotid sheath and trachea/esophagus, place first Caspar pin in a convergent manner to allow leveraged manipulation of the dislocated facet with help of a Cloward spreader, gentle

	Carlos A. Bagley, MD Neurosurgery University of Texas Southwestern Dallas, Texas, United States	Alvaro Camparo, MD Ramiro Barrera, MD Neurosurgery Hospital Padilla – Tucuman Universidad Nacional de Tucuman Tucuman, Argentina	Peter Jarzem, MD Orthopaedic Surgery McGill University Montreal General Hospital Montreal, Canada	Alexander R. Vaccaro, MD, PhD, MBA Orthopaedic Surgery Thomas Jefferson University Philadelphia, Pennsylvania, United States
	screw holes and confirm trajectory with intraoperative x-ray, place T1-2 pedicle screws bilaterally, drill pilot holes and place lateral mass screws in C4-6 using Magerl technique, drill troughs in C7 lamina at junction of lamina and lateral mass, remove spinous process and lamina, widen laminectomy with Kerrison rongeur, ensure satisfactory decompression of canal centrally and both C7 and C8 nerve roots, ensure satisfactory alignment by readjusting Mayfield if necessary, secure contoured rods, irrigate with bacitracin lactate ringers, decorticate remaining cortical surfaces, pack mixture of local autograft and graft extender on decorticated surfaces, disperse vancomycin powder throughout wound, layered closure with subfascial drain		Stage 2 (same day): if reduction still required, awake fiberoptic intubation, position prone with Jackson sandwich and flip onto horseshoe headrest, expose C2-T2, keep muscle attachments to C2, detach muscles to C7/T1/T2, place pedicle screws at T1 and T2 with aid of fluoroscopy, drill lateral mass screws C4-6 and decompress C6 and C7, place screws, realign spine if needed, ensure head position is optimal, attach rods to screws and lock down, close wound over drain	distraction of the interspace, rotate left-sided dislocated facet to allow it to pivot on right facet while distracting and reducing dislocated facet, x-ray to confirm successful reduction, place interbody spacer, shave down anterior surface of C6 vertebral body to make it flush with C7 vertebral body, place C6-7 plate, standard closure, posterior approach if unable to reduce, position prone, midline incision based on x-ray, subperiosteal dissection, confirm level with x-ray, decompress partially reduced facet, place C6 lateral mass and C7 pedicle screws, reduce deformity, instrumentation two levels above and below, standard closure
Complication avoidance	Magerl technique for lateral mass screws, ensure satisfactory decompression of canal centrally and both C7 and C8 nerve roots	Screws under fluoroscopy, limit fusion to two levels	Reduce fracture with traction, posterior reduction if needed, keep muscle attached to C7	Anterior approach if unable to visualize anterior epidural space, use Caspar spin to distract disc space, posterior approach added if necessary
Postoperative				
Admission	Intermediate care	ICU	ICU	Floor
Postoperative complications feared	Wound infection, medical complication, pseudoarthrosis	Implant loosening or migration, pseudoarthrosis	Spinal cord injury, infection, hematoma, C5 palsy	Pseudoarthrosis, neurological worsening
Anticipated length of stay	3 days	3 days	3–5 days	2–3 days
Follow-up testing	C-spine x-rays within 1 day, 6 weeks, 12 weeks, 6 months, 12 months after surgery	Cervical x-ray after surgery, 1 month after surgery Cervical CT 3 months after surgery	Cervical x-rays within 1 day after surgery	Cervical x-rays after surgery, 6 weeks, 3 months, 6 months after surgery

(continued on next page)

	Carlos A. Bagley, MD Neurosurgery University of Texas Southwestern Dallas, Texas, United States	Alvaro Camparo, MD Ramiro Barrera, MD Neurosurgery Hospital Padilla – Tucuman Universidad Nacional de Tucuman Tucuman, Argentina	Peter Jarzem, MD Orthopaedic Surgery McGill University Montreal General Hospital Montreal, Canada	Alexander R. Vaccaro, MD, PhD, MBA Orthopaedic Surgery Thomas Jefferson University Philadelphia, Pennsylvania, United States
Bracing	None	Philadelphia collar for 1 month	None	Hard collar for 6 weeks
Follow-up visits	6 weeks, 12 weeks, 6 months, 12 months after surgery	7 days, 1 month, 3 months after surgery	6 weeks after surgery	2 weeks, 6 weeks, 3 months, 6 months after surgery

ACDF, Anterior cervical decompression and fusion; CT, computed tomography; ICU, intensive care unit; IOM, intraoperative monitoring; MAP, mean arterial pressure; MEP, motor evoked potential; NSAIDs, nonsteroidal antiinflamatory drugs; SSEP, somatosensory evoked potential.

Differential diagnosis

- Cervical facet dislocation
- Acute disc herniation
- Cervical muscle strain
- Cervical stenosis

Important anatomical considerations

The subaxial spine is significantly more flexible than the upper thoracic spine, which allows for unique biomechanical associations. There are also many neurovascular structures that must be accounted for during planning of a surgical procedure in this region. The foramen transversarium runs along the lateral border of the cervical spine from C6 to C2 and houses the vertebral artery. Far lateral dissection of the vertebral bodies in the subaxial spine places this artery at risk because it is mostly unprotected along its course. The spinal sympathetic chain runs along the lateral border of the cervical spine and can be found along the longus colli muscles, thus it must also be considered during far lateral dissection. The facet joint complex accounts for a significant portion of stability in the subaxial cervical spine and needs to be closely evaluated when determining stability of an injury. The orientation of the facet joints transitions from axial in the upper cervical spine to coronal in the thoracic spine. This orientation allows for the significant amount of rotation of the subaxial spine. There are also important neurovascular structures anterior to the subaxial cervical spine. The cervical carotid artery can be found within the carotid sheath running alongside the jugular vein and the vagus nerve. Preoperative imaging can help determine the location of the carotid artery, as the artery may sometimes take a more medial course making an anterior cervical approach more challenging.

Approaches to this lesion

The initial evaluation of any patient with suspected cervical spinal cord injury begins with first evaluating the patient's airway, breathing, and circulation according to the Advanced Trauma Life Support system.[3] Patients should be immobilized and placed into a cervical collar while waiting for radiographic evaluation. The NEXUS criteria were created in 1992 to assist clinicians in determining which patients require thin-cut computed tomography (CT) imaging of the cervical spine and which patients can be cleared of their cervical collar without imaging.[4,5] An alert, oriented patient without intoxication, midline cervical tenderness, neurological deficits, or pain with range of motion can be cleared of the collar without further imaging. The NEXUS criteria were validated by a study involving 34,069 patients in the United States with cervical trauma and found to have a sensitivity of 99.6% and a specificity of 12.9%.[6] The imaging modality of choice for assessment of cervical spine trauma is thin-sliced CT imaging, which has a negative predictive value of a 100% for detecting unstable cervical spine injuries in obtunded or intubated patients.[7] Magnetic resonance imaging (MRI) should be considered in patients with neurological deficits and/or when a more detailed assessment of ligamentous integrity is needed. After imaging is completed, determination must be made as to the need for surgery depending on the fracture morphology and neurological status of the patient. Subaxial fractures can be classified USING the AOSpine Subaxial Cervical Spine Injury Classification System.[8] The subtypes of fractures include compression injuries, tension band injuries to the anterior or posterior tension band, translational injuries, and facet fractures (Table 33.1). The Subaxial Injury Classification and Severity (SLICS) score was developed to create a standardized treatment algorithm to guide decision making for patients with fractures of the subaxial cervical spine.[9] The grading scale has three components: fracture morphology, disco-ligamentous complex integrity, and neurological status (Table 33.2). The disco-ligamentous complex includes the disc space, the posterior longitudinal ligament, and the facets joints and capsules.

Fractures of the subaxial spine can typically be approached via an anterior approach, posterior approach, or a combination of the two. This can be performed via a posterior approach with removal of the dislocated portion of the joint using a high-speed drill to allow for manual reduction. This can be followed with stabilization using lateral mass and pedicle screws, depending on the length of the planned construct. Typically, fractures that cannot be completely reduced prior to surgery need to be approached posteriorly to allow for direct reduction of the dislocated joints, but anterior approaches for facetectomy and reduction have been described.[10] This begins with an anterior cervical discectomy followed by a foraminotomy to identify the nerve root. After the nerve root has been

Table 33.1 AOSpine Subaxial Cervical Spine Injury Classification System	
Injury Subtypes	
A	Compression Injury
O	Isolated lamina or spinous process fractures
A1	Involve a single end plate
A2	Involves both end plates or fracture line splits vertebral body (VB)
A3	Burst fracture extending into posterior wall of VB and one end plate
A4	Burst type involving both end plates
B	Tension band injury
B1	Pure bone involvement
B2	Bone and ligament involvement
B3	Anterior tension band with intact posterior hinge
C	Translation Injury

Table 33.2 The Subaxial Injury Classification and Severity (SLICS) score	
Characteristics	**Points**
Fracture Morphology	
No abnormality	0
Compression	1
Burst	2
Distraction (hyperextension, perched facet)	3
Rotation/translation (jumped facets, unstable teardrop)	4
Disoligamentous Complex (DLC)	
Intact	0
Indeterminate	1
Disrupted	2
Neurological Status	
Intact	0
Root injury	1
Complete injury	2
Incomplete injury	3
Continuous cord compression in setting of neurological deficit	+1

0–3: NONSURGICAL MANAGEMENT; 4: INDETERMINATE, SURGEONS' PREFERENCE, >4 SURGICAL MANAGEMENT

identified, the next step is removal of the uncovertebral joint including the dislocated superior facet to allow for reduction of the dislocation. After fracture reduction, a graft is placed into the disc space and a plate is placed anterior to the vertebral body to be stabilized with screws. A third option is for a combined approach with an anterior discectomy and fusion followed by posterior stabilization. The benefit of this approach would be added stability of the construct, but a combined anterior and posterior approach would subject the patient to the risks associated with both an anterior as well as a posterior approach.

What was actually done

A CT scan obtained at admission revealed anterolisthesis of C6 on C7 and bilateral jumped facets (Fig. 33.1). After admission, the patient was placed into cervical traction to reduce the facet joints into normal alignment prior to instrumentation. Pretraction lateral x-ray and physical examination were performed and then the patient was placed into Gardner-Wells tongs. The patient was given muscle relaxers and 15 lb of weight was applied. The patient was examined again followed by another lateral C-spine x-ray, which showed the facet to be partially reduced. Another 5 lb was added for a total of 20 lb then with a repeat x-ray still showing partial reduction. He remained neurologically intact. Because of incomplete reduction and worsening neck pain, the patient was taken to the operating room for manual reduction and surgical stabilization. The patient was monitored with motor evoked and somatosensory evoked potentials. A skin incision was made from C2 to T2 followed by fluoroscopic confirmation of the level. Using anatomical landmarks, pedicle screws were placed at C2, followed by lateral mass screws from C3 to C5. The superior aspect of the C7 facet joint was drilled. This then allowed the inferior aspect of C6 facet joint to fall into better alignment, thus fully reducing the fracture. Given the fracture at the C6-7 levels, instrumentation was skipped at these levels. Pedicle screws were then placed at T1 and T2 using anatomical landmarks. An O-arm spin was used to

check screw placement. Local autograft was harvested from the spinous processes in the cervical spine and used as autograft for the posterolateral fusion. All the facet joints and laminar surfaces were decorticated and packed off with local autograft as well as corticocancellous allograft and demineralized bone matrix allograft. The rods were then placed and the wound was copiously irrigated. The wound was closed in anatomical layers. The patient returned to the supine position and awoke from general anesthesia in stable condition. Neurophysiologic monitoring remained stable throughout the entire case. The patient was taken to the intensive care unit after awaking from surgery with no new neurological deficits. Postoperative x-rays showed good location of the hardware (Fig. 33.2).

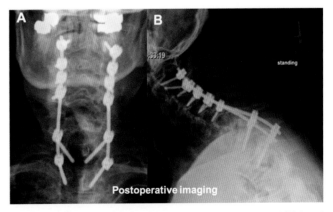

Fig. 33.2 Postoperative cervical spine x-rays. (A), Anteroposterior and **(B),** lateral x-rays demonstrating good positioning of instrumentation extending from C2 to T2.

Commonalities among the experts

There was agreement among the experts as to the initial management strategy for the patient, which involved further imaging including CT of the cervical spine. Half recommended placing the patient into cervical traction prior to surgery to attempt to reduce and realign the facet joints. One of the experts planned for closed reduction in the operating room and another planned for traction as an initial management strategy prior to going to the operating room. The most common procedure planned by the experts was for a posterior cervical approach. Of the experts that planned for a posterior approach, half of them planned for a cervical laminectomy at C7 followed by C4-T2 instrumented fusion. Half of the experts would admit the patient to the intensive care unit following the surgery and half would have used a rigid collar. All recommended imaging after surgery to assess hardware.

SUMMARY OF QUALITY OF EVIDENCE TO GUIDE SPECIFIC INTERVENTIONS FOR THIS CASE

- Surgical management of unilateral facet fractures in the subaxial spine is associated with better outcomes compared with conservative management: level 2A.
- There is no significant benefit of postoperative cervical bracing over no bracing: level 1A.

REFERENCES

1. Goldberg W, et al. Distribution and patterns of blunt traumatic cervical spine injury. *Ann Emerg Med*. 2001;38(1):17–21.
2. Lee BB, et al. The global map for traumatic spinal cord injury epidemiology: update 2011, global incidence rate. *Spinal Cord*. 2014;52(2):110–116.
3. Shakiba H, Dinesh S, Anne MK. Advanced trauma life support training for hospital staff. *Cochrane Database Syst Rev*. 2004(3): CD004173.
4. Hoffman JR, et al. Selective cervical spine radiography in blunt trauma: methodology of the National Emergency X-Radiography Utilization Study (NEXUS). *Ann Emerg Med*. 1998;32(4):461–469.
5. Hoffman JR, et al. Low-risk criteria for cervical-spine radiography in blunt trauma: a prospective study. *Ann Emerg Med*. 1992;21(12): 1454–1460.
6. Hoffman JR, et al. Validity of a set of clinical criteria to rule out injury to the cervical spine in patients with blunt trauma. National Emergency X-Radiography Utilization Study Group. *N Engl J Med*. 2000;343(2):94–99.
7. Panczykowski DM, Tomycz ND, Okonkwo DO. Comparative effectiveness of using computed tomography alone to exclude cervical spine injuries in obtunded or intubated patients: meta-analysis of 14, 327 patients with blunt trauma. *J Neurosurg*. 2011;115(3):541–549.
8. Vaccaro AR, et al. AOSpine Subaxial Cervical Spine Injury Classification System. *Eur Spine J*. 2016;25(7):2173–2184.
9. Vaccaro AR, et al. The Subaxial Cervical Spine Injury Classification System: a novel approach to recognize the importance of morphology, neurology, and integrity of the disco-ligamentous complex. *Spine (Phila Pa 1976)*. 2007;32(21):2365–2374.
10. Zhang Z, et al. Anterior Facetectomy for Reduction of Cervical Facet Dislocation. *Spine (Phila Pa 1976)*. 2016;41(7):E403–E409.

34

Proximal junctional kyphosis after deformity surgery

Kingsley Abode-Iyamah, MD

Introduction

Adult spinal deformity is a prevalent pathology with increasing incidence in the aging population. The correction of this pathology requires multilevel fusion, which unfortunately results in frequent revision. Proximal junctional kyphosis (PJK) and proximal junctional failure (PJF) are common and serious complications following long constructs for spinal deformity. It has been reported to occur in up to 39% of adult spinal deformity cases.[1-9] PJK is defined as a sagittal Cobb angle ≥10 degrees and at least 10 degrees greater than the preoperative measurement, while PJF is defined as any type of symptomatic PJK requiring revision surgery.[10, 11] The etiology is thought to be multifactorial. It can result in symptoms of back pain, kyphotic deformity, and even neurological deficit from spinal cord and/or nerve root compression. Because PJK has broad implications for both symptomatic and asymptomatic patients, two separate classification systems have emerged. In 2012, Yati et al. proposed a classification system that allowed description by type (type 1 = ligamentous failure; type 2 = bone failure; type 3 = implant or bone interface failure), severity (grade A, B, or C corresponding to an increase in the PJA of 10 to 14 degrees, 15 to 19 degrees, or >20 degrees, respectively), and the presence (S) or absence (N) of spondylolisthesis (Table 34.1).[11, 12] Laue et al. proposed a PJK severity scale that integrates six components, which are stratified and assigned a point value and summed for total severity score: neurological deficit, focal pain, instrumentation problems, change in kyphosis/posterior ligament complex integrity, fracture location, and level of upper instrumented vertebrae (UIV) (Table 34.2).[5] Although no known technique exists to prevent PJK, there are factors that may reduce its incidence.

Example case

Chief complaint: back pain

History of present illness: A 67-year-old female who underwent T10 to pelvis instrumented fusion for scoliosis (Figs. 34.1–34.3) repair 7 months prior presents with recurrent back pain. She did well postoperatively with improvement of her back pain, leg pain, and posterior. However, she also presents with increasing worsening upper thoracic back pain and increasing kyphosis. Imaging showed concern for PJK (Fig. 34.4). She denies any weakness, numbness, or bowel/bladder dysfunction.

Medications: rosuvastatin, paroxetine, carvedilol, ramipril, timolol, trazodone

Allergies: no known drug allergies

Past medical and surgical history: T10 to pelvis instrumented fusion for scoliosis repair, osteopenia, diabetes, depression, anxiety, hypertension, hyperlipidemia

Family history: noncontributory

Social history: teacher, no smoking history, occasional alcohol

Physical examination: awake, alert, and oriented to person, place, and time; cranial nerves II–XII intact; bilateral deltoids/triceps/biceps 5/5; interossei 5/5; iliopsoas/knee flexion/knee extension/dorsi, and plantar flexion 5/5

Reflexes: 2+ in bilateral biceps/triceps/brachioradialis with negative Hoffman; 2+ in bilateral patella/ankle; no clonus or Babinski; sensation intact to light touch

Table 34.1 Modified Boachie-Adjei Classification of Proximal Junctional Kyphosis

Type	Definition
1	Ligamentous failure
2	Bone failure
3	Implant and bone interface failure
Grades	Definition
A	Proximal junctional increase 10–19 degrees
B	Proximal junctional increase 20–29 degrees
C	Proximal junctional increase ≥30 degrees
Spondylolisthesis	Definition
N	No obvious spondylolisthesis above UIV
S	Spondylolisthesis above UIV

	Dean Chou, MD Rory Mayer, MD Neurosurgery University of California at San Francisco San Francisco, California, United States	Michael G. Fehlings, MD, PhD Neurosurgery University of Toronto Toronto, Canada	Lawrence G. Lenke, MD Orthopaedic Surgery Columbia University New York City, New York, United States	Susana Nunez-Pereira, MD, PhD Orthopaedic Surgery Hospital Universitario Vall d'Hebron Barcelona, Spain
Preoperative				
Additional tests requested	DEXA Endocrinology evaluation (teriparatide for minimum of 6 months preoperative) MRI thoracic and lumbar spine CT thoracic and lumbar spine Medicine evaluation	DEXA CT complete spine Psychiatry evaluation Medicine evaluation Nutrition evaluation	DEXA CT T/L/S-spine MRI complete spine Endocrinology evaluation	DEXA CT complete spine Scoliosis x-rays for sagittal alignment parameters
Surgical approach selected	If pain is disabling, T4 to pelvis fusion with T9-10 and T10-11 posterior column osteotomies	T9-10, T10-11 Smith-Peterson osteotomies and T2-12 posterior fusion	T9-10 posterior column osteotomy, revision instrumentation from T2, T3, or T4 to L2 or L3	If kyphosis progresses or symptoms are disabling, L4 pedicle subtraction osteotomy and T4-pelvis fusion
Surgical approach if 25 Surgical approach if 80	Similar approach with domino Similar approach with domino	Unlikely to see Same approach	Same approach with increased bone removal at upper lumbar spine Conservative approach or limit upper level to T12	Same approach Conservative management
Goal of surgery	Restoration of sagittal balance, improve pain	Restoration of sagittal balance, obtain solid fusion, improve pain, enhance mobility	Restoration of sagittal balance, minimize chance of proximal junctional kyphosis, improve pain and postural imbalance	Restoration of sagittal balance, improve pain
Perioperative				
Positioning	Prone on Jackson table	Prone on Allen table, with Mayfield pins	Prone with Gardner-Wells tongs	Prone on Jackson table
Surgical equipment	IOM (MEP/SSEP/EMG) Fluoroscopy Surgical navigation Cell saver	IOM (MEP/SSEP) Fluoroscopy O-arm Surgical navigation	IOM (MEP/SSEP/EMG) Fluoroscopy O-arm	IOM (MEP/SSEP) Fluoroscopy Cell saver
Medications	Tranexamic acid	Tranexamic acid, MAP >80	Tranexamic acid, steroids	Tranexamic acid
Anatomical considerations	Dura/spinal cord, interspinous ligaments, facet joints at top of construct	Pedicle anatomy, spinal cord, nerve roots, aorta	Posterior column abnormalities, prior laminectomy defects	L4-5 nerve roots, thecal sac, spinal cord
Complications feared with approach chosen	Proximal junctional kyphosis in upper thoracic spine, pseudoarthrosis, delayed implant fracture	Spinal cord/nerve root injury, excessive bleeding, pedicle fracture, malposition of implants, posterior ischemic optic neuropathy	CSF leak, excessive upper lumbar/lower thoracic lordosis	Spinal cord/nerve root injury, blood loss/hemodynamic instability
Intraoperative				
Anesthesia	General	General	General	General
Exposure	T4-pelvis	T2-L2	T3-L3	T4-pelvis
Levels decompressed	None	None	T9-10	L4
Levels fused	T4-pelvis	T2-L2	T3-L3	T4-pelvis

	Dean Chou, MD Rory Mayer, MD Neurosurgery University of California at San Francisco San Francisco, California, United States	Michael G. Fehlings, MD, PhD Neurosurgery University of Toronto Toronto, Canada	Lawrence G. Lenke, MD Orthopaedic Surgery Columbia University New York City, New York, United States	Susana Nunez-Pereira, MD, PhD Orthopaedic Surgery Hospital Universitario Vall d'Hebron Barcelona, Spain
Surgical narrative	Position prone, expose T4 to pelvis including prior implants, inspect prior fusion, routine soft tissue culture to evaluate for subclinical infection, place pedicle screws from T4-T9, perform T9-T11 posterior column osteotomies, remove set screws down to 2 levels below where domino will be placed, stagger domino placement to avoid stress of two dominoes at same level, use rod bender to bend proximal rod up, remove pedicle screws where dominoes will go, cut rod in situ with rod cutter, place dominoes onto cut ends of rods, bend distal rods back down with new rods placed into dominoes, new rods are bent down into proximal spine to T4, gentle cantilever can be applied to correct kyphosis but ensure proximal rod is kyphotic, set screws are placed, final tighten set screws, decortication of posterior elements across entire exposure, placement of autograft and allograft, layered closure with two subfascial drains	Position prone with Mayfield pins using Allen table sandwich flip, IOM, posterior midline exposure, expose T2-T12, cut rods at T10, evaluate if pedicle screws T10-T12 are solid or loose, replace with bigger screws if loose, clamp reference frame, O-arm spins to cover T2-8 and T8-T12, cannulate pedicles from T2-T9 and likely replace T10 pedicle screws, perform Smith-Peterson osteotomies at T9-10 and T10-11 bilaterally with bur and Kerrison punches, contour rods to desired curvature, decorticate exposed bony surfaces, place rods, use side-to-side connectors to connect new rod to the previous rod at T11 and T12, use manual positioning and gentle compression to reduce kyphosis, final O-arm spine to confirm hardware placement and satisfactory alignment correction, local bone and two units of BMP for fusion, local anesthetic and vancomycin powder, layered closure with subfascial drain	Position prone with Gardner-Wells tongs and avoid hyper lordosis, subperiosteal exposure up to T2, T3, or T4 and minimize tissue disruption and down to prior implants at L2 or L3, place vancomycin powder into muscle and subcutaneous tissue, check fixation from T10 to L3, consider exposing all the way to sacrum/ilium if the hardware is loose or spine not fused, remove inferior facets from T3 to 4 down to T9-10 if T3 chosen as upper level, remove rods from T10 to L3 by cutting short third rod on left side, check screw purchase of remaining screws and replace if not solid, place bilateral pedicle screws up to T3 with freehand technique, posterior column osteotomies at T9-10 and TLIF if unstable or needed for segmental kyphosis correction, O-arm to assess screw and cage placement, reinstrumentation placed from T3 to L2 on left and T3-L3 on right with cantilever and posterior compressive correction of lower thoracic junctional kyphosis and recreate normal kyphosis from T3 to 6, new rods connected to old rods with rod-rod connectors, intraoperative long cassette stitched x-rays to evaluate alignment, fusion with auto/allograft and potentially BMP especially in thoracolumbar junction, layered closure with deep and superficial drain with vancomycin and tobramycin powder into muscle and subcutaneous tissue	Position prone, preferably on Jackson table, incision above the old scar until T4, pedicle instrumentation T4 to T9 with free hand technique, identify previous instrumented area. Remove taps from T10 to L2 or L3, check if it is possible to pull the rod and put it aside. Otherwise, cut the rods below L1 and remove the rod between T10 and L1, remove T12 screw at one side and L1 at the other side, check the purchase of the remaining screws, if any of them is loose or has not a good purchase, change it. Then, perform Smith-Petersen osteotomies T9/T10 and T10/T11. Place hooks at T3, and cut rods and bend them according to previously calculated and desired kyphosis. Place rods, close osteotomies performing local compression, connect rods with more caudal rods with end-to-end connectors. Check fluoroscopy if adequate correction has been obtained. Close the system under slight compression. Add DTT/cross-link at osteotomy site. Add bone graft. Layered wound closure, applying vancomycin at the subcutaneous layer.

	Dean Chou, MD Rory Mayer, MD Neurosurgery University of California at San Francisco San Francisco, California, United States	Michael G. Fehlings, MD, PhD Neurosurgery University of Toronto Toronto, Canada	Lawrence G. Lenke, MD Orthopaedic Surgery Columbia University New York City, New York, United States	Susana Nunez-Pereira, MD, PhD Orthopaedic Surgery Hospital Universitario Vall d'Hebron Barcelona, Spain
Complication avoidance	Evaluate for subclinical infection, domino rod placement that is staggered, cantilever rods to correct kyphosis	Surgical navigation, evaluate previous screws for loosening, Smith-Peterson osteotomies for sagittal correction, domino rods to previous rods, BMP	Avoid hyper lordosis during positioning, avoid tissue mobilization at upper surgical level, extend down to sacrum/ilium if previous hardware loose or not fused during intraoperative evaluation, O-arm to assess hardware, different ending points distally to offset implants, rod-rod connectors to make sure stable, intraoperative long cassette stitched x-rays to evaluate alignment	IONM, careful positioning and check fluoroscopy after positioning, take intraoperative cultures to rule out subclinic infection.
Postoperative				
Admission	ICU	Stepdown unit	ICU	ICU
Postoperative complications feared	Medical complications, wound infection, proximal junctional kyphosis in upper thoracic spine, pseudoarthrosis, delayed implant fracture	Wound infection, screw pullout, early hardware failure, medical complications	Medical complications, CSF leak, excessive upper lumbar/lower thoracic lordosis	Wound infection, CSF leak, Pseudoarthrosis, rod breakage
Anticipated length of stay	5–7 days	5–7 days	4 days	8–9 days
Follow-up testing	Full length standing x-rays prior to discharge, 3 months, 6 months, 1 year, 2 years after surgery	Standing x-rays 6 weeks, 3 months, 6 months, 12 months, 24 months after surgery CT T-L spine 6 months after surgery	Upright x-rays after drains removed	Full-standing x-rays before discharge
Bracing	None	None	None	None
Follow-up visits	2 weeks, 6 weeks, 3 months, 6 months, 1 year, 2 years after surgery	6 weeks, 3 months, 6 months, 12 months, 24 months after surgery	2 weeks, 6–8 weeks after surgery	2 weeks, 6 weeks, 6 months, 1 and 2 years

CSF, Cerebrospinal fluid; CT, computed tomography; BMP, bone morphogenic protein; DEXA, dual-energy x-ray absorptiometry; EMG, electromyography; ICU, intensive care unit; IOM, intraoperative monitoring; MAP, mean arterial pressure; MEP, motor evoked potential; MRI, magnetic resonance imaging; SSEP, somatosensory evoked potential; TLIF, transforaminal lumbar interbody fusion.

Differential diagnosis

- Proximal junctional kyphosis
- Proximal junctional failure
- Adjacent segment disease

Important anatomical considerations

It is well documented that fusion of any two vertebrae increases both the intradiscal pressure and adjacent segment motion leading to adjacent segment disease.[13–16] This is especially magnified following a long construct for spinal deformity leading to transition from a fused to mobile segment, which creates abnormal forces seen in the disc, facet, and surrounding ligaments. Failure occurs when these segments can no longer accommodate these forces leading to vertebral body, disc space, and facet changes. This can ultimately lead to symptoms of pain, kyphotic deformity, and even neurological deficit from spinal cord or nerve root compression. The fact that the cause of PJK/PJF is multifactorial has made it difficult to predict, prevent, and treat. There are known surgical, radiographic, and patient-specific risk factors, which may increase the risk of PJK. Surgical approaches that disrupt the posterior tension band especially when there is disruption of the facet capsule and interspinous tissue have a propensity to cause PJK.[3,10,12,17] Furthermore, combined anterior-posterior approaches may increase the rate of PJK. Additionally, the

Table 34.2 Hart-International Spine Study Group Proximal Junctional Kyphosis Severity Scale	
Characteristic	Severity Score (points)
Neurological Deficit	
None	0
Radicular pain	2
Myelopathy/motor deficit	4
Focal pain	
None	0
VAS ≤4	1
VAS ≥5	3
Instrumentation Problem	
None	0
Partial fixation loss	1
Prominence	1
Complete fixation loss	2
Change in Kyphosis/PLC Integrity	
0–10 degrees	0
10–20 degrees	1
>20 degrees	2
PLC failure	2
UIV/UIV + 1 fracture	
None	0
Compression fracture	1
Burst/chance fracture	2
Translation	3
Level of UIV	
Thoracolumbar junction	0
Upper thoracic	1
VAS, visual analogue scale; PLC, posterios ligamentous complex; UIV, upper instrumented vertebrae	

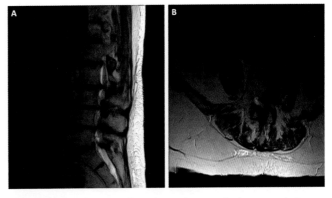

Fig. 34.1 Preoperative magnetic resonance images prior to any surgical intervention. (A) T2 sagittal and **(B)** T2 axial images demonstrating multilevel disc degeneration with foraminal and lateral recess stenosis.

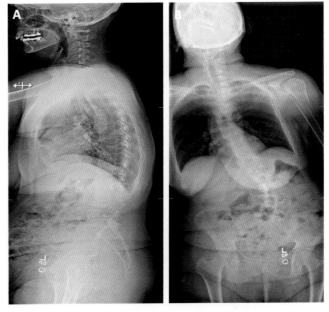

Fig. 34.3 Preoperative x-rays prior to any surgical intervention. (A) Anteroposterior (AP) and **(B)** lateral x-rays showing coronal and sagittal deformity.

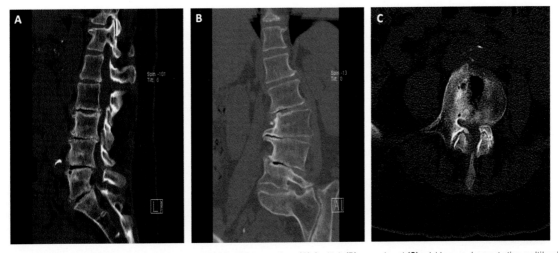

Fig. 34.2 Preoperative computed tomography scans prior to any surgical intervention. (A) Sagittal, **(B)** coronal, and **(C)** axial images demonstrating multilevel disc degeneration, with foraminal and lateral recess stenosis.

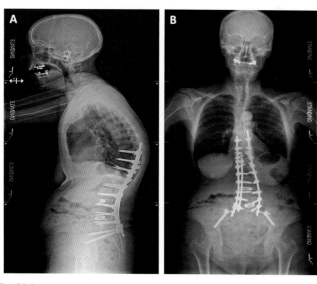

Fig. 34.4 Postoperative x-rays. (A) Lateral and **(B)** AP x-rays showing proximal junctional kyphosis at T9-10 after undergoing T10-pelvis fusion.

rigidity of the construct in addition to the degree of correction may also increase the likelihood of PJK.[12,18–20] Radiographic factors that may increase PJK include high preoperative sagittal vertical axis (SVA), thoracic kyphosis, higher pelvic index, and pelvic retroversion.[20,21] Patient-specific factors such as age, increasing body mass index, smoking, and osteoporosis may also cause PJK.[10,20,22,23]

Approaches to this lesion

The main strategy for approaching PJK is that of prevention. Given the potentially devastating impact of PJK on the patient, all attempts should be made to address any predisposing factors. These include both patient-specific factors and surgical techniques. Patient-specific factors, which can be addressed preoperatively, should be maximized prior to proceeding with extensive fusion whenever possible. This includes smoking cessation, weight loss for reduction of body mass index, and treatment of osteopenia/osteoporosis prior to undertaking surgical treatment. Surgical strategies that help prevent PJK should also be considered. Lau et al. suggest that some strategies to help prevent PJK include (1) extension of fusion to include levels with baseline segmental kyphosis >5 degrees, (2) decreased instrument stiffness, (3) use of composite materials, (4) use of fewer implants, (5) more distal osteotomies, (6) less destruction of the soft tissues at the upper instrumented vertebrae, (7) an attempt to achieve optimal spinal balance, (8) use of transition rods, and (9) optimizing postoperative alignment.[5] When PJK does occur, it is seen within the first 8 weeks in over 60% of patients and those requiring intervention occurs within 10 months in over 85% of patients.[11,20] Initial treatment should involve conservative management with muscle strengthening, pain control, and proper posturing techniques in asymptomatic patients. When surgical treatment is required, this can typically be addressed with posterior extension of the prior instrumentation.

What was actually done

This patient who presented with thoracic back pain approximately 7 months following scoliosis correction noted improvement of her preoperative symptoms but gradually began having back pain. She also reported that she has had progressive worsening kyphosis. Upon detailed questioning, the patient reported that she had not been adherent to her posturing recommendation and lifting restrictions. Her pain was fairly tolerable and improved with muscle relaxants. Additionally, she denied any neurological deficit. Given this history, the patient was first prescribed conservative management with physical therapy. Additionally, she was placed in a thoracic lumbar sacral orthosis (TLSO) brace for 3 months and with posturing advice. With this conservative management, the patient had improvement of the symptoms and did not require surgical intervention. We continue to monitor the patient with scoliosis films every 6 months.

Commonalities among the experts

All experts agreed that additional imaging and consultation were needed to further assess this patient. The most common requested imaging included a dual-energy x-ray absorptiometry scan, computed tomgoraphy scans of the entire spine, and endocrinology consultation. One expert recommended that the patient be placed on teriparatide for a minimum of 6 months prior to any surgical intervention. With all our experts recommending surgical intervention, all recommended surgical intervention in the face of disabling pain or progression of the kyphosis. The most common upper level of extension of the fusion was T2 or T4 and the majority of our surgeons recommended a Smith-Peterson osteotomy at T9-10.[24] One expert also recommended an additional Smith-Peterson osteotomy at T10-11. One surgeon recommended a L4 pedicle subtraction osteotomy followed by a T4-pelvis fusion. The majority of our surgeons also recommended a similar plan when faced with a younger patient, while the majority recommended conservative management in older patients. There was consensus in the use of intraoperative monitoring,[25] fluoroscopy, and tranexamic acid, and the majority also recommended O-arm use intraoperatively to help guide pedicle screw placement. The majority recommend admission to the intensive care unit postperatively with planned imaging at multiple time points postoperatively.

SUMMARY OF QUALITY OF EVIDENCE TO GUIDE SPECIFIC INTERVENTIONS FOR THIS CASE

- Intraoperative monitoring for deformity correction: level II.1
- Smith-Peterson osteotomy for PJK correction: Level II.2
- Hook versus pedicle screw at the upper instrumented vertebral level for PJK prevention: level II.1
- Complication in deformity in patient >80 years of age: level II.1

REFERENCES

1. Denis F, Sun EC, Winter RB. Incidence and risk factors for proximal and distal junctional kyphosis following surgical treatment for Scheuermann kyphosis: minimum five-year follow-up. *Spine (Phila Pa 1976)*. 2009;34(20):E729–E734.
2. DeWald CJ, Stanley T. Instrumentation-related complications of multilevel fusions for adult spinal deformity patients over age 65:

surgical considerations and treatment options in patients with poor bone quality. *Spine (Phila Pa 1976)*. 2006;31(19 Suppl):S144–S151.

3. Kim HJ, Lenke LG, Shaffrey CI, Van Alstyne EM, Skelly AC. Proximal junctional kyphosis as a distinct form of adjacent segment pathology after spinal deformity surgery: a systematic review. *Spine (Phila Pa 1976)*. 2012;37(22 Suppl):S144–S164.

4. Kim YJ, Bridwell KH, Lenke LG, Glattes CR, Rhim S, Cheh G. Proximal junctional kyphosis in adult spinal deformity after segmental posterior spinal instrumentation and fusion: minimum five-year follow-up. *Spine (Phila Pa 1976)*. 2008;33(20):2179–2184.

5. Lau D, Clark AJ, Scheer JK, Daubs MD, Coe JD, Paonessa KJ, et al. Proximal junctional kyphosis and failure after spinal deformity surgery: a systematic review of the literature as a background to classification development. *Spine (Phila Pa 1976)*. 2014;39(25):2093–2102.

6. Lau D, Funao H, Clark AJ, Nicholls F, Smith J, Bess S, et al. The Clinical Correlation of the Hart-ISSG Proximal Junctional Kyphosis Severity Scale With Health-Related Quality-of-life Outcomes and Need for Revision Surgery. *Spine (Phila Pa 1976)*. 2016;41(3):213–223.

7. Yagi M, Akilah KB, Boachie-Adjei O. Incidence, risk factors and classification of proximal junctional kyphosis: surgical outcomes review of adult idiopathic scoliosis. *Spine (Phila Pa 1976)*. 2011;36(1):E60–E68.

8. Yang SH, Chen PQ. Proximal kyphosis after short posterior fusion for thoracolumbar scoliosis. *Clin Orthop Relat Res*. 2003;411:152–158.

9. Yasuda T, Hasegawa T, Yamato Y, Kobayashi S, Togawa D, Oe S, et al. Proximal junctional kyphosis in adult spinal deformity with long spinal fusion from T9/T10 to the ilium. *J Spine Surg*. 2017;3(2):204–211.

10. Glattes RC, Bridwell KH, Lenke LG, Kim YJ, Rinella A, Edwards C. 2nd. Proximal junctional kyphosis in adult spinal deformity following long instrumented posterior spinal fusion: incidence, outcomes, and risk factor analysis. *Spine (Phila Pa 1976)*. 2005;30(14):1643–1649.

11. Yagi M, Rahm M, Gaines R, Maziad A, Ross T, Kim HJ, et al. Characterization and surgical outcomes of proximal junctional failure in surgically treated patients with adult spinal deformity. *Spine (Phila Pa 1976)*. 2014;39(10):E607–E614.

12. Yagi M, King AB, Boachie-Adjei O. Incidence, risk factors, and natural course of proximal junctional kyphosis: surgical outcomes review of adult idiopathic scoliosis. Minimum 5 years of follow-up. *Spine (Phila Pa 1976)*. 2012;37(17):1479–1489.

13. Abode-Iyamah K, Kim SB, Grosland N, Kumar R, Belirgen M, Lim TH, et al. Spinal motion and intradiscal pressure measurements before and after lumbar spine instrumentation with titanium or PEEK rods. *J Clin Neurosci*. 2014;21(4):651–655.

14. Bruner HJ, Guan Y, Yoganandan N, Pintar FA, Maiman DJ, Slivka MA. Biomechanics of polyaryletherketone rod composites and titanium rods for posterior lumbosacral instrumentation. Presented at the 2010 Joint Spine Section Meeting. Laboratory investigation. *J Neurosurg Spine*. 2010;13(6):766–772.

15. Dekutoski MB, Schendel MJ, Ogilvie JW, Olsewski JM, Wallace LJ, Lewis JL. Comparison of in vivo and in vitro adjacent segment motion after lumbar fusion. *Spine (Phila Pa 1976)*. 1994;19(15):1745–1751.

16. Schlegel JD, Smith JA, Schleusener RL. Lumbar motion segment pathology adjacent to thoracolumbar, lumbar, and lumbosacral fusions. *Spine (Phila Pa 1976)*. 1996;21(8):970–981.

17. Lee JH, Kim JU, Jang JS, Lee SH. Analysis of the incidence and risk factors for the progression of proximal junctional kyphosis following surgical treatment for lumbar degenerative kyphosis: minimum 2-year follow-up. *Br J Neurosurg*. 2014;28(2):252–258.

18. Annis P, Lawrence BD, Spiker WR, Zhang Y, Chen W, Daubs MD, et al. Predictive factors for acute proximal junctional failure after adult deformity surgery with upper instrumented vertebrae in the thoracolumbar spine. *Evid Based Spine Care J*. 2014;5(2):160–162.

19. Kim HJ, Bridwell KH, Lenke LG, Park MS, Song KS, Piyaskulkaew C, et al. Patients with proximal junctional kyphosis requiring revision surgery have higher postoperative lumbar lordosis and larger sagittal balance corrections. *Spine (Phila Pa 1976)*. 2014;39(9):E576–E580.

20. Maruo K, Ha Y, Inoue S, Samuel S, Okada E, Hu SS, et al. Predictive factors for proximal junctional kyphosis in long fusions to the sacrum in adult spinal deformity. *Spine (Phila Pa 1976)*. 2013;38(23):E1469–E1476.

21. Mendoza-Lattes S, Ries Z, Gao Y, Weinstein SL. Proximal junctional kyphosis in adult reconstructive spine surgery results from incomplete restoration of the lumbar lordosis relative to the magnitude of the thoracic kyphosis. *Iowa Orthop J*. 2011;31:199–206.

22. Kim HJ, Bridwell KH, Lenke LG, Park MS, Ahmad A, Song KS, et al. Proximal junctional kyphosis results in inferior SRS pain subscores in adult deformity patients. *Spine (Phila Pa 1976)*. 2013;38(11):896–901.

23. Watanabe K, Lenke LG, Bridwell KH, Kim YJ, Koester L, Hensley M. Proximal junctional vertebral fracture in adults after spinal deformity surgery using pedicle screw constructs: analysis of morphological features. *Spine (Phila Pa 1976)*. 2010;35(2):138–145.

24. McClendon Jr. J, O'Shaughnessy BA, Sugrue PA, Neal CJ, Acosta Jr. FL, Koski TR, et al. Techniques for operative correction of proximal junctional kyphosis of the upper thoracic spine. *Spine (Phila Pa 1976)*. 2012;37(4):292–303.

25. Fehlings MG, Brodke DS, Norvell DC, Dettori JR. The evidence for intraoperative neurophysiological monitoring in spine surgery: does it make a difference? *Spine (Phila Pa 1976)*. 2010;35(9 Suppl):S37–S46.

35

Coronal deformity

Fidel Valero-Moreno, MD, Jaime L. Martinez Santos, MD, and Henry Ruiz-Garcia, MD

Introduction

Adult spinal deformities may be caused by progressive degenerative disease, iatrogenic changes, or progression of adolescent curves.[1] It is most commonly seen in patients older than 65 years, which is also the fastest growing population in the United States.[2] The management of adult deformity hinges upon the etiology of the condition.[3] The most common symptom in the adult population is pain.[4,5] The chief complaints of the patient must be taken into consideration, as radicular symptoms may need treatment regimens that differ from those with only back pain.[6,7] The global balance of the patient must also be thoroughly investigated, both in the coronal and sagittal planes. Dynamic radiographic films may be employed to determine the flexibility of the patient's curve(s) and can aid in surgical planning of osteotomies and corrective maneuvers. Even though the effectiveness of conservative management has not been well established, it has been used as the first-line treatment in patients with mild and nonworsening symptoms. However, coronal deformity is a dynamic condition and early identification of patients who may benefit from surgery is crucial for good outcomes and cost-efficiency.[2] Both open and minimally invasive techniques may be used to correct coronal imbalance and decompress neural elements, without a high level of evidence to suggest efficacy of one method of correction over another.[8–10] Within this chapter, we present the case of a 50-year-old female patient with progressive low back pain over the course of a year with a spinal deformity.

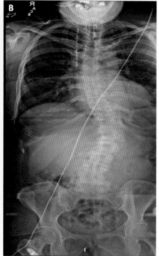

Fig. 35.1 Preoperative standing scoliosis films. (A) Lateral standing scoliosis 36-inch x-ray imaging showing a positive C7-S1 sagittal vertical axis (SVA) of less than 5 cm (blue arrows), because the patient compensated for her sagittal imbalance with pelvic retroversion as evidenced by the positive pelvic tilt (PT) angle of more than 19 degrees. There is also a grade I L5-S1 anterolisthesis. **(B)** Anteroposterior standing scoliosis 36-inch x-ray imaging demonstrating significant thoracolumbar levoscoliosis (B) and widening of sacroiliac joints and sclerosis.

Example case

Chief complaint: neck pain and weakness

History of present illness: This is a 50-year-old female with mid and low back pain that has progressed over the last year. She does not have any leg pain or genitourinary symptoms. Imaging findings are shown in Fig. 35.1 that were concerning for scoliosis.

Medications: acetaminophen, aspirin

Allergies: no known drug allergies

Past medical and surgical history: depression, anxiety

Family history: none

Social history: none

Physical examination: awake, alert, and oriented to person, place, and time; cranial nerves II–XII intact; bilateral deltoids/triceps/biceps 5/5; interossei 5/5; iliopsoas/knee flexion/knee extension/dorsi, and plantar flexion 5/5

Reflexes: 2+ in bilateral biceps/triceps/brachioradialis with negative Hoffman; 2+ in bilateral patella/ankle; no clonus or Babinski; sensation intact to light touch

	Pedro Luis Bazán, MD Spine Surgeon HIGA San Martín La Plata (Chief Orthopaedic) Hospital Italiano La Plata Instituto de Diagnóstico La Plata La Plata, Buenos Aires, Argentina	Esteban F. Espinoza-García, MD, MSc University of Valparaíso San Felipe, Chile	Hamid Hassanzadeh, MD Orthopaedic Surgery University of Virginia Charlottesville, Virginia, United States	Timothy F. Witham, MD Neurosurgery Johns Hopkins Baltimore, Maryland, United States
Preoperative				
Additional tests requested	T-L spine AP/lateral/flexion-extension x-rays T-L spine MRI T-L spine CT	CT and MRI T-spine DEXA No operative: medial branch block	MRI T-L spine Physical therapy evaluation Pain management evaluation for medical brain block and/or radiofrequency ablation	MRI T-L spine Scoliosis x-rays DEXA Calcium, vitamin D, PTH serum levels
Surgical approach selected	Stage 1: L1-2, L2-3, L3-4 LLIF Stage 2: percutaneous L1-4 posterior fusion Hounsfield Units in CT.	T5-S1 posterolateral fusion and correction of deformity	Stage 1: L1-4 LLIF Stage 2: percutaneous L1-4 posterior fusion	After nonsurgical treatments have been maximized, Stage 1: T10-pelvis fusion with multilevel Ponti osteotomies, cement augmentation of T9-10 Stage 2: Retroperitoneal L5-S1 discectomy, L5-S1 ALIF
Surgical approach if 21 Surgical approach if 80	Same approach Same approach	Same approach Nonoperative management	Same approach Same approach	Same approach but stopping at L4 Same approach
Goal of surgery	Relieve pain, avoid progression of deformity	Relieve pain, avoid progression of deformity	Relieve pain, deformity correction	Relieve pain and improve disability, deformity correction, stabilization
Perioperative				
Positioning	Stage 1: lateral decubitus Stage 2: prone	Prone	Stage 1: lateral decubitus Stage 2: prone	Stage 1: prone on Jackson table Stage 2: supine on Jackson table with flat adapter
Surgical equipment	IOM Fluoroscopy	Fluoroscopy	IOM (MEP/SSEP) Fluoroscopy	Stage 1: IOM, fluoroscopy, osteotomes, O-arm, cement augmentation Stage 2: fluoroscopy, sagittal saw
Medications	Maintain MAP	Maintain MAP	None	Tranexamic acid for stage 1
Anatomical considerations	Transverse processes, psoas, disc space, pedicles, vertebral body	Pedicles	Psoas, nerve roots	Neural elements, iliac vessels, iliolumbar vein, ureter, bowels
Complications feared with approach chosen	Progression of deformity	Screw misplacement	Lumbar plexus injury, psoas injury	Proximal and distal junctional failure, pseudoarthrosis, proximal junctional kyphosis
Intraoperative				
Anesthesia	General	General	General	General
Exposure	Stage 1: L1-4 Stage 2: L1-4	T5-S1	L1-4	Stage 1: T9-S2 Stage 2: L5-S1
Levels decompressed	Stage 1: L5-7 Stage 2: L1-2	all levels where ponti osteotomies are completed along the coronal curve	L1-4	Stage 1: None Stage 2: L5-S1
Levels fused	Stage 1: L1-4 Stage 2: L1-4	T5-S1	L1-4	Stage 1: T10-pelvus Stage 2: L5-S1

	Pedro Luis Bazán, MD Spine Surgeon HIGA San Martín La Plata (Chief Orthopaedic) Hospital Italiano La Plata Instituto de Diagnóstico La Plata La Plata, Buenos Aires, Argentina	Esteban F. Espinoza-García, MD, MSc University of Valparaíso San Felipe, Chile	Hamid Hassanzadeh, MD Orthopaedic Surgery University of Virginia Charlottesville, Virginia, United States	Timothy F. Witham, MD Neurosurgery Johns Hopkins Baltimore, Maryland, United States
Surgical narrative	Stage 1: position lateral, preoperative x-ray to determine level, percutaneous discectomy, disc replacement with arthrodesis at L1-L4, x-ray to confirm hardware, standard closure Stage 2 (after 1 week): position prone, preoperative x-ray to determine levels, percutaneous placement of pedicle screws under biplanar fluoroscopy L1-4, possible increase to T10 depending on prestage 2 alignment, placement of rods, system shutdown, standard closure	Intubated, prone positioning, x-ray to confirm localization, midline incision, subperiosteal bilateral dissection from T5-S1, x-ray to confirm levels, thoracic and lumbar pedicle screw placements, rods connected sequentially to each pedicle screw one by one to progressively correct deformity, subfascial drain placement	Position lateral decubitus with left side up, break table in midline, posterolateral accessory incision off of multifidus musculature, sharply incise 3 cm through skin, monopolar cautery down to fascia levels, enter through fascia, bluntly retract down to level of psoas, retract peritoneal contents anteriorly, incise obliquely over L3 vertebral body and dissect down into retroperitoneal space, laterally incise and dock tube over L3-4 disc space, bluntly place all dilators and retractors under EMG of psoas, sweep posteriorly to stay out of lumbar plexus, confirm position on fluoroscopy, stimulate surgical field, annulotomy and discectomy, prepare end plates, dilate disc space and size it starting L3-4 with bone graft, confirm position with x-ray, repeat with L2-3 followed by L1-2, place tube between 11 and 12th ribs, layered closure Stage 2: position prone on Jackson table, stab incision over lateral aspect of each pedicle using fluoroscopy, incise through fascia, insert Jamshidi needle through pedicle and traverse from medial to lateral, perform bilaterally L1-4, place screws under EMG stimulation, insert rods on both sides, layered closure	Stage 1: position prone on Jackson table to promote lumbar lordosis, expose T9-S2, preserve T9-10 facet joints and posterior soft tissue envelope, perform osteotomies along the area of the coronal curve bilaterally, place pedicle screws from T10 to S2AI, leave one screw in T10 out for cement, placement cement at T9-10, O-arm spin to confirm screw and cement placement, place rods and correct deformity, decorticate, layered closure with drain Stage 2 (6–8 weeks after stage 1): position supine, vascular surgeon to expose using retroperitoneal approach to L5-S1, place Syn frame, confirm with x-ray, L5-S1 discectomy, endplate preparation, size and cut femoral ring allograft, fill with demineralized bone matrix and place, place screw and washer at L5-S1, x-ray, layered closure
Complication avoidance	Two-staged approach, percutaneous lateral approach, percutaneous pedicle screw and posterior fixation	Progressive sequential deformity correction	Break table slightly in midline, EMG of psoas for tubular retractor placement, sweep tubular retractor posteriorly to avoid lumbar plexus, percutaneous pedicle screw and posterior fixation	Two-staged procedure, preserve T9-10 facet joints and posterior soft tissue envelope, multilevel osteotomies along coronal curve, cement augmentation, O-arm spin, vascular surgery to expose L5-S1, place screw and washer to prevent kick out
Postoperative				
Admission	Floor	Floor	Floor	Stage 1: ICU Stage 2: floor
Postoperative complications feared	Infection, hardware failure	CSF leak, spinal instability, subcutaneous hemorrhage	Neural injury, lower extremity weakness, pseudoarthrosis	Proximal junctional kyphosis, distal junction pseudoarthrosis, CSF leak, instrument failure

	Pedro Luis Bazán, MD Spine Surgeon HIGA San Martín La Plata (Chief Orthopaedic) Hospital Italiano La Plata Instituto de Diagnóstico La Plata La Plata, Buenos Aires, Argentina	Esteban F. Espinoza-García, MD, MSc University of Valparaíso San Felipe, Chile	Hamid Hassanzadeh, MD Orthopaedic Surgery University of Virginia Charlottesville, Virginia, United States	Timothy F. Witham, MD Neurosurgery Johns Hopkins Baltimore, Maryland, United States
Anticipated length of stay	5–7 days	5 days	2–3 days	7–9 days total
Follow-up testing	T-L spine x-rays within 1 day after surgery T-L flexion-extension x-rays 1 month after surgery T-L spine CT 3 months after surgery	T- and L-spine CT 1 day and 3 months after surgery, x-rays 3 months after surgery	Standing PA and lateral scoliosis x-rays before discharge, 3 weeks, 3 months, 6 months, 12 months after surgery Physical therapy evaluation	CT T-L spine after stage 1 Standing scoliosis x-rays prior to discharge, 6 weeks, 3 months, 6 months, 1 year after surgery
Bracing	None	Jewett brace for 3 months	None	None
Follow-up visits	2 weeks, 1 month, 2 months, 3 months, 6 months, 1 year after surgery	3 weeks, 3 months, 6 months, 1 year after surgery	3 weeks, 3 months, 6 months, 12 months after surgery	2 weeks, 6 weeks, 3 months, 6 months, 1 year after surgery

ALIF, Anterior lumbar interbody fusion; CSF, cerebrospinal fluid; CT, computed tomography; DEXA, dual-energy x-ray absorptiometry; EMG, electromyography; ICU, intensive care unit; IOM, intraoperative monitoring; LLIF, lateral lumbar interbody fusion; MAP, mean arterial pressure; MEP, motor evoked potential; MRI, magnetic resonance imaging; PTH, parathyroid hormone; SSEP, somatosensory evoked potential.

Differential diagnosis

- Adult degenerative scoliosis
- Progression of adolescent scoliosis
- Lumbar spondylolisthesis
- Lumbar stenosis

Important anatomical and preoperative considerations

A spinal deformity in the coronal plane, established by means of the Cobb angle greater than 10 degrees, constitutes the current definition of adult degenerative scoliosis. The development of deformity can be the product of osteoporosis, vertebral fractures, and asymmetrical degeneration of the intervertebral discs and facet joints leading to an asymmetrical load over a determined spinal segment.[11] In general, adult scoliosis can be classified in two groups: (1) patients with scoliosis since childhood or adolescence that became symptomatic or who experienced progression of the curve and (2) patients in whom deformity developed after bone maturity.[12] Despite its etiology, both conditions will eventually develop loss of intersegmental instability and progressive deformity.[12] The apical vertebra has the greatest segmental angulation (rostral and caudal interspaces) and is usually located at the apex of the curve. The segment with minimal or no angulation is defined as the neutral vertebra.[11] Several features such as apical level of the scoliotic deformity, absence of lumbar lordosis, degree of intervertebral subluxation, and sagittal balance can help determine whether or not an invasive approach is necessary and to plan a surgical strategy.[11,13] In the absence of clear neurological deterioration or deformity progression, conservative management has been the initial treatment for many surgeons.[4,11,14] Bracing has not been proven to prevent deformity progression and its stabilizing function may be relevant just for pain relief.[11,14]

Surgical treatment should be considered for every patient with pain-related deformity who failed to improve under conservative treatment or with persistent neurological deficit. Patients harboring deformities greater than 50 to 60 degrees on the thoracic spine and greater than 40 degrees on the lumbar spine are strong candidates for correction.[11] The mainstay of surgery is to establish a solid fusion and stabilization of the deformity. Achieving proper sagittal and coronal balance is crucial for optimal surgical outcome. For this purpose, it is not recommended to terminate an instrumentation at or near the apical vertebra of the curve, but extension to a neutral vertebra is preferred.[11] Ending the fusion in a transitional zone (thoracolumbar) is also not recommended.[11,14] In the other hand, multiple scenarios should be taken into consideration before deciding where to end the caudal instrumentation. Commonly, extension to the sacrum has been recommended in cases of spondylolisthesis, significant L5-S1 stenosis, or postlaminectomy at L5-S1; however, this strategy is related to a higher incidence of postoperative complications.[11] Fusions ending at L5 are not exempt from complications as 61% of patients developed adjacent segment disease in some series.[11] When lumbosacral fusion is performed, interbody fusion at L5-S1 can improve stability and iliac fixation should be considered.[11] Patients presenting with stenosis symptoms, radiculopathy, and/or neurogenic claudication must undergo surgical decompression of the neural elements.[11,14]

What was actually done

The patient underwent dynamic x-rays with side-bending, which demonstrated an approximately 50-degree thoracolumbar/lumbar curve from T10 to L3. There was also approximately 3 cm of left coronal imbalance but no significant sagittal imbalance. The patient also had a grade I L5-S1 spondylolisthesis. Magnetic resonance imaging (MRI) did not show any significant central or foraminal stenosis. Due to these findings and current symptomatology, the decision was made to take the patient to the operating room in order to perform a T3-S1 instrumented fusion, sacropelvic fixation using iliac crest, and an L4-L5 and L5-S1 left-sided transforaminal lumbar interbody fusion (TLIF).

The patient was placed in prone position on the Jackson table, and after general anesthesia was provided, a midline incision was made from T3 to the sacrum. Intraoperative fluoroscopy confirmed the levels, and subperiosteal dissection was used to reflect the paraspinal muscles bilaterally; the bilateral iliac crests were also exposed. Pedicle screws were placed starting at L4 bilaterally and moved sequentially up until T3. Posteriorly, computed tomography images of L5-sacrum were acquired by the O-arm and loaded for navigation. Pedicle screws at L5 and S1 were placed using image guidance. Then bilateral iliac crest autografts were harvested, and iliac crest screws were placed. Thereafter, lateral connectors were positioned. Next, the spinous processes from T7 to S1 were removed to later serve as autograft. A left-sided TLIF was performed using 10 mm cages, bone morphogenic protein (BMP), and local autograft. A cobalt chrome rod was then placed within the screw heads on the left in order to reduce the scoliosis ipsilaterally. After intraoperative x-rays confirmed good positioning of the rod and adequate coronal balance, the second rod was placed on the right side. Later, autografts, allografts chips, and BMP were placed in the facet joins from T3 to the sacrum bilaterally. Vancomycin powder was distributed within the wound before closing in layers. Intraoperative somatosensory and motor evoked potentials were unchanged throughout the case. Postoperatively, the patient had no complications and was discharged home on postoperative day 6. A thoracic lumbar sacral orthosis (TLSO) brace was recommended when out of bed. Follow-up at 1 year demonstrated solid fusion of the construct and adequate correction of her coronal deformity (Fig. 35.2).

Commonalities among the experts

Preoperative thoracolumbar magnetic resonance image was advocated by all the surgeons. In addition, scoliosis x-rays and bone density scans were requested by half of the physicians. Surgical approaches were significantly different, where the majority opted for a two-stage procedure in order to achieve deformity correction. Overall, a similar treatment would be offered to all adult patients regardless of their age. Deformity correction and limitation of progress, as well as pain relief, remained the principal purposes of surgery. Half opted for a long fusion spanning the T5-S1 levels, while the other half recommended a shorter one covering four lumbar

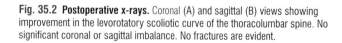

Fig. 35.2 Postoperative x-rays. Coronal (A) and sagittal (B) views showing improvement in the levorotatory scoliotic curve of the thoracolumbar spine. No significant coronal or sagittal imbalance. No fractures are evident.

levels. The most common feared complications were diverse and ranged from psoas and neural injury to screw misplacement and junction failure. Surgery was typically completed with fluoroscopy and intraoperative monitoring. No special perioperative pharmacotherapy was administered. Surgical nuances to avoid complications greatly varied. After surgery, most of the patients continued observation in the floor and all requested imaging before discharge to evaluate for adequate instrumentation and/or for complications. All advocated for a close follow-up during the first year, starting 2 to 3 months after surgery.

SUMMARY OF QUALITY OF EVIDENCE TO GUIDE SPECIFIC INTERVENTIONS FOR THIS CASE

- Adults older than 50 years old with spinal coronal deformity could benefit from surgical intervention: level III.
- A close follow-up during the first postoperative year is recommended: level III.

REFERENCES

1. Aebi M. The adult scoliosis. *Eur Spine J.* 2005;14(10):925–948.
2. Diebo BG, Shah NV, Boachie-Adjei O, et al. Adult spinal deformity. *Lancet.* 2019;394(10193):160–172.
3. Schwab F, Lafage V, Farcy JP, et al. Surgical rates and operative outcome analysis in thoracolumbar and lumbar major adult scoliosis: application of the new adult deformity classification. *Spine (Phila Pa 1976).* 2007;32(24):2723–2730.
4. Graham RB, Sugrue PA, Koski TR. Adult Degenerative Scoliosis. *Clin Spine Surg.* 2016;29(3):95–107.
5. Alanazi MH, Parent EC, Dennett E. Effect of stabilization exercise on back pain, disability and quality of life in adults with scoliosis: a systematic review. *Eur J Phys Rehabil Med.* 2018;54(5): 647–653.

6. Grubb SA, Lipscomb HJ, Suh PB. Results of surgical treatment of painful adult scoliosis. *Spine (Phila Pa 1976)*. 1994;19(14): 1619–1627.

7. Schwab F, Dubey A, Gamez L, et al. Adult scoliosis: prevalence, SF-36, and nutritional parameters in an elderly volunteer population. *Spine (Phila Pa 1976)*. 2005;30(9):1082–1085.

8. Cho KJ, Kim YT, Shin SH, Suk SI. Surgical treatment of adult degenerative scoliosis. *Asian Spine J*. 2014;8(3):371–381.

9. Daffner SD, Vaccaro AR. Adult degenerative lumbar scoliosis. *Am J Orthop (Belle Mead NJ)*. 2003;32(2):77–82. discussion 82.

10. Dakwar E, Cardona RF, Smith DA, Uribe JS. Early outcomes and safety of the minimally invasive, lateral retroperitoneal transpsoas approach for adult degenerative scoliosis. *Neurosurg Focus*. 2010;28(3):E8.

11. Birknes JK, White AP, Albert TJ, Shaffrey CI, Harrop JS. Adult degenerative scoliosis: a review. *Neurosurgery*. 2008;63(3 Suppl): 94–103.

12. Schwab FJ, Smith VA, Biserni M, Gamez L, Farcy JP, Pagala M. Adult scoliosis: a quantitative radiographic and clinical analysis. *Spine (Phila Pa 1976)*. 2002;27(4):387–392.

13. Schwab F, Farcy JP, Bridwell K, et al. A clinical impact classification of scoliosis in the adult. *Spine (Phila Pa 1976)*. 2006;31(18):2109–2114.

14. Faldini C, Di Martino A, De Fine M, et al. Current classification systems for adult degenerative scoliosis. *Musculoskelet Surg*. 2013;97(1):1–8.

36

Coronal and sagittal deformity with back pain (adult idiopathic)

Kingsley Abode-Iyamah, MD

Introduction

Adult degenerative scoliosis (ADS), or de novo degenerative lumbar scoliosis, is a spinal deformity diagnosed in individuals with a coronal curve of >10 degrees, beginning after the age of 50, and without a prior history of scoliosis.[1-3] It differs from adult idiopathic scoliosis in that the latter is a result of unrecognized/untreated adolescent idiopathic scoliosis. ADS develops secondary to degenerative changes occurring over an individual's lifetime, typically presenting at the age of 70.[3,4]

Although not previously recognized, ADS is believed to be more prevalent than previously thought; it is reported to be 68% in asymptomatic individuals and the incidence increases with age.[5] McCarthy et al. have shown an increase in surgeries performed for ADS in the Medicare population, creating

an increasing economic burden.[6] With increasing life expectancy, prevalence and cost are expected to further increase for this condition.

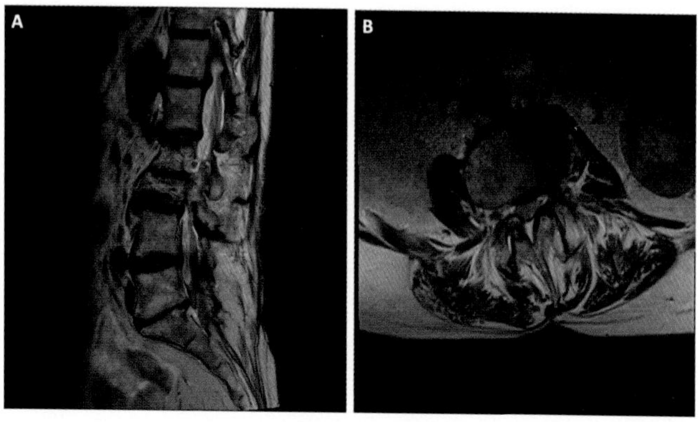

Example case

Chief complaint: back pain

History of present illness: A 63-year-old female presents with back pain and radiculopathy. She underwent a laminectomy approximately 15 years ago but has had back pain for about 25 years. The patient also has right leg pain and left leg numbness that is worsened with standing and walking. More recently, the back pain has become constant over the past 3 months. She has tried physical therapy, epidural steroid injections, and selective nerve root injection without significant improvement. She also notes right leg weakness. She underwent imaging that revealed significant scoliosis (Figs. 36.1–36.3).

Medications: albuterol, omeprazole, temazepam

Allergies: codeine

Past medical and surgical history: hypertension, chronic obstructive pulmonary disease, hypothyroidism, depression, laminectomy

Family history: noncontributory

Social history: previous smoker, occasional alcohol

Physical examination: awake, alert, and oriented to person, place, and time; cranial nerves II–XII intact; bilateral deltoids/triceps/biceps 5/5; interossei 5/5; iliopsoas/knee flexion/knee extension/dorsi, and plantar flexion 5/5

Reflexes: 3+ in bilateral biceps/triceps/brachioradialis with negative Hoffman; 3+ in bilateral patella/ankle; no clonus or Babinski; sensation intact to light touch

Fig. 36.1 Preoperative magnetic resonance images. (A) T2 sagittal and (B) T2 axial images demonstrating multilevel disc degeneration with foraminal and lateral recess stenosis.

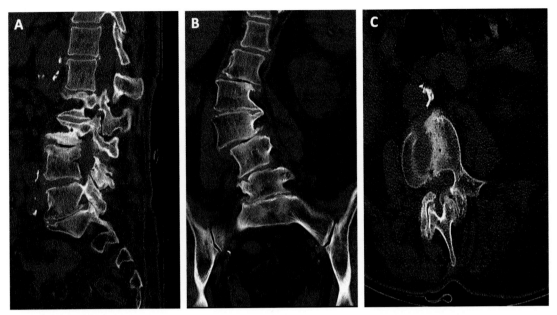

Fig. 36.2 Preoperative computed tomography scans. (A) Sagittal, (B) coronal, and (C) axial images demonstrating dextroscoliosis, multilevel disc degeneration, with foraminal stenosis.

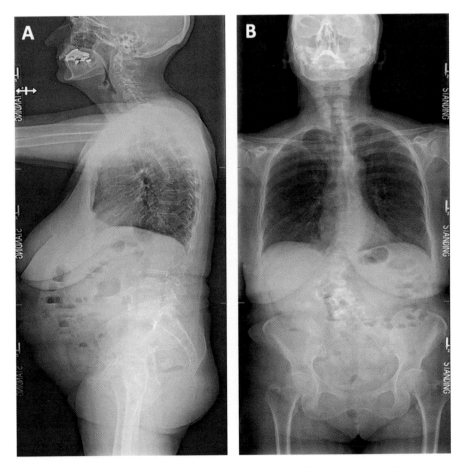

PT: 21, PI: 45, SVA 4, LL:19   Cobb angle: 45

Fig. 36.3 Preoperative x-rays. (A) Anteroposterior (AP) and (B) lateral x-rays demonstrating dextroscoliosis, multilevel disc degeneration with coronal deformity, and loss of lumbar lordosis.

	Ciaran Bolger, MD Royal College of Surgeons Catherine Moran, MD Neurosurgery Tallaght University Hospital Dublin, Ireland	Benjamin D. Elder, MD, PhD Neurosurgery Mayo Clinic Rochester, Minnesota, United States	Hamid Hassanzadeh, MD Orthopaedic Surgery University of Virginia Charlottesville, Virginia, United States	Baron Zarate Kalfopulos, MD Orthopaedic Surgery Instituto Nacional de Rehabilitacion Medica Sur Mexico City, Mexico
Preoperative				
Additional tests requested	MRI C-spine DEXA	MRI C-spine DEXA Supine scoliosis x-rays Vitamin D levels Nicotine tests	MRI C-T spine DEXA L-spine flexion-extension x-rays Nutrition evaluation Anesthesia evaluation Medicine evaluation	L-spine flexion-extension x-rays EMG lower extremities
Surgical approach selected	L3-4 laminectomy based on preop symptoms that locate to nerve root	If meets all criteria (BMI<35, negative nicotine test, pretreatment with anabolic therapy) Stage 1: L5-S1 ALIF Stage 2: T10 vs. 11-sacrum instrumented fusion with pelvic fixation	L4-S1 TLIF, L4-S1 posterior column osteotomies, T10-S1 sublaminar decompression, T10-pelvis fusion	L3-4 and L5-S1 TLIF, L1-5 posterior fusion, L3-S1 laminectomy
Surgical approach if 21 Surgical approach if 80	Correct sagittal imbalance and scoliosis Same approach	Same approach with sparing of some levels Same approach	Same approach L4-S1 TLIF	Same approach Same approach
Goal of surgery	Decompress neural elements, relieve leg pain/paresthesias, relieve stenosis, improve walking distance	Decompress neural elements, correct sagittal and coronal deformities, stabilize spine	Decompress neural elements, correct sagittal and coronal deformities, stabilize spine	Decompress neural elements, correct sagittal and coronal deformities, stabilize spine
Perioperative				
Positioning	Prone	Stage 1: supine on flat Jackson table with arterial line bag inflated transversely across lumbosacral junction Stage 2: prone on Jackson table with pins	Prone	Prone
Surgical equipment	Fluoroscope Surgical microscope	Stage 1: vascular surgery, abdominal retractor system, fluoroscopy, osteotomes, IOM (SSEP/EMG) Stage 2: surgical navigation, osteotomes, BMP-2, allograft, cell saver	IOM (MEP/SSEP/EMG) Fluoroscopy Osteotomes	Fluoroscopy IOM
Medications	None	Tranexamic acid	Tranexamic acid	Tranexamic acid
Anatomical considerations	Thecal sac, nerve roots, pedicles, pars interarticularis, disc space at appropriate levels	Stage 1: ureter, aorta, inferior vena cava, iliac vessels Stage 2: prior laminectomy defect, aorta, inferior vena cava, iliac vessels	Nerve roots, dura, SI joint	Pedicle rotation at apex of deformity, venous plexus
Complications feared with approach chosen	CSF leak, nerve root injury, instability	Anterior expulsion of graft, pseudoarthrosis, proximal junction failure, instrumentation failure, sagittal/coronal imbalance, durotomy	CSF leak, neurological injury, pseudoarthrosis	Nerve root injury, proximal junctional kyphosis, lumbar plexus injury

	Ciaran Bolger, MD Royal College of Surgeons Catherine Moran, MD Neurosurgery Tallaght University Hospital Dublin, Ireland	Benjamin D. Elder, MD, PhD Neurosurgery Mayo Clinic Rochester, Minnesota, United States	Hamid Hassanzadeh, MD Orthopaedic Surgery University of Virginia Charlottesville, Virginia, United States	Baron Zarate Kalfopulos, MD Orthopaedic Surgery Instituto Nacional de Rehabilitacion Medica Sur Mexico City, Mexico
Intraoperative				
Anesthesia	General	General	General	General
Exposure	L3-4	Stage 1: L5-S1 Stage 2: T10-sacrum	T10-S2	L1-S1
Levels decompressed	L3-4	None	T10-S1	L3-S1
Levels fused	None	Stage 1: L5-S1 Stage 2: T10-sacrum	T10-pelvis	L1-S1
Surgical narrative	Position prone, x-ray to guide incision, 3 cm midline incision through previous laminectomy scar at appropriate level, dissect on more affected side to expose ipsilateral facet joint, undercut the joint, expose and decompress ipsilateral traversing root along length from disc space level to ipsilateral pedicle and foramen using high-speed drill with direct visualization, dissect scar free from root using microdissection, extend bone removal superiorly and laterally if needed to expose and decompress exiting nerve root, care is taken to expose and preserve the pars, dissect and excise scar lateral to medial to expose thecal sac to midline and onto contralateral side, contralateral facet undercut to expose and decompress contralateral neural elements from disc space to pedicle and foramen under direct visualized, closure in layers	Stage 1: position supine with arterial line bog transversely across lumbosacral junction, IOM to assess reduced signals with prolonged retraction of great vessels, vascular surgery exposure with left retroperitoneal approach and mobilization of iliac vessels below bifurcation to expose L5-S1 disc space, localization x-rays, resection of L5-S1 disc and anterior/posterior osteophytes, bilateral vertebral body distractors to mobilize segment, preparation of end plates and placement of cage (16–24 degrees), deflate arterial line bag, place integrated fixation screws or buttress screw/washer to prevent anterior expulsion, intraoperative x-ray Stage 2 (1–2 days later): expose T10 vs. T11 to sacrum, maintain supraspinous/interspinous ligament at top two levels and facet capsules at upper instrumented vertebrae, expose S1-2 dorsal foramen, multilevel posterior column osteotomies with sublaminar decompression from L1 to S1, placement of pedicle screw fixation with navigation from T10 to 11 to sacrum with bicortical fixation in sacrum, placement of S2-alar-iliac screws at least 9 x 90 mm, placement of 5.5 titanium rods with use of reduction clamps, in situ bending to correct sagittal and coronal plane deformities with compression/distraction, intraoperative scoliosis x-rays to check correction, pulse lavage, decortication of posterior elements including facet joins and residual lamina, place local autograft and morcellized allograft on decorticated surfaces, closure with incisional wound vac and 2 subfascial drains	Position prone after IOM, x-rays to confirm levels, midline skin incision, enter through fascia paraspinally down to lamina of T10-S2, dissect lateral to pedicles to find transverse process for each level, confirm level, place pedicle screws and S2 alar-iliac screws with fluoroscopy, bilateral inferior facetectomy from L1 to L5, sublaminar decompression and posterior column osteotomies at L5-S1 and L4-5 and place TLIF cages at these levels from left side, continue sublaminar decompression to T12-L1 level, x-ray to check alignment, can perform L2-3 and L3-4 posterior column osteotomies if more correction is needed, place rods, confirm alignment with x-rays, compress left side L4-S1 and right side L2-4, place drains, layered closure	Position prone, standard posterior midline incision, subperiosteal dissection and exposure of L1-S1, pedicle screw placement from L1-S1, initiate decompression by inserting interspinous spreader, decompress with laminectomy/ flavectomy/bilateral facetectomy, identify thecal sac and existing nerve root identification, gentle mobilization of neural structures medially to identify disc space, create a window on the disc and enlarge with box osteotomes, obtain local bone from surgical field and demineralized bone matrix, place in disc space, place banana cage filled with demineralized bone matrix, decorticate articular and transverse processes, enhance with local bone graft and demineralized bone matrix, restore lordosis with rod contouring and compression from caudal to cephalad direction, layered closure with subfascial drain

	Ciaran Bolger, MD Royal College of Surgeons Catherine Moran, MD Neurosurgery Tallaght University Hospital Dublin, Ireland	Benjamin D. Elder, MD, PhD Neurosurgery Mayo Clinic Rochester, Minnesota, United States	Hamid Hassanzadeh, MD Orthopaedic Surgery University of Virginia Charlottesville, Virginia, United States	Baron Zarate Kalfopulos, MD Orthopaedic Surgery Instituto Nacional de Rehabilitacion Medica Sur Mexico City, Mexico
Complication avoidance	Decompress only symptomatic nerve roots, bilateral decompression from a unilateral approach, preserve pars, dissect and excise scar lateral to medial to expose thecal sac, directly visualize decompression	Arterial line bag to maximize L5-S1 lordosis, IOM to assess effects of retraction, vertebral body distractors to maximize lordosis, maintain supraspinous/interspinous ligament, navigation, intraoperative scoliosis x-rays, incisional wound vac	Fuse down to S2 alar-iliac level, sublaminar decompression to T10, increase levels of posterior column osteotomies if more sagittal correction is needed, lateral correction with lateral compression	One stage, avoid lateral approach, identify thecal sac and nerve root early, avoid BMP because of economic constraints, increase lordosis by compression from caudal to cephalad
Postoperative				
Admission	Floor	Stage 1: floor Stage 2: ICU	Intermediate care	Floor
Postoperative complications feared	CSF leak, infection	CSF leak, ileus, urinary retention, early proximal junctional kyphosis	CSF leak, neurological injury, pseudoarthrosis, medical complications, infection	Wound infection, adjacent segment disease, proximal junctional kyphosis, pseudoarthrosis, loosening of pedicle screws especially at S1, cage subsidence
Anticipated length of stay	1 day	6–7 days	3–5 days	3 days
Follow-up testing	None	Supine lumbar spine AP/lateral x-rays after stage 1 Standing scoliosis x-rays after stage 2 Standing scoliosis x-rays 6 weeks, 3 months, 6 months, 1 year after surgery CT 1 year after surgery	T-L spine x-rays after surgery Standing PA and lateral scoliosis x-rays prior to discharge, 3 weeks, 3 months, 6 months, 12 months after surgery	L-spine x-rays 6 weeks and every 3 months for first year after surgery CT L-spine 12 months after surgery
Bracing	None	None	None	None
Follow-up visits	2 weeks, 6 weeks after surgery	6 weeks, 3 months, 6 months, 1 year after surgery	3 weeks, 3 months, 6 months, 12 months after surgery after surgery	2 weeks, 6 weeks, every 3 months for first year after surgery

AP, Anteroposterior; BMP, bone morphogenic protein; CSF, cerebrospinal fluid; CT, computed tomography; DEXA, dual-energy x-ray absorptiometry; EMG, electromyography; ICU, intensive care unit; IOM, intraoperative monitoring; MAP, mean arterial pressure; MEP, motor evoked potential; MRI, magnetic resonance imaging; PA, postero-anterior; SSEP, somatosensory evoked potential.

Differential diagnosis

- Adult degenerative scoliosis
- Iatrogenic scoliosis
- Adolescent idiopathic scoliosis

Important anatomical considerations

Given the increasing prevalence of ADS, understanding the importance of the spinopelvic alignment is essential for all spinal surgeons. The formula PI = PT + SS is integral to understanding the relationship between the spine and pelvis. In this formula pelvic incidence (PI) is a fixed morphogenic parameter with only slight changes during prepubertal development. Pelvic tilt (normal PT = <20 degrees) and sacral slope (SS) are variable parameters with indirect relationships to each other. Additional measurements include sagittal vertical axis (SVA = +/−4 cm), which is a common measurement of global sagittal alignment (SA). The difference between the coronal C7 plumb line and the central sacral vertical line (CSVL) assesses the coronal alignment (CA = +/−2cm).[7]

While multiple classifications have been used for ASD, the most widely accepted is the SRS-Schwab, which includes the curve type with multiple modifiers to describe the deformity.[8] ADS is expected to progress an average of 3 degrees per year due to ongoing degeneration. Known risk factors include Cobb angle of >30 degrees, asymmetrical disc above and below the apical vertebra, subluxation of the apical vertebra

>6 mm, and L5 located above the intercrestal line.[1] Although SRS-Schwab classification suggests a number of thresholds predictive of disability, it should be noted that these parameters may vary with age. The SRS-Schwab classification identifies PT greater than 22 degrees, SVA greater than 46 mm, and PI-LL (pelvic incidence-lumbar lordosis = <10 degrees) more than 11 degrees as factors as predictive of disability.[8,9]

Approaches to this lesion

The key to surgical planning for ADS is addressing both the pain generator and the global and regional imbalance. This can be accomplished with combination anterior/posterior procedure or posterior-only approach. For anterior approach, anterior lumbar interbody fusion (ALIF) alone can provide 5 degrees of correction while ALIF with Smith-Peterson osteotomy (SPO) can provide 15 to 20 degrees of sagittal correction. Oblique lateral interbody fusion (OLIF) with/without SPO can provide 3 to 25 degrees. Not only can OLIF aid in coronal correction, but when combined with anterior column realignment (ACR), it can also provide sagittal correction of up to 30 degrees.[10]

Posteriorly, strategic osteotomy cuts are important for realignment. Incorporating transforaminal interbody fusion (TLIF) with SPO can provide 15 to 20 degrees of correction at a single level. Additionally, performing multilevel SPO allows for further correction. Pedicle subtraction osteotomy (PSO), although not physiological, is necessary when correction is needed through a previously bony-fused level, dispensing 30 degrees of movement. Another osteotomy, vertebral column resection (VCR), delivers 30 to 40 degrees and is beneficial when both sagittal and coronal correction are needed.[10] Combination anterior/posterior procedures may add surgical time, lengthen hospitalization, require access surgeons (particularly for ALIF), and expose the patient to additional complications. Therefore, when possible, it is preferable to perform a single approach for correction if possible.

What was actually done

The patient presented with degenerative scoliosis with back and leg pain. She had failed conservative management and was offered a posterior-only scoliosis repair. The patient was taken to the operating room and positioned on an Orthopedic System Inc (OSI) table. A midline incision was made and the posterior boney elements were exposed. Instrumentation was placed from T10 to pelvis, with confirmation of good instrumentation placement using the intraoperative O-arm. Bone marrow aspiration was obtained at each level to soak the corticocancellous bone graft. Iliac bone was laso during placement of the iliac bolts. Ponte osteotomies were then done from L1 to 5 to decompress each nerve root and for correction of the coronal curvature. A TLIF was performed at L3-4 to aid with correction as this was the apex of the curvature. In addition, a L5-S1 TLIF was also performed to aid with fusion at this location. After all the bony work and decompression were completed, rodding was accomplished with cobalt chrome rods, and a third rod placed for extra support for the construct. A tethering device was then placed at the base of T9 to reduce the risk of proximal junctional kyphosis followed by 3 L of gentamicin-impregnated saline irrigation using a pulse lavage. Arthrodesis was performed with use of bone morphogenic protein, harvested

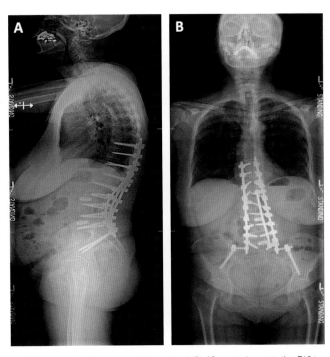

Fig. 36.4 Postoperative x-rays. (A) Lateral and (B) AP x-rays demonstrating T10 to pelvis instrumentation with L3-4 and L5-S1 TLIF with restoration of lumbar lordosis and correction of the coronal deformity.

autograft, and autograft. The wound was closed in layers with two hemovac drains left in place. Intraoperative monitoring was performed throughout the case. The patient was mobilized on postoperative day 1 and discharged on postoperative day 5 with good pain control. X-rays showed good postion of the hardware (Fig. 36.4).

Commonalities among the experts

The majority requested additional imaging including magnetic resonance imaging, dual-energy x-ray absorptiometry scans, and x-rays. Overall, there was a wide variability in what was recommended by the surgeons ranging from laminectomy to scoliosis correction. While half recommended a more focused surgical intervention, one recommended a L3-4 laminectomy and the other recommended a L3-4 and L4-5 TLIF and a Ll-L5 posterior fusion. Half did recommend a more extensive surgical intervention for correction of the scoliosis. While both recommended T10-pelvis instrumentation, one surgeon recommended a staged procedure with L5-S1 ALIF for the first stage. The second surgeon recommended interbody via a TLIF approach at L4-S1 in a single-stage procedure. One surgeon who initially recommend a laminectomy alone suggested a more expensive scoliosis repair if the patient was younger (21 years old), and the others recommended the same approach. In the scenario where the patient was older (80 years old), the same approach was recommended by all but one surgeon who initially recommended a T10-pelvis but would now limit that to a L4-S1 TLIF. The majority agreed on the use of intraoperative monitoring, in addition to the use of tranexamic acid. Only one surgeon recommended admission to the intensive care unit postoperatively. Bracing was recommended again by all surgeons with expected hospitalization ranging from 1 to 7 days.

SUMMARY OF QUALITY OF EVIDENCE TO GUIDE SPECIFIC INTERVENTIONS FOR THIS CASE

- Intraoperative monitoring for deformity correction: level III
- Hook versus pedicle screw at UIV for PJK prevention: level III
- Complication in deformity in patient >80 years old: level III

REFERENCES

1. Pritchett JW, Bortel DT. Degenerative symptomatic lumbar scoliosis. *Spine (Phila Pa 1976)*. 1993;18(6):700–703.
2. Robin GC, Span Y, Steinberg R, Makin M, Menczel J. Scoliosis in the elderly: a follow-up study. *Spine (Phila Pa 1976)*. 1982;7(4): 355–359.
3. Silva FE, Lenke LG. Adult degenerative scoliosis: evaluation and management. *Neurosurg Focus*. 2010;28(3):E1.
4. Phillips FM, Isaacs RE, Rodgers WB, Khajavi K, Tohmeh AG, Deviren V, et al. Adult degenerative scoliosis treated with XLIF: clinical and radiographical results of a prospective multicenter study with 24-month follow-up. *Spine (Phila Pa 1976)*. 2013;38(21): 1853–1861.
5. Schwab F, Dubey A, Gamez L, El Fegoun AB, Hwang K, Pagala M, et al. Adult scoliosis: prevalence, SF-36, and nutritional parameters in an elderly volunteer population. *Spine (Phila Pa 1976)*. 2005;30(9): 1082–1085.
6. McCarthy M. US health spending is expected to rebound with recovering economy. *BMJ*. 2013;346:f2680.
7. Ames CP, Smith JS, Scheer JK, Bess S, Bederman SS, Deviren V, et al. Impact of spinopelvic alignment on decision making in deformity surgery in adults: A review. *J Neurosurg Spine*. 2012;16(6): 547–564.
8. Schwab F, Ungar B, Blondel B, Buchowski J, Coe J, Deinlein D, et al. Scoliosis Research Society-Schwab adult spinal deformity classification: a validation study. *Spine (Phila Pa 1976)*. 2012;37(12): 1077–1082.
9. Lafage R, Schwab F, Challier V, Henry JK, Gum J, Smith J, et al. Defining Spino-Pelvic Alignment Thresholds Should Operative Goals in Adult Spinal Deformity Surgery Account for Age? *Spine*. 2016;41(1):62–68.
10. Uribe JS, Schwab F, Mundis GM, Xu DS, Januszewski J, Kanter AS, et al. The comprehensive anatomical spinal osteotomy and anterior column realignment classification. *J Neurosurg-Spine*. 2018;29(5): 565–575.

37

Adolescent idiopathic deformity

Kingsley Abode-Iyamah, MD

Introduction

Adolescent idiopathic scoliosis (AIS) is the most common type of scoliosis, affecting 2% to 4% of adolescents with an occurrence rate of 0.5 to 5.2%.[1,2] Although the pathophysiology is unclear, there are some studies that suggest a genetic component.[3,4] While smaller curvature is seen in males and females at similar rates, there is a higher prevalence of larger curvature in women.[1] Additionally, around the time of puberty, there is a significant increase in the female-to-male ratio of scoliosis (8.4:1), suggesting there may also be a role of sex hormones in the development of this type of scoliosis.[5,6] Patients typically present with back deformity and shoulder asymmetry, which can also be seen in the waistline and rib prominence.[7] Although the majority of symptoms are cosmetic, patients can occasionally present with back pain and even decreased lung capacity in severe cases.

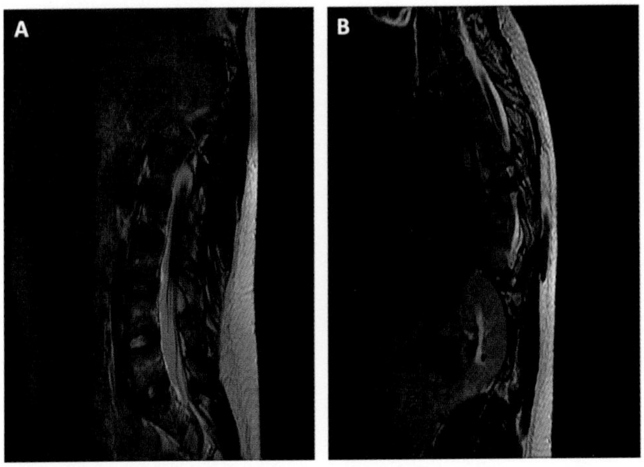

Fig. 37.1 Preoperative magnetic resonance images. (A), T2 sagittal and (B), T2 oblique sagittal images demonstrating severe thoracolumbar scoliosis.

Example Case

Chief complaint: back pain

History of present illness: A 19-year-old male presents with a history of back pain that worsens with activity. He was diagnosed with AIS and has been managed conservatively. Over the past 7 months, he has been having severe back pain with activity that is relieved with rest. He has noted some postural change in this time. His mother has also noted some scapular bulging over the past 3 years. He underwent imaging and this revealed concern for progressive scoliosis (Figs. 37.1–37.2).

Medications: atomoxetine, cetirizine, methylphenidate

Allergies: codeine

Past medical and surgical history: attention-deficit/hyperactivity disorder

Family history: noncontributory

Social history: student, nonsmoker

Physical examination: awake, alert, and oriented to person, place, and time; cranial nerves II–XII intact; bilateral deltoids/triceps/biceps 5/5; interossei 5/5; iliopsoas/knee flexion/knee extension/dorsi, and plantar flexion 5/5

Reflexes: 2+ in bilateral biceps/triceps/brachioradialis with negative Hoffman; 2+ in bilateral patella/ankle; no clonus or Babinski; sensation intact to light touch

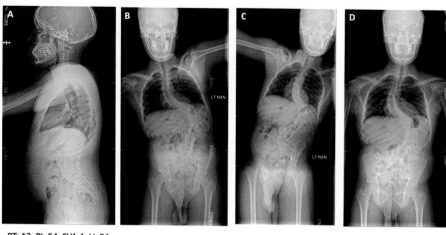

PT: 13, PI: 54, SVA 4, LL:54
Lenke: 6CN   Cobb Major: 84 Minor:56   Cobb Major: 59 Minor:52   Cobb Major: 79 Minor:60

Fig. 37.2 Preoperative x-rays. (A), Lateral, (B), left-bending, (C), right-bending, and (D), anteroposterior x-rays demonstrating a Lenke 6CN thoracolumbar scoliosis.

	Dean Chou, MD Rory Mayer, MD Neurosurgery University of California at San Francisco San Francisco, California, United States	Christopher J. Dewald, MD Orthopaedic Surgery Rush University Medical Center Chicago, Illinois, United States	Takeshi Hara, MD Neurosurgery Juntendo University Hongo, Bunkyo-ku, Tokyo, Japan	Yasuaki Tokuhashi, MD Orthopaedic Surgery Nihon University Oyaguchi Kamicho, Itabashi-ku, Tokyo, Japan
Preoperative				
Additional tests requested	Pulmonary function test Psychosocial assessment Physical therapy evaluation	MRI complete spine	MRI C-spine CT T-L spine	Pulmonary function test Flexion-extension x-rays 3D CT
Surgical approach selected	T3-L4 fusion with posterior column osteotomies at T8-10 and T12-L3	T4-L4 fusion with single posterior column osteotomy	T3-L3 posterior fusion with Ponte osteotomies as needed	Stage 1: T11-L3 posterior release Stage 2: T11-L3/L4 anterior correction and fusion
Surgical approach if 50 Surgical approach if 80	Same approach Same approach	Same approach Same approach	Same approach Same approach	Same approach, minimize levels Stage 1: L2-3 to L4-5 OLIF Stage 2: T6-Iliac (7 days later)
Goal of surgery	Halt curve progression, prevent pulmonary compromise, improve cosmetic deformity, potentially decrease back pain	Halt curve progression, partial correction of deformity, spinal cord safety	Coronal balance	Correct deformity, stabilize spine
Perioperative				
Positioning	Prone on Jackson table, no pins	Prone on Jackson table, Gardner-Wells tongs	Prone, no pins	Stage 1: prone on Hall frame Stage 2: right decubitus position
Surgical equipment	IOM Osteotome	IOM (MEP/SSEP) Fluoroscopy	IOM (MEP) O-arm Surgical navigation	IOM (MEP/SSEP) Osteotome
Medications	Tranexamic acid	Tranexamic acid	Maintain MAP	None
Anatomical considerations	Spinal cord/thecal sac	Spinal cord, nerve roots, dysplastic vertebrae	Aorta, inferior vena cava, spinal cord, nerve roots	Stage 1: facet joints Stage 2: major vessels, ureter, neural structures, pleura

	Dean Chou, MD Rory Mayer, MD Neurosurgery University of California at San Francisco San Francisco, California, United States	Christopher J. Dewald, MD Orthopaedic Surgery Rush University Medical Center Chicago, Illinois, United States	Takeshi Hara, MD Neurosurgery Juntendo University Hongo, Bunkyo-ku, Tokyo, Japan	Yasuaki Tokuhashi, MD Orthopaedic Surgery Nihon University Oyaguchi Kamicho, Itabashi-ku, Tokyo, Japan
Complications feared with approach chosen	Neurological deficit, pseudoarthrosis, adjacent segment disease	Spinal cord injury, blood loss, pseudoarthrosis, adjacent segment degeneration	Spinal cord injury, vascular injury, nerve root injury	Stage 1: paravertebral damage Stage 2: injury to major vessels/ureter, screw malposition, screw back out at correction, neural injury at correction
Intraoperative				
Anesthesia	General	General	General	General
Exposure	T3-L4	T4-L4	T3-L3	T11-L3
Levels decompressed	None	None	None	None
Levels fused	T3-L4	T4-L4	T3-L3	T11-L3/4
Surgical narrative	Position prone, expose posterior elements from T3 to L4, place pedicle screws at T3 to L4 after confirmation of levels with x-ray, reduction screws placed at apex of curve, posterior column osteotomies with facet resection bilaterally from T7-T10 and T12-L3, place working rod that is contoured and placed on concavity of curve and provisionally secured with set screws at cephalad and caudal ends, gradual tightening of the reduction screw to bring spine to the rod, axial derotation as necessary to address rib hump, confirm with IOM stability of signals, release correction if any IOM changes, secure rod with set screws, further coronal correction with coronal plane benders, placement of convexity rod with placement of set screws, further axial derotation done with second rod in place, final tightening of screws after additional distraction/compression maneuvers as necessary to achieve correction, decortication of exposed lamina and placement of local autograft, layered closure with two subfascial drains	Preflip IOM, position prone with Gardner-Wells tongs, add weights to tongs (15 lb), midline posterior incision from T4 to L4, subperiosteal exposure of spinous processes, expose T4-L4 transverse processes using monopolar cautery and Cobb elevator, inferior facetectomies from T4 to L3 bilaterally using osteotome, determine mobility of spinal deformity, place pedicle screws using anatomy with fluoroscopic confirmation starting in lumbar spine and proceeding superiorly, drop screws that are not needed in the middle of construct (pedicles too small or are missed), Ponte osteotomies from T11/12 to L3/4 by removing spinous processes down to ligamentum flavum and exposing superior facets, run MEP, place precontoured rods, utilize rod rotation and cantilever maneuvers to obtain spinal deformity correction in both coronal and sagittal planes, derotation using vertebral derotation tubes, lock correction with set caps and run MEP, decorticate exposed lamina and transverse processed from T4 to L4, place local and allograft bone throughout, use to cross-links, layered closure with drains, neurological check before extubation and leaving the operating room	Position prone, midline incision, remove soft tissue and extend dissection to transverse processes, insert pedicle screws from T3 to L3 with O-arm navigation, use polyethylene cables if pedicles are too small or difficult to insert, place multiaxial reduction screws in apex vertebra in the lumbar curve on concave side and fixed screws on caudal side, attach vertebral column manipulation instruments to fixed screws on concave and convex sides, resect inferior articular processes, perform Ponte osteotomy is necessary for lumbar curve, apply compression force on convex side and apply rotational force in the opposite direction of vertebral body rotation with traction on concave side, apply cobalt chromium alloy rods on both sides once sufficient deformity correction achieved making sure thoracic rods are kyphotic and lumbar spine lordotic, apply pressure to convex side and traction on concave side, final tighten set screws and polyethylene tape, layered closure	Stage 1: position prone, longitudinal midline incision from T11 to L3, expose T11/T12 to L2/3 facet joints, T11-L2 partial inferior facet resection and cartilage curettage by osteotome and diamond bur, standard closure, position change Stage 2: right decubitus position, curved incision along the 10th rib, 10th rib resection, expose T11-L3 vertebral body by incising diaphragm, T11/12 to L2-3 disc resection, T11-L3 anterior plate Snad screws, pack tips of resected rib into disc space, rod and screw fixation from T11-L3 to correct coronal curve slowly, fix anterior rods and screws, compress between posterior screws to correct sagittal lordosis, posterior rods and screws are fixed, closure with chest tube if necessary

	Dean Chou, MD Rory Mayer, MD Neurosurgery University of California at San Francisco San Francisco, California, United States	Christopher J. Dewald, MD Orthopaedic Surgery Rush University Medical Center Chicago, Illinois, United States	Takeshi Hara, MD Neurosurgery Juntendo University Hongo, Bunkyo-ku, Tokyo, Japan	Yasuaki Tokuhashi, MD Orthopaedic Surgery Nihon University Oyaguchi Kamicho, Itabashi-ku, Tokyo, Japan
Complication avoidance	Place reduction screws at apex of curve, axial derotation to address rib hump, IOM while curve correction, coronal plane benders to reduce coronal deformity	Preflip IOM, remove screws in middle of construct that are not needed, utilize rod rotation and cantilever maneuvers to obtain spinal deformity correction in both coronal and sagittal planes	O-arm and surgical navigation for pedicle screws, use polyethylene cables if pedicles are too small or difficult to insert, perform Ponte osteotomy is necessary for lumbar curve	Two stages, dual rods, slow correction of coronal followed by sagittal curves, chest tube if necessary
Postoperative				
Admission	Floor	ICU	ICU	ICU
Postoperative complications feared	Neurological deficit, pseudoarthrosis, adjacent segment disease with potential need to extend fusion to pelvis in future	Neurological deficit, pseudoarthrosis, spinal imbalance, pain	Spinal cord or nerve root injury, CSF leak, spinal instability, aorta or vena cava injury	Hemothorax, ileus, injury to major vessels or ureter
Anticipated length of stay	4–5 days	3–5 days	10–14 days	10–14 days
Follow-up testing	Standing scoliosis x-rays at discharge, 6 weeks, 3 months, 6 months, 1 year, 2 years after surgery	Standing scoliosis x-rays 3 weeks after surgery	CT T-L spine within 24 hours, 3 months after surgery	CT scan 7 days, 6 months after surgery
Bracing	None	None	Corset for 3 months	Hard corset for 6 months
Follow-up visits	2 weeks, 6 weeks, 3 months, 6 months, 1 year, 2 years after surgery	3 weeks after surgery	2 weeks, 3 months after surgery	4 weeks after surgery

APP, Advanced practice provider; BAERs, brainstem auditory evoked responses; CT, computed tomography; DEXA, dual-energy x-ray absorptiometry; ERAS, enhanced recovery after surgery; ESI, epidural spinal injections; ICU, intensive care unit; IOM, intraoperative monitoring; MAP, mean arterial pressure; MEP, motor evoked potential; MRI, magnetic resonance imaging; SSEP, somatosensory evoked potential.

Differential diagnosis

- Adolescent idiopathic scoliosis
- Neuromuscular scoliosis
- Degenerative scoliosis

Important anatomical considerations

Evaluation for AIS should include curvature pattern, shoulder and waist asymmetry, gait, posture, and leg length discrepancy. Forward bending for the assessment of rib rotational deformity and measurement of the vertebral angle with a scoliometer should also be performed. Standard imaging should be obtained, which includes an upright posteroanterior (PA) and lateral view x-rays. With these x-rays, routine measurements can be obtained and the scoliosis classified. Given the serial imaging that young patients must obtain throughout their lifetime to assess their scoliosis and the overall cumulative effects of radiation, it is important to reduce radiation to patients when possible. The EOS slot-scanning two-dimensional/three-dimensional system significantly reduces the radiation dose by 50% to 80% compared with conventional x-ray and has therefore gained popularity in assessing patients with scoliosis.[8,9]

The King classification was first developed in the 1980s to describe five thoracic curve types and gave recommendations on vertebral levels to include during spinal arthrodesis with Harrington rods; however, the classification did not include thoracolumbar, lumbar, or double or triple curves.[10] The King classification was used for many years, despite consensus on a need to consider scoliosis a three-dimensional deformity during consideration or correction. It was not until 2001 that the Lenke classification was published (Table 37.1).[11] This classification system uses six types based on the location of the major curve and whether the curves are structural or nonstructural. Additionally, this classification allows for lumbar modifier as well as thoracic sagittal profile modifiers. This allows for intraobserver consistency in classification of the curve, which was lacking in the King classification.[11]

Approaches to this lesion

Untreated AIS can lead to progressive back pain, cardiopulmonary problems, and even psychosocial problems.[12] Treatment of AIS includes both nonsurgical and surgical management and the treatment approach is somewhat dictated by the curve size, curve progression, and skeletal maturity. Those patients who reach skeletal maturity with a curve less than 30 degrees

Table 37.1 Lenke Classification Of Scoliosis

Curve Type				
Type	Proximal Thoracic	Main Thoracic	Thoracolumar/Lumbar	Description
1	Nonstructural	Structural (Major)[a]	Nonstructural	Main thoracic (MT)
2	Structural	Structural (Major)[a]	Nonstructural	Double thoracic (DT)
3	Nonstructural	Structural (Major)[a]	Structural	Double major (DM)
4	Structural	Structural (Major)[a]	Structural	Triple major (TM)[b]
5	Nonstructural	Nonstructural	Structural (Major)[a]	Thoracolumbar/lumbar (TL/L)
6	Nonstructural	Structural	Structural (Major)[a]	Thoracolumbar/lumbar-main thoracic (TL/L-MT)

Structural Criteria

(Minor Curves)

Proximal Thoracic:

    Side-bending Cobb ≥25 degrees

    T2-T5 kyphosis ≥20 degrees

Main Thoracic:

    Side-bending Cobb ≥25 degrees

    T10-L2 kyphosis ≥20 degrees

Thoracolumbar/Lumbar:

    Side-bending Cobb ≥25 degrees

    T10-L2 kyphosis ≥20 degrees

[a]Major = Largest Cobb measurement, always structural

Minor = All other curves with structural criteria applied

[b]Type IV: MT or TL/L can be major curve

Location of Apex

(SRS Definition)

Curve	Apex
Thoracic	T2-T11/12 disc
Thoracolumbar	T12-L1
Thoracolumbar/lumbar	L1-2 disc-L4

are less likely to see progression of their curves. Those with curve angle of 30 to 50 degrees may have a lifetime change of 10 to 15 degrees, while there is an expected curve progression rate of 1 degree per year in individuals with a curve of >50 degrees.[13] The Scoliosis Research Society (SRS) currently recommends that those without skeletal maturity and a curve of <25 degrees and those with skeletal maturity and a curve of <45 degrees be managed conservatively.[14,15] In the BRAIST study, Weinstein et al. in a multicenter study found that bracing at least 18 hours a day prevented progression to >50 degrees 72% of the time compared with 48% in individuals without bracing.[16–19] While there are multiple bracing options such as the Boston, Milwaukee, and Rigo Cheneau orthosis braces, treatment is initiated for 16 to 20 hours a day and success is defined as less than 5 degrees of progression at the conclusion of the treatment.[15] When patients fail nonsurgical intervention or surgical intervention is deemed necessary from the start, surgical intervention entails a fusion operation. This can be accomplished through an anterior approach, posterior approach, or a combination of both.

What was actually done

This patient presented with back pain worsened with activity, which led to his initial diagnosis of AIS. He had been previously managed conservatively and over time has noted mild postural change. The patient was sent and obtained the side bending images, which revealed a structural main thoracic curve measuring 60 degrees with Lenke 6CN AIS. The patient was offered a T4 to L4 posterior spinal fusion and correction of his scoliosis. The patient was a new college student and surgical intervention needed to be scheduled during semester breaks. On follow-up to determine timing of surgery, the patient was hesitant to proceed with surgical intervention. Repeat scoliosis films at that time did not show progression of his curve. Despite concerns about the large curve and

Modifier		
Lumbar Spine Modifier	Central Sacral Vertical Line in Lumbar Apex	Thoracic Sagittal Profile T5-T12
A	CSVL C between pedicles	– (Hypo) <10 degrees
B	CSVL touches apical body/bodies	N (Normal) 10–40 degrees
C	CSVL completely medial	+ (Hyper) >40 degrees
SVL		
CSVL, central sacral vertical line		

likelihood for progression of his curve, the patient and family elected for nonsurgical intervention and continues with conservative management and close follow-up.

Commonalities among the experts

Half recommended complete magnetic resonance imaging of the spine and the other half recommended a pulmonary function test prior to surgical intervention. All experts agreed that given the large Cobb angle, surgical intervention was necessary to prevent curve progression and prevent pulmonary compromise. There was consensus on pursuing posterior instrumentation with osteotomies. The levels recommended for fusion varied only by one level for the majority of surgeons. Most recommended fusion from T3 or T4 to L3 or L4. One surgeon recommended a T11 to L3 release and T11 to L3 anterior correction and fixation in a staged procedure. These recommendations did not change when presented with a middle-aged patient (50 years old) or and older adult patient (80 years old). All agreed on the use of intraoperative monitoring and half recommended tranexamic acid use during the procedure. The majority recommended admission to the intensive care unit with planned hospitalization of 4 to 14 days. Additionally, half recommended bracing postoperatively.

SUMMARY OF QUALITY OF EVIDENCE TO GUIDE SPECIFIC INTERVENTIONS FOR THIS CASE

- Intraoperative monitoring for deformity correction: level II.1
- Hook versus pedicle screw at upper index level for proximal junctional kyphosis prevention: level II.1
- Bracing following lumbar fusion: level I
- Risk of pulmonary dysfunction with scoliosis: level II.1
- Risk of progression of scoliosis: level II.1

REFERENCES

1. Konieczny MR, Senyurt H, Krauspe R. Epidemiology of adolescent idiopathic scoliosis. *J Child Orthop*. 2013;7(1):3–9.
2. Kikanloo SR, Tarpada SP, Cho W. Etiology of Adolescent Idiopathic Scoliosis: A Literature Review. *Asian Spine J*. 2019;13(3):519–526.
3. Cheng JC, Castelein RM, Chu WC, Danielsson AJ, Dobbs MB, Grivas TB, et al. Adolescent idiopathic scoliosis. *Nat Rev Dis Primers*. 2015;1:15030.
4. Kelly JSN, Freetly T, Dekis J, Hariri O, Walker S, et al. Treatment of adolescent idiopathic scoliosis and evaluation of the adolescent patient. *Current Orthopaedic Practice*. 2018;29:424–429.
5. Esposito T, Uccello R, Caliendo R, Di Martino GF, Gironi Carnevale UA, Cuomo S, et al. Estrogen receptor polymorphism, estrogen content and idiopathic scoliosis in human: a possible genetic linkage. *J Steroid Biochem Mol Biol*. 2009;116(1-2):56–60.
6. Schlosser TP, Vincken KL, Rogers K, Castelein RM, Shah SA. Natural sagittal spino-pelvic alignment in boys and girls before, at and after the adolescent growth spurt. *Eur Spine J*. 2015;24(6):1158–1167.
7. Altaf F, Gibson A, Dannawi Z, Noordeen H. Adolescent idiopathic scoliosis. *BMJ*. 2013;346:f2508.
8. Bagheri A, Liu XC, Tassone C, Thometz J, Tarima S. Reliability of Three-Dimensional Spinal Modeling of Patients With Idiopathic Scoliosis Using EOS System. *Spine Deform*. 2018;6(3):207–212.
9. Lau LCM, Hung ALH, Chau WW, Hu Z, Kumar A, Lam TP, et al. Sequential spine-hand radiography for assessing skeletal maturity with low radiation EOS imaging system for bracing treatment recommendation in adolescent idiopathic scoliosis: a feasibility and validity study. *J Child Orthop*. 2019;13(4):385–392.
10. King HA, Moe JH, Bradford DS, Winter RB. The selection of fusion levels in thoracic idiopathic scoliosis. *J Bone Joint Surg Am*. 1983;65(9):1302–1313.
11. Lenke LG, Betz RR, Harms J, Bridwell KH, Clements DH, Lowe TG, et al. Adolescent idiopathic scoliosis: a new classification to determine extent of spinal arthrodesis. *J Bone Joint Surg Am*. 2001;83(8):1169–1181.
12. Weinstein SL, Dolan LA, Cheng JC, Danielsson A, Morcuende JA. Adolescent idiopathic scoliosis. *Lancet*. 2008;371(9623):1527–1537.
13. Reamy BV, Slakey JB. Adolescent idiopathic scoliosis: review and current concepts. *Am Fam Physician*. 2001;64(1):111–116.
14. Ovadia D. Classification of adolescent idiopathic scoliosis (AIS). *J Child Orthop*. 2013;7(1):25–28.
15. Zheng S, Zhou H, Gao B, Li Y, Liao Z, Zhou T, et al. Estrogen promotes the onset and development of idiopathic scoliosis via disproportionate endochondral ossification of the anterior and posterior column in a bipedal rat model. *Exp Mol Med*. 2018;50(11):1–11.
16. Danielsson AJ. Natural history of adolescent idiopathic scoliosis: a tool for guidance in decision of surgery of curves above 50 degrees. *J Child Orthop*. 2013;7(1):37–41.
17. Nachemson A. A long term follow-up study of non-treated scoliosis. *Acta Orthop Scand*. 1968;39(4):466–476.
18. Nilsonne U, Lundgren KD. Long-term prognosis in idiopathic scoliosis. *Acta Orthop Scand*. 1968;39(4):456–465.
19. Weinstein SL, Dolan LA, Wright JG, Dobbs MB. Effects of bracing in adolescents with idiopathic scoliosis. *N Engl J Med*. 2013;369(16):1512–1521.

38

Flat back after fusion

Kingsley Abode-Iyamah, MD

Introduction

Flat back syndrome is described as loss of lumbar lordosis, which alters the center of gravity, thereby shifting the head anterior to the sacrum causing sagittal imbalance. This is typically seen following multiple lumbar fusions with distraction of the lumbar spine that ultimately lead to loss of lumbar lordosis. It was first described in patients undergoing scoliosis repair with placement of Harrington distraction by Doherty.[1] This resulted in forward inclination of the trunk and inability for upright posture. Patients were unable to stand erect without knee flexion and required cervical extension to maintain horizontal gaze.[2] This ultimately leads to increased energy expenditure when standing upright, leading to back pain. In addition to back pain, patients may also report anterior thigh pain from constant flexion at the hips. While loss of lumbar lordosis can occur from degenerative changes leading to pelvic incidence to lumbar lordosis mismatch, another common cause is iatrogenic during fusion operations. Positioning such as kneeling or knee-chest position causes flexion of the hips and leads to loss of lumbar lordosis, while positioning that fully extends the hips accentuates lumbar lordosis.[3] Other causes of loss of lumbar lordosis include posterior interbody fusion and segmental distraction, which can result in focal kyphosis.[4] Return of normal posture requires the return of normal lumbar lordosis to restore the normal sagittal balance.

Example case

Chief complaint: back pain

History of present illness: A 65-year-old male with a history of multiple lumbar fusions in the past as well as cervical fusion beginning over 20 years ago, with his last surgery being approximately 10 years ago. He has had both decompressive and fusion surgery. He has not been able to lay down flat on his bed for many years. He has severe back and radicular pain and requires high doses of pain medication. He is unable to stand straight and complains of his back fatiguing. He denies weakness. He underwent imaging and was concerning for flat back syndrome (Figs. 38.1–38.3).

Medications: AndroGel, armodafinil, omeprazole, valsartan, ranitidine

Allergies: nickel

Past medical and surgical history: hypertension, back pain, laminectomy, L1-S1 posterior spinal fusion, spinal cord stimulator placement and removal, anterior cervical discectomy and fusion

Family history: noncontributory

Social history: disabled, nonsmoker

Physical examination: awake, alert, and oriented to person, place, and time; cranial nerves II–XII intact; bilateral deltoids/triceps/biceps 5/5; interossei 5/5; iliopsoas/knee flexion/knee extension/dorsi, and plantar flexion 5/5

Reflexes: 2+ in bilateral biceps/triceps/brachioradialis with negative Hoffman; 2+ in bilateral patella/ankle; no clonus or Babinski; sensation intact to light touch

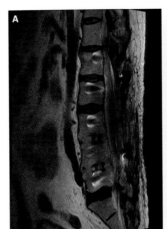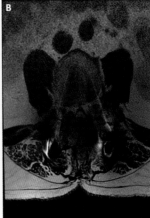

Fig. 38.1 Preoperative magnetic resonance images. (A) T2 sagittal and **(B)** T2 axial images demonstrating postoperative changes with loss of lumbar lordosis.

	Belal Elnady, MD Orthopaedic Surgery Assiut University Assiut, Egypt	Diego F Gómez MD MSc. Neurosurgey Fundación Santafe de Bogotá Bogota, Colombia	John G. Heller, MD Orthopaedic Surgery Emory University Atlanta, Georgia, United States	Daniel M. Sciubba, MD Jeffrey Ehresman, BS Neurosurgery Johns Hopkins Baltimore, Maryland, United States
Preoperative				
Additional tests requested	Conservative measures	SPECT/CT L-spine EMG/NCS DEXA Anesthesiology evaluation	Vitamin D levels and titrate to normal levels if low Pain management evaluation with narcotic titration Medicine evaluation Psychiatry evaluation	DEXA Lumbar flexion-extension x-rays
Surgical approach selected	L4-5 modified pedicle subtraction osteotomy and T10-ileum posterior fusion	T10-S2 posterior fusion with L4 pedicle subtraction osteotomy	If agrees to pain and psychiatric evaluations, Stage 1: posterior removal of L1-S1 instrumentation, T12-L1 laminectomy, redo L5-S1 decompression with facet osteotomies, L2-3 osteotomies, T10-pelvis with iliac bolts Stage 2: L5-S1 ALIF Stage 3: L2-3 XLIF and anterior column release if needed Stage 4: T10-pelvis with posterior T10-L3 fusion and L5-S1 posterolateral fusion	Stage 1: removal of previous S1 screws and rods, placement of bilateral pelvic screws, posterior column osteotomy at L5-S1 Stage 2: ALIF Stage 3: pedicle subtraction osteotomy at L4 (if lumbar lordosis not >40 degrees) followed by rod placement (L1-pelvis)
Surgical approach if 21 Surgical approach if 80	Same Same	Same Conservative management	Same T10-pelvis fusion only	Closely match LL to PI LL substantially less than PI
Goal of surgery	Restore sagittal balance and LL	Restore sagittal balance and LL, spinal cord decompression at L5-S1	Decompress stenosis at L5-S1 and L1-2, repair L5-S1 nonunion, correct sagittal balance (40–45 degrees of correction)	Increase LL in order to decrease PI-LL mismatch, improve overall sagittal balance
Perioperative				
Positioning	Prone, no pins	Prone on Jackson table, no pins	Stage 1: prone, no pins Stage 2: supine, no pins Stage 3: lateral, no pins Stage 4: prone, no pins	Stage 1: prone, no pins on Jackson table Stage 2: supine on Jackson table Stage 3: prone, no pins
Surgical equipment	Fluoroscopy IOM (MEP/SSEP/ EMG) Surgical microscope	Fluoroscopy IOM (MEP/SSEP/ EMG) Plasma blade cautery Aquamantys® bipolar	Fluoroscopy BMP	Fluoroscopy IOM (MEP/SSEP) Ultrasonic bone scalpel
Medications	None	None	None	Tranexamic acid
Anatomical considerations	Dura, nerve root	Aorta, iliac arteries, dura sac, nerve roots	Dura, nerve root, PLL	Dura, spinal cord, iliac vessels, ureter
Complications feared with approach chosen	Dural tear, CSF leak	Excessive blood loss, nerve root injury, pedicle fracture, CSF leak	Dural tear, CSF leak, nerve root injury, cage displacement	Vascular injury, CSF leak
Intraoperative				
Anesthesia	General	General	General	General
Exposure	T10-sacrum	T10-sacrum	Stage 1: T10-pelvis Stage 2: L5-S1 Stage 3: L2-3 Stage 4: T10-pelvis	L1-pelvis

	Belal Elnady, MD Orthopaedic Surgery Assiut University Assiut, Egypt	Diego F Gómez MD MSc. Neurosurgey Fundación Santafe de Bogotá Bogota, Colombia	John G. Heller, MD Orthopaedic Surgery Emory University Atlanta, Georgia, United States	Daniel M. Sciubba, MD Jeffrey Ehresman, BS Neurosurgery Johns Hopkins Baltimore, Maryland, United States
Levels decompressed	L4-5	L5-S1	Stage 1: T12-L1, L5-S1 Stage 2: L5-S1 Stage 3: L2-3 Stage 4: none	
Levels fused	T10-sacrum	T10-sacrum	Stage 1: none Stage 2: L5-S1 Stage 3: L2-3 Stage 4: T10-pelvis	L1-pelvis
Surgical narrative	Position prone, midline incision, subperiosteal dissection, expose from T10 to sacrum, extend previous fusion to T10 with pedicle screws and down to ilium with iliac screws, modified pedicle subtraction osteotomy at L4-5 level with posterior wedge closing osteotomy, rod insertion and compression to restore lumbar lordosis, wound closure in layers with drain	Position prone with transverse rolls to increase LL, midline incision from T10-S2, subperiosteal dissection exposing posterior elements including facet joints and transverse processes, remove previous lumbar instrumentation, implant pedicle screws from T10 to S1 and S2 alar iliac screws, pedicle subtraction osteotomy at L4, closure of osteotomy with extension of hip joints and elevation of trunk, gentle compression between the pedicle screw head, position rod with lordotic contouring avoiding excessive stress on pedicle screws, careful attention to SSEP and MEP at this time, L5-S1 laminectomy with bilateral foraminotomy, apply autograft with bony substitutes along bony surfaces, layered closure with subfascial drain	Stage 1: position prone, posterior midline approach, expose T10-S3, remove all instrumentation from L1-S1, decompress T12-L1 stenosis, dissect out scar at L5-S1 nonunion, generously decompress L5 and S1 nerve roots with partial or complete facetectomies (closing wedge osteotomies), create closing wedge osteotomies at L2-3 bilaterally to facilitate XLIF during stage 2, place pedicles screws from T10-pelvis, layered closure Stage 2 (3–5 days later after obtaining x-rays, CT, MRI): position supine with thick bolster at lumbosacral junction, standard left retroperitoneal approach to L5-S1 disc space, complete L5-S1 discectomy all the way back to posterior annulus but leaving it intact, release anterolateral annulus, insert appropriately sized cage with BMP-2, secure with screws into S1 end plate Stage 3 (same day as stage 2): position lateral, target correction for XLIF depends on amount of correction achieved with L5-S1 ALIF, may be necessary to perform an anterior column release with release of ALL and lateral annular walls if greater correction needed, insert appropriate cage with BMP-2 and secure with either L2 or L3 screw fixation, standard closure Stage 4 (same day as stage 3): position prone, x-ray to confirm anterior devices in place, complete posterior segmental instrumentation, compress across osteotomies to optimize final alignment, confirm adequate space for nerve roots prior to compressing, place bone grafts at L5-S1 and T10-L3, layered closure with drains	Stage 1 (day 1): position prone on Jackson table, skin incision from L1 to pelvis, subperiosteal dissection, previous hardware inspected and S1 screws and rods removed, place bilateral pelvic screws using external landmarks, confirm location with x-ray, stimulate all screws, posterior column osteotomy at L5-S1, wound irrigated and closed Stage 2 (day 1): position supine, transverse incision between umbilicus and pubis down to anterior rectus sheath, retroperitoneal plane followed on left side to common iliac artery making sure to identify ureter/ psoas/lower iliac vessels, dissect common iliac artery off of spine, place retractors, confirm L5-S1 disc space, remove L5-S1, curette edges and decorticate, cut large femoral strut graft using ultrasonic bone scalpel to optimal size, place demineralized bone matrix in disc space, confirm location with x-ray, one screw in L5 and one in S1 to hold graft in place, wound closed, imaging obtained Stage 3 (day 2): position prone on Jackson table, incision and subperiosteal dissection from L1-pelvis exposing instrumentation, if LL was >40 degrees then place rods and compress, if LL <40 degrees then perform pedicle subtraction osteotomy at L4, remove bone above and below L4 pedicle, identify L3 and L4 nerve roots, separate L4 pedicles from L4 transverse processes, tin pedicles down until flush with spinal canal, complete with osteotomy with osteotome while protecting thecal sac and nerve roots, stimulate all screws, place lordotic rods, confirm LL >40 degrees with x-rays, decorticate exposed bone and place allograft and BMP, close in layers with drains

(continued on next page)

	Belal Elnady, MD Orthopaedic Surgery Assiut University Assiut, Egypt	Diego F Gómez MD MSc. Neurosurgey Fundación Santafe de Bogotá Bogota, Colombia	John G. Heller, MD Orthopaedic Surgery Emory University Atlanta, Georgia, United States	Daniel M. Sciubba, MD Jeffrey Ehresman, BS Neurosurgery Johns Hopkins Baltimore, Maryland, United States
Complication avoidance	Good debridement of disc space, gentle compression over pedicles to compress screws, attempt to achieve 360-degree fusion	Position with transverse roll to increase LL, pedicle subtraction osteotomy to increase LL, careful attention to MEP and SSEP during closure of the osteotomy and compression on pedicle screw	Multistage approach, remove scar at nonunion so that area can be properly decorticated, generous facetectomies posteriorly to avoid iatrogenic nerve root injury during anterior correction, imaging between stages, bolster for stage 2 to provide extension, leave posterior annulus at L5-S1 intact, anterior column release if more correction needed, confirm nerve roots decompress before compressing across osteotomies	Three-stage approach, pelvic screws with anatomical landmarks, stimulate screws to confirm location, posterior column osteotomy to increase LL, femoral strut graft, pedicle subtraction osteotomy if needed to increase LL
Postoperative				
Admission	ICU	ICU	ICU	ICU
Postoperative complications feared	CSF leak, wound infection, instrument failure	Neurological deficit, hematoma	Epidural hematoma, wound infection, nerve root injury, medical complications, nonunion, loss of fixation	CSF leak, vascular injury, new neurological deficit, hardware failure/spinal instability, nonunion
Anticipated length of stay	5–7 days	3 days	8–10 days	4–7 days
Follow-up testing	T-L spine x-rays 2 weeks, 2 months, 6 months, 1 year after surgery	CT T-L spine within 48 hours of surgery	Standing full length x-ray prior to discharge, 6 weeks, 3 months, 6 months, 12 months after surgery CT T-L spine 6 or 12 months after surgery	CT T-L spine within 24 hours of surgery
Bracing	None	None	TLSO when out of bed for 12 weeks	None
Follow-up visits	2 weeks, 2 months, 6 months, 1 year after surgery	1 week after surgery	6 weeks, 3 months, 6 months, 12 months after surgery	3 weeks after surgery

ALL, Anterior longitudinal ligament; *BMP*, bone morphogenic protein; *CSF*, cerebrospinal fluid; *CT*, computed tomography; *DEXA*, dual-energy x-ray absorptiometry; *XLIF*, extreme lateral interbody fusion; *EMG*, electromyography; *ICU*, intensive care unit; *IOM*, intraoperative monitoring; *LL*; lumbar lordosis; *MEP*, motor evoked potential; *NCS*, nerve conduction study; *PI*, pelvic index; *PLL*, posterior longitudinal ligament; *SPECT*, single-photon emission computed tomography; *SSEP*, somatosensory evoked potential; *TLSO*, thoracic lumbar sacral orthosis.

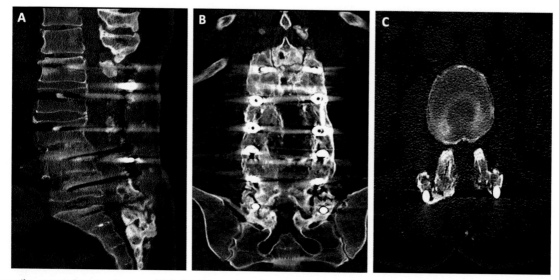

Fig. 38.2 Preoperative computed tomography scans. (A) Sagittal, **(B)** coronal, and **(C)** axial images demonstrating postoperative changes of previous fusion with massive fusion mass.

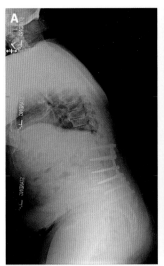 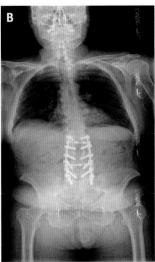

PT: 30, PI: 51, SVA 20, LL:10   Cobb angle: 45

Fig. 38.3 Preoperative x-rays. (A) Anteroposterior (AP) and **(B)** lateral x-rays demonstrating positive sagittal balance with loss of lumbar lordosis.

Differential diagnosis

- Flat back syndrome
- Back pain
- Scoliosis
- Adjacent segment disease
- Proximal junctional kyphosis

Important anatomical considerations

Treatment and prevention of flat back syndrome requires understanding the importance of the spinopelvic alignment. The formula PI = PT + SS is integral to understanding the relationship between the spine and pelvis. In this formula, pelvic incidence (PI) is a fixed morphogenic parameter with only slight changes during prepubertal development. Pelvic tilt (normal PT = <20 degrees) and sacral slope (SS) are variable parameters with indirect relationships to each other. Additional measurements include sagittal vertical axis (SVA = +/−4 cm), which is a common measurement of global sagittal alignment (SA). The difference between the coronal C7 plumb line and the central sacral vertical line (CSVL) assesses the coronal alignment (CA = +/−2 cm).[5] The SRS-Schwab classification identifies PT greater than 22 degrees, SVA greater than 46 mm, and PI-LL (pelvic incidence-lumbar lordosis = <10 degrees) more than 11 degrees as factors as predictive of disability.[6,7]

It is important to understand that given the morbidity and mortality of surgical treatment to correct flat back syndrome, prevention during index surgeries is paramount. Perioperative complication rates up to 60% have been reported while complete resolution of symptoms is rare. La Grone et al. reported that even after correction, up to 47% of patients continued to complain of forward leaning and over 30% continued to have back pain.[8] Preventive measures such as proper positioning and avoiding distracting instrumentation especially in the lower lumbar spine as well as segmental instrumentation in combination with compression can help prevent loss of lumbar lordosis.

Approaches to this lesion

The key to surgical planning is assessing the degree of correction needed to correct the PI-LL mismatch and correcting the sagittal imbalance. This can be accomplished with combination an anterior/posterior procedure or a posterior-only approach (Table 38.1). For anterior approaches, an anterior lumbar interbody fusion (ALIF) alone can provide 5 degrees of correction while an ALIF with Smith-Peterson osteotomy (SPO) can provide 15 to 20 degrees of sagittal correction. At presentation, most patients typically have already undergone fusion of most of the lumbar disc spaces, so interbody placement at other disc spaces is often not an option. When there are additional disc spaces available for correction, direct lateral interbody fusion (DLIF), anterior lateral interbody fusion (ALIF), and oblique lateral interbody fusion (OLIF) are options to consider. Not only can OLIF aid in coronal correction, but when combined with anterior column realignment (ACR), it can also provide sagittal correction of up to 30 degrees.[9]

Pedicle subtraction osteotomy (PSO), although not physiological, is necessary when correction is needed through a previously bony-fused level, allowing up to 30 degrees correction. Another osteotomy, vertebral column resection (VCR), delivers 30 to 40 degrees and is especially beneficial when both sagittal and coronal correction are needed.[9,10] Combined anterior and posterior procedures may add surgical time, lengthen hospitalization, require access surgeons (particularly for ALIF), and expose the patient to additional complications. Although these procedures carry a significant risk, correction can often not be obtained without it. Prior to planning surgical intervention, it is important to assess for iliopsoas contracture, which may prevent the patient's ability to stand erect even after correction. Those patients with concerns for iliopsoas contracture may require aggressive physical therapy or even iliopsoas release prior to undergoing surgical correction.[5]

What was actually done

At the initial evaluation, the patient was found to have flat back syndrome with significant PI-LL mismatch and

Table 38.1 Different Forms of Correcting Sagittal Imbalance and the Degree of Correction They Provide

Expected Degree of Correction per Approach		
Approach	Average Degree of Correction	Average Degree of Correction with SPO
Anterior interbody fusion	5.6	15 to 20
Lateral interbody fusion	1.2 to 3.6	20 to 25
Lateral interbody fusion (with ACR)	10 to 30	10 to 30
Posterior interbody fusion	−6 to 0	15 to 20
Transforaminal lumbar interbody fusion	−6 to 0	15 to 20
Vertebral column resection	30 to 40	30 to 40

sagittal imbalance (Fig. 38.3). Given the extended length of his symptoms and forward bending, he had also developed iliopsoas contracture, which needed correction prior to surgical correction. He was also evaluated by our orthopedic colleagues who recommended physical therapy that improved his contracture. Given the degree of correction needed, a staged procedure was to improve. The patient first underwent an L5-S1 ALIF with access supplied by a vascular surgeon. Following this procedure, the patient was brought back 3 days later to complete the posterior portion of the case. For the posterior portion, the patient was placed on an Orthopedic System Inc (OSI) table. The patient received tranexamic acid bolus at the beginning of the case and continuous infusion during the case. The previous incision was exposed and extended rostral and caudally to expose from T10 to the pelvis. The previous instrumentation was removed and instrumentation was extended to T10 and to the pelvis leaving out the instrumentation at L3. SPO was performed at both T12-L1 and L5-S1 through the fusion mass. We then proceeded with an L3 PSO alternating temporary rods during our cuts. After closure of the PSO, a three-rod system was placed and tethering device was placed at T9. Postoperatively, the patient developed mild right quadriceps weakness, which gradually improved during his hospitalization. He was discharged to inpatient rehabilitation on postoperative day 10. Postoperative imaging showed good location of the instrumentation and correction of the deformity and imbalance (Fig. 38.4).

Commonalities among the experts

The consensus was that this patient required surgical intervention. Some recommended conservative measures first, while others recommended psychiatric evaluation and pain management to titrate his narcotics. Half of the surgeons recommended a single-stage procedure while the other half recommended a three- and four-stage procedure. The majority recommended an L4 PSO,[11] and one surgeon recommended multilevel SPO and XLIF at L2-3. Additionally, half recommended a staged ALIF and all but one recommended a long construct extending to T10. When these surgeons were presented with a younger patient (21 years old), they all recommended the same procedure. When presented with an older patient (80 years old), the majority still recommended surgical intervention although with limited aggressive correction. The majority recommended the use of fluoroscopy and intraoperative monitoring[12] and one recommended the use of bone morphogenic protein. All expected the patient to be admitted to the intensive care until after surgery with hospitalization ranging from 3 to 10 days.

SUMMARY OF QUALITY OF EVIDENCE TO GUIDE SPECIFIC INTERVENTIONS FOR THIS CASE

- Neuromonitoring for PSO: level II.2
- Anterior versus posterior approach for correction of flat back syndrome: level II.2
- Does level of pedicle subtraction osteotomy correlate to degree of correction obtained: level II.2?

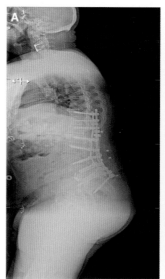
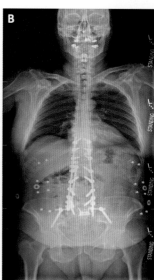

Fig. 38.4 Postoperative x-rays. (A) Lateral and **(B),** AP x-rays demonstrating L3 pedicle subtraction osteotomy and T10-pelvis instrumentation with correction of lumbar lordosis and sagittal imbalance.

REFERENCES

1. JH D. Complications of fusion in lumbar scoliosis. *J Bone Joint Surg Am.* 1973;55:438.
2. DeWald RL. Revision surgery for spinal deformity. *Instr Course Lect.* 1992;41:235–250.
3. Stephens GC, Yoo JU, Wilbur G. Comparison of lumbar sagittal alignment produced by different operative positions. *Spine (Phila Pa 1976).* 1996;21(15):1802–1806. discussion 7.
4. Hsieh PC, Koski TR, O'Shaughnessy BA, Sugrue P, Salehi S, Ondra S, et al. Anterior lumbar interbody fusion in comparison with transforaminal lumbar interbody fusion: implications for the restoration of foraminal height, local disc angle, lumbar lordosis, and sagittal balance. *J Neurosurg Spine.* 2007;7(4):379–386.
5. Ames CP, Smith JS, Scheer JK, Bess S, Bederman SS, Deviren V, et al. Impact of spinopelvic alignment on decision making in deformity surgery in adults: A review. *J Neurosurg Spine.* 2012;16(6):547–564.
6. Lafage R, Schwab F, Challier V, Henry JK, Gum J, Smith J, et al. Defining Spino-Pelvic Alignment Thresholds: Should Operative Goals in Adult Spinal Deformity Surgery Account for Age? *Spine (Phila Pa 1976).* 2016;41(1):62–68.
7. Schwab F, Ungar B, Blondel B, Buchowski J, Coe J, Deinlein D, et al. Scoliosis Research Society-Schwab adult spinal deformity classification: a validation study. *Spine (Phila Pa 1976).* 2012;37(12):1077–1082.
8. Lagrone MO, Bradford DS, Moe JH, Lonstein JE, Winter RB, Ogilvie JW. Treatment of symptomatic flatback after spinal fusion. *J Bone Joint Surg Am.* 1988;70(4):569–580.
9. Uribe JS, Schwab F, Mundis GM, Xu DS, Januszewski J, Kanter AS, et al. The comprehensive anatomical spinal osteotomy and anterior column realignment classification. *J Neurosurg Spine.* 2018;29(5):565–575.
10. Wiggins GC, Ondra SL, Shaffrey CI. Management of iatrogenic flat-back syndrome. *Neurosurg Focus.* 2003;15(3):E8.
11. Lafage V, Schwab F, Vira S, Hart R, Burton D, Smith JS, et al. Does vertebral level of pedicle subtraction osteotomy correlate with degree of spinopelvic parameter correction? *J Neurosurg Spine.* 2011;14(2):184–191.
12. Lau D, Dalle Ore CL, Reid P, Safaee MM, Deviren V, Smith JS, et al. Utility of neuromonitoring during lumbar pedicle subtraction osteotomy for adult spinal deformity. *J Neurosurg Spine.* 2019;31(3):397–407.

39

Cervical kyphosis

Oluwaseun O. Akinduro, MD

Introduction

The cervical spine, which was first described as lordotic by Borden et al. in 1960,[1] is tasked with the responsibility of maintaining a wide range of motion, and allowing proper gaze that is essential for upright gait.[2,3] The cervical spine also absorbs the torsional, axial, and shear loads exerted by the cranium and more rigid thoracic spine, which serves a crucial role in maintaining normal day-to-day function.[4] Although misalignment of spinopelvic parameters may play a role in back pain and disability,[5] there has been less consistent evidence to support similar findings in the cervical spine.[6–10] It is reported that up to 30% of the general population may have kyphosis of the cervical spine although the ramification of this is unclear.[8,11] While there is evidence suggesting a portion of the population may live with cervical kyphosis without adverse symptoms,[6–8,10] many others have reported on the effects of cervical sagittal parameters on axial neck pain and degenerative effects on cervical disks.[9, 12, 13]

Additionally, many authors have found that cervical sagittal misalignment has been found to be an independent predictor of disability, higher neck disability index (NDI), and severity of myelopathy.[14, 15] The role of cervical kyphosis in radicular pain is limited as this is due to focal pathology, which can be addressed by intervention addressing the underlying cause of the radicular pain.

Example case

Chief complaint: neck pain and radiculopathy

History of present illness: A 48-year-old male with progressive neck pain and right arm pain in C5 and C7 distributions that has been unresponsive to physical therapy, steroid injections, and spinal manipulations. This pain has progressed over the past 2 weeks and he underwent imaging of his cervical spine (Figs. 39.1–39.2).

Medications: acetaminophen

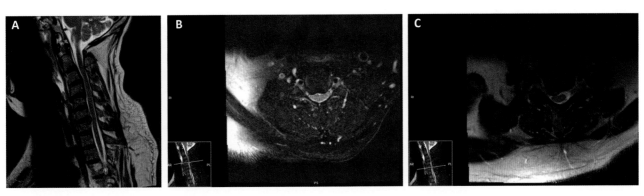

Fig. 39.1 Preoperative magnetic resonance imaging. (A), T2 sagittal and **(B)**, T2 axial images demonstrating disc degeneration and foraminal stenosis at the right C4-5 with a disc herniation at C6-7 causing nerve root compression and cord compression on the right side.

Allergies: no known drug allergies
Past medical and surgical history: depression, anxiety, obesity, appendectomy
Family history: noncontributory
Social history: smokes one pack per day, drinks one alcoholic beverage per day
Physical examination: awake, alert, andoriented to person, place, and time; cranial nerves II–XII intact, decreased cervical range of motion; bilateral deltoids/triceps/biceps 5/5 except right deltoid 4/5; interossei 5/5; iliopsoas/knee flexion/knee extension/dorsi, and plantar flexion 5/5

Reflexes: 2+ in bilateral biceps/triceps/brachioradialis with negative Hoffman; 2+ in bilateral patella/ankle; no clonus or Babinski; sensation intact to light touch

	Benjamin D. Elder, MD, PhD Neurosurgery Mayo Clinic Rochester, Minnesota, United States	Alugolu Rajesh, MD Neurosurgery Nizam's Institute of Medical Sciences Punjagutta, Hyderbad, India	K. Daniel Riew, MD Orthopaedic Surgery Columbia University New York, New York, United States	Luiz Robert Vialle, MD Orthopaedic Surgery Pontifical Catholic University of Parana Curitiba, Brazil
Preoperative				
Additional tests requested	Flexion-extension cervical x-rays DEXA Right C4-5 transforaminal epidural injection Right C5-6 transforaminal epidural injection Physical therapy with traction	CT C-spine Respiratory evaluation Anesthesiology evaluation	CT cervical spine	Physical therapy with cervical traction Nerve root injections
Surgical approach selected	If meets all criteria (fails nonoperative management, negative nicotine test), C4-5 and C6-7 ACDF	C4-5 and C6-7 ACDF	C4-5 ACDF and C6-7 ACDF	If fails with conservative management, C4-5 ACDF with anchored cages
Surgical approach if 21 Surgical approach if 80	Possible cervical arthroplasty Same	Possible cervical arthroplasty Conservative management	C4-5 and C6-7 ACDA C4-7 ACDF	Disc replacement Same
Goal of surgery	Decompress right C5 and C7 nerves, increase lordosis, stabilize spine	Decompress spinal cord at C4-5 and right C7 nerve root, stabilization and fixation	Relief of weakness in arm and pain in arm and neck	Decompress index level
Perioperative				
Positioning	Supine on flat Jackson table with Gardner-Wells tongs and 10 lb of traction	Supine	Supine	Supine
Surgical equipment	Fluoroscopy IOM (MEP/SSEP) Surgical microscope Retractor system Distraction pins	IOM (MEP) Fluoroscopy Surgical microscope	Fluoroscopy Surgical microscope	Wired tracheal tube Nasopharyngeal tube Fluoroscopy
Medications	None	None	Steroids, gabapentin	None
Anatomical considerations	Carotid sheath, recurrent laryngeal nerve, esophagus, vertebral arteries	Carotid sheath, trachea/esophagus, thyroid, recurrent laryngeal nerve, index levels, vertebral arteries, dura, spinal cord	Trachea, esophagus, carotid sheath contents, longus colli, uncinate processes, foramen, vertebral artery, nerve root	Carotid artery, esophagus, vertebral artery
Complications feared with approach chosen	Neck hematoma, hoarseness, swallowing dysfunction, C5 palsy, pseudoarthrosis, degeneration of C5-6 disc space, CSF leak, kyphosis	Injury to carotid sheath contents, trachea/esophagus, thyroid gland, recurrent laryngeal nerve, vertebral arteries, spinal cord	Adjacent level reoperative, pseudoarthrosis	Esophageal fistula

	Benjamin D. Elder, MD, PhD Neurosurgery Mayo Clinic Rochester, Minnesota, United States	Alugolu Rajesh, MD Neurosurgery Nizam's Institute of Medical Sciences Punjagutta, Hyderbad, India	K. Daniel Riew, MD Orthopaedic Surgery Columbia University New York, New York, United States	Luiz Robert Vialle, MD Orthopaedic Surgery Pontifical Catholic University of Parana Curitiba, Brazil
Intraoperative				
Anesthesia	General	General	General	General
Exposure	C4-6	C4-7	C4-7	C4-5
Levels decompressed	C4-6	C4-7	C4-5, C6-7	C4-5
Levels fused	C4-5, C6-7	C4-5, C6-7	C4-5, C6-7	C4-5
Surgical narrative	Position supine on flat Jackson table with gel axillary roll transversely across shoulders, 10 lb of traction, tape shoulders down, fluoroscopy for preoperative localization to position incision over C6 vertebral body in neck crease, left-sided transverse neck incision, mobilize esophagus medially and carotid sheath laterally, place distraction pins into vertebral body for localization, mobilize longus colli off vertebral bodies, place retractor system and 14 mm distraction pins in C4 and C5, remove C4-5 disc and PLL, place frozen structural allograft and anterior plate, repeat procedure at C6-7, obtain final x-rays, leave drain in retropharyngeal space	Position supine in neutral lordosis, oblique skin incision over anterior border of right sternocleidomastoid from C3 to sternal notch, platysma incised along with skin, subplatysmal dissection and identification of fascial plane medial to sternocleidomastoid is developed, retract carotid sheath laterally and trachea/esophagus medially, fascial dissection deepened, inferior belly of digastric is identified and cut sharply and sutured at the end, identify longus colli and midline, identify C4-5 and C6-7 levels with x-ray, incise longus colli and prevertebral fascia at above cranial then caudal levels, disc space distracted with disc space distracted with pins, discectomy with cutting PLL sharply to expose dura, end plate preparation until punctate bleeding noted, spacer filled with cancellous bone graft secured with median screws at both levels, layered wound closure with drain	Position supine, standard Smith-Robinson approach, fluoroscopy to confirm levels, perform discectomy at C4-5 first, right uncinatectomy, maintain PLL, place allograft with BMP and anterior plate, anterior cervical discectomy at C6-7 but go through PLL, place prosthesis, closure in layers	Position supine, approach on right, meticulous dissection, remove nasopharyngeal tube to avoid compression with retractors once esophagus localized, avoid static retractors, use small manual retractors with less pressure over structures, fluoroscopy to determine correct level, C4-5 discectomy using Caspar distractors, open PLL for intracanal disc removal, cage test and size selection, cage filled with allograft bone, place cage and anchor with three or four screws, depending on the model
Complication avoidance	Increase neck extension with gel axillary roll, left-sided approach to decompress right foramen and minimize injury to recurrent laryngeal nerve, distraction pin in vertebral body for localization, start with more symptomatic level	Oblique skin incision to maximize exposure, cut PLL to expose dura, end plate preparation until punctate bleeding noted	Right uncinatectomy at C4-5, BMP to promote fusion, place arthroplasty at C6-7 to preserve motion	Right-sided approach to minimize laryngeal nerve injury, meticulous dissection to avoid laryngeal nerve injury, nasopharyngeal tube to help identify esophagus, avoid static retractors to minimize risk of dysphagia or dysphonia
Postoperative				
Admission	Floor	ICU	Outpatient	Floor
Postoperative complications feared	Swallowing dysfunction, hoarseness, neck hematoma, C5 palsy	Hematoma, neurological deterioration, recurrent laryngeal nerve palsy, wound infection	Pseudoarthrosis, hematoma, swelling, dysphagia, dysphonia	Unlikely but bleeding, dysphagia, dysphonia
Anticipated length of stay	Overnight	1–2 days	Same day	Overnight
Follow-up testing	C-spine AP/lateral x-rays after surgery, 6 weeks, 3 months, 6 months after surgery CT C-spine 12 months after surgery	C-spine x-ray within 6 hours, every 3 months after surgery	Standing AP and lateral x-rays prior to discharge C-spine flexion-extension and neutral lateral x-rays at 6 weeks, 6 months, 12 months after surgery	C-spine x-rays 30 days, every 2 months until 6 months after surgery

	Benjamin D. Elder, MD, PhD Neurosurgery Mayo Clinic Rochester, Minnesota, United States	Alugolu Rajesh, MD Neurosurgery Nizam's Institute of Medical Sciences Punjagutta, Hyderbad, India	K. Daniel Riew, MD Orthopaedic Surgery Columbia University New York, New York, United States	Luiz Robert Vialle, MD Orthopaedic Surgery Pontifical Catholic University of Parana Curitiba, Brazil
Bracing	None	None	Hard collar for 6 weeks	Soft collar for comfort for 2 weeks
Follow-up visits	6 weeks and 12 months after surgery	4 weeks and every 3 months after surgery	6 weeks, 6 months, 12 months after surgery	30 days, every 2 months until 6 months after surgery

ACDF, Anterior cervical decompression and fusion; *AP*, anteroposterior; *BMP*, bone morphogenic protein; *CT*, computed tomography; *DEXA*, dual-energy x-ray absorptiometry; *ICU*, intensive care unit; *IOM*, intraoperative monitoring; *MAP*, mean arterial pressure; *MEP*, motor evoked potential; *PLL*, posterior longitudinal ligament; *SSEP*, somatosensory evoked potential.

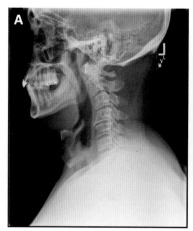
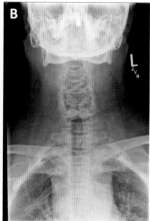

Fig. 39.2 **Preoperative x-rays. (A)**, Lateral and **(B)**, anteroposterior images demonstrating cervical kyphosis and loss of normal cervical lordosis.

Differential diagnosis

- Cervical kyphosis
- Cervical scoliosis
- Torticollis
- Cervical stenosis
- Cervical radiculopathy

Important anatomical considerations

The cervical spine is composed of seven vertebrae. With the exception of the first cervical vertebrae, each vertebra has an associated nerve that exits the foramen above the vertebrae. Additionally, the vertebral artery enters the foramen transversarium typically at the sixth cervical vertebra and exits at C1 prior to entering the foramen magnum. When considering surgical intervention in the cervical spine, especially in individuals with neck pain, it is important to consider the overall regional alignment of the cervical spine as restoration has been shown to impact quality of life, neurological outcome, and adjacent segment disease.[16,17]

The normal cervical spine has a lordotic angle in most individuals with an average angle of approximately 20 to 25 degrees with majority of the lordosis occurring at C1-C2 as reported by Hardacker et al.[18] This angle is measured from the superior end plate of C2 to the lower end plate of C7 and represents the focus on which to determine angulation of the cervical spine. Additionally, the K-line allows surgeons to determine whether the cervical spine is lordodic, neutral, or kyphotic, which is important in deciding the approach, especially in myelopathic disease. The lordosis of the cervical spine can be divided into the high cervical angle represented by occiput to cervical 2 (O-C2) and the low cervical curvature represented by C2-7. These two angles maintain an inverse relationship with one another, increasing and decreasing as the other value changes.[19] Perhaps the most significant factor affecting the lordosis of the cervical spine is the C7 slope, where those with a slope greater than 20 degrees maintain lordotic spine while those with a slope less than 20 degrees have neutral or kyphotic cervical spine. An additional important factor to consider in the assessment of the cervical sagittal alignment is the odontoid to C7 plum line, which is <2 cm in normal adults. Misalignment of these parameters causing kyphosis of the cervical spine is a well documented cause of poor quality of life, neck pain, and neurological dysfunction.[16,17]

Approaches to this lesion

The surgical treatment for cervical radiculopathy is decompression of the affected nerve. Decompression can be accomplished via an anterior or posterior approach. Given the neck pain in the setting of kyphosis, the cervical sagittal alignment should also be taken into consideration and attempted correction may be warranted. Restoration of the cervical lordosis can be accomplished through an anterior approach with an anterior cervical decompression and fusion (ACDF).[20] This approach would also allow for decompression of the effected nerve root. ACDF is one of the most common procedures performed by spine surgeons. It has a low complication rate and a high fusion rate, especially when a single level is fused. As with any fusion surgery, it does carry a risk of adjacent segment degeneration requiring additional surgery.[21] Recently, anterior cervical arthroplasty has been popularized due to its motion preserving characteristics, but conflicting data is available on its ability to restore and maintain cervical alignment and restoration of lordosis.[22-27] A recent meta-analysis comparing ACDF to arthroplasty found increased reoperation rate, adjacent segment disease, and decreased motion in the ACDF group compared with arthroplasty group.[28] Like arthroplasty, a posterior approach is motion-preserving. This includes posterior discectomy and cervical foraminotomy, although this technique serves no value in restoring cervical spinal alignment.

What was actually done

Given the patient's neck pain as well as radicular pain in the setting of cervical kyphosis, the decision was made to proceed with anterior cervical discectomy and fusion after failed conservative therapy. The patient had foraminal stenosis at C4-5 and C6-7 with the C5-6 location being fairly healthy. Given the kyphotic deformity and increased risk of degeneration at C5-6 and the fusion above and below this level, a C4-7 ACDF was offered. Although arthroplasty's ability to restore cervical alignment remains unclear, it was not offered as this would have been an off-label use (it is currently only approved for up to two levels). The patient elected for an ACDF and underwent an anterior cervical discectomy and fusion with placement of a titanium interbody and a cervical plate placement. No monitoring was used during the case, and with thorough hemostasis, a drain was placed. The patient was placed in a cervical collar for 6 weeks with a 10 lb weight restriction. The patient discharged on postoperative day 2 and had significant improvement in his symptoms. Postoperative imaging showed good location of the hardware and good correction of the cervical kyphosis (Fig. 39.3).

Commonalities among the experts

While a number of our experts recommended additional imaging including CT C-spine and flexion-extension x-rays, further conservative management including physical therapy and injection were also recommended. When surgical intervention failed, ACDF was most commonly recommended. The majority of our experts recommended skip level ACDFs at C4-5 and C6-7, although one expert recommended arthroplasty at C6-7 with a ACDF at C4-5. Uniformly, all agreed that disc replacement would be recommended in a younger patient (21 years old) at the same level while the recommendation changed for an older patient (80 years old). The majority recommended the same plan of care for an older patient (80 years old) while only one recommended conservative management. While half of the experts would use intraoperative montiroing for this case, the majority recommended surgical microscope. There was unanimous agreement on the use of fluoroscopy. Half the experts would admit the patient to the floor, and one recommended admission to the intensive care unit and another recommended an outpatient procedure. Follow-up with additional imaging was recommended, although only half our experts recommended bracing for this procedure.

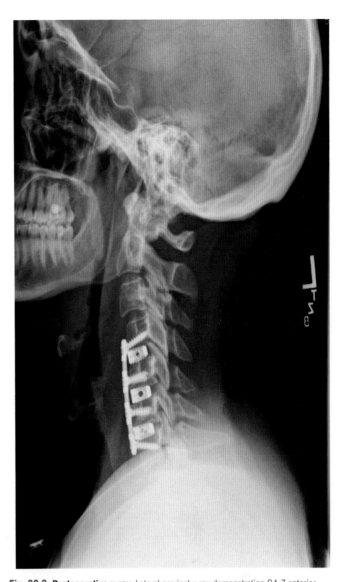

Fig. 39.3 Postoperative x-ray. Lateral cervical x-ray demonstrating C4-7 anterior cervical discectomy and fusion with good correction of the cervical kyphosis.

SUMMARY OF QUALITY OF EVIDENCE TO GUIDE SPECIFIC INTERVENTIONS FOR THIS CASE

- Intraoperative monitoring for spine surgery: level II-1
- Cervical foraminotomy versus ACDF for cervical radiculopathy: level II-2

REFERENCES

1. Borden AG, Rechtman AM, Gershon-Cohen J. The normal cervical lordosis. *Radiology.* 1960;74:806–809.
2. Lafage R, Challier V, Liabaud B, Vira S, Ferrero E, Diebo BG, et al. Natural Head Posture in the Setting of Sagittal Spinal Deformity: Validation of Chin-Brow Vertical Angle, Slope of Line of Sight, and McGregor's Slope With Health-Related Quality of Life. *Neurosurgery.* 2016;79(1):108–115.
3. Patla AE, Prentice SD, Robinson C, Neufeld J. Visual control of locomotion: strategies for changing direction and for going over obstacles. *J Exp Psychol Hum Percept Perform.* 1991;17(3):603–634.

4. White 3rd AA, Johnson RM, Panjabi MM, Southwick WO. Biomechanical analysis of clinical stability in the cervical spine. *Clin Orthop Relat Res*. 1975;109:85–96.

5. Ames CP, Smith JS, Scheer JK, Bess S, Bederman SS, Deviren V, et al. Impact of spinopelvic alignment on decision making in deformity surgery in adults: A review. *J Neurosurg Spine*. 2012;16(6):547–564.

6. Hey HWD, Lau ET, Wong GC, Tan KA, Liu GK, Wong HK. Cervical Alignment Variations in Different Postures and Predictors of Normal Cervical Kyphosis: A New Understanding. *Spine (Phila Pa 1976)*. 2017;42(21):1614–1621.

7. Iorio J, Lafage V, Lafage R, Henry JK, Stein D, Lenke LG, et al. The Effect of Aging on Cervical Parameters in a Normative North American Population. *Global Spine J*. 2018;8(7):709–715.

8. Le Huec JC, Demezon H, Aunoble S. Sagittal parameters of global cervical balance using EOS imaging: normative values from a prospective cohort of asymptomatic volunteers. *Eur Spine J*. 2015;24(1):63–71.

9. Li J, Zhang D, Shen Y. Impact of cervical sagittal parameters on axial neck pain in patients with cervical kyphosis. *J Orthop Surg Res*. 2020;15(1):434.

10. Virk S, Lafage R, Elysee J, Louie P, Kim HJ, Albert T, et al. The 3 Sagittal Morphotypes That Define the Normal Cervical Spine: A Systematic Review of the Literature and an Analysis of Asymptomatic Volunteers. *J Bone Joint Surg Am*. 2020;102(19):e109.

11. Yukawa Y, Kato F, Suda K, Yamagata M, Ueta T. Age-related changes in osseous anatomy, alignment, and range of motion of the cervical spine. Part I: Radiographic data from over 1, 200 asymptomatic subjects. *Eur Spine J*. 2012;21(8):1492–1498.

12. Liu S, Lafage R, Smith JS, Protopsaltis TS, Lafage VC, Challier V, et al. Impact of dynamic alignment, motion, and center of rotation on myelopathy grade and regional disability in cervical spondylotic myelopathy. *J Neurosurg Spine*. 2015;23(6):690–700.

13. Nicholson KJ, Millhouse PW, Pflug E, Woods B, Schroeder GD, Anderson DG, et al. Cervical Sagittal Range of Motion as a Predictor of Symptom Severity in Cervical Spondylotic Myelopathy. *Spine (Phila Pa 1976)*. 2018;43(13):883–889.

14. Lee JS, Youn MS, Shin JK, Goh TS, Kang SS. Relationship between cervical sagittal alignment and quality of life in ankylosing spondylitis. *Eur Spine J*. 2015;24(6):1199–1203.

15. Smith JS, Lafage V, Ryan DJ, Shaffrey CI, Schwab FJ, Patel AA, et al. Association of myelopathy scores with cervical sagittal balance and normalized spinal cord volume: analysis of 56 preoperative cases from the AOSpine North America Myelopathy study. *Spine (Phila Pa 1976)*. 2013;38(22 Suppl 1):S161–S170.

16. Hansen MA, Kim HJ, Van Alstyne EM, Skelly AC, Fehlings MG. Does postsurgical cervical deformity affect the risk of cervical adjacent segment pathology? A systematic review. *Spine (Phila Pa 1976)*. 2012;37(22 Suppl):S75–S84.

17. Shamji MF, Mohanty C, Massicotte EM, Fehlings MG. The Association of Cervical Spine Alignment with Neurologic Recovery in a Prospective Cohort of Patients with Surgical Myelopathy: Analysis of a Series of 124 Cases. *World Neurosurg*. 2016;86:112–119.

18. Hardacker JW, Shuford RF, Capicotto PN, Pryor PW. Radiographic standing cervical segmental alignment in adult volunteers without neck symptoms. *Spine (Phila Pa 1976)*. 1997;22(13):1472–1480. discussion 80.

19. Le Huec JC, Thompson W, Mohsinaly Y, Barrey C, Faundez A. Sagittal balance of the spine. *Eur Spine J*. 2019;28(9):1889–1905.

20. Mummaneni PV, Burkus JK, Haid RW, Traynelis VC, Zdeblick TA. Clinical and radiographic analysis of cervical disc arthroplasty compared with allograft fusion: a randomized controlled clinical trial. *J Neurosurg Spine*. 2007;6(3):198–209.

21. DiAngelo DJ, Foley KT, Vossel KA, Rampersaud YR, Jansen TH. Anterior cervical plating reverses load transfer through multilevel strut-grafts. *Spine (Phila Pa 1976)*. 2000;25(7):783–795.

22. Buchowski JM, Anderson PA, Sekhon L, Riew KD. Cervical disc arthroplasty compared with arthrodesis for the treatment of myelopathy. Surgical technique. *J Bone Joint Surg Am*. 2009;91(Suppl 2):223–232.

23. Goffin J, Van Calenbergh F, van Loon J, Casey A, Kehr P, Liebig K, et al. Intermediate follow-up after treatment of degenerative disc disease with the Bryan Cervical Disc Prosthesis: single-level and bi-level. *Spine (Phila Pa 1976)*. 2003;28(24):2673–2678.

24. Gornet MF, Burkus JK, Shaffrey ME, Argires PJ, Nian H, Harrell Jr. FE. Cervical disc arthroplasty with PRESTIGE LP disc versus anterior cervical discectomy and fusion: a prospective, multicenter investigational device exemption study. *J Neurosurg Spine*. 2015;23(5):558–573.

25. Heller JG, Sasso RC, Papadopoulos SM, Anderson PA, Fessler RG, Hacker RJ, et al. Comparison of BRYAN cervical disc arthroplasty with anterior cervical decompression and fusion: clinical and radiographic results of a randomized, controlled, clinical trial. *Spine (Phila Pa 1976)*. 2009;34(2):101–107.

26. Luo J, Gong M, Huang S, Yu T, Zou X. Incidence of adjacent segment degeneration in cervical disc arthroplasty versus anterior cervical decompression and fusion meta-analysis of prospective studies. *Arch Orthop Trauma Surg*. 2015;135(2):155–160.

27. Wigfield C, Gill S, Nelson R, Langdon I, Metcalf N, Robertson J. Influence of an artificial cervical joint compared with fusion on adjacent-level motion in the treatment of degenerative cervical disc disease. *J Neurosurg*. 2002;96(1 Suppl):17–21.

28. Zou S, Gao J, Xu B, Lu X, Han Y, Meng H. Anterior cervical discectomy and fusion (ACDF) versus cervical disc arthroplasty (CDA) for two contiguous levels cervical disc degenerative disease: a meta-analysis of randomized controlled trials. *Eur Spine J*. 2017;26(4):985–997.

40

Degenerative scoliosis with radiculopathy

Kingsley Abode-Iyamah, MD

Introduction

Adult degenerative scoliosis (ADS), or de novo degenerative lumbar scoliosis, is a form of spinal deformity diagnosed in individuals with a coronal curve of >10 degrees, beginning after the age of 50, and without a prior history of scoliosis.[1-3] Unlike adult idiopathic scoliosis (see Chapter 41), which results from unrecognized/untreated adolescent idiopathic scoliosis, ADS results from degeneration over an individual's lifetime. This condition typically occurs as a result of degenerative changes due to uneven loss of disc height that occurs over an individual's lifetime and results in coronal changes, which is typically recognized after the age of 70.[3,4] Although not previously recognized, ADS is believed to be more prevalent than previously thought and reported to be present in 68% of asymptomatic individuals; this number increases with age.[5] McCarthy et al. have shown an increase in surgeries performed for ADS in the Medicare population, which creates an increasing economic burden.[6] With increasing life expectancy, the prevalence, need for treatment, and overall cost for treatment, ADS is expected to further increase in prevalence and incidence.

Example Case

Chief complaint: mid and low back pain

History of present illness: A 67-year-old female with progressive back pain and new-onset left leg pain when she ambulates that follows an L5 distribution. She underwent imaging that was concerning for adult degenerative scoliosis (Figs. 40.1–40.2).

Medications: oxycodone, gabapentin
Allergies: no known drug allergies
Past medical and surgical history: none
Family history: noncontributory
Social history: retired, no smoking or alcohol
Physical examination: awake, alert, and oriented to person, place, and time; cranial nerves II–XII intact; bilateral deltoids/triceps/biceps 5/5; interossei 5/5; iliopsoas/knee flexion/knee extension/dorsi, and plantar flexion 5/5
Reflexes: 2+ in bilateral biceps/triceps/brachioradialis with negative Hoffman; 2+ in bilateral patella/ankle; no clonus or Babinski; sensation intact to light touch

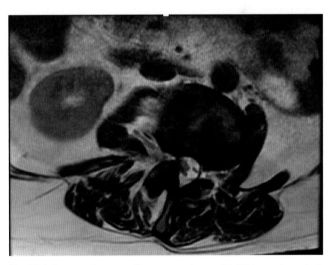

Fig. 40.1 Preoperative magnetic resonance image. Axial T2 image demonstrating.

	Mohamed El-Fiki, MBBCh, MS, MD Neurosurgery Alexandria University Alexandria, Egypt	Hamid Hassanzadeh, MD Orthopaedic Surgery University of Virginia Charlottesville, Virginia, United States	Yasuaki Tokuhashi, MD Orthopaedic Surgery Nihon University Oyaguchi Kamicho, Itabashi-ku, Tokyo, Japan	Michael Y. Wang, MD Yingda Li, MBBS Neurosurgery University of Miami Miami, Florida, United States
Preoperative				
Additional tests requested	L-spine flexion-extension x-rays L-spine supine x-rays with traction Scoliosis x-rays CT L-spine high resolution MRI L-spine Full electrophysiological study	L-spine flexion-extension x-rays DEXA Physical therapy evaluation Pain management evaluation with left L5 steroid injection Nutritional evaluation Anesthesia evaluation Medicine evaluation	L-spine flexion-extension x-rays Right and lateral bending x-rays 3D CT DEXA Echocardiogram	Pain drawing Parasagittal MRI views to assess L5-S1 foramen L-spine lateral flexion-extension x-rays Selective epidural steroid injection, SPECT scan to refine LBP pain generators DEXA if long-segment deformity correction
Surgical approach selected	L4-5 and possibly L3-4 TLIF and possible L3-4 pedicle subtraction osteotomy if needed, and L2-5 posterior fusion	L4-S1 TLIF, L4-S1 posterior column osteotomies, T10-S1 sublaminar decompression, T10-pelvis fusion	Stage 1: L2-5 OLIF Stage 2: T10-iliac posterior correction and fusion	MIS endoscopic transforaminal decompression at L4-5 and/or L5-S1 as incrementalist approach
If patient is 25 years of age	Same approach	L5-S1 fusion	Same approach	Same approach
If patient is 80 years of age	MIS percutaneous surgery	L4-S1 TLIF, T10-pelvis fusion	Same approach with reinforcement of pedicle screws	Same approach
Goal of surgery	Stabilize spine, correction of sagittal alignment, prevent deformity progression	Relief of pain and disability, correction of sagittal alignment, deformity correction	Improve global alignment and lower extremity pain	Decompress neural elements, address stenosis along fractional curve, mitigate/delay long segment deformity correction, incremental approach
Perioperative				
Positioning	Prone	Prone	Stage 1: right decubitus Stage 2: prone on Hall frame	Prone on Jackson table with Wilson frame
Surgical equipment	IOM Fluoroscopy	IOM (MEP/SSEP/EMG) Fluoroscopy Surgical navigation Cell saver	Fluoroscopy OLIF cage IOM (for stage 2) Osteotome Correction device Polyester tape	Fluoroscopy Endoscope
Medications	None	Tranexamic acid, maintain MAP >80	None	None
Anatomical considerations	Dura, nerve roots, end plates	Spinal cord, nerve roots, dura, SI joint	Stage 1: major vessels, intestine, ureter, psoas Stage 2: facet joints, pedicles, iliac bone	Dorsal root ganglion, dura
Complications feared with approach chosen	Durotomy, nerve root injury, extensive blood loss	CSF leak, lower extremity weakness, infection	Stage 1: injury to major vessels, intestines, ureters Stage 2: nerve root injury, facture	DRG irritation, inadequate decompression
Intraoperative				
Anesthesia	General	General	General	Conscious sedation
Exposure	L2-5	T10-S2	Stage 1: L2-5 Stage 2: T10-sacrum	L4-5 and/or L5-S1

	Mohamed El-Fiki, MBBCh, MS, MD Neurosurgery Alexandria University Alexandria, Egypt	Hamid Hassanzadeh, MD Orthopaedic Surgery University of Virginia Charlottesville, Virginia, United States	Yasuaki Tokuhashi, MD Orthopaedic Surgery Nihon University Oyaguchi Kamicho, Itabashi-ku, Tokyo, Japan	Michael Y. Wang, MD Yingda Li, MBBS Neurosurgery University of Miami Miami, Florida, United States
Levels decompressed	L2-5	T10-S1	Stage 1: L2-5 Stage 2: None	L4-5 and/or L5-S1
Levels fused	L2-5	T10-pelvis	Stage 1: L2-5 Stage 2: T10-iliac	None
Surgical narrative	Position prone, confirm levels, midline skin incision with muscular retraction to expose lumbar lamina, insert bilateral L2-5 pedicle screws under fluoroscopy, distract under fluoroscopy to confirm reducibility, may need to extend screws up to T11, TLIF with expandable cage at L4-5 and possible L3-4, perform pedicle subtraction osteotomy at L3-4 as needed, assess if correction is acceptable based on AP and lateral x-rays with distraction on the right-sided screws and compression on the left-sided screws, insert expandable cases, shape rods, rotate the rods to distract and reduce lordosis and translation into acceptable position, tighten screws and remove distractor and compressor, consider connectors, add bone grafts to all fused levels, layered closure	Position prone after IOM, midline posterior incision, enter through fascia paraspinally down to laminas from T10-S2, dissect all the way lateral to find transverse process for each level, posterior column osteotomies and partial facetectomies to release spina and better visualization of anatomical landmarks, pedicle screw placement from T10-pelvis with S2 alar-iliac screws, sublaminar decompression at appropriate levels using osteotome and Kerrison rongeur, TLIF at L5-S1 and L4-5 from left side, x-rays to evaluate alignment, contour rods for correction of sagittal and coronal alignment, x-rays to confirm alignment, segmental compression and distraction at appropriate levels for correction of coronal and sagittal deformity, decorticate posterior element with osteotome/bur/Leksell, bone graft over decorticated area, place drains, layered closure	Stage 1: right decubitus position, check levels with fluoroscopy marking L2-5 vertebral bodies, 7–10 cm incision 6 cm anterior vertebral marking, dissect abdominal muscles and expose retroperitoneal space, retract psoas and expose L2-3 to L4-5 discs, curettage each disc, insert lateral lumbar interbody cage with graft bone, closure with drain Stage 2: 3–7 after stage 1, prone position, midline longitudinal incision from T10-sacrum, expose facets from T10-sacrum, posterior release by fascectomy, T10 transverse hooks, T11-S1 pedicle and iliac screws, left L5 root exposure if pain not improved following stage 1, polyester tape reinforcement if osteoporotic, prebending rod set up by cantilever technique assisting correction device from left T10 hook to left iliac screw, correction with derotation technique, compress between screws, right rod in situ is set up after left corrected rod placed, decorticate lamina and facets, bone tip from fascectomy and hydroxyapatite granule graft is placed, closure with drain	Conscious sedation, position prone on Jackson with Wilson frame, AP fluoroscopy to determine trajectory and entry point usually 10–14 cm from midline, spinal needle to access Kambin triangle, interchange with nitinol wire and then sequential dilation, dock onto superior articular process with AP and lateral fluoroscopy, passage of endoscope, foraminal and lateral recess decompression with endoscopic drill and rongeurs, done while under constant antibiotic irrigation, single-layer tissue closure
Complication avoidance	Distract under fluoroscopy to confirm reducibility, perform pedicle subtraction osteotomy as needed, correct coronal deformity with compression on one side and distraction on another	Early posterior column osteotomies and partial facetectomies to release spina and better visualization of anatomical landmarks, surgical navigation if available, TLIF for anterior column support and fusion, segmental compression and distraction at appropriate levels for correction of coronal and sagittal deformity	OLIF at three levels during first stage, retroperitoneal approach, stages separated by 3–7 days, reevaluate L5 pain after stage 1, polyester tape if osteoporotic, prebending rod with cantilever technique, derotation technique	Conscious sedation to assess dorsal root ganglion irritation, constant AP and lateral fluoroscopy

(continued on next page)

	Mohamed El-Fiki, MBBCh, MS, MD Neurosurgery Alexandria University Alexandria, Egypt	Hamid Hassanzadeh, MD Orthopaedic Surgery University of Virginia Charlottesville, Virginia, United States	Yasuaki Tokuhashi, MD Orthopaedic Surgery Nihon University Oyaguchi Kamicho, Itabashi-ku, Tokyo, Japan	Michael Y. Wang, MD Yingda Li, MBBS Neurosurgery University of Miami Miami, Florida, United States
Postoperative				
Admission	Floor	ICU	Floor	Floor
Postoperative complications feared	CSF leak, neurological injury, vascular injury, wound infection	CSF leak, lower extremity weakness, infection	Stage 1: injury to intestines, ureters, or vasculature Stage 2: CSF leak, pedicle screw malposition, pedicle fracture	Failure to improve, DRG/nerve root injury
Anticipated length of stay	3–6 days	5–7 days	2–3 weeks	4 hours
Follow-up testing	L-spine x-rays 2 weeks, 1 month, every 3 months for 1–2 years after surgery CT L-spine 3 months after surgery	Standing scoliosis PA and lateral x-rays before discharge, 3 weeks, 3 months, 6 months, 12 months after surgery	CT 7 days and 6 months after surgery Bending x-rays 6 months after surgery	Physical therapy as needed
Bracing	None	None	Hard corset for 6 months	None
Follow-up visits	2 weeks, every 3 months for 1–2 years after surgery	3 weeks, 3 months, 6 months, 12 months after surgery after surgery	4 weeks after surgery	2 and 6 weeks after surgery

AP, Anteroposterior; *BMP*, bone morphogenic protein; *CSF*, cerebrospinal fluid; *CT*, computed tomography; *DEXA*, dual-energy x-ray absorptiometry; *EMG*, electromyography; *ICU*, intensive care unit; *IOM*, intraoperative monitoring; *MAP*, mean arterial pressure; *MEP*, motor evoked potential; *MIS*, minimally invasive surgery; *MRI*, magnetic resonance imaging; *OLIF*, oblique lateral interbody fusion; *PA*, posteroanterior; *SI*, sacroiliac; *SSEP*, somatosensory evoked potential; *TLIF*, transforaminal lumbar interbody fusion.

Differential diagnosis

- Lumbar stenosis
- Lumbar foraminal stenosis
- Peripheral neuropathy
- Adult degenerative scoliosis
- Iatrogenic scoliosis

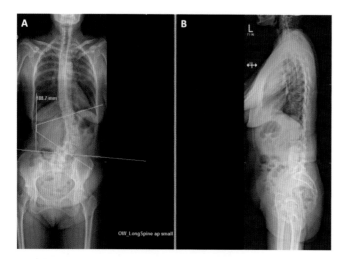

Fig. 40.2 Preoperative x-rays. (A) Anteroposterior and **(B)** lateral images demonstrating coronal and sagittal deformity with the apex of the curvature at L2-3.

Important anatomical considerations

Given the increasing prevalence of ADS, an understanding the importance of the spinopelvic alignment is essential for all spinal surgeons. The formula PI = PT + SS is integral to understanding the relationship between the spine and pelvis. In this formula, pelvic incidence (PI) is a fixed morphogenic parameter with only slight changes during prepubertal development. Pelvic tilt (normal PT = <20 degrees) and sacral slope (SS) are variable parameters with indirect relationships to each other. In addition, the sagittal vertical axis (SVA = +/− 4 cm), which is a common measurement of global sagittal alignment (SA), is also important to evaluate. Moreover, coronal alignment (CA) can be assessed by calculating the difference between the coronal C7 plumb line and the central sacral vertical line (CSVL), where the CA should be +/−2 cm.[7]

While multiple classifications have been used for ASD, the most widely accepted is the SRS-Schwab, which includes the curve type with multiple modifiers to describe the deformity.[8] ADS is expected to progress an average of 3 degrees per year due to ongoing degeneration. Known risk factors include Cobb angle of >30 degrees, asymmetrical disc above and below the apical vertebra, subluxation of the apical vertebra >6 mm, and L5 located above the intercrestal line.[1] Although SRS-Schwab classifications suggest a number of thresholds predictive of disability, it should be noted that these parameters may vary with age. The SRS-Schwab classification identifies PT greater than 22 degrees, SVA greater than 46 mm, and PI-LL (pelvic incidence-lumbar lordosis = <10 degrees) more than 11 degrees as factors that are predictive of disability.[8,9]

Approaches to this lesion

For successful treatment of ASD when patients present with back pain and lumbar radiculopathy, the pain generator in addition to sagittal and coronal imbalance must be addressed to restore global balance. This can be accomplished with combination anterior/posterior or posterior-only approaches (see Chapter 38, Table 1). For anterior approaches, anterior lumbar interbody fusion (ALIF) alone can provide 5 degrees of correction while ALIF with Smith-Peterson osteotomy (SPO) and provide 15 to 20 degrees of sagittal correction. Oblique lateral interbody fusion (OLIF) with/without SPO can provide 3 to 25 degrees. Not only can OLIF aid in coronal correction, but when combined with anterior column realignment (ACR), it can also provide sagittal correction of up to 30 degrees.[10] Posteriorly, strategic osteotomy cuts are important for realignment. Incorporating transforaminal interbody fusion (TLIF) with SPO can provide 15 to 20 degrees of correction at a single level. Additionally, performing multilevel SPO allows for further correction. Pedicle subtraction osteotomy (PSO), although not physiological, is necessary when correction is needed through a previously bony-fused level, dispensing 30 degrees of movement. Another osteotomy, vertebral column resection (VCR), delivers 30 to 40 degrees and is beneficial when both sagittal and coronal correction is needed.[10] Combination anterior/posterior procedures may add surgical time, lengthen hospitalization, require access surgeons (particularly for ALIF), and expose the patient to additional complications. Therefore, when possible, a single approach for correction is ideal.

What was actually done

The patient presented with degenerative scoliosis with back and leg pain. The patient had failed conservative management and was offered a posterior-only scoliosis repair. The patient was taken to the operating room and positioned prone on an Orthopedic system Inc (OSI) table. A midline incision was made and the posterior bony elements were exposed. Instrumentation was placed from T10 to pelvis, and good instrumentation placement was confirmed with intraoperative O-arm. Bone marrow aspiration was obtained at each level to soak the corticocancellous bone graft. Iliac bone graft was also harvested during placement of the iliac bolts. Ponte osteotomies were then made from L1-5 to decompress each nerve root and for correction of the coronal curvature. A transforaminal interbody fusion was performed at L2-3 to aid with correction as this was the apex of the curvature. An L5-S1 transforaminal interbody fusion was also done to aid with fusion at this location. After all the bony work and decompression was completed, rodding was done with cobalt chrome rods, as well as placement of a third rod for extra support of the construct. A tethering device was placed at the base of T9 to reduce the risk of proximal junctional kyphosis followed by gentamicin saline irrigation using a pulse lavage. Arthrodesis was then performed with use of bone morphogenic protein, harvested autograft, and allograft. The wound was closed in layers with two hemovac drains left in place. Intraoperative monitoring was performed throughout the case. The patient was mobilized on postoperative day 1 and discharged on postoperative day 5 with good pain control. Postoperative x-rays showed good sagittal and coronal alignment and good location of the hardware (Fig. 40.3).

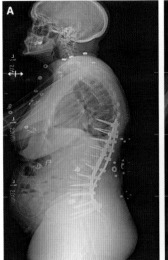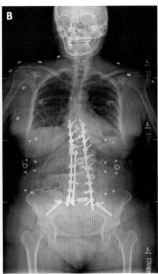

Fig. 40.3 Postoperative x-rays. (A) Lateral and **(B)** anteroposterior standing images demonstrating good location of the hardware and good sagittal and coronal balance.

Commonalities among the experts

The majority of our experts requested additional testing prior to surgical intervention, which included computed tomography (CT), x-rays, bone density scans, physical therapy, and pain clinic consult. Medical clearance was also recommended in addition to nutritional consult. When surgical intervention was recommended, the majority recommended posterior-only approach. Half recommended T10 to pelvis fusion, one recommended L4-S1 TLIF with posterior osteotomies at these levels, and the other surgeon recommended a staged L2-5 OLIF followed by T10 to pelvis instrumentation. Of the other two surgeons, one recommended L4-5 and possible L3-4 TLIF with L2-5 instrumentation with possible PSO at L3, while the other recommended a minimally invasive surgery endoscopic transforaminal decompression at L4-5 or L5-S1 only. All who recommended a fusion operation also requested the use of intraoperative monitoring in addition to intraoperative fluoroscopy. Transexamic acid and mean arterial blood pressure goals were only recommended by one surgeon while the others did not recommend either. The majority expressed the patient be transferred to the floor postoperatively after surgery, and the recommended hospitalization stay ranged from 3 days to 3 weeks in the fusion patients. Routine follow-up was recommended by all surgeons with additional imaging recommended by those who recommended instrumented fusion.

SUMMARY OF QUALITY OF EVIDENCE TO GUIDE SPECIFIC INTERVENTIONS FOR THIS CASE

- Intraoperative monitoring for deformity correction: level III
- Hook versus pedicle screw at upper instrumented vertebrae for proximal junctional kyphosis prevention: level III
- Complication in deformity in patient >80 years of age: level III

REFERENCES

1. Pritchett JW, Bortel DT. Degenerative symptomatic lumbar scoliosis. *Spine (Phila Pa 1976)*. 1993;18(6):700–703.
2. Robin GC, Span Y, Steinberg R, Makin M, Menczel J. Scoliosis in the elderly: a follow-up study. *Spine (Phila Pa 1976)*. 1982;7(4):355–359.
3. Silva FE, Lenke LG. Adult degenerative scoliosis: evaluation and management. *Neurosurg Focus*. 2010;28(3):E1.
4. Phillips FM, Isaacs RE, Rodgers WB, Khajavi K, Tohmeh AG, Deviren V, et al. Adult degenerative scoliosis treated with XLIF: clinical and radiographical results of a prospective multicenter study with 24-month follow-up. *Spine (Phila Pa 1976)*. 2013;38(21):1853–1861.
5. Schwab F, Dubey A, Gamez L, El Fegoun AB, Hwang K, Pagala M, et al. Adult scoliosis: prevalence, SF-36, and nutritional parameters in an elderly volunteer population. *Spine (Phila Pa 1976)*. 2005;30(9):1082–1085.
6. McCarthy M. US health spending is expected to rebound with recovering economy. *BMJ*. 2013;346:f2680.
7. Ames CP, Smith JS, Scheer JK, Bess S, Bederman SS, Deviren V, et al. Impact of spinopelvic alignment on decision making in deformity surgery in adults: A review. *J Neurosurg Spine*. 2012;16(6):547–564.
8. Schwab F, Ungar B, Blondel B, Buchowski J, Coe J, Deinlein D, et al. Scoliosis Research Society-Schwab adult spinal deformity classification: a validation study. *Spine (Phila Pa 1976)*. 2012;37(12):1077–1082.
9. Lafage R, Schwab F, Challier V, Henry JK, Gum J, Smith J, et al. Defining Spino-Pelvic Alignment Thresholds: Should Operative Goals in Adult Spinal Deformity Surgery Account for Age? *Spine (Phila Pa 1976)*. 2016;41(1):62–68.
10. Uribe JS, Schwab F, Mundis GM, Xu DS, Januszewski J, Kanter AS, et al. The comprehensive anatomical spinal osteotomy and anterior column realignment classification. *J Neurosurg Spine*. 2018;29(5):565–575.

41

Iatrogenic deformity after Harrington rod

Kingsley Abode-Iyamah, MD

Introduction

Adolescent idiopathic scoliosis (AIS) is the most common type of scoliosis, affecting 2% to 4% of adolescents with an occurrence rate of 0.5 to 5.2%.[1,2] Although the pathophysiology is unclear, there are some studies that suggest a genetic component.[3,4] While the presence of smaller curvature is similar in males and female at similar rates, there is a higher prevalence of larger curvatures seen in women.[2]

The treatment of AIS has been significantly advanced since the introduction of Harrington rods in the 1960s. While this technique represented a significant development during its time, it was limited in its ability to correct overall scoliosis and has led to a large number of patients who suffer from flat back syndrome and back pain as they have matured.[5,6] The introduction of pedicle screws has led to better outcomes and correction of the three-dimensional deformity associated with AIS and improving upon the pitfalls of Harrington rods including neurological deficit and infection.[6] As AIS patients mature into adulthood, many symptoms develop as a result of flat back resulting from Harrington rods, as well as progression of deformity and adjacent level degeneration at the lower levels, including back and radicular pain due to degenerative changes leading to foraminal stenosis and lateral recess stenosis.[7,8] Treatment of these complex patients involves innovative thinking and treatment options to address the patient's symptoms and correction of any progressive deformity.

Example case

Chief complaint: back pain

History of present illness: This is a 45-year-old female with a history of Harrington rods for spinal deformity as a teenager who presents with progressive back pain for several months. She denies any leg pain or genitourinary symptoms. She unfortunately has had no response to pain medications and/or physical therapy. She underwent imaging that was concerning for flat back syndrome (Figs. 41.1–41.2).

Medications: oxycodone, prednisone, antidepressants
Allergies: no known drug allergies
Past medical and surgical history: Harrington rod placement as a teenager
Family history: noncontributory
Social history: none
Physical examination: awake, alert, and oriented to person, place, and time; cranial nerves II–XII intact; bilateral deltoids/triceps/biceps 5/5; interossei 5/5; iliopsoas/knee flexion/knee extension/dorsi, and plantar flexion 5/5
Reflexes: 2+ in bilateral biceps/triceps/brachioradialis with negative Hoffman; 2+ in bilateral patella/ankle; no clonus or Babinski; sensation intact to light touch

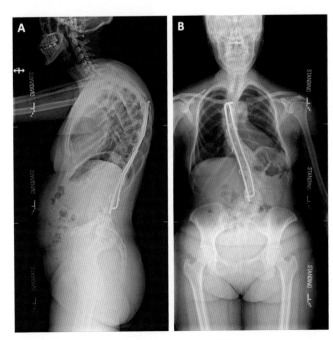

Fig. 41.1 Preoperative x-rays. (A) Anterioposterior and **(B)** lateral x-ray demonstrating previously placed Harrington rods with hyperkyphosis of the thoracic spine.

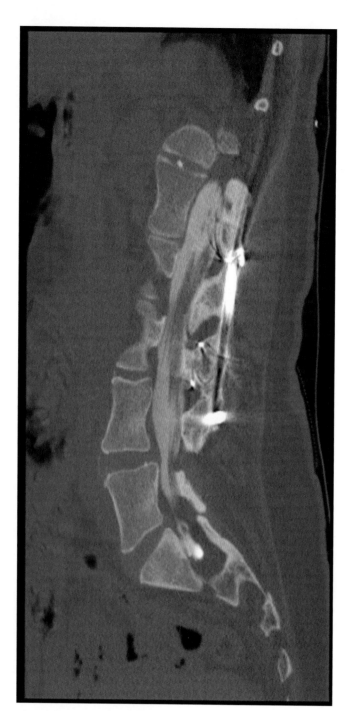

Fig. 41.2 Preoperative computed tomography myelogram. (A) Sagittal image demonstrating postoperative changes of previous fusion with massive fusion mass.

	Lorin M. Benneker, MD Orthopaedic Surgery Spine Unit Sonnenhofspital, Bern, Switzerland	Scott Daffner, MD Orthopaedic Surgery West Virginia University Morgantown, West Virginia, United States	Rodrigo Navarro-Ramirez, MD Neurosurgery McGill University Montreal, Quebec, Canada	Justin S. Smith, MD, PhD Neurosurgery University of Virginia Charlottesville, Virginia, United States
Preoperative				
Additional tests requested	Preoperative complete spine x-rays if available MRI T- and L-spine DEXA Orthoradiogram SI joint steroid injections	Sagittal CT L-spine through L4-5 and L5-S1 levels L-spine flexion-extension x-rays Pain management evaluation	Recumbent T-spine x-rays DEXA Pain management evaluation Psychology evaluation Nutrition evaluation	CT myelogram of T- and L-spine Lumbar flexion-extension x-rays
Surgical approach selected No implant removal	Stage 1: L4-5 and L5-S1 ALIF Stage 2: MIS posterior implant removal and percutaneous L2-pelvis fusion	If pain localizes to lumbar spine and pseudoarthrosis at L3-4, Stage 1: L3-4 lateral lumbar interbody fusion Stage 2: L1-pelvis fusion	If pain localizes to lumbar spine and pseudoarthrosis at L3-4, L3-S2/Iliac fusion with connection to previous fusion	If pseudarthrosis detected, L2-ilium posterior instrumented arthrodesis, L4-5 and L5-S1 transforaminal lumbar interbody fusion
Surgical approach if 21 Surgical approach if 80	Same approach Same approach	Same approach Same approach	Same approach Same approach	Same approach Same approach
Goal of surgery	Pain control and fusion	Solid bony arthrodesis	Solid bony arthrodesis	Solid bony arthrodesis
Perioperative				
Positioning	Stage 1: supine Stage 2: prone on carbon table	Stage 1: lateral decubitus on flat Jackson table Stage 2: prone on Jackson frame	Prone on Jackson table	Prone on Jackson table
Surgical equipment	Fluoroscopy	Stage 1: IOM (EMG), fluoroscopy, cell saver, MIS retractor system Stage 2: IOM (MEP/SSEP), fluoroscopy, surgical robot	Fluoroscopy Surgical navigation O-arm Cell saver BMP	IOM (MEP/SSEP/EMG) Fluoroscopy Cell saver
Medications	None	None	Tranexamic acid	Tranexamic acid
Anatomical considerations	Left iliac vein	Stage 1: peritoneum, aorta, vena cava, lumbar plexus Stage 2: pedicles, nerve roots, SI joints	S1-2 foramen, S2 venous plexus	Spinal cord and conus, nerve roots, cauda equina
Complications feared with approach chosen	Coronal imbalance, Ogilvy syndrome		Iliac or gluteal artery injury	Global coronal malalignment
Intraoperative				
Anesthesia	General	General	General	General
Exposure	Stage 1: L4-S1 Stage 2: L2-pelvis	Stage 1: L3-4 Stage 2: L2-pelvis	L3-pelvis	L2-pelvis
Levels decompressed	Stage 1: L4-S1 Stage 2: none	Stage 1: L3-4 Stage 2: none	None	None
Levels fused	Stage 1: L4-S1 Stage 2: L2-pelvis	Stage 1: L3-4 Stage 2: L2-pelvis	L3-pelvis	L2-ilium

	Lorin M. Benneker, MD Orthopaedic Surgery Spine Unit Sonnenhofspital, Bern, Switzerland	Scott Daffner, MD Orthopaedic Surgery West Virginia University Morgantown, West Virginia, United States	Rodrigo Navarro-Ramirez, MD Neurosurgery McGill University Montreal, Quebec, Canada	Justin S. Smith, MD, PhD Neurosurgery University of Virginia Charlottesville, Virginia, United States
Surgical narrative	Stage 1: position supine, horizontal skin incision, split rectus, retroperitoneal exposure of L5-S1 and L4-L5, discectomy and decompression through disc scape after sequential distraction and reposition of the segment, insert trial cages under fluoroscopy control, cage should have lordotic angle according to preoperative calculations, insertion of final cage filled with allo/autograft and angular-stable screw fixation, x-ray to confirm hardware location, soft drain placement and closure Stage 2 (same day): position prone, stab incisions, transpedicular placement of k-wires with fluoroscopic control in L2-5 bilaterally and for SI screws, thread and insert poly axial screws, rod insertion, in situ fixation	Stage 1: position lateral with left side up, axillary roll under right chest wall, hip and knee flexed to relax psoas muscle, x-ray to localize incision and able to obtain true AP and lateral projection, 8–10 cm oblique incision centered over L3-4 disc, bluntly split each muscular layer in line with fibers, carefully split transversalis fascia, identify peritoneum, bluntly dissect peritoneum off lateral and posterior abdominal wall, identify psoas, confirm level of exposure, gently elevate psoas, confirm level with x-ray, dock MIS retractor system at middle to anterior 1/3 of disc space, L3-4 discectomy making sure to release contralateral annulus, clean cartilage from end plates and leveled with rasp to punctate bleeding subchondral bone, fluoroscopy to confirm instruments do not pass beyond contralateral annulus, size and place neutral or slightly lordotic cage filled with allograft wrapped in rhBMP-2, impact disc space under fluoroscopy, remove retractor, layered closure Stage 2 (same day): sandwich in Jackson frame and position prone, x-ray to confirm location of lateral cage, standard posterior midline exposure, using robot and navigation place pedicle screws bilaterally from L1-5 and bilateral iliac bolts over wire, cut with bur and remove if prior instrumentation in the way otherwise leave intact, contour and insert rods, decorticate exposed bone, spinous processes harvested for autograft and combined with allograft or other extender and placed over decorticated bone, layered closure with drain	Position prone, place reference ray over iliac crest, posterior midline incision from L3-S2, work in different areas and pack to minimize blood loss, identify previous hardware and confirm quality of posterolateral fusion, cut previous rods and leave 5 mm segment free of rod to allow connection, pack this area and work on placing pedicle screws from L4-S2, advance S2 screw through iliac cancellous bone using fluoroscopy with tear drop landmark or navigation guidance, place cobalt chrome rod and connect to previous Luque rod using dominoes, decorticate exposed bony elements (laminas, facets, transverse processes, sacrum), irrigate surgical site, remove L4-5 spinous processes and mix with allograft and vancomycin and pack along decorticated site, layered closure with subfascial drain	Position prone on Jackson table, fluoroscopy to mark incision, expose upper lumbar spine to sacrum, expose PSIS bilaterally, confirm levels with fluoroscopy once exposed, place pedicle screws L4-S1 bilaterally and on left L2 and L3, place bilateral iliac bolts, L4-5 and L5-S1 transforaminal lumbar interbody fusions place rods bilaterally and connect rod on the right (and possible rod on the left) directly to Luque rods with connectors for added stability, intraoperative long-cassette AP x-ray to assess global coronal alignment and adjust with coronal in situ benders as needed, placement of graft material for arthrodesis, wound closure with two subfascial drains

	Lorin M. Benneker, MD Orthopaedic Surgery Spine Unit Sonnenhofspital, Bern, Switzerland	Scott Daffner, MD Orthopaedic Surgery West Virginia University Morgantown, West Virginia, United States	Rodrigo Navarro-Ramirez, MD Neurosurgery McGill University Montreal, Quebec, Canada	Justin S. Smith, MD, PhD Neurosurgery University of Virginia Charlottesville, Virginia, United States
Complication avoidance	Two-staged approach, anterior lordotic cage based on preoperative angle, percutaneous minimally invasive pedicle screw placement	Two-staged approach, MIS retractor system, make sure to release contralateral annulus during discectomy, BMP, cut with bur and remove if prior instrumentation in the way	Work in different areas and pack to minimize blood loss, domino to previous fusion construct, surgical navigation to guide pedicle screw placement, endovascular team on standby if vascular injury	Intraoperative long-cassette x-rays to assess coronal alignment, anchoring of rods to Luque rods for added stability, BMP for arthrodesis
Postoperative				
Admission	Floor	Stepdown unit	Floor	ICU
Postoperative complications feared	Coronal imbalance, Ogilvy syndrome	Pseudoarthrosis, overcorrection of sagittal balance, loss of fixation, infection, incisional hernia	Pseudoarthrosis, adjacent segment disease, hardware failure, infection	Pseudarthrosis, rod fracture, global coronal malalignment
Anticipated length of stay	6–7 days	3 days	4 days	6–7 days
Follow-up testing	Standing full spine x-rays prior to discharge, 2 months, 6 months, 12 months after surgery	CT L-spine prior to discharge Standing scoliosis x-rays prior to discharge, 6 weeks, 6 months, 12 months, 24 months after surgery	Standing AP/lateral L-spine and scoliosis x-rays prior to discharge, 1 month, 3 months after surgery	Supine x-rays after surgery Full-length standing x-rays before discharge X-rays at 6 weeks, 1 year, 2 years after surgery
Bracing	None	None	None	None
Follow-up visits	2 months, 6 months, 12 months after surgery	2 weeks, 6 weeks, 3 months, 6 months, 12 months, 24 months after surgery	2 weeks, 1 month, 3 months after surgery	10–14 days, 6 weeks, 1 year, 2 years after surgery

ALIF, Anterior lumbar interbody fusion; *AP*, anteroposterior; *BMP*, bone morphogenic protein; *CT*, computed tomography; *DEXA*, dual-energy x-ray absorptiometry; *ESI*, epidural spinal injections; *IOM*, intraoperative monitoring; *MAP*, mean arterial pressure; *MEP*, motor evoked potential; *MIS*, minimally invasive surgery; *PLL*, posterior longitudinal ligament; *PSIS*, posterior superior iliac spine; *SI*, sacroiliac; *SSEP*, somatosensory evoked potential.

Differential diagnosis

- Iatrogenic scoliosis
- Degenerative scoliosis
- Adolescent idiopathic scoliosis
- Adjacent segment disease
- Hardware failure
- Lumbar stenosis

Important anatomical considerations

The approach to progressive degeneration following Harrington rod placement should involve assessing not only the pain generator but also the overall global balance for patients who present with back pain. The formula $PI = PT + SS$ is integral to understanding the relationship between the spine and pelvis. In this formula, pelvic incidence (PI) is a fixed morphogenic parameter with only slight changes during pre-pubertal development. Pelvic tilt (normal $PT = <20$ degrees) and sacral slope (SS) are variable parameters with indirect relationships to each other. These parameters are important to ensure global balance has been achieved in those selected patients who undergo spine surgery to ensure symptom resolution. Additional measurements include sagittal vertical axis ($SVA = +/- 4$ cm), which is a common measurement of global sagittal alignment (SA). The difference between the coronal C7 plumb line and the central sacral vertical line (CSVL) assesses the coronal alignment ($CA = +/-2$ cm) (see Chapter 37, Table 1).[9]

Scoliosis repair with Harrington rods are typically associated with robust fusion mass, which should be assessed prior to undertaking any surgical intervention. Additionally, due to the imaging artifact from the Harrington rod that limit radiographic visualization, a computed tomography (CT) myelogram may prove more useful in assessing the spinal canal in addition to the foramen (Fig. 41.2). Furthermore, depending on the degree of correction that must be obtained, pedicle screw placement at the levels of the Harrington rods may be required. In some cases, cutting and removal of the Harrington rod maybe needed, although this is a very difficult task, especially when the lamina has been removed in some areas.

Table 41.1 Coronal Curve Types With Sagittal Modifier

Coronal Curve Types	Sagittal Modifier
T: Thoracic only with lumbar curve <30 degrees L: TL/lumbar only with thoracic curve <30 degrees D: Double curve with T and TL/L curve >30 degrees N: No major coronal deformity all coronal curves <30 degrees	PI minus LL 0: With 10 degrees +: Moderate = 10–20 degrees ++: Marked >20 degrees <u>Global Alignment</u> 0: SVA <4 cm +: SVA 2–9.5 cm ++: SVA > 9.5 cm <u>Pelvic Tilt</u> 0: PT <20 degrees +: PT = 20–30 degrees ++: PT >30 degrees

LL: lumbar lordosis; *PI*: Pelvic incidence; *PT*: pelvic tilt; *SVA*: sagittal vertical axis

Approaches to this lesion

As with degenerative scoliosis, progressive degeneration of AIS with Harrington rod should address the pain generator as well as the global and regional imbalance (Table 41.1). This can be accomplished with combination anterior/posterior procedure or posterior-only approach. For a detailed description of what each surgical technique corrects, see Chapter 38, Table 1. For anterior approach, anterior lumbar interbody fusion (ALIF) alone can provide 5 degrees of correction while ALIF with Smith-Peterson osteotomy (SPO) can provide 15 to 20 degrees of sagittal correction. Oblique lateral interbody fusion (OLIF) with/without SPO can provide 3 to 25 degrees. Not only can OLIF aid in coronal correction, but when combined with anterior column realignment (ACR), it can also provide sagittal correction of up to 30 degrees.[10] Posteriorly, strategic osteotomy cuts are important for realignment. Incorporating transforaminal interbody fusion (TLIF) with SPO can provide 15 to 20 degrees of correction at a single level. Additionally, performing multilevel SPO allows for further correction. Pedicle subtraction osteotomy (PSO), although not physiological, is necessary when correction is needed through a previously bony-fused level, dispensing 30 degrees of movement. Another osteotomy, vertebral column resection (VCR), delivers 30 to 40 degrees and is beneficial when both sagittal and coronal correction is needed.[10] Combination anterior/posterior procedures may add surgical time, lengthen hospitalization, require access surgeons (particularly for ALIF), and expose the patient to additional complications. Therefore, when possible, a single approach for correction is favored.

What was actually done

The patient initially underwent a Harrington rod placement for progressive AIS at 13 years of age in 1987. Although she initially did well with pause of her scoliosis progression, she presented at the age of 44 with symptoms of back pain and severe left leg radiculopathy. Scoliosis images revealed hyperkyphosis of the thoracic spine in addition to adjacent segment degeneration with foraminal stenosis at L4-5 and a positive sagittal balance. The decision was therefore made to proceed with correction of the imbalance addressing the lumbar and lower thoracic and avoiding additional intervention in the upper thoracic spine. She was offered a staged procedure of L4-5 and L5-S1 ALIF followed by T10 to pelvis instrumentation. In the first stage of

the procedure, the patient was brought to the operating room and, following exposure by the vascular surgery team, the neurosurgical team proceeded with L4-S1 ALIF. Bone morphogenetic protein was used for interbody arthrodesis and fluoroscopy was used for ensuring proper placement of the instrumentation. Five days following the ALIF, the patient was brought back to the operating room for the posterior portion of the procedure, which involved a T10 to pelvis instrumentation. Following positioning on an OSI table, the previous incision was reopened. Exposure from T10 to the pelvis was completed and intraoperative OR was brought in place and imaging acquisition was obtained for stealth neuronavigation for instrumentation placement. Following placement of the instrumentation and rodding, the exposed bone was decorticated and local autograft and autograft was used for arthrodesis. Intraoperative neuromonitoring was used for the case and the patient admitted to the intensive care unit postoperatively. Bracing was instituted for mobilization with weight restriction. The patient was discharged on postoperative day 7 following the second stage. Postoperative imaging showed good location of the instrumentation with correction of the global imbalance (Figs. 41.3–41.4).

Commonalities among the experts

The majority of our experts requested additional testing prior to surgical intervention, which included CT, x-rays, bone density scans, and pain clinic consult. All our experts recommended surgical intervention involving a fusion, although their approach significantly varied. While half recommend a staged procedure, the other half recommend posterior-only approach. Of the two surgeons who recommended a posterior-only approach, one recommended an L3 to pelvis instrumentation while the other recommended an L2 to pelvis instrumentation and

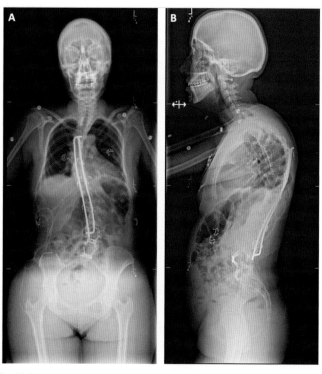

Fig. 41.3 Postoperative x-rays. (A) Anteroposterior and **(B)** lateral images demonstrating postoperative changes of L4-5 and L5-S1 ALIF with some restoration of the lumbar lordosis, however, the thoracic hyperkyphosis is still present after the anterior or first stage of the procedure.

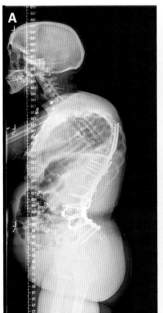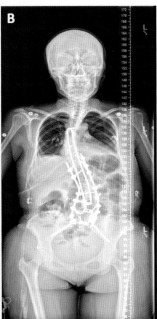

Fig. 41.4 Postoperative x-rays. (A) Lateral and **(B)** anteroposterior images demonstrating a T10 to pelvis instrumentation with significant improvement of the lumbar lordosis and global balance.

arthrodesis. Although the other two surgeons recommended a staged procedure with first performing an interbody fusion either lateral or anteriorly, the levels varied for recommended interbody. One surgeon recommended an L4-S1 ALIF and the other recommended an L3-4 lateral interbody fusion. Both recommended L1 versus L2 to pelvis instrumentation, although one expert recommended this be done percutaneously. All surgeons recommended the use of intraoperative fluoroscopy, but only half recommended the use of intraoperative monitoring. All patients were recommended to the stepdown unit or floor with the exception of one patient who was recommended to the intensive care unit with expected hospital stay ranging from 3 to 7 days. None of the experts recommended bracing and all recommended routine follow-up with screening imaging.

SUMMARY OF QUALITY OF EVIDENCE TO GUIDE SPECIFIC INTERVENTIONS FOR THIS CASE

- Intraoperative monitoring for deformity correction: level II-1
- Bracing following lumbar fusion: level I
- Risk of progression of scoliosis with Harrington rod placement: level II-1

REFERENCES

1. Kikanloo SR, Tarpada SP, Cho W. Etiology of Adolescent Idiopathic Scoliosis: A Literature Review. *Asian Spine J.* 2019;13(3):519–526.
2. Konieczny MR, Senyurt H, Krauspe R. Epidemiology of adolescent idiopathic scoliosis. *J Child Orthop.* 2013;7(1):3–9.
3. Cheng JC, Castelein RM, Chu WC, Danielsson AJ, Dobbs MB, Grivas TB, et al. Adolescent idiopathic scoliosis. *Nat Rev Dis Primers.* 2015;1:15030.
4. Kelly JSN FT, Dekis J, Hariri O, Walker S, et al. Treatment of adolescent idiopathic scoliosis and evaluation of the adolescent patient. *Current Orthopaedic Practice.* 2018;29:424–429.
5. de Jonge T, Dubousset JF, Illes T. Sagittal plane correction in idiopathic scoliosis. *Spine (Phila Pa 1976).* 2002;27(7):754–760.
6. Lykissas MG, Jain VV, Nathan ST, Pawar V, Eismann EA, Sturm PF, et al. Mid- to long-term outcomes in adolescent idiopathic scoliosis after instrumented posterior spinal fusion: a meta-analysis. *Spine (Phila Pa 1976).* 2013;38(2):E113–E119.
7. Bartie BJ, Lonstein JE, Winter RB. Long-term follow-up of adolescent idiopathic scoliosis patients who had Harrington instrumentation and fusion to the lower lumbar vertebrae: is low back pain a problem? *Spine (Phila Pa 1976).* 2009;34(24):E873–E878.
8. Connolly PJ, Von Schroeder HP, Johnson GE, Kostuik JP. Adolescent idiopathic scoliosis. Long-term effect of instrumentation extending to the lumbar spine. *J Bone Joint Surg Am.* 1995;77(8):1210–1216.
9. Ames CP, Smith JS, Scheer JK, Bess S, Bederman SS, Deviren V, et al. Impact of spinopelvic alignment on decision making in deformity surgery in adults: A review. *J Neurosurg Spine.* 2012;16(6):547–564.
10. Uribe JS, Schwab F, Mundis GM, Xu DS, Januszewski J, Kanter AS, et al. The comprehensive anatomical spinal osteotomy and anterior column realignment classification. *J Neurosurg Spine.* 2018;29(5):565–575.

42

Iatrogenic kyphoscoliosis

Kingsley Abode-Iyamah, MD

Introduction

Kyphoscoliosis is the loss of the normal thoracolumbar curvature resulting in increased kyphosis as a result of either increased thoracic kyphosis or thoracolumbar kyphosis. This can result in significant amount of disability due to pain drastically altering the patient's quality of life. Many present with back pain, inability to stand erect, and leg pain. The pain is the result of loss of normal posture requiring more expenditure of energy to stay upright. The causes of kyphoscoliosis can be varied but iatrogenic causes are frequently seen following decompressive thoracic/lumbar surgery or failed surgical fusion. Patient can also develop kyphoscoliosis following a traumatic event that results in compression or burst fractures that have been managed with decompression alone or with fusion. A significant number of these patients typically also have underlying osteoporosis that was undiagnosed at their index surgery. Hardware failure as a result of poor bone

quality, loss of anterior column support, and/or loss of the posterior column integrity begins to propagate iatrogenic kyphoscoliosis, which ultimately results in severe deformity.

Example case

Chief complaint: back pain and postural change

History of present illness: This is a 58-year-old female with a history of motor vehicle accident a few years prior. She suffered a fracture and underwent a T10-L3 decompression and instrumentation. The instrumentation was removed due to hardware complications. She ultimately developed kyphosis. She has now severe back pain with kyphosis focused with the apex at T12-L1. She is on oral pain medication and has a spinal cord stimulator without significant improvement of her symptoms. She has a history of osteoporosis and has been on pain medications for 5 months. She underwent imaging that was concerning for progressive kyphoscoliosis (Figs. 42.1–42.3).

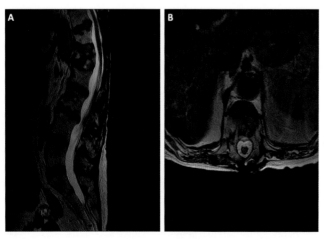

Fig. 42.1 Preoperative magnetic resonance images. (A) T2 sagittal and **(B)** T2 axial images demonstrating thoracolumbar kyphosis and T12 compression fracture and a L1 burst fracture.

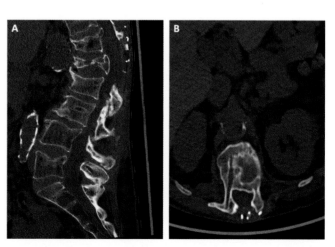

Fig. 42.2 Preoperative computed tomography scans. (A) Sagittal and **(B)** axial images demonstrating thoracolumbar kyphosis and T12 compression fracture and a L1 burst fracture.

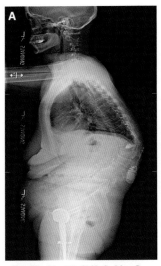 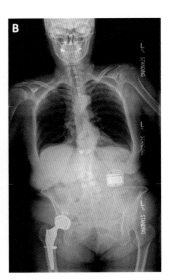

Medications: amlodipine, levothyroxine, Xanax

Allergies: no known drug allergies

Past medical and surgical history: osteoporosis, fracture, hypothyroidism, hypertension, laminectomy, fusion with hardware removal, spinal cord stimulator placement

Family history: noncontributory

Social history: disabled, nonsmoker

Physical examination: awake, alert, and oriented to person, place, and time; cranial nerves II–XII intact; bilateral deltoids/triceps/biceps 5/5; interossei 5/5; iliopsoas/knee flexion/knee extension/dorsi, and plantar flexion 5/5

Reflexes: 2+ in bilateral biceps/triceps/brachioradialis with negative Hoffman; 2+ in bilateral patella/ankle; no clonus or Babinski; sensation intact to light touch

PT: 46, PI: 47, SVA 8, LL:+3

T9-L3 kyphotic angle: 67

Fig. 42.3 Preoperative x-rays. (A) Anteroposterior (AP) and **(B)** lateral x-rays demonstrating regional and global sagittal imbalance.

	Ahmed S. Barakat, MD Orthopaedic Surgery University of Cairo Cairo, Egypt	Fabio Cofano, MD Neurosurgery University of Turin Spine Surgery Unit Humanitas Gradenigo Hospital Turin, Italy	James S. Harrop, MD Neurosurgery Jefferson University Philadelphia, Pennsylvania, United States	Lawrence G. Lenke, MD Orthopaedic Surgery Columbia University New York City, New York, United States
Preoperative				
Additional tests requested	T- and L-spine dynamic x-rays CTA T-L spine	Endocrinology evaluation for osteoporosis	DEXA, optimize bone density (i.e., teriparatide) Lumbar flexion-extension x-rays Supine x-rays while laying on bump Nonoperative management: PT, acupuncture, chiropractor, pain management	CT C-T spine with 3D reformat MRI C-T spine Supine long cassette AP/lateral x-rays Cardiology evaluation Lower extremity dopplers
Surgical approach selected	T12-L1 corpectomy, T6-sacroiliac fusion	Stage 1: T4-Pelvis posterior fusion with T12-L1 osteotomy Stage 2: T11-L2 lateral plate and discectomy for interbody fusion	L1 VCR, T4-iliac fusion	Revision T4-sacrum/ilium with T12/L1 VCR and T11-L2 anterior spinal fusion with cage, L5-S1 TLIF
Surgical approach if 21 Surgical approach if 80	Same approach Conservative management	T12-L1 corpectomy with expandable cage with T4-L4 posterior fusion Same approach	Same approach Same approach	T9-L3 or L4 Same approach except no VCR, with four rods and posterior column osteotomies
Goal of surgery	Correct sagittal and coronal imbalance	Restore alignment, achieve solid fusion	Correct thoracolumbar kyphosis	Realign sagittal and coronal regional and global malalignment, relieve current symptoms
Perioperative				
Positioning	Left lateral up, then prone	Stage 1: prone on Jackson table, no pins Stage 2: lateral approach	Prone on Jackson table	Prone on Jackson table, with Gardner-Wells tongs
Surgical equipment	Fluoroscopy Surgical navigation	IOM Fluoroscopy	IOM (MEP/SSEP) Aquamantys® bipolar O-arm Surgical navigation Instrumentation	IOM (MEP/SSEP/EMG) Fluoroscopy O-arm

	Ahmed S. Barakat, MD Orthopaedic Surgery University of Cairo Cairo, Egypt	Fabio Cofano, MD Neurosurgery University of Turin Spine Surgery Unit Humanitas Gradenigo Hospital Turin, Italy	James S. Harrop, MD Neurosurgery Jefferson University Philadelphia, Pennsylvania, United States	Lawrence G. Lenke, MD Orthopaedic Surgery Columbia University New York City, New York, United States
Medications	Tranexamic acid	I think this equipment is not strictly considered a medication according to the english term, then probably better cancel. Write please tranexamic acid as well	Tranexamic acid	Tranexamic acid, steroids
Anatomical considerations	Aorta, segmental vessels, dura, lung	Posterior bony anatomy, ribs, pleura, lung, diaphragm, vascular structures	Aorta, spinal cord	Prior distorted anatomy
Complications feared with approach chosen	Vascular injury, lung injury, neurological injury	Durotomy, excessive bleeding, inadequate correction, neurological injury, pleural injury, spinal cord infarct	Paralysis, adjacent level disease, medical complications	Nerve root injury, adjacent segment disease, medical complications
Intraoperative				
Anesthesia	General	General	General	General
Exposure	T6-sacrum	Stage 1: T4-Pelvis Stage 2: T11-L2	T4-sacrum	T4-sacrum
Levels decompressed	T12-L1	T11-12	L1	T12-L1
Levels fused	T6-pelvis	Stage 1: T4-Pelvis Stage 2: T11-L2	T4-pelvis	T4-sacrum
Surgical narrative	Stage 1: position lateral with left-side up, Hogden's approach, preserve latissimus dorsi, V-shaped osteotomy of the left 10 rib or removal, blunt dissection of peritoneum, sharp bow-shaped dissection of diaphragm, identify T12 and L1 with x-ray, identify segmental vessels and securely suture, T11-12 and T12-L1 and L1-2 discectomies, T12 and L1 corpectomies, preserve ALL, place appropriately sized expandable cage filled with autograft from ribs and excised vertebral bodies, careful correction of kyphosis, anterior lumbar plate from T11-L3, closure of wound with drain and vancomycin powder, chest tube applied	Stage 1: position prone with hips extended to reduce kyphosis, posterior incision, place T4-Ilium screws screws, placement of T12-L1 pedicle screws to increase posterior support or adding T12-L1 pedicles to osteotomy to enhance correction with table bending, check IOM during correction maneuvers, fluoroscopy to confirm global sagittal alignment, grafting, possible screw augmentation with cement Stage 2 (same day): left lateral approach with flexion of table to increase working space, incision after fluoroscopy check, dissect and remove rib on its superior border, dissect retropleural space and avoid visceral and pleural damage, possible lung deflation, fluoroscopy to identify T12-L1 level, place tubular retractor, ligation of segmental vessels with temporary clamps to observe for IOM changes, T11-12 discectomy with bone graft from rib, plate and fix with screws, careful check of pleural integrity and use drainage if necessary, reconstruct chest wall	Baseline (SSEP/MEP), place prone, incision and exposure with Aquamantys,® screws from T4-pelvis and not in L1, L1 laminectomy and drill down L1 pedicles, placement of temporary rods, vertebrectomy and discectomy to achieve enough correction, L1 vertebral body cage, close down deficit, lock rods, two subfascial drains	Position prone, posterior midline incision, subperiosteal exposure from T4-sacrum/ilium, place vancomycin powder into muscle and subcutaneous tissues, L5-S1 inferior face excision except T4-5, place bilateral or dual S2 alar-iliac screws/dual headed S1 screw/reduction L5 pedicle screw, L5-S1 TLIF with lordotic cage, place pedicle screws segmentally up to T4 skipping T12 and L1 with dual-headed screws at T10-11 and L2-3 on left and T11 and L2 on right. O-arm to check hardware, temporary rods on right T10-L3

Ahmed S. Barakat, MD Orthopaedic Surgery University of Cairo Cairo, Egypt	Fabio Cofano, MD Neurosurgery University of Turin Spine Surgery Unit Humanitas Gradenigo Hospital Turin, Italy	James S. Harrop, MD Neurosurgery Jefferson University Philadelphia, Pennsylvania, United States	Lawrence G. Lenke, MD Orthopaedic Surgery Columbia University New York City, New York, United States
Stage 2: position prone, expose from T6-S1, insert pedicle screws from T6-L5 followed by sacroiliac screws, vertebroplasty to T11 and L2, fix rods with correct curvature, place remainder of autograft/BMP/TCP in posterolateral space from T11 to L2, vancomycin powder, closure over drains			VCR of T12 and L1 with complete laminectomy of T12 and L1 to expose inferior pedicle of T11 and superior pedicle of L2, left-sided VCR with T12-L1 pedicle excision and T11-12/T12-L1/L1-2 discs excision with care to remain endplate integrity, excise majority of left-sided T12 and L1 vertebral body with remnant of anterior T12 and L1 left body for stability and fusion, temporary rods on left side and repeat T12 and L1 VCR, dural temporary rods placed with compressive shortening of the spine at T12-L1 to remove tension of ventral thecal sac, posterior wall impact or used to push dorsal cortex off ventral dura, multiple posterior compressions to shorten spine and remove segmental kyphosis, place titanium expandable cage from posterior to anterior with further posterior compression and expansion of cage to distract again end plates, place copious autograft into anterior defect prior to cage placement and then in and around cage, remove left temporary rod and place permanent rod, repeat on right, AP/lateral x-rays, structural rib allograft over laminectomy defect from decorticated T11-L2 remaining lamina, decortication from T4-sacrum with auto/allograft and two large BMP kits, two additional rods that are staggered proximally where two rods span T2-9/#3 rod T9-11/#4 rod T11-sacrum, layered closure with a deep and superficial drain after applying tobramycin to tissues

	Ahmed S. Barakat, MD Orthopaedic Surgery University of Cairo Cairo, Egypt	Fabio Cofano, MD Neurosurgery University of Turin Spine Surgery Unit Humanitas Gradenigo Hospital Turin, Italy	James S. Harrop, MD Neurosurgery Jefferson University Philadelphia, Pennsylvania, United States	Lawrence G. Lenke, MD Orthopaedic Surgery Columbia University New York City, New York, United States
Complication avoidance	Two-staged approach, two-level corpectomy to correct kyphosis, chest tube, vertebroplasty to augment pedicle screws, place rods with correct curvature	T12-L1 pedicle screws vs. osteotomy in stage 1, check neuro monitoring during correction maneuvers, possible screw augmentation, dissect along superior border of rib, temporarily clamp segmental vessels to observe for IOM changes	Baseline IOM, Aquamantys,® vertebrectomy if needed to achieve deformity correction	All screws placed freehand, place bilateral or dual S2 alar-iliac screws freehand, L5-S1 TLIF with lordotic cage, intraoperative O-arm, maintain end plate disc integrity during VCR, save all nerve roots, keep anterior vertebral body for fusion, staggered rod construct
Postoperative				
Admission	ICU, then floor	ICU, then floor	ICU, then spine unit	ICU
Postoperative complications feared	Osteoporosis, neurological deficits, respiratory dysfunction	CSF leak, neurological deficits, inadequate correction, infection	Paralysis, neurological deficit, adjacent level disease, medical problems	Medical complications
Anticipated length of stay	6–8 days	4–5 days	4–6 days	6 days
Follow-up testing	Thoracolumbar x-rays within 24 hours, 2 weeks, 6 weeks, 6 months, every 2 years after surgery	Standing x-rays within 24 hours after surgery, 1 month, 3 months, 6 months, 12 months after surgery	Plain x-rays prior to discharge Standing scoliosis x-rays prior to discharge	Upright x-rays when drains removed
Bracing	None	Semirigid thoracolumbar brace for 30 days	6 weeks	None
Follow-up visits	2 weeks, 3 months, 6 months, 12 months, 24 months after discharge	1 month, 3 months, 6 months, 12 months after surgery	2 weeks with APP, 6 weeks after surgery	2 weeks, 6–8 weeks after surgery

AP, Anteroposterior; *BMP*, bone morphogenic protein; *CSF*, cerebrospinal fluid; *CT*, computed tomography; *CTA*, computed tomography angiogram; *DEXA*, dual-energy x-ray absorptiometry; *EMG*, electromyogram; *ICU*, intensive care unit; *IOM*, intraoperative monitoring; *MEP*, motor evoked potential; *SSEP*, somatosensory evoked potential; *TCP*, tricalcium phosphate; *TLIF*, transforaminal lumbar interbody fusion; *VCR*, vertebral column resection.

Differential diagnosis

- Proximal junctional kyphosis
- Proximal junctional failure
- Adjacent segment disease

Important anatomical considerations

Iatrogenic kyphoscoliosis is typically the result of loss of anterior column integrity followed by destruction of the posterior column during surgical intervention for the initial injury. This is typically followed by instrumentation failure and/or progressive kyphosis, which lead to the deformity. It is important to note that those patients with hardware failure from screw pullout should undergo bone density scan to look for osteoporosis. In fact, it is believed that 50% of the population 50 years and older are at risk for osteoporosis and therefore should be evaluated with bone density imaging for prior to any fusion surgery in this population.[1] The focal kyphosis resulting from loss of both anterior and posterior column is often the driving force behind formation of the kyphoscoliosis, which must be addressed during correction

of the deformity. Just like all other deformities, the spinopelvic parameters must be assessed to address the deformity that exists in these patients. Although the patient may sometimes be globally balanced, evaluating the pelvic index (PI) based on the formula PI = pelvic tilt (PT) + sacral slope (SS) is integral to understanding the relationship between the spine and pelvis; specifically, how the parameters have allowed the patient to compensate. In this formula, the PI is a fixed morphogenic parameter with only slight changes during prepubertal development. PT (normal PT = <20 degrees) and SS are variable parameters with indirect relationships to each other.

Additional measurements include sagittal vertical axis (SVA = +/− 4 cm), which is a common measurement of global sagittal alignment (SA). The difference between the coronal C7 plumb line and the central sacral vertical line (CSVL) is used to assesses the coronal alignment (CA = +/−2 cm).[2] The SRS-Schwab classification identifies PT greater than 22 degrees, SVA greater than 46 mm, and PI-LL (pelvic incidence-lumbar lordosis = <10 degrees) more than 11 degrees as factors, which are predictive of disability[3,4] (see Chapter 40, Table 1). Additionally, understanding the normal curvature of the thoracic and lumbar spine, as well as maintaining a thoracolumbar junction degree of less than 10 degrees, helps understand optimal correction goals for this condition.

Full 36-inch cassette scoliosis imaging, magnetic resonance imaging (MRI) involving the entirety of the deformity, and computed tomography (CT) scans are important for assessing the neural elements. Additionally, the CT scan allows the surgeon to determine the bony component, assess for fusion mass, and assess the local bone quality using Hounsfield units. Although these are typically rigid deformity, occasionally supine scoliosis films maybe helpful in determining how much movement is present within the deformity.

Approaches to this lesion

The management of kyphoscoliosis truly depends on the degree of correction needed for both global and focal correction. Depending on the degree of correction that is needed, in addition to flexibility of the deformity, when less correction is needed, typically a posterior-only approach is preferred. When more aggressive correction is needed, as with the need for vertebrectomy to obtain proper correction, a posterior versus and anterior-posterior approach are more likely to be considered (see Chapter 38, Table 1).

Pedicle subtraction osteotomy (PSO), although not physiological, is necessary when correction is needed through a previously bony-fused level, allowing up to 30 degrees correction. Another osteotomy, vertebral column resection (VCR), delivers 30 to 40 degrees and is especially beneficial when both sagittal and coronal correction are needed.[5] Combination anterior/posterior procedures may add surgical time, lengthen hospitalization, require access to surgeons, and expose the patient to additional complications; however, this may sometimes be needed. Although these procedures carry a significant risk, correction can often not be obtained without it. Prior to planning surgical intervention, it is important to assess for iliopsoas contracture, which may prevent the patient's ability to stand erect even after correction. Those patients with concerns for iliopsoas contracture may require aggressive physical therapy or even iliopsoas release prior to undergoing surgical correction.[2]

The length of the construct is another fundamental concern that will determine the success of the correction. Attempt to get away with smaller constructs especially those with poor bone quality will most likely result in failure of the construct. Good bony purchase above and below the correction is needed. When osteoporosis is identified, anabolic treatment is required for months prior to attempted correction. In addition, augmentation with methylmethacrylate cement through fenestrated screws may be helpful in increasing screw pullout strength.[6,7]

What was actually done

At the initial evaluation, the patient was noted to have osteoporosis with a T-score of −2.8. The patient underwent treatment with anabolic osteoporosis medication for 6 months prior to surgical intervention. After completing this treatment, the patient was then offered a staged procedure to undergo a lateral T12-L1 corpectomy to correct the anterior column deformity followed by a T4 to pelvis instrumentation with multilevel Smither-Peterson osteotomies (SPOs). The patient underwent lateral corpectomy with assistant from

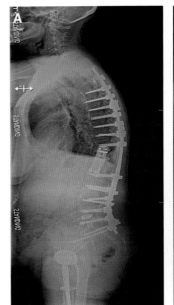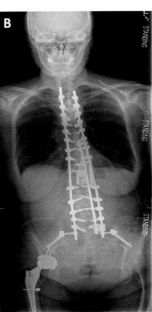

Fig. 42.4 Postoperative x-rays. (A) Lateral and **(B)** AP x-rays after surgery demonstrating T4 to pelvis instrumentation with T12-L1 anterior cage placement and correction of sagittal imbalance.

the cardiothoracic surgeons in order to gain access. These levels had prior cement placement for vertebroplasty, which had to be drilled out. A cage was placed along with a lateral plate and screws. Following this procedure, the patient was brought back 3 days later to complete the posterior portion of the case. For the posterior portion, the patient was placed on an OSI table. The patient received tranexamic acid bolus at the beginning of the case and continuous infusion throughout the case. The previous incision was exposed and extended rostral and caudally to expose from T4 to the pelvis. T4 to pelvis instrumentation was performed. SPOs were performed at both T11-12 and L1-2. An L5-S1 transforaminal lumbar interbody fusion (TLIF) was then performed followed by tethering to T3. The patient tolerated both procedures well without complication. She ambulated postoperatively with a brace and was discharged to inpatient rehabilitation on postoperative day 10. Imaging showed good location of the hardware (Fig. 42.4).

Commonalities among the experts

There was consensus among our surgeons that surgical intervention was warranted after additional testing. Half recommended endocrinology workup and bone density scans, while others requested dynamic imaging, computed tomography angiography (CTA), and cardiology consult. It was also widely agreed that anterior reconstruction was needed by corpectomy or VCR at T12-L1. All but one surgeon recommended instrumentation from T4 to pelvis except one who recommended instrumentation only to T6. The majority planned on a single-staged procedure, and one expert recommended a staged procedure. Intraoperative monitoring was recommended by the majority as well as tranexamic acid intraoperatively. Uniformly it was recommended that the patient be admitted to the intensive care unit, with hospitalization that ranged from 4 to 8 days. Half recommended bracing for a period of time. All recommended postoperative imaging.

SUMMARY OF QUALITY OF EVIDENCE TO GUIDE SPECIFIC INTERVENTIONS FOR THIS CASE

- Intraoperative monitoring for deformity correction: level II.1
- Hook versus pedicle screw at upper index vertebral level for proximal junctional kyphosis prevention: level II.1
- Bracing following lumbar fusion: level I
- Cement augmentation of pedicle screws in osteoporosis: level II.2

REFERENCES

1. Lewiecki EM, Leader D, Weiss R, Williams SA. Challenges in osteoporosis awareness and management: results from a survey of US postmenopausal women. *J Drug Assess.* 2019;8(1):25–31.
2. Ames CP, Smith JS, Scheer JK, Bess S, Bederman SS, Deviren V, et al. Impact of spinopelvic alignment on decision making in deformity surgery in adults: A review. *J Neurosurg Spine.* 2012; 16(6):547–564.
3. Lafage R, Schwab F, Challier V, Henry JK, Gum J, Smith J, et al. Defining Spino-Pelvic Alignment Thresholds: Should Operative Goals in Adult Spinal Deformity Surgery Account for Age? *Spine (Phila Pa 1976).* 2016;41(1):62–68.
4. Schwab F, Ungar B, Blondel B, Buchowski J, Coe J, Deinlein D, et al. Scoliosis Research Society-Schwab adult spinal deformity classification: a validation study. *Spine (Phila Pa 1976).* 2012;37(12): 1077–1082.
5. Uribe JS, Schwab F, Mundis GM, Xu DS, Januszewski J, Kanter AS, et al. The comprehensive anatomical spinal osteotomy and anterior column realignment classification. *J Neurosurg Spine.* 2018;29(5): 565–575.
6. Elder BD, Lo SF, Holmes C, Goodwin CR, Kosztowski TA, Lina IA, et al. The biomechanics of pedicle screw augmentation with cement. *Spine J.* 2015;15(6):1432–1445.
7. Liu MY, Tsai TT, Lai PL, Hsieh MK, Chen LH, Tai CL. Biomechanical comparison of pedicle screw fixation strength in synthetic bones: Effects of screw shape, core/thread profile and cement augmentation. *PLoS One.* 2020;15(2):e0229328.

43

Broken rod after scoliosis correction with back pain

Kingsley Abode-Iyamah, MD

Introduction

Rod fracture following complex spinal deformity correction is a common problem occurring in up to 15% of cases.[1,2] Following deformity correction, the rods act as struts that allow the bony fusion to occur. The rods during this time period undergo stress, which may ultimately lead to metal fatigue resulting in rod fracture before solid bony fusion has occurred.[3–5] While this may be identified during routine follow-up imaging, most patients who have had a rod fracture typically notice a loud pop, which may result in pain. In addition to back and radicular pain, fracture of the rod prior to solid bony fusion may also lead to new deformity from loss of prior deformity correction. The decision on surgical intervention for a fracture rod is one that is dependent on the patient's symptoms and presence of instability.

Example case

Chief complaint: back pain and postural change
History of present illness: This is a 70-year-old female with a history of multiple spinal fusion. She is now fused from occiput to pelvic. She had been having multiple falls and now complains of increasing back pain. Additionally, she had noticed she was no longer able to stand straight. Computed tomography scans and x-rays were obtained, which showed a rod fracture (Figs. 43.1–43.2). She attempted conservative management but continued to have severe back pain.
Medications: atorvastatin, Xanax
Allergies: ketamine, naproxen, ciprofloxacin
Past medical and surgical history: chronic pain, glaucoma, pack pain, chronic kidney disease, hyperlipidemia, laminectomy, fusion, anterior cervical decompression and fusion
Family history: noncontributory

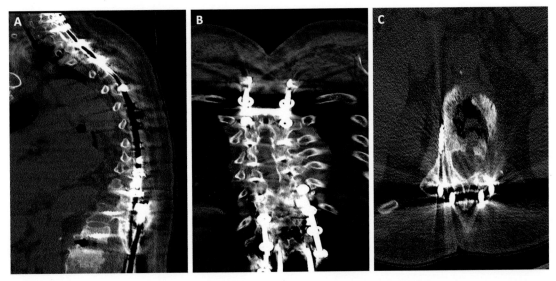

Fig. 43.1 Preoperative computed tomography scans. (A) Sagittal, **(B)** coronal, and **(C)** axial images demonstrating rod fracture and a vacuum disc at T12-L1.

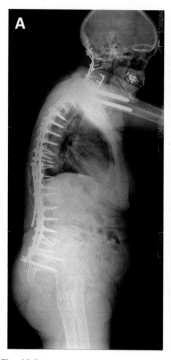
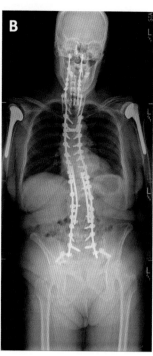

Fig. 43.2 Preoperative standing x-rays. (A) Lateral and **(B)** anteroposterior (AP) standing x-rays demonstrating rod fracture with progressive sagittal imbalance.

Social history: nonsmoker

Physical examination: awake, alert, and oriented to person, place, and time; cranial nerves II–XII intact; bilateral deltoids/triceps/biceps 5/5; interossei 5/5; iliopsoas/knee flexion/knee extension/dorsi, and plantar flexion 5/5

Reflexes: 2+ in bilateral biceps/triceps/brachioradialis with negative Hoffman; 2+ in bilateral patella/ankle; no clonus or Babinski; sensation intact to light touch

	Jason Cheung, MD Orthopaedic Surgery The University of Hong Kong Queen Mary Hospital Pokfulam, Hong Kong SAR, China	Hazem Eltahawy, MD Neurosurgery St. Mary Mercy Hospital Ain Shams University Livonia, Michigan, United States	Lawrence G. Lenke, MD Orthopaedic Surgery Columbia University New York City, New York, United States	Timothy F. Witham, MD Neurosurgery Johns Hopkins Baltimore, Maryland, United States
Preoperative				
Additional tests requested	Obtain older x-rays and operative notes MRI complete spine Nephrology evaluation	CT myelogram T-L spine DEXA Cardiopulmonary evaluation Ophthalmology evaluation	CT complete spine (occiput-pelvis) DEXA Cardiac evaluation Lower extremity dopplers Pulmonary function test	CT myelogram T-L spine DEXA Calcium, vitamin D, PTH serum levels Medicine evaluation
Surgical approach selected	C5-T4 revision instrumentation and fusion	L3 pedicle subtraction osteotomy, TLIF at pseudoarthrosed levels, revision of right-sided screws, correction of kyphosis, T3-L4 fusion	If patient elected to pursue, revision T6-sacrum/ilium, possible TLIF, several posterior column osteotomies	After weight reduction and osteoporotic management, T10 three-column osteotomy and thoracolumbar fusion with possible reinstrumentation
Surgical approach if 25 Surgical approach if 50	Revision osteotomy at lumbar spine, possible interbody fusion Revision osteotomy at lumbar spine, possible interbody fusion, possibly in staged fashion	Same approach Same approach, but osteoporosis management may not be necessary and the correction of kyphosis may need to be more aggressive	Same approach Same approach, but osteoporosis management may not be necessary and the correction of kyphosis may need to be more aggressive	Same approach except osteoporotic management and more aggressive kyphosis correction Same approach but more aggressive with kyphosis correction
Goal of surgery	Stabilize segment, enhance fusion	Correction of sagittal imbalance, repair of pseudoarthrosis, hardware replacement	Repair pseudoarthrosis, realign sagittal global malalignment	Correct deformity, stabilize spine, revise arthrodesis

	Jason Cheung, MD Orthopaedic Surgery The University of Hong Kong Queen Mary Hospital Pokfulam, Hong Kong SAR, China	Hazem Eltahawy, MD Neurosurgery St. Mary Mercy Hospital Ain Shams University Livonia, Michigan, United States	Lawrence G. Lenke, MD Orthopaedic Surgery Columbia University New York City, New York, United States	Timothy F. Witham, MD Neurosurgery Johns Hopkins Baltimore, Maryland, United States
Perioperative				
Positioning	Prone, with Mayfield pins	Prone, with Mayfield pins	Prone on OSI frame, with Gardner-Wells tongs	Prone on Jackson table, no pins
Surgical equipment	IOM (MEP/SSEP) Ultrasonic bone scalpel Cables and wires Bone saw	IOM (MEP/SSEP) Cell saver Pedicle osteotomy set Surgical navigation	IOM (MEP/SSEP/EMG) Fluoroscopy	IOM Fluoroscopy Osteotomes
Medications	Tranexamic acid, BMP	MAP >80	Tranexamic acid, steroids	Tranexamic acid
Anatomical considerations	Spinal cord, pedicle integrity	Dura, nerve roots, segmental vessels, great vessels	Prior laminectomy defects	Spinal cord, segmental vessels, aorta, inferior vena cava
Complications feared with approach chosen	Spinal cord injury, implant failure, prolonged ventilation, renal failure	CSF leak, medical complications, wound breakdown	Nerve root injury, CSF leak, medical complications	Instability, failed fusion, recurrent deformity
Intraoperative				
Anesthesia	General	General	General	General
Exposure	C5-T4	T3-L4	T5-sacrum	T-L
Levels decompressed	None	L2-4	T10-L3	T10
Levels fused	C5-T4	T3-L4	T6-sacrum	T-L
Surgical narrative	Preflip IOM, position prone with Mayfield pins to stabilize skull, expose cervicothoracic spine, remove cross-link at T5-6, loosen caps and disengage rod, check screws at C5-6 to see if loosened, likely replace T2-4 screws with bigger caliber screws except T4 screws where the fracture is located, pack bone graft through pedicle hole, tapered rod to connect entire segment or use cross connectors to connect upper and lower segments with two additional rods, possible laminar wires if no screws can be inserted, try to move expeditiously to avoid blood loss, four-rod construct, promote fusion with fibula allograft to span unstable segment with cancellous bone and BMP, vancomycin powder before closure	Position prone, baseline SSEP and MEP, place iliac crest reference frame for spin navigation, skin incision centered over lumbar and thoracic midline using old scar, thorough hemostasis during exposure of bone and hardware, unlock set screws and remove rods, cut rod at T4 and reconnect later, O-arm spine, L2-4 laminectomy with bilateral facetectomy and excision of scar on top of dura, replace L2 and L4 screws with dual head screws, L3 pedicle osteotomy with removing L2-3 disc, TLIF at thoracolumbar pseudoarthrosed level, revise right-sided screw confirm anatomical alignment with x-ray or O-arm, insert bilateral contoured rods, connect to rest of construct at T3, supplement with dual rods across thoracolumbar junction, insert one submuscular and one subcutaneous drain, layered closure	Position prone, subperiosteal dissection from T5 to sacrum/iliac, place vancomycin powder into muscles and subcutaneous tissue, check for implant failure, removal all rods from T6 to scrum/ilium, check for fusion status level by level, clean up scar over suspected pseudoarthrosis level, perform posterior column osteotomies from T10-L3, check all pedicle screws and replace with larger diameter if needed, reinstrument T6 bilaterally, cantilever placement of correcting rods to maximize lordosis, construct-construct compression to close osteotomies and pseudoarthrosis sites, two rods in upper T-spine going to three rods at lower T-spine to four rods covering TL junction to sacrum/lilium, intraoperative long cassette coronal and sagittal x-rays, adjust as needed, revision posterior fusion at all pseudoarthrosis and osteotomy sites with auto/allograft and potentially BMP, layered closure with one deep and one superficial drain, place vancomycin and tobramycin powder into muscles and subcutaneous tissue prior to closure	Position prone, localizing x-rays and establishment of on-table alignment, exposure of levels deemed necessary for revision, cut rods, remove instrumentation as needed, reinstrument if needed, laminectomy at level of osteotomy likely around T10, perform extended pedicle subtraction osteotomy, place small Harms cage, close osteotomy with instrumentation and continuous IOM, x-ray to confirm hardware and alignment, decortication, place BMP, layered closure with drain

(continued on next page)

	Jason Cheung, MD Orthopaedic Surgery The University of Hong Kong Queen Mary Hospital Pokfulam, Hong Kong SAR, China	Hazem Eltahawy, MD Neurosurgery St. Mary Mercy Hospital Ain Shams University Livonia, Michigan, United States	Lawrence G. Lenke, MD Orthopaedic Surgery Columbia University New York City, New York, United States	Timothy F. Witham, MD Neurosurgery Johns Hopkins Baltimore, Maryland, United States
Complication avoidance	Preflip IOM, check previous hardware for loosening, bone graft in pedicle where the fracture is located, possible laminar wires if screws cannot be inserted, four-rod construct, BMP to promote fusion	Cut rod at T4 to connect to later, L3 pedicle osteotomy for deformity correction, connect to construct at T3, supplement with dual rods across thoracolumbar junction	Check for implant failure, check fusion status level by level, check all pedicle screws and replace with larger diameter if needed, cantilever placement of correcting rods to maximize lordosis	Revise instrumentation as needed, three column pedicle subtraction osteotomy, revise instrumentation as needed based on intraoperative determination
Postoperative				
Admission	ICU	ICU	ICU	ICU
Postoperative complications feared	Spinal cord injury, implant failure, prolonged ventilation, renal failure	Wound healing issues, CSF leak, neurological deficits, medical complications	Nerve root injury, CSF leak, medical complications	Spinal cord injury, CSF leak, recurrent pseudoarthrosis, instrumentation failure
Anticipated length of stay	2 weeks	5–7 days	6 days	5–7 days
Follow-up testing	Cervicothoracic x-rays every 3 months for first year after surgery CT C-T spine 6 months after surgery	36-inch standing x-rays 3 months, 6 months, 1 year after surgery CT C-T-L spine 1 year after surgery	Upright x-rays after drain removed	CT T-L spine prior to discharge Scoliosis x-rays prior to discharge, 6 weeks, 3 months, 6 months, 1 year after surgery
Bracing	Body jacket with cervical component for at least 6 months until union achieved	None	None	None
Follow-up visits	Every 3 months for 1 year after surgery	2 weeks, 6 weeks, 3 months 6 months, 1 year after surgery	2 weeks, 6-8 weeks after surgery	2 weeks, 6 weeks, 3 months, 6 months, 1 year after surgery

BMP, Bone morphogenic protein; *CSF,* cerebrospinal fluid; *CT,* computed tomography; *DEXA,* dual-energy x-ray absorptiometry; *EMG,* electromyography; *ICU,* intensive care unit; *IOM,* intraoperative monitoring; *MAP,* mean arterial pressure; *MEP,* motor evoked potential; *OSI,* orthopedic system Inc; *PTH,* parathyroid hormone; *SSEP,* somatosensory evoked potential; *TLIF,* transforaminal lumbar interbody fusion.

Differential diagnosis

- Rod fracture
- Pseudoarthrosis
- Osteomyelitis

Important anatomical considerations

Over the years, there have been changes to the metal available for rod fixation. Once commonly used, steel rods are no longer the norm and today titanium and cobalt-chrome rods are most popular. These titanium and cobalt-chrome rods are available in various stiffness. The most important factor in determination of the type of rod to be used is the patient's own bone quality. With poor bone quality, the stiffer rod places additional stress at the bone-metal interface with the screw and can lead to haloing of the screw.[6-9] It is clear that all metal reach a point of failure if bony fusion does not occur in a timely fashion, and the rods that act as a strut for the correction will

ultimately lead to failure or "rod fracture." Those with poor bone quality would most likely benefit from less stiff rods, which causes less stress on the bone metal interface. Those with good bone quality may benefit from stiffer rods, which helps in preventing rod failure and ultimately fracture. Additionally, the degree of correction needed also influences the type of rod needed, as those with larger curve correction may require a stiffer rod to help maintain the correction.[10,11]

Approaches to this lesion

Treatment of rod fracture can be accomplished by multiple strategies. Rod fracture is the result of pseudoarthrosis, and therefore the treatment strategy should include addressing the underlying pseudoarthrosis. When failure of arthrodesis is posterior, this can be addressed by replacement of the fractured rods and arthrodesis. Recombinant bone morphogenetic protein (rhBMP) is a synthetic protein that has been shown to induce bone formation and is currently U.S. Food and Drug Administration (FDA)-approved for anterior lumbar interbody fusion (rhBMP-2) and revision posterolateral surgery (rhBMP-7).[12] The use of RhBMP has been shown to increase arthrodesis, although it is associated with various complications including seroma formation and ectopic bone formation at high doses.[12-16] A meta-analysis completed by Papakostidis and colleagues demonstrated a fusion failure rate of 14.5% versus 39% for rhBMP versus autologous bone graft in the setting of posterolateral spinal fusion, respectively.[17] Additionally, the use of interbody fusion across an area with pseudoarthrosis may also help accomplish fusion across that area. In many cases, interbody fusion can be accomplished posteriorly, although in some cases a lateral or anterior approach may be appropriate. Additional considerations following reoperation for rod fracture are the diameter of the rods and placement of three- and four-rod constructs to minimize fractures in the future. This should be balanced with the bone quality of the patient in order to minimize risk of failure at the bone-metal interface.

What was actually done

This patient had a history of a previous rod fracture and presented with another fracture in the thoracolumbar spine. On computed tomography scans, there was a vacuumed disc noted at T12-L1. The patient was therefore offered a staged T12-L1 lateral interbody placement through a thoracotomy approach from the left side followed by a cervical to lumbar replacement of her rods and arthrodesis. The patient was brought to the operating room for a left-sided approach via a thoracotomy. After exposure by the cardiothoracic team, an T12-L1 discectomy and interbody cage placement was done. The rib was harvested at this location and used for arthrodesis. A chest tube was placed and the wound closed. The patient was brought back for the second stage of the procedure on postoperative day 3. They were positioned on a Jackson table and underwent exposure of the cervical to lumbar spine. The previous rods and satellite rods were removed and the site of the fracture identified. Tapered cobalt-chrome rods were then placed and connected to the cervical rods with side connectors. A Smith-Peterson osteotomy was done at T12-L1 to allow compression on the interbody. Arthrodesis was performed and two hemovacs were placed. Postoperatively, the patient was place in a thoracic lumbar sacral orthosis (TLSO) brace and was discharged on postoperative day 10 to rehabilitation. Postoperative imaging showed good location of the instrumentation and correction of the sagittal deformity (Fig. 43.3).

Commonalities among the experts

Among our surgeons, there was a consensus on obtaining further imaging including computed tomography myelogram, magnetic resonance imaging, bone density scans, and medicine consult. After thorough evaluation, surgical intervention was offered by all surgeons, but their levels of surgery varied. One surgeon offered a C5-T4 revision and fusion, and another recommended a T6 to ilium revision with multilevel osteotomies and interbody at the level of pseudoarthrosis. Half recommended a three-column osteotomy (L3 vs. T10) with differing levels of instrumentation. When presented with younger patients (25 and 50 years old), the majority of surgeons offered a similar surgical plan. Universally, all surgeons recommended the use of intraoperative monitoring and fluoroscopy. The majority also recommended the use of tranexamic acid during surgical correction. All expected

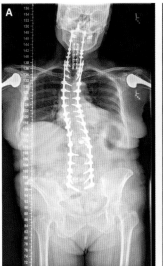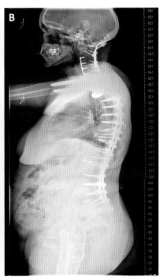

Fig. 43.3 Postoperative x-rays. (A) AP and **(B)** lateral x-rays demonstrating placement of a T12-L1 interbody as well as repair of the rod fracture and restoration of the sagittal alignment.

intensive care unit admission after surgery with hospitalization times of 5 to 14 days. The majority did not recommend bracing, but routine follow-up with postoperative additional imaging was recommended.

SUMMARY OF QUALITY OF EVIDENCE TO GUIDE SPECIFIC INTERVENTIONS FOR THIS CASE

- Intraoperative monitoring for deformity correction: level II.1
- Hook versus pedicle screw at upper index level for proximal junctional kyphosis prevention: level II.1
- Bracing following lumbar fusion: level I

REFERENCES

1. Bridwell KH, Lewis SJ, Edwards C, Lenke LG, Iffrig TM, Berra A, et al. Complications and outcomes of pedicle subtraction osteotomies for fixed sagittal imbalance. *Spine (Phila Pa 1976)*. 2003;28(18):2093–2101.
2. Buchowski JM, Bridwell KH, Lenke LG, Kuhns CA, Lehman Jr. RA, Kim YJ, et al. Neurologic complications of lumbar pedicle subtraction osteotomy: a 10-year assessment. *Spine (Phila Pa 1976)*. 2007;32(20):2245–2252.
3. Barton C, Noshchenko A, Patel V, Cain C, Kleck C, Burger E. Risk factors for rod fracture after posterior correction of adult spinal deformity with osteotomy: a retrospective case-series. *Scoliosis*. 2015;10:30.
4. Charosky S, Guigui P, Blamoutier A, Roussouly P, Chopin D. Study Group on S. Complications and risk factors of primary adult scoliosis surgery: a multicenter study of 306 patients. *Spine (Phila Pa 1976)*. 2012;37(8):693–700.
5. Hamilton DK, Buza 3rd JA, Passias P, Jalai C, Kim HJ, Ailon T, et al. The Fate of Patients with Adult Spinal Deformity Incurring Rod Fracture After Thoracolumbar Fusion. *World Neurosurg*. 2017;106:905–911.
6. Halvorson TL, Kelley LA, Thomas KA, Whitecloud 3rd TS, Cook SD. Effects of bone mineral density on pedicle screw fixation. *Spine (Phila Pa 1976)*. 1994;19(21):2415–2420.
7. McLain RF, McKinley TO, Yerby SA, Smith TS, Sarigul-Klijn N. The effect of bone quality on pedicle screw loading in axial instability. A synthetic model. *Spine (Phila Pa 1976)*. 1997;22(13):1454–1460.

8. Pfeifer BA, Krag MH, Johnson C. Repair of failed transpedicle screw fixation. A biomechanical study comparing polymethyl-methacrylate, milled bone, and matchstick bone reconstruction. *Spine (Phila Pa 1976)*. 1994;19(3):350–353.

9. Snider RK, Krumwiede NK, Snider LJ, Jurist JM, Lew RA, Katz JN. Factors affecting lumbar spinal fusion. *J Spinal Disord*. 1999;12(2):107–114.

10. Angelliaume A, Ferrero E, Mazda K, Le Hanneur M, Accabled F, de Gauzy JS, et al. Titanium vs cobalt chromium: what is the best rod material to enhance adolescent idiopathic scoliosis correction with sublaminar bands? *Eur Spine J*. 2017;26(6):1732–1738.

11. Han S, Hyun SJ, Kim KJ, Jahng TA, Kim HJ. Comparative Study Between Cobalt Chrome and Titanium Alloy Rods for Multilevel Spinal Fusion: Proximal Junctional Kyphosis More Frequently Occurred in Patients Having Cobalt Chrome Rods. *World Neurosurg*. 2017;103:404–409.

12. Garrett MP, Kakarla UK, Porter RW, Sonntag VK. Formation of painful seroma and edema after the use of recombinant human bone morphogenetic protein-2 in posterolateral lumbar spine fusions. *Neurosurgery*. 2010;66(6):1044–1049. discussion 9.

13. Lindley TE, Dahdaleh NS, Menezes AH, Abode-Iyamah KO. Complications associated with recombinant human bone morphogenetic protein use in pediatric craniocervical arthrodesis. *J Neurosurg Pediatr*. 2011;7(5):468–474.

14. Meyer Jr. RA, Gruber HE, Howard BA, Tabor Jr. OB, Murakami T, Kwiatkowski TC, et al. Safety of recombinant human bone morphogenetic protein-2 after spinal laminectomy in the dog. *Spine (Phila Pa 1976)*. 1999;24(8):747–754.

15. Mimatsu K, Kishi S, Hashizume Y. Experimental chronic compression on the spinal cord of the rabbit by ectopic bone formation in the ligamentum flavum with bone morphogenetic protein. *Spinal Cord*. 1997;35(11):740–746.

16. Miyamoto S, Takaoka K, Yonenobu K, Ono K. Ossification of the ligamentum flavum induced by bone morphogenetic protein. An experimental study in mice. *J Bone Joint Surg Br*. 1992;74(2):279–283.

17. Papakostidis C, Kontakis G, Bhandari M, Giannoudis PV. Efficacy of autologous iliac crest bone graft and bone morphogenetic proteins for posterolateral fusion of lumbar spine: a meta-analysis of the results. *Spine (Phila Pa 1976)*. 2008;33(19):E680–E692.

44

Spine metastasis

Oluwaseun O. Akinduro, MD and Kingsley Abode-Iyamah, MD

Introduction

Metastatic spine disease occurs in approximately 20% of cancer patients, with an estimated 20,000 new cases each year.[1,2] Most malignancies have the ability to spread to the spine, but the most common primary sites are lung, breast, prostate, and kidney.[3] Chemotherapy and immunotherapies have become more efficacious; thus cancer patients are living longer, leading to an ever-growing number of patients with spinal metastasis.[4] Historically, surgical management of spinal metastatic disease was controversial, with typical treatment paradigms consisting of steroids and radiation.[5] The Patchell et al. trial that was published in 2005 provided level 1 evidence that surgical decompression plus radiotherapy is superior to radiotherapy alone for patients with spinal cord compression secondary to metastatic disease.[2] This trial excluded patients with radiosensitive tumors, complete paraplegia for >48 hours, and multiple noncontiguous levels of disease; therefore, these patients are typically not considered for surgery. Radiation is a critical component of treatment, and there have been significant advances in the delivery methods for these tumors. The advent of stereotactic body radiotherapy (SBRT) has revolutionized the treatment of these lesions, allowing for excellent conformality and precision of treatment doses with minimal spillover to the spinal cord.[6,7] Despite advances in surgical and radiation treatment, decision making for patients with spinal metastatic disease remains controversial. The neurological, oncological, mechanical, and systemic (NOMS) framework can be used to help guide this decision making.[8] NOMS is an acronym for neurological, oncological, mechanical, and systemic disease. Each component of this framework must be considered when deciding which treatment strategy would be most ideal for a particular patient. The International Spine Oncology Consortium also published an algorithm to assist with decision

making for these patients.[4] Algorithms and guidelines like these must be used when deciding which treatment strategy would be best for cases like the one presented below.

Example case

Chief complaint: neck pain and radiculopathy

History of present illness: This is a 75-year-old male with a history of cholangiocarcinoma diagnosed 6 months ago and status post chemoradiation. He started having incapacitating left shoulder and neck pain. The pain radiates into his scapula and is not relieved with pain medications. He also has mild left-hand weakness and paresthesia and denies bowel/bladder dysfunction. He underwent imaging that was concerning for metastatic spine disease (Figs. 44.1–44.2).

Medications: amlodipine, apixaban, lorazepam, mirtazapine, oxycodone

Allergies: iodinated contrast

Past medical history: reflux, cholangiocarcinoma, hypertension, deep vein thrombosis, Barrett's esophagus, hyperlidpiemia, back pain

Family history: noncontributory

Social history: nonsmoker

Physical examination: awake, alert, and oriented x 3; cranial nerves CNII–XII intact

Motor: Bilateral deltoids/triceps/biceps 5/5; right interossei 5/5; left interossei 4+/5. iliopsoas/knee flexion/knee extension/dorsi, and plantar flexion 5/5

Reflexes: 2+ in bilateral biceps/triceps/brachioradialis with negative Hoffman; 2+ in bilateral patella/ankle no clonus or Babinski; sensation intact to light touch

Laboratories: basic metabolic panel, heme-8, coags all within normal limits

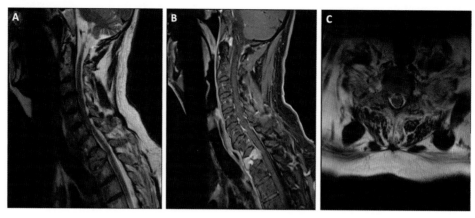

Fig. 44.1 Preoperative magnetic resonance images. (A) T2 sagittal, **(B)** T1 sagittal with contrast, and **(C)** T2 axial with contrast images demonstrating pathological involvement of the T1 vertebral body and inferior half of C7 vertebral body with slight ventral cord compression.

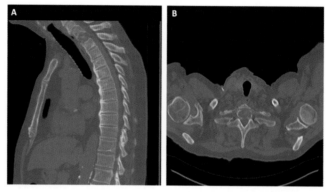

Fig. 44.2 Preoperative computed tomography scans. (A) Sagittal and **(B)** axial images demonstrating pathological fracture of the T1 vertebral body.

	Ali A. Baaj, MD Neurological & Orthopedic Surgery University of Arizona Banner – University Medical Center Phoenix, AZ, United States	Ilya Laufer, MD Neurosurgery Memorial Sloan Kettering New York, New York, United States	Aron Lazary, MD, PhD Orthopaedic Surgery Buda Health Center Semmelweis University Budapest, Hungary	Clemens Weber, MD, PhD Neurosurgery Stavanager University Hospital Stavanager, Norway
Preoperative				
Additional tests requested	PET or CT chest/ abdomen/pelvis Medical oncology evaluation for prognosis Medicine evaluation	CT chest/abdomen/pelvis Medical oncology evaluation for prognosis Medicine evaluation Lower extremity dopplers	C-spine x-rays	Anesthesia evaluation
Surgical approach selected	Posterior C5-T4 instrumented fusion, T1 decompression if survival expected greater than 6 months	Minimally invasive T1 hemilaminectomy, left facetectomy, percutaneous C7-T2 fusion	T1 corpectomy and C7-T2 anterior plate	T1 corpectomy
Goal of surgery	Decompress C7-T1 and stabilize across cervicothoracic junction	Decompress left T1 nerve root, stabilization	Tumor debulking, stabilization	Decompression of spinal cord, tumor resection
Perioperative				
Positioning	Prone with Mayfield clamps	Prone with Mayfield clamps	Supine, no pins	Supine, no pins
Surgical equipment	IOM Surgical microscope Surgical navigation	Surgical navigation Tubular retractors Surgical microscope	Fluoroscopy	Fluoroscopy Surgical microscope

	Ali A. Baaj, MD Neurological & Orthopedic Surgery University of Arizona Banner – University Medical Center Phoenix, AZ, United States	Ilya Laufer, MD Neurosurgery Memorial Sloan Kettering New York, New York, United States	Aron Lazary, MD, PhD Orthopaedic Surgery Buda Health Center Semmelweis University Budapest, Hungary	Clemens Weber, MD, PhD Neurosurgery Stavanager University Hospital Stavanager, Norway
Medications	Antibiotics Steroids	Preoperative celecoxib and gabapentin Liposomal bupivacaine	None	None
Anatomical considerations	Traversing and exiting nerve roots Central canal	C7 and T2 pedicles, left T1 facet and pedicle, left T1 nerve root	Right sternocleidomastoid, carotid sheath, thyroid gland	Carotid artery, esophagus/trachea
Complications feared with approach chosen	Pseudoarthrosis, CSF leak	Postoperative pain, wound infection	Recurrent laryngeal nerve injury, thyroid gland injury, esophageal injury, carotid injury	Nerve root injury
Intraoperative				
Anesthesia	General	General	General	General
Exposure	C5-T4	C7-T2	C7-T2	C7-T2
Levels decompressed	C7-T2 laminectomy	T1	T1	T1
Levels fused	C5-T4	C7-T2	C7-T2	C7-T2
Surgical narrative	Head is pinned, placed prone, incision, subperiosteal dissection from C5 to T4, bilateral lateral mass screws from C5 to 7 and pedicle screws T2-4 with navigation is available, secure with rods, wide laminectomy from C7-T2, posterolateral fusion with allograft, subfascial drain	Position prone with Mayfield pins, neck in neutral position, place spinous clamp and register navigation, intraoperative CT, percutaneous placement of C7 and T2 pedicle screws, connect rods, place expandable retractor through left C7 screw incision and doc on left T1 lamina, hemilaminectomy/ facetectomy/pedicle removal under microscopic visualization, full decompress left T1 nerve root, standard closure	Position supine, lower anterior skin incision above medial border of right sternocleidomastoid muscle, approach anterior spinal column in standard fashion based on preoperative CT, limited manubriotomy with 1 cm of the central part of the manubrium with preservation of muscle attachment if needed after gentle mobilization of thyroid gland, ligate significant thyroid vessels on one side, T1 corpectomy, remove all tumor until thecal sac, remove cartilaginous end plates of C7 and T2, place PMMA spacer with plate fixed to spacer with two screws, augment C7 and T2 vertebral body with PMMA through the holes in the plate, fix screws quickly into cemented vertebral body, place synthetic strip-like bone substitute to promote lateral fusion laterally to plate, wound closure with drain	Right-sided incision at C6-7 level, blunt dissection between vessels and trachea/ esophagus, confirm level with fluoroscopy, black belt retractor, continue with microscope, incision of C7-T1 and T1-T2 discs, removal of the uncus bilaterally, insertion of expandable PEEK cage, plate from C7 to T2
Complication avoidance	Several levels above and below to prevent instability, neuronavigation	Surgical navigation, percutaneous screw placement, minimally invasive laminectomy	Avoid posterior approach, limited manubriotomy, use of PMMA spacer, augment C7 and T2 vertebral bodies, place synthetic strip-like bone substitute to promote fusion	Anterior approach, blunt dissection between vessels and trachea/ esophagus
Postoperative				
Admission	ICU	Floor	ICU	Floor
Postoperative complications feared	Hematoma, hardware failure, medical complications	Tumor recurrence, misplaced screws, pain control	Vessel injury, laryngeal nerve paresis, thyroid gland and esophageal injury	Bleeding, hardware failure, tumor progression
Anticipated length of stay	3–4 days	2–3 days	3–5 days	23 hours
Follow-up testing	C-spine upright AP/ lateral x-rays	C-spine x-rays prior to discharge MRI C-spine 2–3 months after radiation therapy	C-spine x-rays after drain removal	CT C-spine after surgery and per oncology

	Ali A. Baaj, MD Neurological & Orthopedic Surgery University of Arizona Banner – University Medical Center Phoenix, AZ, United States	Ilya Laufer, MD Neurosurgery Memorial Sloan Kettering New York, New York, United States	Aron Lazary, MD, PhD Orthopaedic Surgery Buda Health Center Semmelweis University Budapest, Hungary	Clemens Weber, MD, PhD Neurosurgery Stavanager University Hospital Stavanager, Norway
Bracing	Cervical collar when out of bed	None	Hard collar for 6 weeks	None
Follow-up visits	2 weeks for wound check; 3, 12, and 24 months	3–4 weeks, 3 months after surgery	3 months, 6 months, 12 months, 18 months, 24 months after surgery	3 months after surgery

AP, Anteroposterior; *CSF*, cerebrospinal fluid; *CT*, computed tomography; *ICU*, intensive care unit; *IOM*, intraoperative monitoring; *MRI*, magnetic resonance imaging; *PEEK*, polyetheretherketone; *PET*, positron emission tomography; *PMMA*, polymethylmethacralate.

Differential diagnosis

- Metastatic disease
- Multiple myeloma
- Primary bone tumor such as chordoma
- Osteomyelitis

Important anatomical considerations

This tumor has completely eroded the T1 vertebral body and partially eroded the vertebral body of C7. There are multiple neurovascular structures in this region that must be considered when planning an operation. The primary structures anterior to the cervical vertebral bodies are the common carotid artery, esophagus, and trachea. The primary vascular structures of interest are the carotid arteries and jugular veins anteriorly and the vertebral arteries laterally. Nerves to be mindful of are the recurrent laryngeal and vagal nerves. An anterior approach in the lower cervical and upper thoracic spine may be obstructed by the sternum and clavicle. Funakoshi et al. suggested using a line from the suprasternal notch to the vertebral body (SV line) to help determine the ideal surgical approach for ventral lesions of the upper thoracic spine.[9] They suggested use of a sternotomy when the caudal edge of the tumor was below the SV line or considering a posterior approach. With this in mind, patients with a high riding sternum may require sternotomy and involvement of a thoracic surgeon to gain access. When considering a surgical procedure that will require removal of a vertebral body, the vertebral artery must be taken into consideration. If there is involvement of the vertebral artery with a tumor, or if vertebral artery sacrifice is deemed necessary, surgeons should consider performing a preoperative angiogram with a balloon occlusion test to determine whether the patient would tolerate sacrifice of the vessel. A preoperative angiogram may also be beneficial in hypervascular tumors, as embolization may lead to decreased intraoperative blood loss.[10–12]

Approaches to this lesion

Patients with cervical epidural spinal cord compression primarily ventral in location may be treated with an anterior approach, with or without posterior stabilization, whereas patients with posterior-only disease typically undergo a posterior decompression with or without instrumentation. An anterior approach would provide direct access to a ventrally located lesion and avoid subjecting the spinal cord to manipulation during surgery. This will typically require a corpectomy of the involved levels followed by reconstruction of the anterior column with instrumentation. Patients with circumferential disease may be treated with a combination of the two, and due to the location of the spinal cord, a posterior-only approach can be challenging and may require nerve sacrifice. Although there is a risk for neurological decline secondary to inadvertent compression of the spinal cord during surgery, there have been multiple reports of posterior-only approaches for circumferential disease.[13,14] The primary hindrance to a posterior-only approach is the need for nerve root sacrifice to place a graft, but Shaaya et al. reported use of a chest tube filled with polymethylmethacrylate (PMMA) for anterior reconstruction only from a posterior approach.[13]

What was actually done

The surgical plan for this patient was a T1 anterior cervical corpectomy with anterior instrumented fusion from C7 to T2. Following intubation with general anesthesia, the patient was placed in the supine position and then placed into traction with Gardner-Wells tongs. After fluoroscopic localization, a skin incision was made and dissection was carried medial to the sternocleidomastoid. The carotid was identified and lateralized. The diseased vertebral body of T1 was identified and resected in a piecemeal fashion. A T1 corpectomy was then completed and also a C7 corpectomy was then done because there was confirmation of tumor invasion into the C7 vertebral body based on preoperative imaging. After the C7 corpectomy, the superior end plate of T2 and inferior end plate of C6 were prepared by removing all of the cartilaginous material. An expandable corpectomy cage followed by a plate was then placed, which was secured in place with screws at C6 and T2. A Jackson-Pratt drain was placed and the wound was closed in layers. The patient's diet was advanced appropriately, and he was discharged from the hospital on postoperative day 3 with a hard-cervical collar. Postoperative imaging showed good location of the instrumentation and decompression of the spinal canal (Fig. 44.3).

Commonalities among the experts

Half opted for an anterior approach with corpectomy of T1 and half opted for a posterior approach for decompression of the spinal cord with instrumented fusion. This split highlights the fact that a lesion such as this may be amenable to either an anterior or a posterior approach depending on the goal of surgery, surgeon comfort, and patient-specific anatomical considerations. Despite the differing opinions on the choice of approach, there was a general consensus that the patient

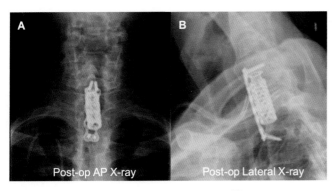

Fig. 44.3 Postoperative x-rays. (A) Anteroposterior and **(B)** lateral x-rays demonstrating partial C7 and complete T1 corpectomy with expandable cage and plate placement.

would require stabilization including at least C7 to T2. Other areas of disagreement were the postoperative management and use of postoperative cervical bracing. Half planned for immediate postoperative care to be completed in the intensive care unit, while the other half planned for care on the neurosurgical floor.

SUMMARY OF QUALITY OF EVIDENCE TO GUIDE SPECIFIC INTERVENTIONS FOR THIS CASE

- Surgical decompression and radiation improve outcomes over radiation alone for patients with spinal compression: level IA[15]
- Spinal radiosurgery is safe and efficacious for treatment of spinal metastasis compared with conventional radiation: level IIA[16–19]
- Hypofractionated radiotherapy is safe and efficacious and has the advantage of shortened treatment course: level IIB[20]

REFERENCES

1. Lee BH, Kim TH, Chong HS, et al. Prognostic factor analysis in patients with metastatic spine disease depending on surgery and conservative treatment: review of 577 cases. *Ann Surg Oncol.* Jan 2013;20(1):40–46.
2. Patchell RA, Tibbs PA, Regine WF, et al. Direct decompressive surgical resection in the treatment of spinal cord compression caused by metastatic cancer: a randomised trial. *Lancet.* Aug 20-26 2005;366(9486):643–648.
3. Choi D, Bilsky M, Fehlings M, Fisher C, Gokaslan Z. Spine Oncology-Metastatic Spine Tumors. *Neurosurgery.* Mar 1, 2017;80(3S):S131–S137.
4. Spratt DE, Beeler WH, de Moraes FY, et al. An integrated multidisciplinary algorithm for the management of spinal metastases: an International Spine Oncology Consortium report. *Lancet Oncol.* Dec 2017;18(12):e720–e730.
5. Ryu S, Yoon H, Stessin A, Gutman F, Rosiello A, Davis R. Contemporary treatment with radiosurgery for spine metastasis and spinal cord compression in 2015. *Radiat Oncol J. Mar.* 2015; 33(1):1–11.
6. Bhatt AD, Schuler JC, Boakye M, Woo SY. Current and emerging concepts in non-invasive and minimally invasive management of spine metastasis. *Cancer Treat Rev.* Apr 2013;39(2):142–152.
7. Zhang HR, Li JK, Yang XG, Qiao RQ, Hu YC. Conventional Radiotherapy and Stereotactic Radiosurgery in the Management of Metastatic Spine Disease. *Technol Cancer Res Treat.* Jan-Dec 2020;19 1533033820945798.
8. Laufer I, Rubin DG, Lis E, et al. The NOMS framework: approach to the treatment of spinal metastatic tumors. *Oncologist.* Jun 2013; 18(6):744–751.
9. Funakoshi Y, Hanakita J, Takahashi T, et al. Investigation of Radiologic Landmarks Used to Decide the Appropriate Surgical Approach for Upper Thoracic Ventral Degenerative Disorders. *World Neurosurg.* May 2019;125:e856–e862.
10. Ma J, Tullius T, Van Ha TG. Update on Preoperative Embolization of Bone Metastases. *Semin Intervent Radiol.* Aug 2019;36(3):241–248.
11. Clausen C, Dahl B, Frevert SC, Hansen LV, Nielsen MB, Lonn L. Preoperative embolization in surgical treatment of spinal metastases: single-blind, randomized controlled clinical trial of efficacy in decreasing intraoperative blood loss. *J Vasc Interv Radiol.* Mar 2015;26(3):402–412. e401.
12. Pazionis TJ, Papanastassiou ID, Maybody M, Healey JH. Embolization of hypervascular bone metastases reduces intraoperative blood loss: a case-control study. *Clin Orthop Relat Res.* Oct 2014;472(10):3179–3187.
13. Shaaya E, Fridley J, Barber SM, et al. Posterior Nerve-Sparing Multilevel Cervical Corpectomy and Reconstruction for Metastatic Cervical Spine Tumors: Case Report and Literature Review. *World Neurosurg.* Feb 2019;122:298–302.
14. Bydon M, De la Garza-Ramos R, Suk I, et al. Single-Staged Multilevel Spondylectomy for En Bloc Resection of an Epithelioid Sarcoma With Intradural Extension in the Cervical Spine: Technical Case Report. *Oper Neurosurg (Hagerstown).* Dec 1, 2015;11(4):E585–E593.
15. Hunter RE, Wigfield CC. Direct decompressive surgical resection in the treatment of spinal cord compression caused by metastatic cancer: a randomized trial. *Br J Neurosurg.* Oct 2008;22(5):713–714.
16. Amdur RJ, Bennett J, Olivier K, et al. A prospective, phase II study demonstrating the potential value and limitation of radiosurgery for spine metastases. *Am J Clin Oncol.* Oct 2009;32(5):515–520.
17. Gerszten PC, Burton SA, Belani CP, et al. Radiosurgery for the treatment of spinal lung metastases. *Cancer.* Dec 1, 2006;107(11): 2653–2661.
18. Gerszten PC, Burton SA, Ozhasoglu C, Welch WC. Radiosurgery for spinal metastases: clinical experience in 500 cases from a single institution. *Spine (Phila Pa 1976).* Jan 15, 2007;32(2):193–199.
19. Chang EL, Shiu AS, Mendel E, et al. Phase I/II study of stereotactic body radiotherapy for spinal metastasis and its pattern of failure. *J Neurosurg Spine.* Aug 2007;7(2):151–160.
20. Maranzano E, Bellavita R, Rossi R, et al. Short-course versus split-course radiotherapy in metastatic spinal cord compression: results of a phase III, randomized, multicenter trial. *J Clin Oncol.* May 20, 2005;23(15):3358–3365.

45

Diffuse mets to spine with lumbar stenosis

Oluwaseun O. Akinduro, MD

Introduction

The skeleton is the third most common site of metastatic disease, with the spinal column being the most common location.[1,2] Metastatic spinal disease can be found in 20% to 30% of patients with primary malignancies and leads to significant morbidity secondary to compression of the spinal cord, pain related to spinal instability, or neural compression.[3–5] Concomitant degenerative spinal disease will be found in a significant portion of patients with spinal metastasis, as it tends to occur in patients over 60 years of age. In addition, many patients with symptomatic degenerative spine disease will have radiographic evidence of spinal metastasis as primary cancers are becoming more common.[6] Thus, it is not uncommon to have patients with symptomatic spinal stenosis secondary to degenerative changes and concomitant spinal metastatic disease, which may or may not be symptomatic. The decision-making strategy should be derived from a multidisciplinary discussion including the oncology team to determine the overall disease status of the patient. Patients with well-controlled systemic disease and a life expectancy of at least 3 months will likely benefit from surgical decompression of their symptomatic stenosis. Consideration can sometimes be made for palliative, minimally invasive decompression for patients who may have poor life expectancy but are still able to tolerate surgery. Although there is no high-level evidence for management of patients with spinal metastatic disease and concomitant stenosis, this chapter presents a patient with these concomitant pathologies.

Example case

Chief complaint: leg pain

History of present illness: This is a 73-year-old male with a history of prostate cancer and known spinal metastasis presenting with bilateral leg pain when walking. He denies any weakness or bowel or bladder incontinence. Metastatic disease has been controlled after chemotherapy and spinal radiation. The patient underwent magnetic resonance imaging (MRI), which revealed evidence of known metastatic disease but with lumbar stenosis (Fig. 45.1).

Medications: aspirin 81 mg

Allergies: no known drug allergies

Past medical history: prostate cancer s/p chemotherapy and spinal radiation

Past surgical history: transurethral resection of the prostate (TURP), IR-guided vertebral body biopsy

Family history: none

Social history: former smoker

Physical examination: awake, alert, and oriented x 3; CNII–XII intact; bilateral deltoids/triceps/biceps 5/5; interossei 5/5; iliopsoas/knee flexion/knee extension/dorsi, and plantar flexion 5/5

Reflexes: 2+ in bilateral, biceps/triceps/brachioradialis with negative Hoffman; 2+ in bilateral patella/ankle; no clonus or Babinski; sensation is intact to light touch

Laboratories: all within normal limits

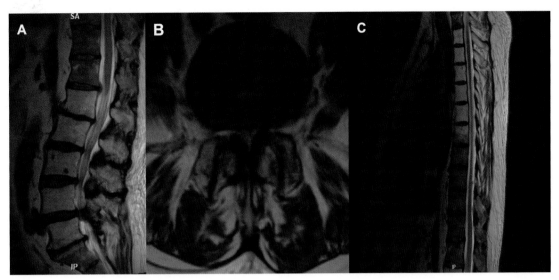

Fig. 45.1 Preoperative magnetic resonance imaging (MRI). (A) Sagittal T2, **(B)** axial T2 at the level of L4/5, and **(C)** sagittal T2 thoracic images demonstrating postradiation T2 hyperintensity at L1-5 and T2-7. There is evidence of multilevel lumbar spondylosis with severe L4-5 central canal stenosis secondary to disc bulge, ligamentum flavum thickening, and facet hypertrophy.

	Carlos A. Bagley, MD Neurosurgery University of Texas Southwestern Dallas, Texas, United States	Mohamed El-Fiki, MBBCh, MS, MD Neurosurgery Alexandria University Alexandria, Egypt	Tong Meng, MD Orthopaedic Surgery Shanghai General Hospital Shanghai Jiaotong University Shanghai, China	Meic H. Schmidt, MD, MBA Neurosurgery University of New Mexico Albuquerque, New Mexico, United States
Preoperative				
Additional tests requested	L-spine standing x-rays Physical therapy Physiatrist of lumbar injections Geriatrics evaluation	PET CT chest Creatinine level Lower extremity Dopplers Electrophysiological evaluation	MRI L-spine CT L-spine PET Oncology evaluation Urology evaluation	Anesthesia evaluation
Surgical approach selected	If fails conservative measures, L4 laminectomy and bilateral foraminotomies	L4-5 endoscopic discectomy and bilateral foraminotomy	If survival greater than a year, L4-5 TLIF	Left MIS L4-5 bilateral decompression
Goal of surgery	Nerve root decompression	Nerve root decompression	Nerve root decompression	Nerve root decompression
Perioperative				
Positioning	Prone on Jackson table	Prone	Prone	Prone on Wilson frame
Surgical equipment	Fluoroscopy	Fluoroscopy Surgical microscope Endoscope	Ultrasonic bone scalpel Electrical drill Fluoroscopy	Fluoroscopy Surgical microscope Electric drill Tubular retraction system
Medications	Pregabalin	None	Steroids	None
Anatomical considerations	Thecal sac, nerve roots, facet joints	Lumbar nerve roots	Lumbar nerve roots	Lumbar nerve roots, dura
Complications feared with approach chosen	Spinal instability	CSF leak, nerve root injury	CSF leak, nerve root injury	CSF leak, spinal instability
Intraoperative				
Anesthesia	General	General	General	General
Exposure	L4-5	L4-5	L4-5	Left L4-5 lamina
Levels decompressed	L4-5	L4-5	L4-5	Left L4-5 lamina and bilateral foraminotomies

	Carlos A. Bagley, MD Neurosurgery University of Texas Southwestern Dallas, Texas, United States	Mohamed El-Fiki, MBBCh, MS, MD Neurosurgery Alexandria University Alexandria, Egypt	Tong Meng, MD Orthopaedic Surgery Shanghai General Hospital Shanghai Jiaotong University Shanghai, China	Meic H. Schmidt, MD, MBA Neurosurgery University of New Mexico Albuquerque, New Mexico, United States
Levels fused	None	None	L4-5	None
Surgical narrative	Position prone, localize intercristal line, make 1-inch incision at intercristal line, subperiosteal dissection to expose spinous process and proximal lamina, x-ray to confirm level, adjust incision ½ or less if necessary, place retractors, remove spinous process and superficial lamina of L4 with Leksell rongeur, drill away remnants of L4 lamina, define plane between dura and ligamentum flavum, remove ligamentum and wide laminectomy with Kerrison rongeur, undercut overgrown facets with Kerrison, generous foraminotomies bilaterally, probe foramen and obtain final x-ray in L4-5 foramen, irrigate with bacitracin lactated ringers, multilayer closure	Position prone, confirm level with x-ray, midline skin incision over L4-5 space and dissect down to lamina, confirm level with x-ray, introduce microscope or use endoscopy with tube directed toward inferior border of L4, sequential dilation, then lock endoscope, remove soft tissue from posterior border of laminofacet junction, proceed to base of spinous process, drill lower 1.5cm of the L4 lamina until junction with inferior articular facet, remove ligamentum flavum on inner surface of L4, remove 0.5cm of lower L5 lamina, remove ligamentum until expose shoulder of nerve root, perform adequate foraminotomy so annulus seen with slight medial retraction of nerve root, open annulus and evacuate disc material, additional foraminotomy until nerve root is lax and pulsating, maintain integrity of facets, continue drilling medially to remove base of spinous process and cross to opposite side, decompress contralateral root, contralateral foraminotomy, apply vancomycin in wound, layered closure with drain	Position prone, posterior midline incision, place L4-5 pedicle screws, L4-5 laminectomy, expose and remove ligamentum flavum, facetectomy, resect posterior bony elements, mobilize dural and neural elements to access posterior annulus and disc space without any dural tension, distract with triple distraction technique, enlarge a window on the disc to protect exiting and traversing nerve roots, resect disc, place appropriate sized interbody cage packed with bone graft, confirm location by fluoroscopy, restore lordosis, perform contralateral facetectomy, closure in layers	Position prone with maximum lumbar flexion, fluoroscopy to determine level, left paraspinal muscle dissection down to lamina, place tubular retractor, laminectomy to ligamentum flavum under microscope, ipsilateral ligamentum flavum removed, ipsilateral foraminotomy, view contralateral side and resect contralateral ligamentum flavum, contralateral foraminotomy
Complication avoidance	No fusion, target radicular nerve pain, undercut overgrown facets, generous foraminotomies	MIS, endoscopy, partial laminectomy, additional foraminotomy until nerve root is lax and pulsating, maintain integrity of facets, unilateral approach to decompress bilaterally	Mobilize dura and neural elements, distract with triple distraction technique, bilateral facetectomy	Ipsilateral approach for bilateral decompression
Postoperative				
Admission	Floor	Floor	Floor	Floor
Postoperative complications feared	Infection, hematoma, medical complication	CSF leak, neurological deficit, infection, medical complication	CSF leak, neurological deficit	CSF leak, spinal instability
Anticipated length of stay	1 day	1–2 days	4–5 days	23 hours
Follow-up testing	None	L-spine x-ray every 3 months for 1 year after surgery	Lumbar x-rays 1 day, 3 months, 6 months after surgery MRI L-spine 3 days after surgery	Upright AP/lateral L-spine x-rays
Bracing	None	None	Lumbar support for 3–4 weeks	None
Follow-up visits	6 weeks after surgery	2 weeks, every 1 month for 1 year after surgery	3 and 6 months after surgery	3, 6, 12 months with x-rays after surgery

AP, Anteroposterior; *CSF*, cerebrospinal fluid; *CT*, computed tomography; *ICU*, intensive care unit; *IOM*, intraoperative monitoring; *MIS*, minimally invasive surgery; *MRI*, magnetic resonance imaging; *PET*, positron emission tomography.

Differential diagnosis

- Lumbar spinal stenosis
- Metastatic spine disease with possible epidural compression
- Synovial cyst
- Postradiation myelopathy

Important anatomical considerations

The lumbar spine has significantly more mobility than the semirigid thoracic spine and the rigid sacral spine, which allows for unique biomechanical properties that must be considered when planning surgery in this region. The lumbar facet joints are oriented in the sagittal plane unlike the joints in the thoracic spine, which are oriented in the coronal plane. It is important to determine whether the symptomatology of the patient is secondary to compression of the exiting nerve root at the corresponding neural foramen or whether the compression is of the traversing nerve root in the lateral recess. Lateral recess stenosis is typically secondary to hypertrophy of the superior articulating process and ligamentum flavum, thus a medial facetectomy is typically required to adequately address this form of compression. When the compression is at the level of the neural foramen, this can be identified by first finding the pedicle of the level of interest, as the corresponding foramen will be immediately caudal to the pedicle. When performing a laminectomy, consideration must be made to avoid destabilization of the spinal column. Removing more than the medial one-third of the facet join will increase the risk of instability. Also, identification of the lateral border of the pars interarticularis will prevent inadvertently causing a pars defect during the laminectomy. The location of the lumbar nerve roots should also be considered. The lumbar nerve roots will be immediately caudal to the corresponding pedicle. For example, the left L5 nerve root will be located at the inferior surface of the left L5 pedicle.

Approaches to this lesion

In this patient with spinal stenosis secondary to degenerative spondylosis and concomitant spinal metastatic disease, the two primary approaches are nonsurgical and surgical management. Nonsurgical approaches to treatment of this patient include pain medications, physical therapy with core strengthening, and epidural or transforaminal injections. For patients with significant medical comorbidities, conservative management strategies may be favored to decrease risk of adverse events during the surgical procedure. If the decision is made to proceed with surgery, the next decision is to determine whether the patient would be best managed with a decompressive surgery alone or decompression plus fusion.[7,8] The factors that determine this include the presence of dynamic instability on flexion-extension imaging, the presence of grade II or higher spondylolisthesis, and mechanical pain due to instability. There has been a surge in the use of minimally invasive surgeries for both decompression and instrumentation of the spine, with studies showing anywhere from noninferiority to superiority of minimally invasive procedure for treatment of spinal pathologies.[9,10,11] Endoscopy is an emerging minimally invasive approach that could also be employed, but there is an initial learning curve that must be overcome. Studies have shown good outcomes using the endoscope for patients with lumbar spinal stenosis.[12]

What was actually done

The patient had a history of metastatic prostate cancer with metastasis to multiple vertebral bodies including C6, T1, T2, and T9 and multiple liver metastases. He was seen by the oncology department to determine his estimated life capacity. He was given an estimated survival of over 6 months, and thus surgical decompression of his L4-5 level to address his progressively worsening pain and weakness was offered. The patient was positioned prone on a Wilson frame, with the spine placed into a lordotic position to open the interlaminar spaces. Using a vertical midline incision, the spinous processes and lamina of L4-L5 were exposed bilaterally. An intraoperative x-ray was taken to identify the proper level. A decompressive laminectomy was performed at L4-L5 using a high-speed drill and a Leksell rongeur. The superior portion of the L5 lamina was removed and the lamina of L4 was removed well beyond the distal border of the ligamentum flavum. The medial border of the L4-L5 facets was then removed. The ligamentum flavum was removed and foraminotomy was performed over the L5 nerve roots bilaterally. Thorough exploration was performed to assure that the thecal sac and L5 nerve roots were well decompressed. The surgical bed was irrigated with bacitracin irrigation and the incision closed in layers. The patient had significant improvement in his lower extremity symptoms and was discharged on postoperative day 2. Follow-up imaging showed good decompression (Fig. 45.2). The patient unfortunately succumbed to his systemic disease 1 year after surgery.

Commonalities among the experts

There was general consensus as to the overall goals of surgery in this case being decompression of the neural foramen in a patient with symptomatic spinal stenosis. Half opted for a minimally invasive approach, with one surgeon planning for endoscopic decompression of the neural foramen. There is no high-level evidence to support or refute the use of minimally invasive procedures over conventional open procedures, but there may be an added benefit in situations where a more minimal approach is preferred due to patient-specific

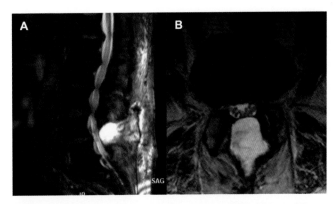

Fig. 45.2 Postoperative magnetic resonance imaging (MRI). (A) Sagittal T2 weighted and **(B)** axial T2 at the level of L4-5 images displaying evidence of L4-5 laminotomy defect. There is evidence of a small postoperative seroma with minimal effacement of the thecal sac.

factors. Half also recommended use of medications to help with pain and swelling, with one surgeon planning for pregabalin use and another for use of steroids. Only one surgeon opted for fusion of the level of interest, with the added caveat that this would be considered only if the life expectancy for the patient was greater than 1 year. All were cognizant of the thecal sac and nerve root, and the most common feared complications were cerebrospinal fluid leak, nerve root injury, and instability. All would admit to the floor, and most advocated for follow-up lumbar x-rays.

SUMMARY OF QUALITY OF EVIDENCE TO GUIDE SPECIFIC INTERVENTIONS FOR THIS CASE

- In patients with lumbar spinal stenosis, with or without degenerative spondylolisthesis, decompression surgery plus fusion surgery did not result in better clinical outcomes at 2 years and 5 years than did decompression surgery alone: level I A
- Surgery results in improved outcomes compared with nonsurgical management for patients with symptomatic lumbar stenosis without spondylolisthesis: level I A
- Minimally invasive decompression resulted in lower reoperation and need for fusion compared with open surgery for patients with lumbar spinal stenosis and low-grade spondylolisthesis: level II A
- Endoscopy microdiscectomy showed favorable clinical outcomes, less pain, and a shorter hospital stay compared with microscopic surgery in patients with lumbar spinal stenosis: level I B

REFERENCES

1. Abrams HL, Spiro R, Goldstein N. Metastases in carcinoma; analysis of 1000 autopsied cases. *Cancer*. 1950;3(1):74–85.
2. Disibio G, French SW. Metastatic patterns of cancers: results from a large autopsy study. *Arch Pathol Lab Med*. 2008;132(6):931–939.
3. Klimo Jr. P, Schmidt MH. Surgical management of spinal metastases. *Oncologist*. 2004;9(2):188–196.
4. Galgano M, et al. Surgical management of spinal metastases. *Expert Rev Anticancer Ther*. 2018;18(5):463–472.
5. Cobb 3rd CA, Leavens ME, Eckles N. Indications for nonoperative treatment of spinal cord compression due to breast cancer. *J Neurosurg*. 1977;47(5):653–658.
6. Kanna RM, et al. The impact of routine whole spine MRI screening in the evaluation of spinal degenerative diseases. *Eur Spine J*. 2017; 26(8):1993–1998.
7. Forsth P, et al. A Randomized, Controlled Trial of Fusion Surgery for Lumbar Spinal Stenosis. *N Engl J Med*. 2016;374(15):1413–1423.
8. Weinstein JN, et al. Surgical versus nonsurgical therapy for lumbar spinal stenosis. *N Engl J Med*. 2008;358(8):794–810.
9. Mobbs RJ, et al. Outcomes after decompressive laminectomy for lumbar spinal stenosis: comparison between minimally invasive unilateral laminectomy for bilateral decompression and open laminectomy: clinical article. *J Neurosurg Spine*. 2014;21(2):179–186.
10. Ang CL, et al. Minimally invasive compared with open lumbar laminotomy: no functional benefits at 6 or 24 months after surgery. *Spine J*. 2015;15(8):1705–1712.
11. Akinduro OO, et al. Open Versus Minimally Invasive Surgery for Extraforaminal Lumbar Disk Herniation: A Systematic Review and Meta-Analysis. *World Neurosurg*. 2017;108:924–938. e3.
12. Kim JE, Choi DJ, Park EJ. Clinical and Radiological Outcomes of Foraminal Decompression Using Unilateral Biportal Endoscopic Spine Surgery for Lumbar Foraminal Stenosis. *Clin Orthop Surg*. 2018;10(4):439–447.

46

Spinal chondrosarcoma

Oluwaseun O. Akinduro, MD and Tito Vivas-Buitrago, MD

Introduction

Chondrosarcomas are primary malignant tumors that may arise from the cranial skull base or axial skeleton and are characterized by neoplastic growth of hyaline cartilaginous tissue.[1] Primary spinal tumors such as chondrosarcoma only account for about 4% to 13% of all primary bone tumors, but their ability to cause compression of the spinal cord and propensity to recur make them difficult to manage.[2] Primary malignant bone tumors include chordoma, osteosarcoma, and chondrosarcomas, with chondrosarcomas being the most infrequent of these. Chondrosarcomas are a heterogeneous group of tumors with five known subtypes, as follows: conventional, dedifferentiated, clear-cell, mesenchymal, and myxoid.[1] An analysis of the SEER database found that the dedifferentiated subtype had the highest rate of metastasis and shortest progression-free survival among all of the subtypes.[3,4] There are no U.S. Food and Drug Administration (FDA)-approved drugs to combat this aggressive tumor, and unresectable chondrosarcomas have a 5-year survival rate of just 2%.[5] In the past decade there has been a surge of interest in identifying molecular targets for various tumors including chondrosarcoma. Many mutations and pathways have been studied for their role in development and progression of oncogenesis in patients with chondrosarcoma, including isocitrate dehydrogenase (IDH) mutations, sonic hedgehog (SHH) pathway, and the PI3K–Akt–mTOR pathway.[5] Despite an increased understanding of potential targets for chondrosarcoma treatment, patients must all undergo staging of their tumor with consideration of potential en bloc curative resection. Enneking developed a system for staging of sarcomatous tumors that incorporates tumor grading and compartment.[6]

This system divides benign tumors into three stages and malignant tumors into four stages. Although the Enneking staging system was created for long bone tumors, it has been applied to tumors of the mobile and fixed spine (Table 46.1).[7] The *sin qua non* of surgical management for these tumors is en bloc curative resection, but due to the rarity of these lesions, few surgeons have adequate expertise to complete these challenging surgeries. These cases are typically referred to academic tertiary care institutions with multidisciplinary teams able to manage these complex patients.

Example case

Chief complaint: back and leg pain

History of present illness: This is a 65-year-old female with back pain who presents after a computed tomography (CT)-guided biopsy of a T10 lesion that demonstrated chondrosarcoma (Fig. 46.1).

Medications: acetaminophen

Allergies: no known drug allergies

Past medical history: none

Past surgical history: none

Family history: no history of malignances

Social history: none

Physical examination: awake, alert, and oriented to person, place, and time; cranial nerves II–XII intact; bilateral deltoids/triceps/biceps 5/5; interossei 5/5; iliopsoas/knee flexion/knee extension/dorsi, and plantar flexion 5/5

Reflexes: 2+ in bilateral biceps/triceps/brachioradialis with negative Hoffman; 2+ in bilateral patella/ankle; no clonus or Babinski; sensation is intact to light touch

Laboratories: all within normal limits

Table 46.1 Summary of Enneking Surgical Staging Score

Surgical Grade (G)		Surgical Sites (T)	
Low G1	High G2	Intracompartmental (T1)	Extracompartmental (T2)
Secondary chondrosarcoma	Primary chondrosarcoma	Intraosseous	Soft-tissue extension
Chordoma	Classic	Intraarticular	Extrafascial planes or spaces
Fibrosarcoma	Pleomorphic liposarcoma	Superficial to deep fascia	Deep fascial extension Intraosseous or extrafascial
Giant cell tumor, bone	Hemangiopericytoma	Paraosseous	
Hemangiopericytoma	Osteosarcoma	Intrafascial compartments	
Kaposi sarcoma	Radiation sarcoma		
Atypical malignant fibrous histiocytoma	Paget sarcoma		
Myxoid liposarcoma	Neurofibrosarcoma Synovial sarcoma Rhabdomyosarcoma		
Surgical Stages			
IA	G_1		T_1
IB	G_1		T_2
IIA	G_2		T_1
IIB	G_2		T_2
III	Any G with metastasis		Any T

Adapted from Enneking WF, Spanier SS, Goodman MA. A system for the surgical staging of musculoskeletal sarcoma. *Clin Orthop Relat Res*. 1980;106-120.

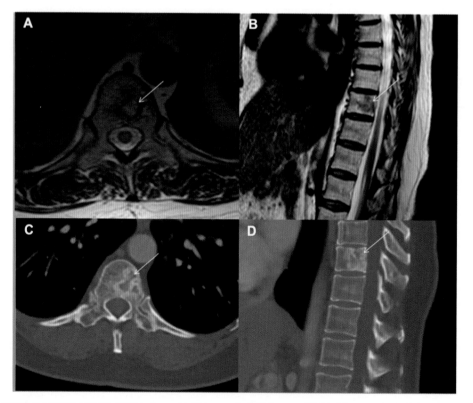

Fig. 46.1 Preoperative magnetic resonance imaging (MRI) and computed tomography (CT) images. (A) Axial T2 centered at the T10 vertebral body demonstrating an area of T2 hyperintensity within the bone with surrounding hypointensity; **(B)** sagittal T2 demonstrating an abnormal lesion within the T10 vertebral body, **(C)** axial CT of the T1 vertebral body, with an arrow highlighting a lytic lesion with surrounding sclerosis; and **(D)** sagittal CT demonstrating sclerosis of the T10 vertebral body.

	Ziya L. Gokaslan, MD Tianyi Niu, MD Brown University Providence, Rhode Island, United States	Tong Meng, MD Orthopaedic Surgery Shanghai General Hospital Shanghai Jiaotong University Shanghai, China	Mohamed A.R. Soliman, MD MSc, PhD Neurosurgery Cairo University Cairo, Egypt	Daniel M. Sciubba, MD Jeffrey Ehresman, BS Neurosurgery Johns Hopkins Baltimore, Maryland, United States
Preoperative				
Additional tests requested	MRI brain and complete spine CT head and complete spine PET	MRI thoracic and lumbar spine to evaluate blood supply Lumbar x-rays Thoracic CT and pulmonary function test Possible PET	MRI cervical spine CT chest/abdomen/pelvis PET DEXA Oncology and anesthesia evaluation	CT chest/abdomen/pelvis Standing 36-inch scoliosis x-rays DEXA
Surgical approach selected	En bloc T10 spondylectomy, T7-L2 posterior instrumentation and fusion	En bloc T10 spondylectomy, T8-12 posterior fusion	En bloc T10 posterolateral extracavitary resection with T9-T11 posterior fusion	En bloc T10 vertebrectomy via bilateral extracavitary approach with anterior reconstruction and T8 12 fusion
Goal of surgery	En bloc resection, reconstruction of the spine, stabilization	En bloc resection	En bloc resection, spinal fusion	En bloc resection, stabilization
Perioperative				
Positioning	Prone on Jackson table	Prone	Prone on Jackson table	Prone on Jackson table
Surgical equipment	Fluoroscopy Surgical navigation IOM (MEP/SSEP) Tomita saw Silastic sheath	Threadwire saws Ultrasonic bone scalpel Fluoroscopy	Surgical navigation Fluoroscopy IOM Surgical microscope	IOM (MEP/SSEP) Fenestrated screws with PMMA
Medications	Maintain MAP	Steroids, cisplatin (1:1 with distilled water)	Steroids, maintain MAP, osteoporotic medication if needed	Tranexamic acid, MAP >90
Anatomical considerations	Pleura, spinal cord	T10 vertebral level, T10 nerve roots, great vessels	T10 vertebral level, Aorta, azygous vein, spinal cord, dura, pleura	Aorta, pleura, dura/spinal cord, inferior vena cava
Complications feared with approach chosen	Violation of the tumor, spinal cord injury	Injury to spinal cord/great vessels/dura	Vascular injury, spinal cord injury, dural tear and CSF leak, pneumothorax, lung injury	CSF leak, pleural injury, spinal cord injury/ infarction, vascular injury
Intraoperative				
Anesthesia	General	General	General	General
Exposure	T7-L2	T8-12	T9-T11	T8-12
Levels decompressed	T9-10	T10	T10	T10
Levels fused	T7-L2	T8-T12	T9-11	T8-12

	Ziya L. Gokaslan, MD Tianyi Niu, MD Brown University Providence, Rhode Island, United States	Tong Meng, MD Orthopaedic Surgery Shanghai General Hospital Shanghai Jiaotong University Shanghai, China	Mohamed A.R. Soliman, MD MSc, PhD Neurosurgery Cairo University Cairo, Egypt	Daniel M. Sciubba, MD Jeffrey Ehresman, BS Neurosurgery Johns Hopkins Baltimore, Maryland, United States
Surgical narrative	Positioned prone, reference array attached and intraoperative CT once appropriate levels exposed, fuse CT with preoperative MRI, place pedicle screws from T7-L2 with navigation but skip T10 pedicles, expose bilateral 3–4 cm of T9-T10 ribs, dissect bilateral T10 ribs from pleura, cut 3 cm of the body of bilateral T10 ribs, bilateral facetectomy at T9-10 and T10-T11, complete T10 laminectomy and inferior T9 laminectomy, cut bilateral T10 pedicles flush with vertebral body, cut T10 nerves after tying with silk ties, dissect between pleural and vertebral body until ventral vertebral body reached bilaterally to create circumferential plane between vertebral body and great vessels anteriorly and lungs laterally, pass Silastic sheath around vertebral body from one side to other to protect vital structures, separate ventral dura from PLL, pass Tomita saw around disc space underneath ventral dura from one side to the other and then around ventral vertebral body back to side, discectomy using Tomita saw at T9-10 and T10-11, place temporary rod on one side, completely disconnect T10 vertebral body using #15 blade to disconnect discs/PLL/ALL, rotate and deliver T10 vertebral body away from temporary rod, inspect that no end plate violation occurred and tumor was not entered, place expandable cage, ensure position and size with fluoroscopy, place permanent rods on contralateral side and secure in place, connect two additional side rods onto primary rods to achieve four-rod construct, final tighten screws, split fibula graft placed in posterior defect to protect spinal cord and enhance fusion, place cross-link connectors between rods and final tighten, decorticate and place morselized allograft over all exposed bony surfaces, pulse lavage, place vancomycin powder, close in anatomical layers with plastic surgery with subfascial drains	Positioned prone, posterior median longitudinal incision, pedicle screws from T8 to 9 and T11-12 bilaterally, place right titanium rod, remove posterior structures of T10 with ultrasonic bone scalpel, ligate left T10 nerve root with nonabsorbable suture and section with scalpel, protect paravertebral muscles with saline-soaked gauze, resect part of the T10 rib, monitor for pleural defect, dissect bluntly between vertebral body and surround tissues including great vessels, place drain between vertebral body and great vessels, pass threadwire saw through the drain, divide T10 vertebral body with saws after confirming appropriate location of saws, remove vertebral body from left side by rotating the dissociative vertebral body, place titanium mesh cage filled with allograft bone, place contralateral rod with cross connectors, confirm location of internal fixation with x-ray, close in layers	Preoperative level marking using medical markers followed by AP and lateral x-rays to confirm level, position prone, confirm level with fluoroscopy, midline incision from one level above and below tumor site, subperiosteal dissection to exposure posterior elements including facet capsule/ transverse processes/ costovertebral joints/medial 4 cm of ribs, register navigation, place drill holes under navigation guidance one level above and below, decorticate spinous process/lamina/facet joints, T10 laminectomy as well as bottom of T9 and top of T11, resect ligamentum flavum and bilateral transverse processes of T10, preserve T10 nerve root if possible, remove bilateral T10 pedicles and superior articular facets with Leksell rongeur, remove T9-T10 and T10-T11 discs with annulotomy followed by discectomy using osteotome and pituitary rongeurs, slide surgical gauze to anterior aspect of vertebral body, separate the vertebral body using a 0.25-inch osteotome and high-speed drill, place screws on ipsilateral side with slightly kyphotic rod, same technique on opposite side until vertebral body separated, completely dissect PLL at T10 level, curettage inferior end plate of T9 and superior end plate of T11, separated 10th rib head from underlying pleura, resect rib 4 cm lateral to costovertebral junction using Kerrison rongeur, remove vertebral body en bloc by pushing it laterally and backward and avoid tension on the cord, place expandable cage of appropriate size filled with bone graft, place screws and rods on this side, intraoperative spin and fluoroscopy to confirm hardware location, place autograft on decorticated bone, closure in layers with subfascial drain	Position prone, plan incision with intraoperative x-ray, midline incision from T8 to 12, subperiosteal dissection, confirm levels with x-ray, cannulate pedicle screws T8-9 and T11-12 using anatomical landmarks, place screws in T8 and T12 for temporary rod, dissect laterally to expose T9 and T10 ribs and resect T10 ribs at angle by disarticulating from joint, transect bilateral T10 nerve roots proximal to dorsal root ganglion by first temporarily ligating nerve root containing radicular artery and running baseline MEP, circumferential dissection around T10 vertebral body paying attention to aorta and pleura, place remainder of screws, check position on x-rays, vertebroplasty trough fenestrated screws if poor bone quality, rods placed and distract, radical discectomies at T9-10 and T10-11, remove entire T10 vertebrae, prepare end plates, place titanium expandable cage with fibular allograft that is sized and in midline of anterior column, confirm position with x-ray, place final rods and compress, closure in layers with drain

	Ziya L. Gokaslan, MD Tianyi Niu, MD Brown University Providence, Rhode Island, United States	Tong Meng, MD Orthopaedic Surgery Shanghai General Hospital Shanghai Jiaotong University Shanghai, China	Mohamed A.R. Soliman, MD MSc, PhD Neurosurgery Cairo University Cairo, Egypt	Daniel M. Sciubba, MD Jeffrey Ehresman, BS Neurosurgery Johns Hopkins Baltimore, Maryland, United States
Complication avoidance	Surgical navigation, fuse intraoperative CT with preoperative MRI, sacrifice T10 nerve roots, Silastic sheath to protect vital structures before using saw, discectomy with Tomita saw, temporary rods to stabilize spine, inspect for tumor violation, en bloc resection, four-rod construct, use split fibular graft, plastics surgery closure	Placement of temporary unilateral rod, ligate T10 nerve roots retract paraspinal muscles with saline-soaked gauze, use of a drain to safely place wired saws, en bloc resection	Preoperative level marking, surgical navigation, attempt to save T10 nerve root, protect anterior structures with surgical gauze, alternate rod placement to prevent spine translation after corpectomy, use rib for graft material, en bloc resection	Anatomical placement of pedicle screws, temporary rod, transect bilateral T10 nerve roots after confirming by temporarily ligating and running MEP, vertebroplasty if necessary, en bloc resection
Postoperative				
Admission	ICU	ICU	Floor	ICU
Postoperative complications feared	Pleura violation, hardware migration, wound infection	CSF leak, neurological deficit, spinal instability	CSF leak, neurological deficit, hardware malposition, pneumothorax	CSF leak, spinal instability, nonunion
Anticipated length of stay	3–4 days	10 days	3–4 days	3–5 days
Follow-up testing	Standing x-rays before discharge and 3 months after surgery	Thoracolumbar x-rays within 1 day of surgery MRI and CT thoracolumbar spine within 3 days of surgery	CT thoracic spine within 1 day of surgery and 6 months after surgery MRI thoracic spine within 3 days of surgery	CT T-spine within 1 day of surgery
Bracing	None	Thoracic brace for 3-4 weeks	None	None
Follow-up visits	2 weeks, 3 months after surgery	CT and MRI at 3 and 6 months after surgery, followed by 6 month intervals for next 2 years, then annually	10–14 days, 4 weeks, 3 months, 6 months, 1 year after surgery	3 weeks after surgery

ALL, Anterior longitudinal ligament; *AP*, anteroposterior; *CSF*, cerebrospinal fluid; *CT*, computed tomography; *DEXA*, dual-energy x-ray absorptiometry; *ICU*, intensive care unit; *IOM*, intraoperative monitoring; *MEP*, motor evoked potential; *MIS*, minimally invasive surgery; *MRI*, magnetic resonance imaging; *PET*, positron emission tomography; *PLL*, posterior longitudinal ligament; *SSEP*, somatosensory evoked potential.

Differential diagnosis

- Primary bone tumors (chordoma, chondrosarcoma)
- Metastasis
- Multiple myeloma
- Infection

Important anatomical considerations

When surgical resection of a primary bone tumor such as chondrosarcoma is planned, a full systemic workup is required for staging purposes, as these tumors are known to metastasize from their primary location. The margin of resection should be wide in order to limit the potential for recurrence; however, wide excisional margins are not always a feasible and dependent on tumor location and involvement of adjacent structures.[8] The most important anatomical considerations at the T10 level will be the aorta, artery of Adamkiewicz, and the lung pleura, as injuries to any of these structures can have catastrophic effects on patients. The other anatomical consideration is the T10 nerve roots. A posterior-only approach will likely require sacrifice of the T10 nerve roots to have adequate space for placement of a graft. The roots can typically be sacrificed at this level with no clinical sequelae except for numbness along the T10 distribution. Care must be taken to transect the roots proximal to the dorsal root ganglion, to prevent a postoperative pain syndrome in that distribution. The aorta will typically be located anterior-lateral to the vertebral body on the left side with the vena cava located on the right. Care must be taken when dissecting on the lateral border of the vertebral body, as this maneuver may place the aorta at risk. Performing a preoperative angiogram is advantageous for locating the artery of Adamkiewicz, which is the primary blood supply to the spinal cord in this region. This artery is typically located between T8 and L3, with T9 or T10 being the most common, and 65% to 75% of them being noted on the left side.[9,10]

Approaches to this lesion

Surgical planning of primary spine tumors should include a biopsy for confirmation of diagnosis. The trajectory of the biopsy is of utmost importance, as this trajectory must be incorporated into the surgical trajectory to prevent seeding of tumor into the biopsy tract. For this reason, the ideal trajectory is typically transpedicular, as the pedicle can be removed during the procedure. The WBB (Weinstein, Boriani, Biagnini) surgical staging system is the primary method for determining the ideal surgical approach in primary bone tumors of the spinal column (Fig. 46.2). En bloc resection of tumors in the thoracic spine is associated with significant morbidity, but many studies have shown en bloc resection results in significantly improved progression-free survival for patients with primary tumors of the spine such as chondrosarcoma.[11–13] En bloc resection with wide margins can typically be performed safely for tumors that are confined to either zones 4 to 8 or 5 to 9, indicating that at least one pedicle is free of tumor. A posterior-only approach may be performed for tumors that involve only zones 3 to 10, but involvement of zones 5 to 8 may require a combined approach that includes removal of the posterior elements followed by an anterior or lateral approach for addressing the segmental vessels.

What was actually done

The patient was referred to our institution after a computed tomography (CT)-guided biopsy at an outside institution returned as chondrosarcoma of T10. She was taken for a bilateral T10 costotransversectomy, T9 and T10 laminectomy, and T7-L1 instrumented fusion. Prior to surgery, a spinal angiogram was performed to identify the location of the artery of Adamkiewicz, which was noted to originate from T9 on the left. The patient was taken to the operating room and placed into the prone position with use of motor evoked and somatosensory evoked potentials. A midline incision was used, with a subperiosteal dissection. After placement of pedicle screws

from T7-L1, skipping screws at T10, a laminectomy and facetectomies at T9-10 and T10-11 were performed, exposing the T10 nerve roots and skeletonizing the pedicles bilaterally. The T10 rib was then transected about 3cm distal to its origin, followed by removal of this portion of the rib to give visualization of the lateral aspect of the vertebral body. The T9-T10 and T10-11 disks were then removed along with the posterior longitudinal ligament. Using finger dissection anteriorly, the aorta was gently dissected away from the vertebral bodies. The azygos vein was identified on the preoperative imaging; however, it was somewhat adherent to the ventral vertebral body. The procedure was then staged with a transthoracic approach rather than resection of the anterior longitudinal ligament in a blind fashion for mobilization of the azygos vein. Stage two was completed with the assistance of a cardiothoracic surgeon for the approach. After identification of the T10 vertebral body, the anterior longitudinal ligament was divided, which allowed for en bloc removal of the vertebral body. The end plates were prepared with removal of cartilaginous material and an expandable cage was placed and packed with iliac crest autograft. The pathology returned as chondrosarcoma with confirmation of negative margins. The patient was taken to the intensive care unit after surgery with an intact neurological examination except for T10 distribution numbness. Postoperative x-rays revealed excellent hardware location (Fig. 46.3). The patient was discharged on postoperative day 5.

Commonalities among the experts

There was a general consensus that en bloc resection of the T10 vertebral body would be the ideal approach for this patient. All of the experts planned for preoperative imaging of the tumor, as well as imaging for staging purposes, although the modality for staging varied from surgeon to surgeon. There was also consensus as to the surgical approach for en bloc spondylectomy, as the experts all

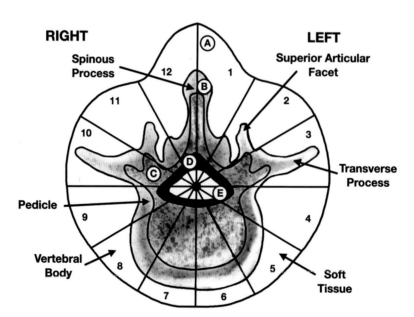

Fig. 46.2 Artist adaptation of the WBB (Weinstein, Boriani, Biagnini) surgical staging system. There are 12 radiating zones numbered 1 to 12 and five concentric layers A to E. A corresponds to the extraosseous soft tissues, B to the superficial intraosseous compartment, C to the deep intraosseous compartment, D to the extradural extraosseous compartment, and E to the intradural extraosseous compartment.

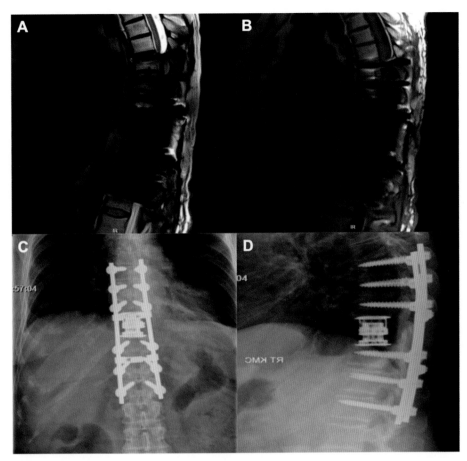

Fig. 46.3 Postoperative MRI and x-rays. (A) Sagittal T2 MRI demonstrating artifact from the instrumentation, **(B)** sagittal T1 with contrast MRI demonstrating no evidence of residual tumor, **(C)** anteroposterior x-ray demonstrating intact instrumentation from T7 to L1 and expandable cage at T10, and **(D)** lateral x-ray demonstrating good alignment and positioning of the hardware.

opted for a posterior approach with instrumented fusion, although there was mild variation in the levels of instrumentation. There was a split among the surgeons concerning the use of perioperative steroids, with two experts opting for steroid use and two surgeons not planning to use steroids. All surgeons opted for removal of 3 to 4 cm of the T10 ribs to allow for a posterior-lateral approach to the vertebral body. There was a wide variation in the planned postoperative imaging modality. Half planned to perform a CT of the construct during the admission, and half planned to perform magnetic resonance imaging (MRI) within 3 days of surgery.

SUMMARY OF QUALITY OF EVIDENCE TO GUIDE SPECIFIC INTERVENTIONS FOR THIS CASE

- En bloc resection is associated with improved prognosis and lower local recurrence: level IIA
- Proton radiation results in favorable local control, survival, and toxicity: level IIB
- Surgical resection followed by high-dose focused radiotherapy is effective in long-term control of spinal chondrosarcoma: level IIB
- Low-grade chondrosarcoma of the osseous spine is resistant to RT, while high-grade chondrosarcoma may have a better response to radiation: level IIA

- Patients referred early for primary adjuvant radiation therapy after surgery had higher rates of disease control than those referred for salvage treatment of recurrent disease: level IIA

REFERENCES

1. Chow WA. Chondrosarcoma: biology, genetics, and epigenetics. *F1000Res*. 2018;7
2. Kelley SP, Ashford RU, Rao AS, Dickson RA. Primary bone tumours of the spine: a 42-year survey from the Leeds Regional Bone Tumour Registry. *Eur Spine J*. 2007;16:405–409.
3. Amer KM, Munn M, Congiusta D, Abraham JA, Basu Mallick A. Survival and Prognosis of Chondrosarcoma Subtypes: SEER Database Analysis. *J Orthop Res*. 2020;38:311–319.
4. Arshi A, Sharim J, Park DY, Park HY, Bernthal NM, Yazdanshenas H, et al. Chondrosarcoma of the Osseous Spine: An Analysis of Epidemiology, Patient Outcomes, and Prognostic Factors Using the SEER Registry From 1973 to 2012. *Spine (Phila Pa 1976)*. 2017;42:644–652.
5. Speetjens FM, de Jong Y, Gelderblom H, Bovee JV. Molecular oncogenesis of chondrosarcoma: impact for targeted treatment. *Curr Opin Oncol*. 2016;28:314–322.
6. Enneking WF, Spanier SS, Goodman MA. A system for the surgical staging of musculoskeletal sarcoma. *Clin Orthop Relat Res*. 1980: 106–120.
7. Boriani S, Amendola L, Bandiera S, Simoes CE, Alberghini M, Di Fiore M, et al. Staging and treatment of osteoblastoma in the mobile spine: a review of 51 cases. *Eur Spine J*. 2012;21:2003–2010.

8. Oluwaseun OA, Diogo PG, Ricardo AD, Tito V-B, Bernardo S-P, Mohamad B, et al. Cervical chordomas: multicenter case series and meta-analysis. *J Neurooncol.* 2021;153(1):65–77.

9. Bley TA, Duffek CC, Francois CJ, Schiebler ML, Acher CW, Mell M, et al. Presurgical localization of the artery of Adamkiewicz with time-resolved 3.0-T MR angiography. *Radiology.* 2010;255:873–881.

10. Charles YP, Barbe B, Beaujeux R, Boujan F, Steib JP. Relevance of the anatomical location of the Adamkiewicz artery in spine surgery. *Surg Radiol Anat.* 2011;33:3–9.

11. Boriani S, Bandiera S, Colangeli S, Ghermandi R, Gasbarrini A. En bloc resection of primary tumors of the thoracic spine: indications, planning, morbidity. *Neurol Res.* 2014;36:566–576.

12. Yamazaki T, McLoughlin GS, Patel S, Rhines LD, Fourney DR. Feasibility and safety of en bloc resection for primary spine tumors: a systematic review by the Spine Oncology Study Group. Spine (Phila Pa 1976). 2009;34:S31–38.

13. Zhang XM, Fournel L, Lupo A, Canny E, Bobbio A, Lasry S, et al. En Bloc Resection of Thoracic Tumors Invading the Spine: A Single-Center Experience. *Ann Thorac Surg.* 2019;108:227–234.

47

Intradural extramedullary tumor

Oluwaseun O. Akinduro, MD and Kingsley Abode-Iyamah, MD

Introduction

Intradural extramedullary (IDEM) tumors arise within the confines of the dura mater but are not intrinsic to the spinal cord itself. Epidemiological studies have reported an incidence of approximately 0.74 per 100,000 person years.[1] These tumors are typically considered benign, with the most common being meningiomas, followed by nerve sheath tumors.[2] Despite being benign, IDEM tumors can lead to significant morbidity secondary to direct compression of the spinal cord, also leading to debilitating weakness. These tumors may be seen in conjunction with syndromes such as neurofibromatosis and schwannomatosis, which will likely alter the management strategy, as these patients tend to be younger in age with multiple tumors growing at different rates.[3,4] The most common presentation for these tumors is pain, which may be radicular or axial back pain, and since these tumors grow slowly over time, they may present with progressively worsening myelopathy from spinal cord compression. It is rare for these tumors to present with spinal instability, and when

instability is present, one should include more aggressive tumors in the differential diagnosis. In this chapter, we will discuss the management and surgical tenets for a patient with a large ventral IDEM tumor.

Example case

Chief complaint: weakness

History of present illness: This is a 69-year-old male with a history of weight loss as well as atrophy of his upper extremity. In addition, he has had difficulty with ambulation and increasing loss of dexterity over the past couple of weeks. This has progressively worsened, and he has significantly deteriorated over this period of time. He underwent imaging concerning for a spinal cord tumor (Fig. 47.1).

Medications: tamsulosin

Allergies: no known drug allergies

Past medical history: weight loss, prostate cancer status post radiation

Past surgical history: none

Family history: noncontributory

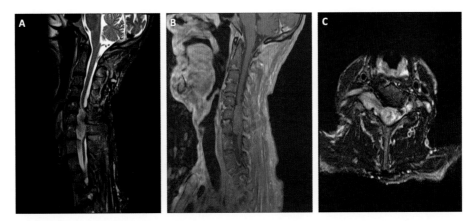

Fig. 47.1 Preoperative magnetic resonance images. (A) T2 sagittal, **(B)** T1 sagittal with contrast, and **(C)** T2 axial images demonstrating an intradural extramedullary lesion that extends from C5 to 7 that is ventral and paracentric to the right of the spinal cord.

Social history: nonsmoker

Physical examination: awake, alert, and oriented x 3; cranial nerves CNII–XII intact

Motor: right: deltoids/triceps/biceps/interossei 3/5; left: deltoids/triceps/biceps/interossei 4/5; bilateral iliopsoas/knee flexion/knee extension/dorsi, and plantar flexion 4/5

Reflexes: 2+ in bilateral biceps/triceps/brachioradialis with negative Hoffman; 2+ in bilateral patella/ankle; no clonus or Babinski; sensation intact to light touch

Laboratories: basic metabolic panel, heme-8, coagulation all within normal limits

	Mark H. Bilsky, MD Neurosurgery Memorial Sloan Kettering Cancer Center New York, New York, United States	Ciaran Bolger, MD Royal College of Surgeons Catherine Moran, MD Neurosurgery Tallaght University Hospital Dublin, Ireland	Nicolas Dea, MD, MSc Neurosurgery Vancouver Spine Surgery Institute Vancouver, Canada	Maziyar A. Kalani, MD Neurosurgery Mayo Clinic Phoenix, Arizona, United States
Preoperative				
Additional tests requested	CTA C-spine MRI brain and complete spine Bilateral lower extremity Dopplers Medical evaluation	MRI brain and complete spine CT chest/abdomen/pelvis PSA Vertebral angiogram	Flexion-extension C-spine x-rays CT/CTA C-spine Oncology evaluation Chest/abdomen/pelvis CT for staging	CT/CTA C-spine MRI brain and complete spine ENT evaluation
Surgical approach selected	C5-T1 laminectomy and resection of tumor with C5-T1 posterior fusion	C5-C7 laminectomy and resection of tumor with possible C5-C7 posterior fusion	C5-T1 laminectomy and resection of tumor with C4-T2 posterior fusion	
Goal of surgery	Spinal cord decompression	Spinal cord decompression, gross total resection	Diagnosis, spinal cord decompression, tumor removal, spinal fusion	Diagnosis, spinal cord decompression, tumor removal, spinal fusion
Perioperative				
Positioning	Prone with Mayfield pins	Prone with Mayfield pins	Prone on Jackson table with Mayfield pins	Prone with Mayfield pins
Surgical equipment	IOM (SSEP/MEP/EMG) Fluoroscopy Surgical microscope Ultrasound Nerve stimulator Ultrasonic aspirator	IOM Fluoroscopy Surgical microscope Ultrasonic aspirator Doppler	IOM (SSEP/MEP/EMG) Surgical navigation Ultrasound Ultrasonic aspirator	IOM Fluoroscopy Ultrasound Ultrasonic aspirator
Medications	Steroids	Steroids, mannitol, MAP >80	Steroids, MAP 85	Steroids, MAP >85
Anatomical considerations	Spinal cord, right C6, C7-C8 motor nerve roots	Spinal cord, nerve roots, vertebral artery, right-side facet joint	Spinal cord, C6 and C7 nerve roots, vertebral arteries	Spinal cord, right C6, C7-C8 motor nerve roots, dentate ligaments
Complications feared with approach chosen	Progressive neurological decline	Instability, spinal cord/nerve root injury, vertebral artery injury, dysphagia	Nerve root injury	New weakness, pseudomeningocele, spinal cord infarct
Intraoperative				
Anesthesia	General	General	General	General
Exposure	C5-T1	C5-T1	C4-T2	C4-T1
Levels decompressed	C5-T1	C5-C7	C5-T1	C5-7
Levels fused	C5-T1	C5-C7 if needed	C4-T2	C4-T1

	Mark H. Bilsky, MD Neurosurgery Memorial Sloan Kettering Cancer Center New York, New York, United States	Ciaran Bolger, MD Royal College of Surgeons Catherine Moran, MD Neurosurgery Tallaght University Hospital Dublin, Ireland	Nicolas Dea, MD, MSc Neurosurgery Vancouver Spine Surgery Institute Vancouver, Canada	Maziyar A. Kalani, MD Neurosurgery Mayo Clinic Phoenix, Arizona, United States
Surgical narrative	Position prone, IOM, fluoroscopy to confirm levels, placement of C5-7 lateral mass and T1 pedicle screws, delay right rod placement until end of case, spinous process resection C5-7 and partial T1 with Leksell rongeur, laminectomy with 3 mm matchstick, resect ligamentum flavum with a #15 blade, ultrasound to confirm laminectomy sufficient, operating microscope brought in, dura opened and tacked back, arachnoid opened sharply, identify tumor/ spinal cord interface, nerve stimulator on posterior capsule of tumor, sharp opening in pia with #11 blade, intralesional debulking with ultrasonic aspirator, frozen section for diagnosis, sequential debulking of tumor away from spinal cord, fascicles giving rise to the tumor are sacrificed, great care to preserve functional motor nerve fascicles at 0.1 mA, dural closure with running nonlocking suture, thrombin glue and Gelfoam are placed over durotomy, drain placed in epidural space, suction for 24 hours and then straight drainage	Position prone, midline incision exposing spinous process of C5-T1, midline laminectomy removing spinous processes and lamina C5-C7, undercut facet joint and expose involved foramen on right side, identify tumor in the foramen and fully expose medial dura, right-side T-shaped with limb extending laterally to involved nerve root, tack dura, arachnoid opened and tacked with clips, expose tumor along its length, dissect tumor away from cord medial to lateral and develop plane along its length, debulk with ultrasonic aspirator to allow tumor retraction away from cord toward foramen, lateral tumor may be delivered medially after sufficient debulking, attempt to preserve nerve as long as nonfunctional, care is taken to identify vertebral artery laterally with use of Doppler if needed, water-tight dural closure with patch if necessary, if risk of instability consider fusion from C5-7 with lateral mass screws and bone graft, layered closure	Position prone, expose C4-T2, predrill screw holes from C4 to T2 except C6-7 on the right with surgical navigation. C5-T1 laminectomy, intraoperative ultrasound to confirm tumor location, right lateral bony resection to reach extraforaminal component of the tumor, remove inferior facet of C6 and superior facet of C7, follow C7 nerve root laterally, midline durotomy under microscope, tack up dura, coagulate tumor capsule, intralesional tumor debulking with ultrasonic aspirator, frozen section, find arachnoid plane within spinal cord, debulk more tumor if necessary to decrease spinal cord manipulation, find rootlet origin of tumor and stimulate if necessary, remove if no stimulation, remove tumor laterally while constant nerve stimulation, water tight dural closure with onlay and glue if necessary, screws from C4 to T2, decorticate bone, layered closure with water tight facial closure	Position prone, Trendelenburg position, x-ray to plan incision from C4 to T1, midline incision, subperiosteal dissection, intraoperative x-ray to confirm levels, place lateral mass holes at C4 bilaterally/ left C5-6 using Magrel technique, place T1 pedicle screws bilaterally, en bloc laminectomy from C5 to 7, intraoperative ultrasound to assess exposure, midline dura opening and dura tacked up with arachnoid, plane is created medially between tumor and spinal cord bluntly and extended cranially and caudally, dentate ligaments identified and sectioned after stimulating, tumor mobilized form medial to lateral to identify neural structures entering tumor and stimulated, internally debulk tumor after confirming lack of stimulation using ultrasonic aspirator to fold in tumor and identify en passage nerve roots, potential facetectomy to identify right nerve roots if needed, dural closure with GoreTex suture and fibrin glue, Valsalva to assess for leakage, place lateral mass screws at C4-6 bilaterally, secure rods, x-ray to assess instrumentation, final tighten, layered closure
Complication avoidance	Instrumentation prior to decompression, avoid Kerrison punches to avoid neurological injury, ultrasound, nerve stimulation to guide resection	Extend exposure on right side to identify foramen, right-side T-shaped with limb extending laterally to involved nerve root, expose tumor along its length and dissect from medial to lateral away from cord, debulk tumor to allow mobilization, identify vertebral artery	Lateral cord exposure, debulk tumor to minimize spinal cord manipulation, nerve stimulation to guide resection	Trendelenburg position to help with venous drainage, Magerl technique for lateral mass screws, en bloc laminectomy, intraoperative ultrasound to assess exposure, section dentate ligaments to mobilize spinal cord, stimulate structures to identify neural structures

	Mark H. Bilsky, MD Neurosurgery Memorial Sloan Kettering Cancer Center New York, New York, United States	Ciaran Bolger, MD Royal College of Surgeons Catherine Moran, MD Neurosurgery Tallaght University Hospital Dublin, Ireland	Nicolas Dea, MD, MSc Neurosurgery Vancouver Spine Surgery Institute Vancouver, Canada	Maziyar A. Kalani, MD Neurosurgery Mayo Clinic Phoenix, Arizona, United States
Postoperative				
Admission	ICU	ICU	Floor	Floor
Postoperative complications feared	Progressive myelopathy or functional radiculopathy	CSF leak, spinal instability, infection	New weakness from cord or root injury, CSF leak	New weakness, pseudomeningocele, spinal cord infarct
Anticipated length of stay	4 days	5–7 days	3–5 days	2–3 days
Follow-up testing	MRI 72 hours after surgery, prone with Mayfield pins	MRI C-spine prior to discharge	Cervical x-rays on discharge MRI C-spine 2–3 months after surgery	MRI C-spine 3 months after surgery CT C-spine 6 months after surgery
Bracing	None	None	None	None
Follow-up visits	3 weeks after surgery	2 weeks, 6 weeks, 6 months, 1 year after surgery	2 months after surgery	2 weeks, 6 weeks, 6 months, 1 year after surgery

CT, Computed tomography; *CTA*, computed tomography angiography; *EMG*, electromyography; *ENT*, ear, nose, and throat; *ICU*, intensive care unit; *IOM*, intraoperative monitoring; *MAP*, mean arterial pressure; *MEP*, motor evoked potential; *MRI*, magnetic resonance imaging; *PSA*, prostate specific antigen; *SSEP*, somatosensory evoked potential.

Differential diagnosis

- Schwannoma
- Meningioma
- Metastasis

Important anatomical considerations

There are multiple vascular and neurological structures to consider when planning surgery in the cervical spine. The nerve roots of the cervical spinal exit above the corresponding levels, which is especially important when decompression of a particular dermatomal distribution is needed for pain relief. Anterior to the spinal column lies the esophagus, trachea, and carotid arteries, which must be protected when approaching the cervical spine from an anterior approach. Lateral to the spinal cord, within the foramen transversarium, lay both vertebral arteries, which are often involved with tumor and may need to be sacrificed to obtain a gross total or en bloc resection of a cervical tumor.[5,6] If vertebral artery sacrifice is considered, patients should be evaluated with balloon occlusion of the vessel with concomitant clinical evaluation to confirm that the vessel may be sacrificed without clinical sequelae.[7,8] Tumors that are ventral to the spinal cord may require manipulation of the spinal cord when approaching the lesion posteriorly. The dentate ligaments are evaginations of pia that attach laterally to the dura mater to help stabilize the spinal cord.[9] Ligation of the dentate ligaments is safe and can assist with rotation of the spinal cord to minimize spinal cord manipulation during decompression of a ventrally located tumor. Many reports have shown the safety and efficacy of dentate ligament ligation for accessing the ventral spinal cord from a posterior approach.[10,11] The facet joints can also be removed to provide a more lateral access during posterior approach.

Although biomechanical study found that unilateral facetectomy only increased the intersegmental motion slightly after a laminectomy,[12] one must consider fusion of the spine when completing facetectomies, as these patients may be at increased risk for postlaminectomy kyphosis.[13–15]

Approaches to this lesion

The tumor depicted in this case is ventral to the cervical spinal cord, which presents as a challenge when considering the optimal surgical approach to resect this tumor and minimize the risk of further iatrogenic neurological decline. Deciding on the ideal approach may be challenging because there are significant risks to accessing this region anteriorly as well as posteriorly. One consideration is for an anterior approach, which would require one or more corpectomies to gain adequate visualization of the lesion. There have been reports describing the approach to the anterior cervical spinal cord with removal of the vertebral bodies to gain access to ventral tumors.[10,11,16–18] Dural repair may be challenging from this approach especially for IDEM tumors.

A posterior only approach may also be undertaken to access ventral cervical lesions. Surgeons are typically more comfortable with posterior approaches, and the risks associated with the esophagus, trachea, and carotid arteries are avoided. However, posterior approaches to the ventral spine may be associated with more risk of damage to the spinal cord. The primary things to consider when determining whether a tumor is amenable to posterior approach is whether the tumor has an en plaque ventral base, heavy calcifications, excessive bleeding, or significant bilateral extension, as these factors will make this a more difficult undertaking. A posterior approach to the ventral spinal cord includes performing a wide laminectomy and

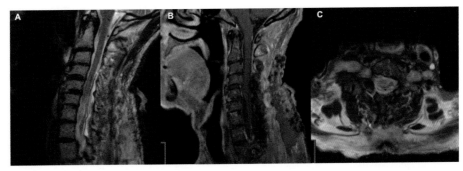

Fig. 47.2 Postoperative magnetic resonance images. (A) T2 sagittal, **(B)** T1 sagittal with contrast, and **(C)** T1 axial with contrast images demonstrating gross total resection of the intradural extramedullary lesion.

typically requires sectioning of multiple dentate ligaments to partially rotate the spinal cord. Tumors that are amenable to a posterior approach are easily internally debulked and eccentric to one side, as bilateral tumors would place patients at higher risk for postoperative neurological deficits.

What was actually done

The patient was positioned prone and secured to the operating room table using rigid fixation with a Mayfield headframe. During the procedure, intraoperative monitoring consisting of somatosensory and motor evoked potentials was used. A posterior midline approach was performed and a high-speed bur was used to perform a laminectomy from C4 down to T1. The lamina was elevated in an en bloc fashion after drilling bilateral troughs. The intraoperative ultrasound was used to confirm adequate exposure of the tumor prior to the midline durotomy. The tumor was identified and removed in a piecemeal fashion. There were nerve roots noted to be attached to the tumor, which raised suspicion for a neurofibroma. These were noted to be sensory in nature based on their exit from the spinal cord. Resection was completed up to the exiting portion of the foramina. The dura was closed in a watertight fashion. The lamina was secured back in place with a plating system. The patient tolerated the procedure well without any immediate postoperative complication. Postoperative imaging showed gross total resection of the lesion (Fig. 47.2).

Commonalities among the experts

All experts agreed with completion of further imaging, including vascular imaging. The majority recommended computed tomography angiography images of the cervical spine, and one recommended an angiogram to assess the vertebral artery for planning the surgical approach. There was consensus for approaching the lesion posteriorly with laminectomy from C5 to T1, with only slight variation in the suggested levels for fusion. All surgeons also opted for use of intraoperative neuromonitoring and perioperative steroids. The majority planned to use intraoperative ultrasound for lesion localization and three planned to use the ultrasonic aspirator to for internal decompression of the tumor. There was disagreement about the postoperative management with half opting for postoperative care in the intensive care unit and the other half opting for postoperative transfer to the floor.

SUMMARY OF QUALITY OF EVIDENCE TO GUIDE SPECIFIC INTERVENTIONS FOR THIS CASE

- Electromyography (EMG) should be considered during resection of IDEM tumors: level IIB[19]
- Radiosurgery is safe and efficacious for benign intramedullary tumors: level IIB[20,21]
- Gross total resection of spinal nerve sheath tumors results in excellent long-term control: level IC[22]
- Anterior approaches to the ventral spinal cord can be performed safely with an anterior corpectomy: level IIC[23]
- Posterior approaches to the ventral spinal cord can be performed safely via a laminectomy with or without instrumented fusion: level IIC

REFERENCES

1. Schellinger KA, Propp JM, Villano JL, McCarthy BJ. Descriptive epidemiology of primary spinal cord tumors. *J Neurooncol.* Apr 2008;87(2):173–179.
2. Duong LM, McCarthy BJ, McLendon RE, et al. Descriptive epidemiology of malignant and nonmalignant primary spinal cord, spinal meninges, and cauda equina tumors, United States, 2004-2007. *Cancer.* Sep 1 2012;118(17):4220–4227.
3. National Institutes of Health Consensus Development Conference Statement: neurofibromatosis. Bethesda, Md., USA, July 13–15, 1987. *Neurofibromatosis.* 1988;1(3):172-178.
4. Holland K, Kaye AH. Spinal tumors in neurofibromatosis-2: management considerations - a review. *J Clin Neurosci.* Feb 2009; 16(2):169–177.
5. George B. Management of the vertebral artery in excision of extradural tumors of the cervical spine. *Neurosurgery.* Oct 1995; 37(4):844–845.
6. Westbroek EM, Pennington Z, Ehresman J, Ahmed AK, Gailloud P, Sciubba DM. Vertebral Artery Sacrifice versus Skeletonization in the Setting of Cervical Spine Tumor Resection: Case Series. *World Neurosurg.* Jul 2020;139:e601–e607.
7. Lunardini DJ, Eskander MS, Even JL, et al. Vertebral artery injuries in cervical spine surgery. *Spine J.* Aug 1, 2014;14(8):1520–1525.
8. Akinduro OO, Baum GR, Howard BM, et al. Neurological outcomes following iatrogenic vascular injury during posterior atlanto-axial instrumentation. *Clin Neurol Neurosurg.* Nov 2016;150:110–116.
9. McCormick PC, Stein BM. Functional anatomy of the spinal cord and related structures. *Neurosurg Clin N Am.* Jul 1990;1(3):469–489.
10. Angevine PD, Kellner C, Haque RM, McCormick PC. Surgical management of ventral intradural spinal lesions. *J Neurosurg Spine.* Jul 2011;15(1):28–37.
11. Martin NA, Khanna RK, Batzdorf U. Posterolateral cervical or thoracic approach with spinal cord rotation for vascular malformations or tumors of the ventrolateral spinal cord. *J Neurosurg.* Aug 1995;83(2):254–261.

12. Hong-Wan N, Ee-Chon T, Qing-Hang Z. Biomechanical effects of C2-C7 intersegmental stability due to laminectomy with unilateral and bilateral facetectomy. *Spine (Phila Pa 1976)*. Aug 15, 2004;29(16):1737–1745. discussion 1746.

13. Heller JG, Edwards 2nd CC, Murakami H, Rodts GE. Laminoplasty versus laminectomy and fusion for multilevel cervical myelopathy: an independent matched cohort analysis. *Spine (Phila Pa 1976)*. Jun 15, 2001;26(12):1330–1336.

14. Herkowitz HN. A comparison of anterior cervical fusion, cervical laminectomy, and cervical laminoplasty for the surgical management of multiple level spondylotic radiculopathy. *Spine (Phila Pa 1976)*. Jul 1988;13(7):774 780.

15. Gok B, McLoughlin GS, Sciubba DM, et al. Surgical management of cervical spondylotic myelopathy with laminectomy and instrumented fusion. *Neurol Res*. Dec 2009;31(10):1097–1101.

16. Funakoshi Y, Hanakita J, Takahashi T, et al. Investigation of Radiologic Landmarks Used to Decide the Appropriate Surgical Approach for Upper Thoracic Ventral Degenerative Disorders. *World Neurosurg*. May 2019;125:e856–e862.

17. Fraioli MF, Marciani MG, Umana GE, Fraioli B. Anterior Microsurgical Approach to Ventral Lower Cervical Spine Meningiomas: Indications, Surgical Technique and Long Term Outcome. *Technol Cancer Res Treat*. Aug 2015;14(4):505–510.

18. Eroglu U, Bahadir B, Tomlinson SB, et al. Microsurgical Management of Ventral Intradural-Extramedullary Cervical Meningiomas: Technical Considerations and Outcomes. *World Neurosurg*. Mar 2020;135:e748–e753.

19. Guo L, Quinones-Hinojosa A, Yingling CD, Weinstein PR. Continuous EMG recordings and intraoperative electrical stimulation for identification and protection of cervical nerve roots during foraminal tumor surgery. *J Spinal Disord Tech*. Feb 2006;19(1):37–42.

20. Sachdev S, Dodd RL, Chang SD, et al. Stereotactic radiosurgery yields long-term control for benign intradural, extramedullary spinal tumors. *Neurosurgery*. Sep 2011;69(3):533–539. discussion 539.

21. Gerszten PC, Burton SA, Ozhasoglu C, McCue KJ, Quinn AE. Radiosurgery for benign intradural spinal tumors. *Neurosurgery*. Apr 2008;62(4):887–895. discussion 895-886.

22. Conti P, Pansini G, Mouchaty H, Capuano C, Conti R. Spinal neurinomas: retrospective analysis and long-term outcome of 179 consecutively operated cases and review of the literature. *Surg Neurol*. Jan 2004;61(1):34–43. discussion 44.

23. O'Toole JE, McCormick PC. Midline ventral intradural schwannoma of the cervical spinal cord resected via anterior corpectomy with reconstruction: technical case report and review of the literature. *Neurosurgery*. Jun 2003;52(6):1482–1485. discussion 1485-1486.

48

Spinal metastasis with kyphotic deformity

Oluwaseun O. Akinduro, MD and Kingsley Abode-Iyamah, MD

Introduction

Primary tumors may spread to the spine in 20% to 40% of cancer patients, and approximately 20% of these patients will be symptomatic from their tumors.[1–3] Their symptomatology may be related to compression of the spinal cord, leading to pain and weakness, mechanical back pain from spinal instability, or a combination of these two. The presence of mechanical back pain should prompt consideration for stabilization of the spine, as this pain may be partially or completely resolved if instability is the true etiology of their pain. There is ample evidence to suggest that surgical decompression plus radiation is the management of choice for patients with spinal metastatic disease and epidural compression.[4,5] However, there is no clear consensus as to when patients undergoing surgery will require stabilization. These decisions were typically made according to factors such as patient symptoms, patient health and life expectancy, and tumor histology, but there was a lack of evidence-based guidelines for determination of spinal stability. The Spinal Instability in Neoplastic disease Score (SINS) is a tool to guide clinicians who are evaluating patients with spinal metastatic disease to help determine the need for surgical stabilization (Table 48.1).[6] There are six components to this scoring system, including location, presence of mechanical pain, spinal alignment, whether the tumor is lytic or blastic, amount of vertebral body collapse, and tumor involvement of posterior elements. A score is given according to each component, and the cumulative score determines whether the patient will require stabilization. In this chapter, we present a patient with metastatic disease for which this score may be applied.

Table 48.1 Spinal Instability in Neoplastic disease Score (SINS)

LOCATION	Junctional (occiput-C2, C7-T2, T11-L1, L5-S1)	3
	Mobile spine (C3-C6, L2-L4)	2
	Semirigid (T3-T10)	1
	Rigid (S2-S5)	0
MECHANICAL PAIN	Yes	3
	Pain present but not mechanical	1
	No pain	0
TYPE OF BONE LESION	Lytic	2
	Mixed	1
	Blastic	0
SPINAL ALIGNMENT	Subluxation/translation	4
	Kyphosis/scoliosis	2
	Normal alignment	0
VERTEBRAL BODY COLAPSE	>50% collapse	3
	<50% collapse	2
	No collapse with >50% body involved	1
	None of the above	0
INVOLVEMENT OF POSTEROLATERAL ELEMENTS	Bilateral	3
	Unilateral	1
	None	0
0 TO 6 INDICATES STABILITY, SCORES OF 7 AND GREATER WARRANT SURGICAL INTERVENTION		

Example case

Chief complaint: neck pain and radiculopathy

History of present illness: This is a 65-year-old female with a history of breast cancer status post chemoradiation on remission. She presents with several months of back pain. Over the past few days, she reports worsening pain, balance dysfunction, leg weakness, and numbness. She underwent imaging and there was concern for cord compression (Figs. 48.1–48.2).

Medications: melatonin, metoprolol

Allergies: iodinated contrast

Past medical history: breast cancer, hypertension

Family history: noncontributory

Social history: nonsmoker

Physical examination: awake, alert, and oriented x 3; cranial nerves CNII–XII intact; bilateral deltoids/triceps/biceps/interossei 5/5; iliopsoas 4/5; knee flexion/knee extension/dorsi, and plantar flexion 5/5

Reflexes: 3+ in bilateral biceps/triceps/brachioradialis with positive Hoffman; 3+ in bilateral patella/ankle; positive clonus and Babinski; sensation intact to light touch

Laboratories: basic metabolic panel, heme-8, coagulation all within normal limits

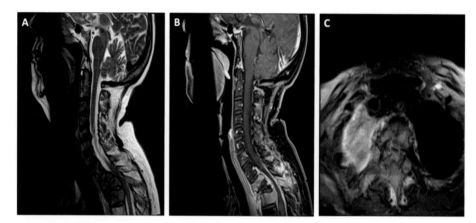

Fig. 48.1 Preoperative magnetic resonance images. (A) T2 sagittal, **(B)** T1 sagittal with contrast, and **(C)** T1 axial with contrast images demonstrating pathological involvement of the T2 and T3 vertebral body and circumferential cord compression.

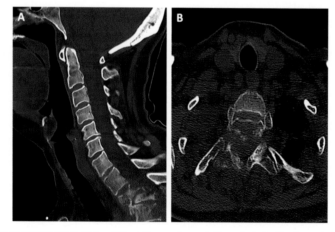

Fig. 48.2 Preoperative computed tomography images. (A) Sagittal and **(B)** axial images demonstrating pathological involvement of the T2 and T3 vertebral body.

	Andres Almendral, MD Neurosurgery Clinica Hospital San Fernando Panama City, Panama	Takeshi Hara, MD Neurosurgery Juntendo University Hongo, Bunkyo-ku, Tokyo, Japan	Maziyar A. Kalani, MD Neurosurgery Mayo Clinic Phoenix, Arizona, United States	Khoi D. Than, MD Neurosurgery Duke University Durham, North Carolina, United States
Preoperative				
Additional tests requested	DEXA Cardiothoracic surgery Oncology evaluation Radiation oncology evaluation Anesthesia evaluation	CTA C-spine CT T-spine MRI T-spine Bone scintigram	MRI complete spine CT T-spine Cardiothoracic surgery Oncology evaluation Radiation oncology evaluation	MRI complete spine Oncology evaluation Radiation oncology evaluation CT chest/abdomen/pelvis
Surgical approach selected	Stage 1: T3-4 laminectomy and C5-T7 posterior fusion Stage 2: T2-4 corpectomy via midline sternotomy		Stage 1: T2-4 corpectomy via midline sternotomy Stage 2: T2-4 posterior decompression and C7-T6 posterior fusion	If prognosis is reasonable (> several months), C6-T6 posterior instrumented fusion with T2-4 laminectomy, possible T2-3 corpectomies with T1-4 interbody fusion
Goal of surgery	Decompress the spinal cord, stabilize spine	Relieve neck pain, improve quality of life	Decompress the spinal cord, correction of kyphosis, stabilize the spine	Decompress the spinal cord, stabilize the spine
Perioperative				
Positioning	Prone with pins	Prone with pins	Stage 1: supine Stage 2: prone on Jackson table, no pins	Prone with pins
Surgical equipment	IOM (MEP/SSEP) Fluoroscopy Surgical navigation	IOM (MEP) Fluoroscopy O-arm Surgical navigation	IOM Fluoroscopy Cardiothoracic surgery Chest tube	IOM (MEP/SSEP/EMG) Fluoroscopy O-arm/surgical navigation
Medications	Steroids, maintain MAP	None	Steroids, MAP >85	MAP >80
Anatomical considerations	Vertebral bone anatomy	Vertebral arteries, aorta	Stage 1: heart, great vessels, trachea, lungs, esophagus Stage 2: spinal cord	Spinal cord, T2-3 nerve roots, pleura
Complications feared with approach chosen	Blood loss, spinal compression, spinal instability	Major vessel injury, spinal cord and/or nerve root injury	Major vessel injury, spinal cord injury, injury to artery of Adamkiewicz	Neurological deficit
Intraoperative				
Anesthesia	General	General	General	General
Exposure	C4-T6	C7-T7	Stage 1: anterior T2-4 Stage 2: C7-T6	C6-T6
Levels decompressed	Stage 1: T3-4 Stage 2: T2-4	T2-4	Stage 1: T2-4 Stage 2: T2-4	T2-4
Levels fused	Stage 1: C5-T7 Stage 2: T2-4	C6-T7	Stage 1: T2-4 Stage 2: C7-T6	C6-T6

	Andres Almendral, MD Neurosurgery Clinica Hospital San Fernando Panama City, Panama	Takeshi Hara, MD Neurosurgery Juntendo University Hongo, Bunkyo-ku, Tokyo, Japan	Maziyar A. Kalani, MD Neurosurgery Mayo Clinic Phoenix, Arizona, United States	Khoi D. Than, MD Neurosurgery Duke University Durham, North Carolina, United States
Surgical narrative	Stage 1: Preflip IOM, position prone after placing Mayfield pins, keep in neutral position, postflip IOM to confirm stability, midline incision, subperiosteal dissection exposing C4 to T6, fluoroscopic or surgical navigation guidance to place pedicle screws at T1-T2/T5-7/C7 and lateral mass screws at C5-6, T3-4 laminectomy, epidural tumor resection, layered closure with drain Stage 2 (same day): cardiothoracic surgery to perform midline sternotomy, T2-4 corpectomy, insertion of expandable cage and plate, layered closure	Preflip IOM, position prone with pin, keep neutral position, midline incision, subperiosteal dissection exposing from C7 to T7, place C7 pedicle pilot holes with surgical navigation as well as T1/T4-6 pedicles, T2-3 laminectomy, place C7/T1/T4-5 pedicle screws, confirm placement with x-rays, place cobalt chromium alloy rods, layered closure	Stage 1: position supine, cardiothoracic surgery to perform exposure via midline sternotomy, intraoperative x-ray to identify correct level, annulotomy at T1-2 and T4-5, discectomy to remove cartilaginous end plates off inferior end plate of T1 and superior end plate of T5, midline marked based on where discs drop off laterally, corpectomy in piecemeal fashion, use discectomies to evaluate depth, remove posterior cortex of bone with upgoing curettes, remove any soft tissue from epidural space, titanium cage filled with allograft and place in space, apply buttress screws to secure cage into end plates of T1 and T5, cardiothoracic closure with chest tube Stage 2 (3 days later): preflip IOM, position prone, postflip IOM, x-ray to confirm anterior cage is not dislodged, midline incision from C7 to T6, subperiosteal dissection, intraoperative x-ray to confirm levels, freehand placement of bilateral pedicle screws at C7/T1/T5/T6, final rods placed to avoid spinal translation and movement of cage, T2-4 laminectomy, final x-rays, closure in layers with subfascial drain	Positioned prone with Mayfield pins, neutral anatomical alignment, fluoroscopy to localize level, midline incision, subperiosteal dissection, instrumentation with lateral mass screws at C6, pedicle screws at C7/T1/T4-T6, T2-4 en bloc laminectomy with high-speed drill, removal of ligamentum flavum, wide bony removal at T2-3 similar to costotransversectomy, bilateral T2-3 nerve roots are identified and ligated, T2-3 corpectomies with osteotome and curettage working lateral to the spinal cord, tissue sent to pathology, size corpectomy defect, insertion of appropriate sized interbody device filled with allograft, O-arm spin to confirm accuracy of instrumentation, rods contoured appropriated and placed in screw heads, set screws placed and final tightened after fluoroscopy, remained bone between C6 and T6 decorticated and allograft is laid, wound closed in layers with drain
Complication avoidance	Preflip IOM, possible surgical navigation, two-staged approach, cardiothoracic for anterior exposure	Preflip IOM, surgical navigation for pedicle screws	Two-staged approach, cardiothoracic for anterior exposure, use discectomies to evaluate depth, preflip IOM prior to starting second stage, early placement of rods to prevent spinal translation and dislodgement of cage	En bloc laminectomy, work lateral to spinal cord for corpectomy
Postoperative				
Admission	ICU	ICU	ICU	ICU
Postoperative complications feared	Blood loss, spinal compression, spinal instability	Infection, instrument failure, aortic injury	Major vessel injury, spinal cord injury, injury to artery of Adamkiewicz	Neurological deficit
Anticipated length of stay	4–6 days	10 days	5–7 days	5 days
Follow-up testing	CT C-T spine within 48 hours of surgery Oncology evaluation	Radiation oncology evaluation	Standing AP/lateral scoliosis x-rays 6 weeks, 6 months, 1 year after surgery Radiation oncology evaluation	Scoliosis films CT myelogram for radiation planning
Bracing	None	Soft collar for 3 months	TLSO for 6 weeks	CTO for 6 weeks
Follow-up visits	2 weeks, monthly after surgery	1 week, every 1–2 months after surgery	2 weeks, 6 weeks, 6 months, 1 year after surgery	3 weeks after surgery

AP, Anteroposterior; *CT*, Computed tomography; *CTA*, computed tomography angiography; *CTO*, cervical thoracic orthosis; *DEXA*, duel-energy x-ray absoprtiometry; *EMG*, electromyography; *ESI*, epidural spinal injections; *ICU*, intensive care unit; *IOM*, intraoperative monitoring; *MAP*, mean arterial pressure; *MEP*, motor evoked potentials; *MIS*, minimally invasive surgery; *SSEP*, somatosensory evoked potentials; *TLSO*, thoracic lumbar sacral orthosis.

Differential diagnosis

- Metastatic disease
- Multiple myeloma
- Primary bone tumor such as chordoma
- Osteomyelitis

Important anatomical considerations

The cervicothoracic junction contains many neurovascular structures that must be considered when planning surgery within this region. The thoracic spine is dorsal to the heart and lungs; thus planning of anterior approaches to this region must be strategic and thorough. The aortic arch will typically be found around T4, and the great vessels will be found emanating from the rostral aspect of the arch, so anterior approaches to this area may be very challenging. The esophagus and trachea will also be encountered anteriorly in the cervicothoracic junction. Another consideration of an anterior approach to the cervicothoracic junction is the location of the sternum, as the location of the sternum may prohibit access to the region during an anterior approach. The biomechanical properties of the cervicothoracic junction must also be taken into consideration. This region is the junction of the subaxial cervical spine and the upper thoracic spine. The subaxial spine is straight to mildly lordotic, and the obliquely oriented facets in this region allow for flexion, rotation, and lateral bending.[7] The upper thoracic spine is kyphotic, and the rib cage resists flexion, rotation, and lateral bending, so the cervicothoracic junction tends to be under significant stress, which should be considered when stabilizing this region.[8] Due to the transition from lordosis to kyphosis, the orientation of the C7-T1 disc space may be highly variable. When the thoracic kyphosis is steep or the sagittal balance is significantly positive, the C7-T1 disc space angle will also be steep, often making an anterior approach very difficult.[8] The thoracic spine could be considered a long lever arm, as the ribs make this segment semirigid, and therefore places significant stress on the thoracolumbar junction, thus making this region prone to injury from trauma. These factors must all be considered when planning stabilization of the cervicothoracic junction to ensure ample strength of the construct.

Approaches to this lesion

The tumor described in this case may be amenable to either a posterior-only approach, anterior-only approach, or a combination of the two, depending on patient-related factors, goals of surgery, and surgeon preference. Multiple options would grant access to tumors in this region, but the tumor location determines the optimal approach. Tumors that are primarily posterior in location would be amenable to a posterior or posterolateral approach. A posterolateral approach may include resection of the proximal portion of the rib and the pedicle at the levels of interest to avoid manipulation of the spinal cord. Posterior approaches are generally more familiar to surgeons and are often preferred if both approaches are reasonable choices. An anterior approach to the cervicothoracic junction will require thorough evaluation of the preoperative imaging. Vascular imaging may be beneficial to determine the location of the great vessels branching from the aortic arch. Bifurcations of these vessels may preclude an anterior approach to the upper thoracic spine. The other major predictor of the ability to approach this region anteriorly is the location of the sternum in relation to the pathology of interest. A high riding sternum may preclude an approach to the anterior cervicothoracic junction and will require assistance of a thoracic surgeon for splitting of the sternum to allow access.

What was actually done

The patient was placed in the prone position and secured with a Mayfield headrest. Mean arterial pressures greater than 85 were maintained throughout the procedure, and the patient received 10 mg of dexamethasone. Intraoperative somatosensory and motor evoked potentials were recorded throughout the entire case. Exposure was carried out from C4 all the way down to T8 followed by intraoperative fluoroscopy for confirmation. Lateral mass screws were placed bilaterally from C4 to 6. Pedicle screws were placed bilaterally from T5 down to T8. No instrumentation was placed at C7, T1, T2, T3, and T4, as this was the location of the disease. After satisfactory placement of the instrumentation, temporary rods were placed and decompression from T1 down to T4 was done. After hemostasis was obtained, a tapered titanium rod was placed and contoured to our instrumentation. Intraoperative O-arm was used to confirm accurate placement of the instrumentation. Arthrodesis was then done in the lateral gutters from C4 down to T8 using a high-speed bur followed by placement of corticocancellous bone to obtain a solid fusion mass. The incision was then closed in layers. The patient woke up with no intra or postoperative complications. Postoperative imaging showed good location of the instrumentation (Fig. 48.3).

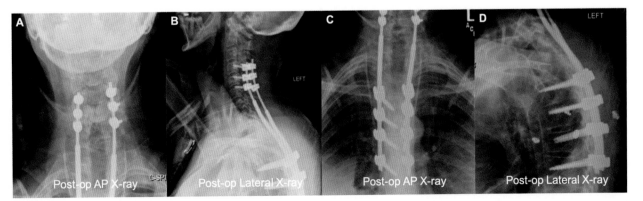

Fig. 48.3 Postoperative x-rays. (A) Cervical anteroposterior, **(B)** cervical lateral, **(C)** thoracic anteroposterior, and **(D)** thoracic lateral x-rays demonstrating T1-4 decompression and C4-T8 instrumentation.

Commonalities among the experts

All experts agreed with obtaining a more thorough evaluation including oncology evaluation and further imaging. The majority planned for a two-staged approach to the lesion, as long as the patient had a reasonable life expectancy. This included an anterior thoracic corpectomy from either T2-3 or T2-4, with interbody grafting and plating. The second stage included a posterior cervical decompression and fusion with mild variation in the chosen levels of fusion. Two of the three surgeons with planned two-staged approach opted for starting with the posterior cervical component, while one surgeon planned to perform the anterior cervical procedure first. Half were concerned with injury to one of the great vessels. The majority opted for use of postoperative bracing. All agreed on postoperative imaging.

SUMMARY OF QUALITY OF EVIDENCE TO GUIDE SPECIFIC INTERVENTIONS FOR THIS CASE

- Surgical decompression and radiation improve outcomes over radiation alone for patients with spinal compression: level IA[9]
- Spinal radiosurgery is safe and efficacious for treatment of spinal metastasis compared with conventional radiation: level IIA[10–13]
- Hypofractionated radiotherapy is safe, efficacious, and has the advantage of shortened treatment course: level IIB[14]

REFERENCES

1. Klimo P, Jr., Schmidt MH. Surgical management of spinal metastases. *Oncologist*. 2004;9(2):188–196.
2. Galgano M, Fridley J, Oyelese A, et al. Surgical management of spinal metastases. *Expert Rev Anticancer Ther*. May 2018; 18(5):463–472.
3. Cobb CA, 3rd, Leavens ME, Eckles N. Indications for nonoperative treatment of spinal cord compression due to breast cancer. *J Neurosurg*. Nov 1977;47(5):653–658.
4. Lee BH, Kim TH, Chong HS, et al. Prognostic factor analysis in patients with metastatic spine disease depending on surgery and conservative treatment: review of 577 cases. *Ann Surg Oncol*. Jan 2013;20(1):40–46.
5. Patchell RA, Tibbs PA, Regine WF, et al. Direct decompressive surgical resection in the treatment of spinal cord compression caused by metastatic cancer: a randomised trial. *Lancet*. Aug 20–26 2005;366(9486):643–648.
6. Fisher CG, DiPaola CP, Ryken TC, et al. A novel classification system for spinal instability in neoplastic disease: an evidence-based approach and expert consensus from the Spine Oncology Study Group. *Spine (Phila Pa 1976)*. Oct 15, 2010;35(22):E1221–1229.
7. Tan LA, Riew KD, Traynelis VC. Cervical Spine Deformity-Part 1: Biomechanics, Radiographic Parameters, and Classification. *Neurosurgery*. Aug 1, 2017;81(2):197–203.
8. Maiman DJ, Pintar FA. Anatomy and clinical biomechanics of the thoracic spine. *Clin Neurosurg*. 1992;38:296–324.
9. Hunter RE, Wigfield CC. Direct decompressive surgical resection in the treatment of spinal cord compression caused by metastatic cancer: a randomized trial. *Br J Neurosurg*. Oct 2008;22(5):713–714.
10. Amdur RJ, Bennett J, Olivier K, et al. A prospective, phase II study demonstrating the potential value and limitation of radiosurgery for spine metastases. *Am J Clin Oncol*. Oct 2009;32(5):515–520.
11. Gerszten PC, Burton SA, Belani CP, et al. Radiosurgery for the treatment of spinal lung metastases. *Cancer*. Dec 1, 2006; 107(11):2653–2661.
12. Gerszten PC, Burton SA, Ozhasoglu C, Welch WC. Radiosurgery for spinal metastases: clinical experience in 500 cases from a single institution. *Spine (Phila Pa 1976)*. Jan 15, 2007;32(2):193–199.
13. Chang EL, Shiu AS, Mendel E, et al. Phase I/II study of stereotactic body radiotherapy for spinal metastasis and its pattern of failure. *J Neurosurg Spine*. Aug 2007;7(2):151–160.
14. Maranzano E, Bellavita R, Rossi R, et al. Short-course versus split-course radiotherapy in metastatic spinal cord compression: results of a phase III, randomized, multicenter trial. *J Clin Oncol*. May 20, 2005;23(15):3358–3365.

49

Multiple spine metastasis with one level symptomatic

Oluwaseun O. Akinduro, MD

Introduction

Spinal metastatic disease is seen in almost 40% of cancer patients, and up to 20% of those patients will have spinal cord compression.[1] The American Cancer Society found that there were 1.7 million new cases of cancer diagnosed in the United States in 2017.[2] As patients are living longer due to improved cancer therapies, there has been an increased incidence of metastatic disease. The treatment of patients with solitary spinal metastasis and compression of the spinal cord has been validated with level 1 data and there is a clear consensus on the benefit of surgery for this group of patients. However, the guidelines are not as clear when patients have multiple noncontiguous areas of disease.[3] The randomized clinical trial by Patchell et al. excluded patients with multiple noncontiguous levels of tumor, so there is no high-level evidence for this group of patients.[3] The treatment goal for these patients with multiple spinal metastases has primarily been centered around the goal of palliation. However, there have been multiple reports and series showing that tumor resection in these patients can lead to improvement in quality of life, although

the surgery itself will not be curative.[4] A prospective multicenter study found that surgical treatment of patients with oligometastatic disease will have improved survival compared with survival management of patients with polymetastatic disease.[5] Both groups, however, had improved quality of life after surgical decompression of the symptomatic lesion. Prior to consideration for surgery, patients should be assessed by a multidisciplinary team to determine their estimated survival, as patients with a short life expectancy may not benefit from surgical management of their tumors and may be better served by less invasive strategies for pain control.[6]

Example case

Chief complaint: back and leg pain with leg weakness
History of present illness: This is a 78-year-old male with a history of renal cell carcinoma who presents with a 3-month history of back pain and 3 weeks of leg pain. He has not been ambulatory due to leg weakness and pain. The patient had magnetic resonance imaging (MRI), which revealed evidence of a tumor compressing his thecal sac at L2, as well as evidence of disease elsewhere (Fig. 49.1).

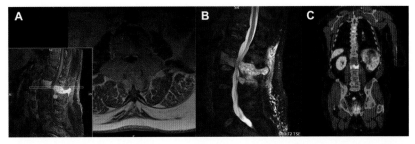

Fig. 49.1 Preoperative imaging. (A), Axial T1 with contrast magnetic resonance imaging (MRI); (B), sagittal T2 MRI demonstrating an expansile destructive L2 metastasis with involvement of the spinous process, lamina, pedicles, and majority of the vertebral body. The vertebral body demonstrates mild pathological collapse of the superior end plate on the left side. There is marked expansion of the pedicles and posterior elements by the soft tissue involvement with posterolateral epidural extension producing severe compression of the thecal sac and crowding of the cauda equina roots. (C), Positron emission tomography/computed tomography scans of the whole body demonstrating a hypermetabolic right upper lobe pulmonary nodule and multiple mediastinal and hilar lymph nodes with increased metabolic activity, concerning for neoplastic processes. There is also evidence of multiple lytic lesions seen within the sternum, spine, and left parietal calvarium, some of which demonstrate increased metabolic activity suggestive of metastatic lesions from patient's known left renal primary.

Medications: aspirin 325 mg
Allergies: no known drug allergies
Past medical history: renal cell carcinoma
Past surgical history: nephrectomy
Family history: noncontributory
Social history: previous smoker
Physical examination: awake, alert, and oriented to person, place, and time; cranial nerves II–XII intact; bilateral deltoids/triceps/biceps 5/5; interossei 5/5; iliopsoas/knee flexion/knee extension 3/5, dorsi and plantar flexion 5/5

Reflexes: 2+ in bilateral biceps/triceps/brachioradialis with negative Hoffman; 2+ in bilateral patella/ankle; no clonus or Babinski; sensation intact to light touch

Laboratories: all within normal limits

	Rafid Al-Mahfoudh, MBChBh Neurosurgery Brighton and Sussex University Hospitals Brighton, United Kingdom	Manoj Phalak, MCh Neurosurgery All India Institute of Medical Sciences New Delhi, India	Khoi D. Than, MD Neurosurgery Duke University Durham, North Carolina, United States	Anand Veeravagu, MD Neurosurgery Stanford University Palo Alto, California, United States
Preoperative				
Additional tests requested	MRI complete spine CT lumbar spine CT chest/abdomen/pelvis CT Oncology evaluation Cerebral angiogram with embolization	DEXA CT lumbar spine Oncology evaluation Radiation oncology evaluation Anesthesia evaluation	CT lumbar spine Oncology evaluation Radiation oncology evaluation	MRI complete spine Standing lumbar spine x-rays (AP and lateral)
Surgical approach selected	L2 decompression and fusion and resection of tumor	L1-3 decompression and tumor resection with T10-L4 posterior fusion	If prognosis is reasonable (> several weeks), minimally invasive L2 laminectomy	If patient has minimal systemic disease, L2 corpectomy, L2-3 laminectomy, T11-L5 instrumented fusion
Goal of surgery	Decompress neural elements, stabilize spine	Maximal tumor resection, stabilization to reduce pain	Decompress neural elements	Decompress neural elements, separate neurological elements to allow for radiotherapy
Perioperative				
Positioning	Prone on Jackson or Allan table	Prone on Allan table	Prone on Wilson frame	Prone on Jackson table
Surgical equipment	Fluoroscopy Surgical microscope Ultrasonic bone scalpel	IOM (MEP/SSEP) Surgical navigation Ultrasonic aspirator	Fluoroscopy Tubular retractor Surgical microscope	Fluoroscopy IOM Surgical navigation
Medications	Tranexamic acid, steroids	Maintain MAP	None	Possible tranexamic acid, steroids
Anatomical considerations	Thecal sac, pedicles	Iliopsoas, lumbar plexus, aorta, renal artery, inferior vena cava, ureter	Thecal sac, nerve roots	Thecal sac, nerve roots
Complications feared with approach chosen	Blood loss, prolonged hospital stay	Injury to blood vessels, ureteral injury, pseudoarthrosis, CSF leak, infection	CSF leak, recurrent stenosis	Conus injury, nerve root injury, CSF leak
Intraoperative				
Anesthesia	General	General	General	General
Exposure	L2	T10-L4	L2	T11-L4
Levels decompressed	L2	L1-3	L2	L2-3
Levels fused	T12-L4	T10-L4	None	T11-L4

	Rafid Al-Mahfoudh, MBChBh Neurosurgery Brighton and Sussex University Hospitals Brighton, United Kingdom	Manoj Phalak, MCh Neurosurgery All India Institute of Medical Sciences New Delhi, India	Khoi D. Than, MD Neurosurgery Duke University Durham, North Carolina, United States	Anand Veeravagu, MD Neurosurgery Stanford University Palo Alto, California, United States
Surgical narrative	Position prone, AP x-ray to ensure good visualization of pedicles using K-wire held against skin, paramedian stab incisions, Jamshidi needles progressed through pedicles with x-ray control, two levels above and below, K-wire inserted through Jamshidi needles, Jamshidi needles removed, percutaneous dilators, tap then pedicle screws inserted under x-ray, rods measured and tunneled, rods reduced and set screws applied, midline incision at L2, bilateral muscle dissection with tranexamic soaked swabs, McCulloch retractors placed, microscope brought in, L2 spinous process removed, laminectomy with high-speed drill, remove remained of thinned lamina with upcuts with flavectomy, lateral recess decompression with ultrasonic bone scalpel, debulk the extradural portion of tumor to achieve good clearance from the theca, pedicle removal to gain and aid access to lateral/ anterolateral aspect of theca, apply hemostatic agent to reduce excessive blood loss, closure in layers with vancomycin and subfascial drain if necessary	Position prone on Allen table, baseline IOM, preparation of iliac crest for bone graft, T10-L4 incision, subperiosteal dissection making sure to not violate tumor, place pedicle screws T10-L4 and including T10-11 because of assumed compression fracture, place temporary rod on right, L1-3 laminectomy with excision of transverse process and intralesional resection, gently create lateral and ventral plane to vertebral body with malleable retractor, detach psoas and crus of diaphragm, excision L1-2 and L2-3 discs, remove pedicle off of tumor, mobilize remaining tumor, maximal tumor removal and decompression, place titanium mesh with iliac crest autograft, decorticate exposed bone posteriorly and use remaining iliac crest graft to help with fusion, layered wound closure with drains	Position prone on Wilson frame, Wilson frame cranked open to provide kyphosis to open interlaminar spaces, midline spinous process marked, 1 cm lateral to midline planned, spinal needle placed aimed directly at L2-3 disc space based on lateral fluoroscopy, 2 cm incision made where needle enters skin, dissect through lumbar muscular fascia with cauterization, gradually increased dilator tubes docked to inferior L2 lamina, 18 mm wide tubular retractor and location confirmed with fluoroscopy, microdissection with microscope, muscles overlying L2 lamina removed, L2 laminectomy down to ligamentum flavum, rostral attachment dissected from underlying thecal sac with curved curette, ligamentum flavum is removed with Kerrison rongeurs, tumor sent to pathology, contralateral decompression with angled tubular retractor, remove bone/ligamentum flavum/ tumor as needed, confirm adequate decompression with Woodson elevator, wound closed in layers	Position prone, O-arm for intraoperative navigation, place pedicle screws T11-12 and L1 and L3–4, perform L2-3 laminectomy, transpedicular decompression, resect L1-2 and L2-3 discs, place temporary rod, complete L2 corpectomy, place expandable titanium cage, insert final rods from T11 to L4, fusion with allograft across laminectomy defect site, multilayer closure with two subfascial drains
Complication avoidance	Embolization, AP x-ray to confirm location of pedicles, percutaneous screws under fluoroscopy, tranexamic soaked swabs, remove tumor to good clearance from dura, remove pedicle if necessary to gain better visualization	Possible staged procedure for blood loss or hemodynamic instability, if this occurs, iliac crest for bone grafting, avoid violating tumor during dissection, incorporate compression fracture levels into construct	Minimally invasive laminectomy, confirm adequacy of decompression with Woodson elevator	Surgical navigation, incorporate T12 vertebral body fracture, separation surgery
Postoperative				
Admission	Floor	ICU	Floor	Floor
Postoperative complications feared	Excessive bleeding	Injury to blood vessels, ureteral injury, pseudoarthrosis, CSF leak, infection	CSF leak, wound infection, recurrent stenosis	Wound complication, CSF leak, failure of fusion
Anticipated length of stay	3–5 days	10 days	2–3 days	4 days

(continued on next page)

	Rafid Al-Mahfoudh, MBChBh Neurosurgery Brighton and Sussex University Hospitals Brighton, United Kingdom	Manoj Phalak, MCh Neurosurgery All India Institute of Medical Sciences New Delhi, India	Khoi D. Than, MD Neurosurgery Duke University Durham, North Carolina, United States	Anand Veeravagu, MD Neurosurgery Stanford University Palo Alto, California, United States
Follow-up testing	Lumbar x-rays within 24 hours of surgery Oncology evaluation	T-L spine x-ray after surgery CT T-L spine 3 months after surgery	MRI lumbar spine after surgery Chemoradiation per oncology 3 weeks after surgery	MRI and CT lumbar spine within 1 month of surgery Lumbar x-rays 1 month, 3 months, 6 months, 12 months after surgery
Bracing	None	None	None	TLSO for 8 weeks
Follow-up visits	6–8 weeks after surgery	14 days and 3 months after surgery	2 weeks after surgery	2 weeks, 1 month, 3 months, 6 months, 1 year after surgery

AP, Anteroposterior; *CSF*, cerebrospinal fluid; *CT*, computed tomography; *DEXA*, dual-energy x-ray absorptiometry; *EMG*, electromyography; *ICU*, intensive care unit; *IOM*, intraoperative monitoring; *MAP*, mean arterial pressure; *MEP*, motor evoked potentials; *MIS*, minimally invasive surgery; *MRI*, magnetic resonance imaging; *SSEP*, somatosensory evoked potential; *TLSO*, thoracic lumbar sacral orthosis.

Differential diagnosis

- Metastatic disease
- Lumbar stenosis
- Multiple myeloma
- Primary bone tumor such as chordoma
- Osteomyelitis

Important anatomical considerations

The thoracolumbar junction has unique biomechanical properties due to the close relation of the semirigid thoracic spine above and the more flexible lumbar spine below. There are also important neurovascular structures to consider when planning surgical approaches to this region. An anterior or lateral approach would place the aorta and inferior vena cava at risk, and therefore the assistance of an access surgeon could be beneficial to diminish this risk. Each spinal level has an associated segmental vessel emanating from the aorta, and the artery of Adamkiewicz is the most important of these in the lower thoracic or upper lumbar region. It is most commonly found on the left around T8-L1.[7] During decompression of the spinal cord, the thecal sac will need to be identified to prevent inadvertent durotomy. The upper lumbar nerve roots will likely be encountered during a posterior-lateral approach, especially if placement of a graft will be required. The nerve roots can be identified immediately caudal to the corresponding pedicle. The placement of a graft may require sacrifice of one of the nerve roots, which can normally be completed safely in the thoracic levels, with nothing more than a postoperative sensory deficit. Sacrifice of nerve roots is typically contraindicated in the lumbar levels as these nerve roots supply motor as well as sensory function.

Approaches to this lesion

Surgical approaches to tumors of the lower thoracolumbar junction must be carefully planned with consideration of all of the neurovascular structures that will be at risk, depending on the approach. There must be a clear understanding of the surgical goal, as the ideal surgical approach will typically be the one that will have the ability to provide adequate access to perform this surgical goal, while minimizing the risk to the patient. The tumor in this case can be approached from a posterior approach, posterior lateral approach, lateral extracavitary approach, or an anterior approach. One primary consideration is whether the patient will require stabilization in addition to decompression. When there is evidence of mechanical pain, destruction of the posterior bony elements, kyphotic deformity, or significant vertebral body collapse, patients will likely require instrumentation to stabilize the spine.[8] The Spinal Instability in Neoplastic disease Score (SINS) is a tool to guide clinicians who are evaluating patients with spinal metastatic disease to help determine the need for surgical stabilization (see Chapter 48, Table 1).[9] Up to 9% of patients with laminectomy without instrumentation will develop spinal instability.[10] The prognosis of the patient must also be considered, as patients with a short life expectancy may not be the best candidates for surgical instrumentation.

What was actually done

This is a patient with known metastatic renal cell carcinoma and metastatic lesions to T5, T12, and L5 with previous chemotherapy and radiation. The patient had significant spinal cord compression at L2 and required surgical decompression with stabilization. A preoperative angiogram was performed, and bilateral embolization was performed through the L2 segmental arteries with >90% reduction in tumor blush. The artery of Ademkiewicz was noted at the left T11. The patient was then taken to the operating room the following day. A midline incision was performed and the paraspinal musculature was then reflected in a subperiosteal fashion from the caudal aspect of T9 to the superior aspect of the sacrum. It became obvious that the spinous process and laminal arches at L2 and superiorly at L3 were completely infiltrated with fleshy hypervascular tumor. After exposure, a localizing device was placed at T9 for an O-arm spin. Pedicle screws were then placed under image gudiance, skipping the L2 pedicles bilaterally and the left L3 pedicle. At the L1 level, the left pedicle was extremely small, particularly on axial imaging, and a screw was not placed at this level. After all screws were placed, the patient underwent resection of his tumor. An Adson rongeur and rib cutters were used to remove the involved spinous process and posterior elements of L1 and L3 as well as the fleshy hypervascular tumor at the L2 level. The high-speed bur was used to remove the lamina of L1 and L3. The ligamentum flavum was then removed, identifying normal dura above and below the compressed region. A wide decompression was obtained and the exiting nerve roots were skeletonized. A separate fascial incision was made overlying the left iliac crest, and using osteotomes and gouges, a moderate amount of autologous bone was harvested. Bilateral iliac crest were evaluated with preoperative imaging including MRI and CT to ensure the absence of tumor. This area was then back-filled with corticocancellous chips, and the overlying fascia was closed with 0 Vicryl. The facet joints and transverse processes were decorticated bilaterally, prior to placement of cobalt chromium rods. A gentle lordotic curve was positioned in order to place the distal rod into the L4 and L5 screw heads with a minimal amount of in situ sagittal bending. After copiously irrigating the wound, the bone graft was placed into the facet joints, which had been drilled out and decorticated. A cross connector was placed at the L2 level. Vancomycin powder was applied over the fusion construct. The wound was then closed in anatomical layers. Postoperative x-rays revealed good location of the hardware (Fig. 49.2). The patient tolerated the procedure well and was discharged on postoperative day 4 after good pain control and ambulation.

Commonalities among the experts

Our panel of expert surgeons were all in agreement that more imaging would be required, including imaging modalities such as magnetic resonance imaging, computed tomography, dual-energy x-ray absorptiometry, and x-rays. All of the surgeons planned for surgical decompression of the tumor, and three of the four surgeons planned instrumentation for stabilization as well. The planned positioning was prone on either a Jackson, Wilson, or Allen frame for all of the surgeons. Two of the four surgeons discussed possible use of tranexamic acid and steroids. Other areas of disagreement were regarding use of embolization, postoperative disposition, and bracing, with only one surgeon planning for preoperative embolization, one surgeon planning for admission to the intensive care unit after surgery, and one surgeon planning for use of a postoperative TLSO brace.

SUMMARY OF QUALITY OF EVIDENCE TO GUIDE SPECIFIC INTERVENTIONS FOR THIS CASE

- Surgical decompression and radiation improve outcomes over radiation alone for patients with spinal compression: level IA
- Laminectomy alone is poor for spinal metastasis when the primary pathology is anterior to the spinal cord, especially with significant destruction of the vertebral body: level III
- The treatment of oligometastatic disease appears to offer a significant survival advantage compared with polymetastatic disease: level IIA

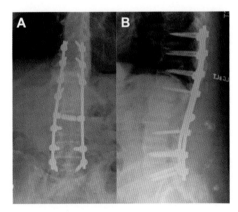

Fig. 49.2 Postoperative x-rays. (A), Anteroposterior and **(B)**, lateral images demonstrating T10-L5 fusion with paired pedicle screws at the T10-T12, L4, and L5 levels. There are right-sided pedicle screws at L1 and L3. There is a single cross-link seen at the L2 level.

REFERENCES

1. Sinson GP, Zager EL. *Metastases and spinal cord compression. N Engl J Med.* 1992;327(27):1953–1954. author reply 1954-5.
2. Siegel RL, Miller KD, Jemal A. *Cancer Statistics, 2017. CA Cancer J Clin.* 2017;67(1):7–30.
3. Patchell RA, et al. *Direct decompressive surgical resection in the treatment of spinal cord compression caused by metastatic cancer: a randomised trial. Lancet.* 2005;366(9486):643–648.
4. Crabtree KL, et al. *Surgical treatment of multiple spine metastases from gastrinoma. Evid Based Spine Care J.* 2011;2(4):45–50.
5. Barzilai O, et al. *Survival, local control, and health-related quality of life in patients with oligometastatic and polymetastatic spinal tumors: A multicenter, international study. Cancer.* 2019;125(5):770–778.
6. Tokuhashi Y, et al. *A revised scoring system for preoperative evaluation of metastatic spine tumor prognosis. Spine (Phila Pa 1976).* 2005;30(19):2186–2191.
7. Taterra D, et al. *Artery of Adamkiewicz: a meta-analysis of anatomical characteristics. Neuroradiology.* 2019;61(8):869–880.
8. Maurer PK. *Systemic approach to spinal reconstruction after anterior decompression for neoplastic disease of the thoracic and lumbar spine. Neurosurgery.* 1993;33(3):533–534.
9. Fisher CG, et al. *A novel classification system for spinal instability in neoplastic disease: an evidence-based approach and expert consensus from the Spine Oncology Study Group. Spine (Phila Pa 1976).* 2010;35(22):E1221–E1229.
10. Findlay GF. *Adverse effects of the management of malignant spinal cord compression. J Neurol Neurosurg Psychiatry.* 1984;47(8):761–768.

50

Sacral schwannoma

Oluwaseun O. Akinduro, MD

Introduction

Intradural extramedullary (IDEM) tumors are tumors of the neuro-axis that grow within the confines of the dura mater but are extrinsic to the spinal cord itself. Epidemiological studies have estimated the incidence of IDEM tumors to be approximately 0.74 per 100,000 persons.[1,2] Although a variety of tumor types may be found within this compartment, the most common are benign tumors such as meningiomas or schwannomas. Meningiomas are benign tumors arising from arachnoid cap cells of the dura; thus, they are typically attached to the dura with a broad base. Their histology is identical to their intracranial counterpart. Schwannomas arise from the dorsal or ventral nerve root, with the dorsal roots being more common. These tumors are hypothesized to originate in the Obersteiner-Redlich zone, which is the transition point between oligodendrocytes of the central nervous system and Schwann cells of the peripheral nervous system.[3] Schwannomas typically arise from a single-nerve fascicle and displace the surrounding roots, causing compression and leading to pain, sensory loss, and weakness. Although these tumors arise from the nerve fascicle itself, this involved fascicle rarely contains functional tissue and thus can typically be ligated without clinical sequelae.[4]

The most common tumors to be found in the sacrum are metastases or a primary tumor such as chordoma, but other tumor types can also be found originating in the sacral region. Schwannomas of the sacrum are rare and account for approximately 1% to 5% of all spinal schwannomas.[5,6] There have been limited reports discussing the surgical management of these cases.[5] In this chapter, we discuss the management of a patient with a sacral tumor and discuss the anatomical associations to be considered when approaching this region.

Example case

Chief complaint: urinary retention, buttock pain

History of present illness: This is a 43-year-old female with right-sided buttock pain and urinary retention for 1 year. She has no pain in her legs. She reports subjective decrease in sensation in her genitals. Magnetic resonance imaging (MRI) of the sacrum raises concern for a nerve sheath tumor (Fig. 50.1).

Medications: gabapentin, antidepressants

Allergies: no known drug allergies

Past medical history: none

Past surgical history: hysterectomy, C-section

Family history: no history of malignancies

Social history: none

Physical examination: awake, alert, and oriented to person, place, and time; cranial nerves II–XII intact; bilateral deltoids/triceps/biceps 5/5; interossei 5/5; iliopsoas/knee flexion/knee extension/dorsi, and plantar flexion 5/5

Reflexes: 2+ in bilateral biceps/triceps/brachioradialis with negative Hoffman; 2+ in bilateral patella/ankle and no clonus or Babinski; sensation intact to light touch

Laboratories: all within normal limits

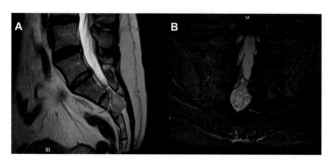

Fig. 50.1 Preoperative T2 magnetic resonance imaging (MRI) of the sacrum. (A) Mid sagittal and (B) coronal images demonstrating a sacral tumor emanating from the right S2 nerve root. There is enlargement of the S2 foramen as the tumor is seen traveling along the nerve. Red arrow highlights the tumor.

	Jorge Eduardo Guzman Prenk, MD Neurosurgery Pontificia Universidad Javeriana Bogota, Colombia	Daniel J. Hoh, MD Neurosurgery University of Florida Gainesville, Florida, United States	Adrian Casey, MD Neurosurgery National Hospital for Neurology and Neurosurgery Queen Square, Holborn, London, United Kingdom	Jean-Paul Wolinsky, MD Neurosurgery Northwestern University Chicago, Illinois, United States
Preoperative				
Additional tests requested	None	CT lumbar spine Urodynamic testing Possible CT-guided biopsy	MRI brain and complete spine CT chest/abdomen/pelvis Urodynamic testing Neurophysiology assessment PET if diagnosis uncertain	Urodynamic testing
Surgical approach selected	S1-2 laminectomy for resection of tumor	S1-2 laminectomy for resection of tumor	S2 laminectomy for resection of tumor	S2-4 laminectomy for resection of tumor
Goal of surgery	Diagnosis, decompression of nerve roots	Diagnosis, gross total resection	Diagnosis, maximal safe resection, prevent further deterioration	Decompression of nerve roots, resection of lesion
Perioperative				
Positioning	Prone	Prone	Pone	Prone
Surgical equipment	Fluoroscopy IOM (EMG sphincter/bladder) Surgical microscope	Fluoroscopy Surgical microscope	Fluoroscopy IOM (EMG sphincter/bladder) Surgical microscope Ultrasonic bone cutter	IOM (EMG sphincter/bladder) Fluoroscopy
Medications	None	Ketorolac 48 hours after surgery	+/– steroids	None
Anatomical considerations	Sacral nerve roots namely sciatic and pudendal	Sacral nerve roots SI joints	Sacral nerve roots, dura	S2-S4 sacral nerve roots
Complications feared with approach chosen	Nerve root injury, CSF leak	S2 nerve root injury, CSF leak	Residual lesion, CSF leak, nerve root injury causing urinary incontinence	Nerve root injury
Intraoperative				
Anesthesia	General	General	General	General
Exposure	S1-3	S1-2	S2	S2-4
Levels decompressed	S1-2	S1-2	S2	S2-4
Levels fused	None	None	None	None
Surgical narrative	Position prone, medial incision from S1-3, subperiosteal dissection of muscles, transverse angled retractors locked in place, mainly right S2 laminectomy with high-speed drill, dissect nerve root from distal to proximal, monopolar stimulation for EMG or relay on CMAP recording, dissect and remove tumor, layered closure	Position prone, vertical midline incision over sacrum, fluoroscopy to confirm S1-2 level, drill and rongeurs to perform right-sided S1-2 laminectomy, identify right S1 nerve root within canal and exiting out S1-2 foramen, open dura overlying nerve root sleeve under microscope, follow tumor proximally to nerve root axilla to evaluate for intrathecal extension, internally debulk tumor and follow distally through S1-2 foramen, may need to unroof foramen to full extent, dissection and	Position prone, x-ray level check, midline incision at S2, subperiosteal muscle dissection to expose laminae, x-ray level check, S2 laminectomy using high-speed drill or ultrasonic bone cutter under microscopic visualization, dissection of presumed nerve sheath tumor, identify lesion and delimitation of edges, excision of lesion +/– nerve root sacrifice, send tissue for histology, dural closure with clips, dura	Position prone, IOM, localization x-ray, midline incision from S2-S4, subperiosteal exposure of S2-4 spinous process and lamina, localization x-ray, S2-4 laminectomies, dissection and identification of bilateral S2-4 nerve roots and tumor, isolate likely S4 nerve root, identify nerve proximal and distal to the tumor, ligate proximal aspect of S4 nerve root below thecal sac with 2-0 silk suture and then cut, cut S4 nerve root distal to tumor, deliver

	Jorge Eduardo Guzman Prenk, MD Neurosurgery Pontificia Universidad Javeriana Bogota, Colombia	Daniel J. Hoh, MD Neurosurgery University of Florida Gainesville, Florida, United States	Adrian Casey, MD Neurosurgery National Hospital for Neurology and Neurosurgery Queen Square, Holborn, London, United Kingdom	Jean-Paul Wolinsky, MD Neurosurgery Northwestern University Chicago, Illinois, United States
		peel tumor capsule off of remaining fascicles, meticulous dural closure with fibrin glue, multilayer closure, horizontal mattress sutures in skin, immediate mobilization after surgery	repair with glue, layered closure, flat for 48 hours if CSF encountered	entire tumor in one piece, hemostasis with gentle irrigation, layered closure with attention to lumbosacral and Scarpa's fascia with subfascial drain tunneled below lumbosacral fascia in rostral direction away from incision and carried out through separate stage incision, skin closure with glue
Complication avoidance	Right hemilaminectomy, follow course of entire nerve from distal to proximal, monopolar stimulation and CMAP to identify nerve roots	Right hemilaminectomy, follow course of entire nerve, assess for intradural tumor, internally debulk tumor before peeling tumor from fascicles, fibrin glue, immediate mobilization after surgery	Follow course of entire nerve, identify beginning and termination, determine whether nerve needs to be sacrificed, flat for 48 hours if CSF encountered	Isolate nerve root where tumor is coming from, ligate and cut proximal nerve root first, en bloc tumor removal
Postoperative				
Admission	Floor	Floor	Floor	Floor
Postoperative complications feared	Nerve root injury, CSF leak, epidural hematoma, infection	Nerve root palsy, pain, CSF leak, urinary retention, paralytic ileus	Nerve root injury causing incontinence or sexual dysfunction, CSF leak, infection	Urinary retention, persistent urinary tract infections, wound infection, CSF leak
Anticipated length of stay	2 days	2–4 days	5–7 days	1–3 days
Follow-up testing	MRI 4 months after surgery Possible genetics evalaution pending histology	MRI 3–4 months after surgery, then annually for 5 years	MRI 3 months, yearly for 2 years	MRI 6 weeks after surgery if en bloc achieved (<48 hours if subtotal resection), 6 months, 12 months, 24 months, 36 months after surgery
Bracing	None	None	None	None
Follow-up visits	2 weeks, 4 months after surgery	3 weeks, 6 weeks, 3–4 months after surgery	6 weeks, 3 months, yearly for 2 years after surgery	2 weeks, 6 weeks, 3 months, 6 months, 12 months, then annually after surgery

CMAP, Compound muscle action potential; *CSF*, cerebrospinal fluid; *CT*, computed tomography; *EMG*, electromyography; *IOM*, intraoperative monitoring; *MRI*, magnetic resonance imaging; *PET*, positron emission tomography; *SSEP*, somatosensory evoked potentials.

Differential diagnosis

- Nerve sheath tumor
- Metastasis
- Chordoma
- Tarlov cyst
- Other primary bone tumor

Important anatomical considerations

Tumors that arise from the sacral nerve roots may be particularly problematic for patients because the sacral nerve roots are involved in critical functions such as bowel and bladder control. Roots S2-4 innervate the intrinsic muscles of the foot and provide sensation for the anus in concentric rings. The anal sphincter is supplied by S2-4 and can be monitored intraoperatively with electromyography.[7] Tumors in this region have a propensity to become large prior to detection because they typically do not cause a significant amount of pain or functional limitations for patients until they are large in size. Giant sacral tumors may require an anterior or combined anterior and posterior approach for safe resection. If an anterior approach is needed, the close association of the great veins will likely require the assistance of a vascular surgeon. The internal iliac veins can be identified ventral to the sacrum prior to joining to form the common iliac vein, which drains into the inferior vena cava. Because of the close relation to bowel and the rectum, the assistance of a colorectal surgeon should also be considered.

Approaches to this lesion

The vast majority of intradural tumors can be adequately addressed with a standard posterior midline approach.[8–10] This approach is typically favored due to its familiarity and the relative ease of dural repair.[8–10] The ideal approach to a tumor of the sacrum is determined by the location of the tumor itself. Most tumors of this region can be safely accessed with a posterior approach, but extradural extension of the tumor into the presacral space may require an anterior approach. Because of the lack of familiarity with the presacral region for most neurosurgeons, an access surgeon is typically used when an anterior approach is required. In the case of a nerve sheath tumor, the involved fascicles are rarely functional, and bowel and bladder functions are typically preserved as long as S2-4 roots are preserved on one side.

What was actually done

The patient was brought to the operating room and placed under general endotracheal anesthesia and then placed into the prone position. The back was prepped and draped in usual sterile fashion. Following confirmatory pause, the C-arm was brought into the field for localization purposes. A midline incision was made over the midportion of the sacrum and dissection was carried down to the dorsal aspect of the sacrum. There was no obvious dorsal violation by the tumor. A sacral laminectomy was done primarily with a Kerrison rongeur beginning at the right S2 dorsal foramen. There was a thin shell of bone over the tumor itself, which was removed. The proximal and distal ends of the schwannoma were identified. The capsule was opened and dissected around the mass. A small fascicle was identified at the proximal and distal end, which seemed to lead into the schwannoma itself. This was divided and the tumor was removed in one piece. The proximal and distal ends were inspected and no additional tumor was identified. There was no evidence of cerebrospinal fluid (CSF) egress. The capsule was then coagulated and hemostasis was assured. A Valsalva maneuver was performed and again no CSF egress was identified. The wound was copiously irrigated with bacitracin irrigation solution and then then closed in anatomical layers. The patient was admitted to the intensive care unit after surgery with an intact neurological exam. They were kept flat overnight and then elevated. They were discharged home on postoperative day 3 with an intact neurological exam. A postoperative magnetic resonance imaging (MRI) revealed gross total resection of the tumor (Fig. 50.2).

Commonalities among the experts

Our panel of expert surgeons all agreed that this patient would require surgical resection of the symptomatic tumor depicted in the MRI. They also agreed with a standard midline posterior approach with sacral laminectomy to access the tumor, where half favored a hemilaminectomy. The majority planned for preoperative urodynamic testing for the patient in order to establish a baseline. The surgeons also agreed with the use of electrophysiological monitoring, especially using electromyography (EMG) to monitor sphincter and bladder function. The majority discussed the need to isolate the entire nerve root. All were concerned about postoperative CSF leak and nerve root injury. There was consensus regarding the postoperative care for the patient. All planned for transfer of the patient to the floor after surgery and also planned to schedule a postoperative MRI approximately 3 months after surgery.

SUMMARY OF QUALITY OF EVIDENCE TO GUIDE SPECIFIC INTERVENTIONS FOR THIS CASE

- Combined monitoring with somatosensory and motor evoked potentials appears superior to monomodal monitoring: level IIA
- Electromyography and intraoperative direct stimulation are efficacious for safe resection of nerve sheath tumors: level III
- The ideal approach to intradural extramedullary tumors is primarily based on the location of the lesion and surgeon preference: level III

REFERENCES

1. Duong LM, McCarthy BJ, McLendon RE, Dolecek TA, Kruchko C, Douglas LL, et al. Descriptive epidemiology of malignant and nonmalignant primary spinal cord, spinal meninges, and cauda equina tumors, United States, 2004-2007. *Cancer.* 2012;118:4220–4227.
2. Schellinger KA, Propp JM, Villano JL, McCarthy BJ. Descriptive epidemiology of primary spinal cord tumors. *J Neuro-Oncol.* 2008;87:173–179.
3. Alfieri A, Fleischhammer J, Strauss C, Peschke E. The central myelin-peripheral myelin transitional zone of the nervus intermedius and its implications for microsurgery in the cerebellopontine angle. *Clin Anat.* 2012;25:882–888.

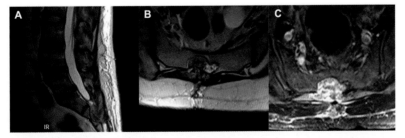

Fig. 50.2 Postoperative magnetic resonance imaging (MRI) of sacrum. (A) Sagittal T2, (B) axial T2, and (C) axial T1 postcontrast images demonstrating gross total resection of the tumor. The surgical cavity can be seen with no obvious tumor remnants.

4. Kim P, Ebersold MJ, Onofrio BM, Quast LM. Surgery of spinal nerve schwannoma. Risk of neurological deficit after resection of involved root. *J Neurosurg*. 1989;71:810–814.

5. Handa K, Ozawa H, Aizawa T, Hashimoto K, Kanno H, Tateda S, et al. Surgical Management of Giant Sacral Schwannoma: A Case Series and Literature Review. *World Neurosurg*. 2019;129:e216–e223.

6. Yu NH, Lee SE, Jahng TA, Chung CK. Giant invasive spinal schwannoma: its clinical features and surgical management. *Neurosurgery*. 2012;71:58–66.

7. Jahangiri FR, Silverstein JW, Trausch C, Al Eissa S, George ZM, DeWal H, et al. Motor Evoked Potential Recordings from the Urethral Sphincter Muscles (USMEPs) during Spine Surgeries. *Neurodiagn J*. 2019;59:34–44.

8. Angevine PD, Kellner C, Haque RM, McCormick PC. Surgical management of ventral intradural spinal lesions. *J Neurosurg Spine*. 2011;15:28–37.

9. Guo L, Quinones-Hinojosa A, Yingling CD, Weinstein PR. Continuous EMG recordings and intraoperative electrical stimulation for identification and protection of cervical nerve roots during foraminal tumor surgery. *J Spinal Disord Tech*. 2006;19:37–42.

10. Pelosi L, Lamb J, Grevitt M, Mehdian SM, Webb JK, Blumhardt LD. Combined monitoring of motor and somatosensory evoked potentials in orthopedic spinal surgery. *Clin Neurophysiol*. 2002;113:1082–1091.

Thoracic spine metastasis with acute myelopathy

Jaime L. Martínez Santos, MD

Introduction

Metastatic spine disease is one of the most feared complications of cancer with serious sequelae such as torturous pain, paralysis, and sphincter and sexual dysfunction. Approximately 30% of cancer patients develop symptomatic metastatic epidural spinal cord compression (MESCC)[1-3] and a timely surgical decompression is the gold standard treatment.[4] In this chapter, we present a case example to illustrate the clinical presentation and management of a patient with acute MESCC.

Example case

Chief complaint: new weakness
History of present illness: The patient is a 61-year-old male who presents to the emergency department with new-onset back pain and sudden-onset severe lower extremity weakness, sensory loss, and bowel and bladder incontinence. Thoracolumbar spine imaging showed a contrast-enhancing lesion involving the vertebral bodies of T8–10 and right pedicle and transverse process of T9, causing a T9 pathological fracture and severe spinal cord compression (Fig. 51.1). The patient was afebrile and denies recent infection, renal insufficiency, or immune deficiency.
Medications: none
Allergies: no known drug allergies
Past medical history: hypertension, thyroid carcinoma, and squamous cell carcinoma of the lung
Past surgical history: none
Family history: noncontributory
Social history: none
Physical examination: awake, alert, and oriented to person, place, and time; cranial nerves II–XII intact; full strength in bilateral upper extremities deltoids/triceps/biceps 5/5; interossei 5/5. Paraplegia with 0/5 strength in all lower extremity muscle groups. Sensory level at T11. No response on deep tendon reflex testing in patellar and Achilles tendons. Absent rectal tone.
Laboratories: all within normal limits

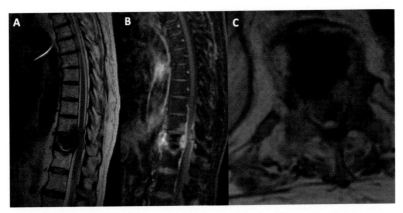

Fig. 51.1 Preoperative magnetic resonance imaging (MRI). (A) Sagittal T2, (B) sagittal T1 with contrast, and (C) axial T2 images demonstrating a contrast-enhancing lesion involving the vertebral bodies of T8-10 (mostly T9) and causing a T9 vertebral body collapse. This extradural tumor causing significant ventral spinal cord compression and displacing the spinal cord to the left.

	Amro F. Al-Habib, MD, MPH Neurosurgery King Khalid University Hospital King Saud University Riyadh, Saudi Arabia	Mark H. Bilsky, MD Neurosurgery Memorial Sloan Kettering Cancer Center New York, New York, United States	Stefano Boriani, MD Orthopaedic Surgery IRCCS Istituto Ortopedico Galeazzi, Milan, Italy	Jang Yoon, MD Neurosurgery University of Pennsylvania Philadelphia, Pennsylvania, United States
Preoperative				
Additional tests requested	CT T-spine Chest x-ray Blood cultures Anesthesia evaluation	MRI complete spine Bilateral lower extremity dopplers Oncology evaluation Family discussion	PET CT C/T/L-spine Spinal angiogram and selective arterial embolization	CT C/T/L-spine CT chest/abdomen/pelvis ESR/CRP Blood cultures Bence-Jones protein in urine
Surgical approach selected	T8–9 laminectomy and costo-transversectomy and fusion	T8–9 laminectomy, resection of epidural disease, PMMA augmentation, T8–9 fusion	T8–9 laminectomy with posterior fusion and possible corpectomy pending preliminary pathology	T8 partial corpectomy, T8–9 laminectomy, T6–11 posterior fusion
Goal of surgery	Diagnosis, decompress neural elements, achieve adequate spinal stabilization	Diagnosis, decompress spinal cord, stabilize spine, separation surgery for radiation treatment	Diagnosis, decompress spinal cord	Diagnosis, decompress spinal cord, stabilize spine
Perioperative				
Positioning	Prone on Jackson table, no pins	Prone in pins	Prone, no pins	Prone on Jackson table, no pins
Surgical equipment	IOM (SSEP/MEP) Surgical navigation Fluoroscopy Ultrasound	IOM (MEP/SSEP/EMG) Fluoroscopy Surgical navigation Ultrasound	Fluoroscopy	Fluoroscopy
Medications	MAP >80	Steroids, maintain MAP	None	Steroids
Anatomical considerations	Pedicles	Spinal cord	Spinal cord	Aorta, segmental vessels, artery of Adamkiewicz, thoracic spinal cord, lungs
Complications feared with approach chosen	Spinal cord injury, neurological worsening	Spinal cord injury	Durotomy, bleeding from epidural veins	Acute blood loss, wound complications, neurological worsening
Intraoperative				
Anesthesia	General	General	General	General
Exposure	T7–11	T8–9	T7-T11	T6-L2
Levels decompressed	T8–9	T8–9	T8–9	T8-T10
Levels fused	T7–11	T8–9	T8–9	T6-T11
Surgical narrative	Position prone, level marking using anatomy landmarks and intraoperative navigation, adequate exposure, placement of navigation reference frame on most proximal spinous process, acquisition of images and connect them to the navigation system, placement of pedicle screws two levels above and below target segment, perform O-arm to confirm screw position, laminectomy and bilateral	Position prone, fluoroscopy to confirm levels, incision, subperiosteal dissection, muscle retraction with forceps to avoid entering tumor, placement of pedicle screws with PMMA augmentation of pedicles, decompression by resecting entire spinous process of the index level and 50% of superior spinous process sparing interspinous ligament, matchstick is used to drill laminae to thin shell, ligamentum flavum	Position prone, midline incision two levels above and below index level, wide T8-T9 laminectomy, sample tissue for frozen section, hemostasis of epidural vessels as soon as thecal sac fully exposed, place pedicle screws two levels above and below, complete fixation and graft if tumor	Position prone, midline incision, subperiosteal dissection of paraspinal muscles and minimize charring of muscles, expose T6-T11, do not violate posterior tension band as well as facets, place bilateral pedicle screw at T6–7 and T10-T11 using anatomical landmarks, confirm position of screws with fluoroscopy, T8–9 laminectomy with medical facetectomy until pedicles can be palpated with a dissector, T8 transpedicular approach with removing both pedicles, confirm disease location, T7–8 and T8–9 discectomy, partial corpectomy

	Amro F. Al-Habib, MD, MPH Neurosurgery King Khalid University Hospital King Saud University Riyadh, Saudi Arabia	Mark H. Bilsky, MD Neurosurgery Memorial Sloan Kettering Cancer Center New York, New York, United States	Stefano Boriani, MD Orthopaedic Surgery IRCCS Istituto Ortopedico Galeazzi, Milan, Italy	Jang Yoon, MD Neurosurgery University of Pennsylvania Philadelphia, Pennsylvania, United States
	facetectomy of involved segment, intraoperative ultrasound to confirm level and assess spinal cord compression, removal of pedicle and rib head and achieve adequate decompression, send tissue for pathology and microbiology examination, another ultrasound to confirm decompression, apply rods and crosslink, close in layers with subfascial drain	resected with #15 blade, medial bilateral pedicles and superior and inferior facet joints at index levels and superior joint at inferior level resected with drill to expose lateral dura, resection of tumor starting from normal dural planes, identify and spare nerve roots, partial resection of epidural tumor creating a defect in vertebral body, PLL-dural interface identified and PLL cut with scissors to create margin, ultrasound to confirm adequate decompression, decortication, placement of autograft, vancomycin in the wound, drain in epidural space, suprafascial flaps	is radiosensitive, complete transpedicular corpectomy for gross total resection and reconstruction with PMMA or expandable cage if radioresistant, layered closure with subfascial drain	and removal of the lesion with drill/curettes/osteotomes as needed, leave anterior cortex intact to minimize risk of vascular injury and pleural injury, remove cartilate from T7–8 and T8–9 to expose bony end plates, placement of expandable cage, preserve segmental vessel if concerned it is the artery of Adamkiewicz, confirm position of cage with fluoroscopy, place titanium rods bilaterally, vancomycin powder in the cavity, close with two subfascial drains
Complication avoidance	Intraoperative navigation, two levels above and below fusion, ultrasound to assess level and decompression, costotransversectomy to achieve adequate decompression, crosslink for rods	Muscle retraction with forceps, PMMA pedicle augmentation, spare interspinous ligament, avoid Kerrison punches, start tumor dissection from normal dural planes, identify and spare nerve roots, ultrasound to evaluate decompression, suprafascial flaps to minimize tension	Hemostasis of epidural veins as soon as thecal sac fully exposed, avoid corpectomy and expandable cage if tumor is radiosensitive based on frozen pathology	Minimize charring of muscles, maintain posterior tension band and facet capsules, bilateral transpedicular approach, leave anterior cortex of vertebral body intact to minimize risk of vascular injury, angiography to study artery of Adamkiewicz
Postoperative				
Admission	Stepdown unit	ICU	ICU	ICU
Postoperative complications feared	Neurological deterioration, infection	Pseudoarthrosis, medical complications	CSF leak, wound healing problems	Instrumentation migration/failure, adjacent segment disease, medical complications
Anticipated length of stay	4 weeks	6 days	7 days	5–7 days
Follow-up testing	Physical therapy MRI T-L spine 1 month after surgery X-rays 1 month after surgery	MRI T-L spine 72 hours after surgery Plain x-rays Radiation oncology evaluation	MRI T-spine every 3–4 months for 2 years depending on pathology Multidisciplinary team discussion pending pathology	Upright thoracic and lumbar x-rays 6 weeks after surgery Radiation oncology evaluation
Bracing	TLSO for 2 months	None	None	None
Follow-up visits	1 month after surgery	3 weeks after surgery	Every 3–4 months for 2 years depending on pathology	2 weeks, 6 weeks, 3 months, 6 months, 12 months, 24 months after surgery

CRP, C-reactive protein; CSF, cerebrospinal fluid; CT, computed tomography; EMG, electromyography; ESR, erythrocyte sedimentation rate; ICU, intensive care unit; IOM, intraoperative monitoring; MAP, mean arterial pressure; MEP, motor evoked potential; MRI, magnetic resonance imaging; PET, positron emission tomography; PLL, posterior longitudinal ligament; PMMA, polymethylmethacrylate; SSEP, somatosensory evoked potential; TLSO, thoracic lumbar sacral orthosis.

Differential diagnosis

- Metastatic spine disease
- Spinal stenosis
- Osteomyelitis
- Primary extradural spinal tumor
- Traumatic fracture

Important anatomical and preoperative considerations

Cancer is prevalent worldwide and 70% of patients with cancer have spinal metastases on postmortem examination.[5] Spinal metastatic disease is the most common type of spine tumor and currently affects approximately 1 million North Americans.[2] Spinal metastases more commonly involve the thoracic spine and locate in the extradural compartment,[3,6] and up to 30% of patients develop symptomatic MESCC.[1–3] Patients usually have a known cancer diagnosis, but MESCC can be the initial clinical manifestation of cancer in about 20%.[7] Prostate, breast, and lung cancers each account for 15% to 20% of MESCC, and non-Hodgkin lymphoma, renal cell carcinoma, and multiple myeloma account for about 5% to 10%.[3,6] Tumor metastases to the vertebral bodies occur mostly through the hematogenous route (85%) via arterial embolization or via the valveless internal vertebral venous plexus (of Batson).[5] Another route is through a direct spread of paravertebral tumors via the intervertebral foramina.[3,5]

The spinal cord compression usually develops at a slow pace; however, vertebral metastases could extend into the cortical bone and precipitate pathological fractures with or without spinal instability causing fragment retropulsion into the canal and sudden onset of pain and neurological deficit.[3] The pathophysiologic mechanism causing the myelopathy may involve direct spinal cord compression resulting in axonal damage and demyelination. It can occur in combination with vascular compromise that is venous in the initial stages with collapse or stenosis of venous tributaries of Batson's plexus that disrupt the blood–spinal cord barrier and result in vasogenic edema (potentially reversible with corticosteroids) and arterial in the final stages with diminished spinal cord perfusion, oxidative stress and ischemia, and eventually infarction (irreversible).[3,8] The most common presentation of MESCC is with local back pain (95%) that is usually worse with Valsalva maneuvers and worse at night with recumbency, as this position stretches the spine and engorges Batson's plexus.[3] Mechanical back pain is worse with movement and is suggestive of spinal instability.[9] The second most common presentation of MESCC is weakness (35%–75%) that usually starts with clumsiness and "heaviness" but progresses to inability to walk in up to 80% of patients at presentation.[3,6,10,11] Sensory loss also occurs and starts distally in the lower extremities and ascends with disease progression. A diminished or abnormal pinprick sensation (sharp vs. dull discrimination) or sensory level is often an early sign of spinal cord compression and should be emphasized as part of a thorough physical examination. Sphincter disturbance is a poor prognostic indicator for preservation or recovery of ambulatory status.[3,6]

Progressive or sudden spinal cord compression with neurological decline requires urgent surgical decompression. The initial diagnostic workup should include at least a whole spine magnetic resonance imaging (MRI) with and without contrast (or a computed tomography myelogram if MRI is contraindicated) to assess the spinal metastatic burden and localize the compressed spinal level that correlate with the patient's symptoms. Standing lateral x-rays or dynamic flexion-extension x-rays should be obtained if tolerated by the patient to assess for dynamic instability. Additionally, metastatic workup with computed tomography of the chest, abdomen, and pelvis should be performed (the spine can be readily visualized and the hardware planned using bone windows) to assess for disease burden. Multiple myeloma and other radiosensitive tumors (e.g., lymphoma) should be identified early. The overall prognosis of patients with spinal metastasis depends on the aggressiveness of the primary tumor pathology, the number of visceral and spinal metastases, and the patient's functional status, including physical reserve (poor if sarcopenic and cachectic),[2] ability to walk, and length of survival, which is usually around 3 to 6 months.[3,6,12–15] Therefore, treatment is mostly palliative and aimed at pain relief and quality of life improvement. Scoring systems have been developed to predict the length of survival of patients with spinal metastasis and determine which patients would survive long enough to benefit from surgery.[16–18] An accepted system is the revised Tokuhashi score,[16] which is a 15-point score consisting of six predictors: (1) Karnofsky's performance status, (2) number of extraspinal bone metastases, (3) number of spinal bone metastases, (4) metastases to major internal organs (e.g., suitable or not for resection), (5) primary site of the cancer (e.g., lung, osteosarcoma, stomach, bladder, esophagus, and pancreas are of worst prognosis), and (6) spinal cord function (Table 51.1). Patients with scores of 8 or less have an estimated survival of less than 3 to 6 months; therefore, palliative management has traditionally taken precedence.[16,19] More recently, however, the 3 to 6 months minimum survival requirement for surgical candidacy is being challenged as some patients experience statistically significant quality of life improvements in as little as 6 weeks after surgery.[20]

The goals of treatment for patients with metastatic spine disease are palliative and include pain control, health-related quality of life improvement, local tumor control, neurological function preservation or restoration, and spinal alignment and stability preservation or restoration.[21,22] Management is an orchestrated effort by a multidisciplinary team involving oncologists, neurooncologists, radiation oncologists, radiologists, internists, anesthesiologists, neurosurgeons, and palliative care and pain control specialists. Indications for surgery include acute or progressive neurological decline, mechanical pain from spinal instability, vertebral body collapse with bony compression or kyphotic deformity, and patients in which the maximal spinal cord radiation dose tolerance has been reached.[22,23] The goals of surgery are decompressing the spinal cord, obtaining a histological diagnosis, and stabilizing the spine. "Separation" surgery is an option for patients with high-grade MESCC who are poor surgical candidates or have inaccessible tumors or a known radiosensitive histology and consists of creating a 1 to 2 mm space between the tumor and the spinal cord to optimize the radiotherapy dose distribution.[22] An important consideration is that 80% of spine metastases involve the vertebral bodies,[24] which normally withstand around 80% of the axial load[25] and cancer tissue lacks the weight-bearing properties of bone, thus predisposed to instability from anterior and middle spine column

Table 51.1 Revised Tokuhashi Score[16]	
Characteristic	Score
General Condition (Karnofsky's performance status [KPS]).	
• Poor (KPS 10%–40%)	0
• Moderate (KPS 50%–70%)	1
• Good (KPS 80%–100%)	1
Number of Extraspinal Bone Metastases	
• ≥3	0
• 1–2	1
• 0	2
Number of Spinal Metastases	
• ≥3	0
• 1–2	1
• 0	2
Metastases to Major Internal Organs	
• Unremovable	0
• Removable	1
• None	2
Primary Cancer	
• Lung, osteosarcoma, stomach, bladder, esophagus, or pancreas	0
• Liver, gallbladder, or unidentified	1
• Others	2
• Kidney or uterus	3
• Rectum	4
• Thyroid, breast, prostate, or carcinoid tumor	5
Spinal Cord Injury	
• Complete (Frankel A or B)	0
• Incomplete (Frankel C or D)	1
• None (Frankel E)	2
Tokuhashi Prognosis	
• Poor (<6 months)	• 0–8
• Intermediate (6–12 months)	• 9–11
• Good (≥12 months)	• 12–15
Tokuhashi score used to predict survival for patients with metastatic spine disease.	

strategies, are discussed in Chapter 44 and Chapter 48, Table 1, respectively. Spine stereotactic radiosurgery (SSRS) is currently the preferred modality of radiotherapy for spinal metastasis. SSRS can provide durable symptomatic response and high local-control rates regardless of tumor histology.[21] General indications for SSRS are (1) initial treatment of spinal metastasis for patients with oligometastatic disease without spinal cord compression (or Bilsky score of <2)[33] and without instability (SINS <10),[31] (2) therapy to residual tumor, and (3) tumor progression or recurrence.[21,22] Evidence suggest waiting at least 1 week between surgery and SSRS or vice versa.[34]

What was actually done

The patient was taken emergently to the operating room with the goals of decompressing the spinal cord and obtaining a diagnosis. Ten mg of dexamethasone was administered and mean arterial pressures (MAPs) were maintained 10% to 20% higher than his baseline. The posterior elements from T10–12 were exposed in the usual subperiosteal fashion and levels were confirmed using fluoroscopy. The spinous processes, laminae, and medial facets of T10 and 11 and the cranial edge of the T12 spinous process and lamina were removed bilaterally. There were no abnormal fluid collections or any macroscopic sign of infection; however, swab cultures were sent for microbiologic analysis. Distinct epidural tumor was visualized and pieces were sent for frozen histopathologic analysis, which returned as metastatic carcinoma of likely lung primary. The tumor was soft and aspirated easily. The intraoperative ultrasound was utilized to confirm adequate spinal cord decompression.[35,36] A Valsalva maneuver was used to identify bleeding points and confirm no durotomy. Complete hemostasis ensued, the wound was irrigated thoroughly with antibiotic solution, a subfascial drain was placed, and the wound was closed in anatomical layers. The patient had an uneventful postoperative course and was discharged to rehabilitation on postoperative day 6. The patient's lower extremity strength improved significantly with 3 to 4/5 in proximal muscle groups and 4 to 5/5 in distal muscle groups. The patient was scheduled for outpatient radiotherapy once his wound healed completely. Postoperative imaging showed good decompression (Fig. 51.2).

Commonalities among experts

Most surgeons would obtain a computed tomography for evaluating bone quality and bony involvement by this tumor and for planning the pedicle screw instrumentation.

failure.[22,26] Extensive posterior decompression without fusion may further destabilize the spine by disrupting the posterior column. The approach selection is not standardized and depends on tumor type and consistency, spinal level, location, and surgeon's preference.[27] Circumferential spinal cord decompression and reconstruction, however, decreases tumor recurrence[27] and may be associated with improved clinical and radiological outcomes.[28] Overall surgery-related morbidity and mortality rates are high with reported complication rates approximately 29% (5%–65%) and 30-day postoperative mortality rates approximately 5% (0%–22%).[22,28,29] The uses of the NOMS (neurological, oncologic, mechanic and systemic disease assessments) framework[30] and Spinal Instability Neoplastic Score (SINS),[17,31,32] which can help guide treatment

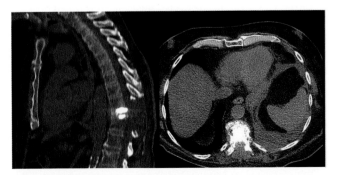

Fig. 51.2 Postoperative computed tomography (CT) scans. (A) Sagittal and (B) axial images demonstrating T9-10 laminectomy and good decompression of the thecal sac.

Half of surgeons would also obtain an infection workup including blood cultures. All of the surgeons would perform a thorough T10–11 posterior decompression with laminectomy, facetectomy, and pediculectomy, and half would also perform a more extensive anterior tumor resection and corpectomy. All surgeons felt that spinal stabilization was indicated, and most surgeons selected pedicle screw instrumentation two (50%) or three levels above and below the pathological fracture. Most surgeons would use freehand technique with fluoroscopic guidance. Half of the surgeons advocated for the use of intraoperative ultrasound and neurophysiologic monitoring and maintaining high MAPs. Feared complications included spinal cord injury, excessive bleeding, durotomy, infection, wound dehiscence, and cord infarction from coagulation of segmental arteries and Adamkiewicz. There was no consensus on postoperative imaging, but most surgeons agreed on obtaining x-rays in the immediate postoperative period and magnetic resonance imaging within 3 to 28 days of the operation, and on following the patient closely with surveillance imaging. Most surgeons would also consult oncology and radiation oncology for adjuvant therapy. Most surgeons recommended no bracing. Follow-up was scheduled 2 to 4 weeks postoperatively.

SUMMARY OF QUALITY OF EVIDENCE TO GUIDE SPECIFIC INTERVENTIONS FOR THIS CASE

- Surgical decompression is recommended for patients with MESCC (especially if high-grade) and neurological deficit: class I[4]

REFERENCES

1. Sciubba DM, Gokaslan ZL. Diagnosis and management of metastatic spine disease. *Surg Oncol.* 2006;15(3):141–151.
2. Pennington Z, Ehresman J, Cottrill E, et al. To operate, or not to operate? Narrative review of the role of survival predictors in patient selection for operative management of patients with metastatic spine disease. *J Neurosurg Spine.* 2020:1–15.
3. Cole JS, Patchell RA. Metastatic epidural spinal cord compression. *Lancet Neurol.* 2008;7(5):459–466.
4. Patchell RA, Tibbs PA, Regine WF, et al. Direct decompressive surgical resection in the treatment of spinal cord compression caused by metastatic cancer: a randomised trial. *The Lancet.* 2005;366(9486):643–648.
5. Arguello F, Baggs RB, Duerst RE, Johnstone L, McQueen K, Frantz CN. Pathogenesis of vertebral metastasis and epidural spinal cord compression. *Cancer.* 1990;65(1):98–106.
6. Bach F, Larsen BH, Rohde K, et al. Metastatic spinal cord compression. Occurrence, symptoms, clinical presentations and prognosis in 398 patients with spinal cord compression. *Acta Neurochir (Wien).* 1990;107(1-2):37–43.
7. Schiff D, O'Neill BP, Suman VJ. Spinal epidural metastasis as the initial manifestation of malignancy: clinical features and diagnostic approach. *Neurology.* 1997;49(2):452–456.
8. Ushio Y, Posner R, Posner JB, Shapiro WR. Experimental spinal cord compression by epidural neoplasm. *Neurology.* 1977;27(5):422–429.
9. Martinez Santos JL, Dmytriw AA, Fermin S. Neurosurgical management of a large meningocele in Jarcho-Levin syndrome: clinical and radiological pearls. *BMJ case reports.* 2015: bcr2015210240.
10. Levack P, Graham J, Collie D, et al. Don't wait for a sensory level-listen to the symptoms: a prospective audit of the delays in diagnosis of malignant cord compression. *Clin Oncol (R Coll Radiol).* 2002;14(6):472–480.
11. Helweg-Larsen S, Sørensen PS. Symptoms and signs in metastatic spinal cord compression: a study of progression from first symptom until diagnosis in 153 patients. *Eur J Cancer.* 1994;30a(3):396–398.
12. Rades D, Fehlauer F, Schulte R, et al. Prognostic factors for local control and survival after radiotherapy of metastatic spinal cord compression. *J Clin Oncol.* 2006;24(21):3388–3393.
13. Switlyk MD, Kongsgaard U, Skjeldal S, et al. Prognostic factors in patients with symptomatic spinal metastases and normal neurological function. *Clin Oncol (R Coll Radiol).* 2015; 27(4):213–221.
14. Tokuhashi Y, Uei H, Oshima M. Classification and scoring systems for metastatic spine tumors: a literature review. *Spine Surg Relat Res.* 2017;1(2):44–55.
15. Oliveira MF, Rotta JM, Botelho RV. Survival analysis in patients with metastatic spinal disease: the influence of surgery, histology, clinical and neurologic status. *Arq Neuropsiquiatr.* 2015;73(4):330–335.
16. Tokuhashi Y, Matsuzaki H, Oda H, Oshima M, Ryu J. A revised scoring system for preoperative evaluation of metastatic spine tumor prognosis. *Spine (Phila Pa 1976).* 2005;30(19):2186–2191.
17. Fisher CG, DiPaola CP, Ryken TC, et al. A novel classification system for spinal instability in neoplastic disease: an evidence-based approach and expert consensus from the Spine Oncology Study Group. *Spine (Phila Pa 1976).* 2010;35(22):E1221–E1229.
18. Bilsky MH, Laufer I, Fourney DR, et al. Reliability analysis of the epidural spinal cord compression scale. *J Neurosurg Spine.* 2010;13(3):324–328.
19. Tokuhashi Y, Uei H, Oshima M. Classification and scoring systems for metastatic spine tumors: a literature review. *Spine Surg Relat Res.* 2017;1(2):44–55.
20. Dea N, Versteeg AL, Sahgal A, et al. Metastatic Spine Disease: Should Patients With Short Life Expectancy Be Denied Surgical Care? An International Retrospective Cohort Study. *Neurosurgery.* 2020;87(2):303–311.
21. Barzilai O, Fisher CG, Bilsky MH. State of the Art Treatment of Spinal Metastatic Disease. *Neurosurgery.* 2018;82(6):757–769.
22. Nater A, Sahgal A, Fehlings M. Management spinal metastases. *Handb Clin Neurol.* 2018;149:239–255.
23. Prasad D, Schiff D. Malignant spinal-cord compression. *The Lancet Oncology.* 2005;6(1):15–24.
24. White AP, Kwon BK, Lindskog DM, Friedlaender GE, Grauer JN. Metastatic disease of the spine. *J Am Acad Orthop Surg.* 2006;14(11):587–598.
25. Ecker RD, Endo T, Wetjen NM, Krauss WE. Diagnosis and treatment of vertebral column metastases. *Mayo Clin Proc.* 2005;80(9):1177–1186.
26. Jacobs WB, Perrin RG. Evaluation and treatment of spinal metastases: an overview. *Neurosurgical focus.* 2001;11(6).
27. Molina C, Goodwin CR, Abu-Bonsrah N, Elder BD, De la Garza Ramos R, Sciubba DM. Posterior approaches for symptomatic metastatic spinal cord compression. *Neurosurg Focus.* 2016;41(2):E11.
28. Rustagi T, Mashaly H, Ganguly R, Akhter A, Mendel E. Transpedicular Vertebrectomy With Circumferential Spinal Cord Decompression and Reconstruction for Thoracic Spine Metastasis: A Consecutive Case Series. *Spine (Phila Pa 1976).* 2020;45(14): E820–e828.
29. Kim JM, Losina E, Bono CM, et al. Clinical Outcome of Metastatic Spinal Cord Compression Treated With Surgical Excision ± Radiation Versus Radiation Therapy Alone: A Systematic Review of Literature. *Spine.* 2012;37(1).
30. Laufer I, Rubin DG, Lis E, et al. The NOMS framework: approach to the treatment of spinal metastatic tumors. *Oncologist.* 2013;18(6):744–751.
31. Pennington Z, Ahmed AK, Westbroek EM, et al. SINS Score and Stability: Evaluating the Need for Stabilization Within the Uncertain Category. *World Neurosurg.* 2019;128:e1034–e1047.
32. Masuda K, Ebata K, Yasuhara Y, Enomoto A, Saito T. Outcomes and Prognosis of Neurological Decompression and Stabilization for Spinal Metastasis: Is Assessment with the Spinal Instability Neoplastic Score Useful for Predicting Surgical Results? *Asian Spine J.* 2018;12(5):846–853.

33. Kim YJ, Kim JH, Kim K, et al. The Feasibility of Spinal Stereotactic Radiosurgery for Spinal Metastasis with Epidural Cord Compression. *Cancer Res Treat.* 2019;51(4):1324–1335.

34. Itshayek E, Cohen JE, Yamada Y, et al. Timing of stereotactic radiosurgery and surgery and wound healing in patients with spinal tumors: a systematic review and expert opinions. *Neurol Res.* 2014;36(6):510–523.

35. Martinez Santos JLWJE, Kalhorn SP. Microsurgical Management of a Primary Neuroendocrine Tumor of the Filum Terminale: A Surgical Technique. *Cureus.* 2020;12(8):e10080.

36. Martinez Santos JL, Alshareef M, Kalhorn SP. Back Pain and Radiculopathy from Non-Steroidal Anti-Inflammatory Drug-induced Dorsal Epidural Haematoma. *BMJ Case Reports.* 2019;12(3):e229015.

52

Thoracic intramedullary lesions

Fidel Valero-Moreno, MD, Henry Ruiz-Garcia, MD and William Clifton, MD

Introduction

The thoracic spine, which includes attachments to the rib cage, is one of the most challenging regions for surgical interventions. Intramedullary cord thoracic lesions are not common, where intramedullary spinal cord tumors (IMSCTs) only account for 20% to 30% of the primary spinal cord neoplasms[1-3] and approximately 2% to 4% of all central nervous system (CNS) lesions.[4] In respect to primary tumors, gliomas are the most frequent neoplasms that involve the cord and account for up to 80% of these cases.[3] Ependymomas represent the highest occurrence in adults (50%–60%), followed by astrocytomas and hemangioblastoma, respectively.[1-6] IMSCTs can be found at any level of the spinal cord; however, IMSCTs show a predilection for the cervical (33%) and the thoracic (26%) levels.[6] The thoracic spinal cord is a high-complexity network of eloquent tissue that produces severe neurological deficit and comorbidities when partially or completely disconnected from the rest of the CNS. Thus optimal treatment must find a balance between extent of resection and adjuvant therapies while minimizing neurological deficits. In this chapter, we present a case of a 24-year-old woman presenting with lower limb weakness and back pain with a thoracic IMSCT.

Example case

Chief complaint: lower limb weakness
History of present illness: This is a 24-year-old healthy female who presented with a 3-month history of lower limb weakness and back pain. In addition, she reported numbness and tingling in both inner thighs for the past 2 weeks with difficulty climbing up stairs and occasional difficulty voiding. The patient was thoroughly evaluated including magnetic resonance image (MRI) of the thoracic spine that

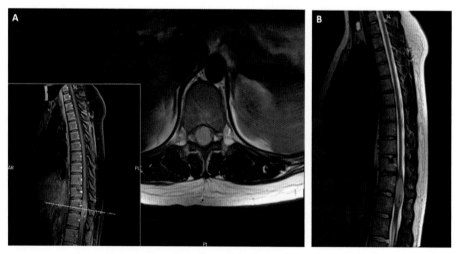

Fig. 52.1. Preoperative magnetic resonance image (MRI) of the thoracic spine. (A) Sagittal and axial T1 with contrast image demonstrating an intraaxial heterogeneous mass with well-demarcated borders at the level of T11-T12. The mass is centrally located and is exerting significant mass effect on the spinal cord. (B) Sagittal T2 image demonstrating a heterogenous mass causing significant radial elongation of the spinal cord. The lesion measures approximately 4 cm in craniocaudal length. No significant cord edema or syrinx is noted.

showed a T11-T12 well-defined intramedullary mass with heterogenous enhancement (Fig. 52.1).

Medications: none
Allergies: no known drug allergies
Past medical and surgical history: none
Family history: no history of malignancies
Social history: none

Physical examination: awake, alert, and oriented to person, place, and time; cranial nerves II–XII intact; bilateral deltoids/triceps/biceps 5/5; interossei 5/5; iliopsoas/knee flexion/knee extension 3/5; dorsi, and plantar flexion 4/5
Reflexes: 2+ in bilateral biceps/triceps/brachioradialis with negative Hoffman; 3+ in bilateral patella/ankle; with bilateral positive Babinski; sensation diffusely decreased in left leg

	Diego F Gómez MD MSc. Neurosurgery Fundación Santafe de Bogotá Bogota, Colombia	George I. Jallo, MD Neurosurgery Johns Hopkins All Children's Tampa, Florida, United States	Allan D. Levi, MD, PhD Meng Huang, MD Neurosurgery University of Miami Miami, Florida, United States	Sheng-Fu Lo, MD Neurosurgery Johns Hopkins Baltimore, Maryland, United States
Preoperative				
Additional tests requested	MRI brain and complete spine EMG/NCS/SSEP	MRI brain and complete spine Neurology evaluation Oncology evaluation	CT chest/abdomen/pelvis CT Lumbar spine MRI Upright AP/lateral flexion-extension x-rays	MRI brain and complete spine MRI T-spine with CISS and DTI
Surgical approach selected	T11–12 laminoplasty and intramedullary tumor resection	T11–12 laminectomy possible laminoplasty and intramedullary tumor resection	T11–12 laminoplasty and intramedullary tumor resection	T11-T12 laminoplasty for en bloc resection of intramedullary tumor
Goal of surgery	Tumor resection, diagnosis, spinal cord decompression	Radical resection with preservation of neurological function	Complete tumor resection	Diagnosis, complete tumor resection with preservation of neurological function
Perioperative				
Positioning	Prone, no pins	Prone	Prone on Jackson table	Prone on Jackson table
Surgical equipment	IOM (MEP/SSEP) Fluoroscopy Ultrasonic bone cutter Ultrasound	IOM (MEP/SSEP) Fluoroscopy Ultrasound Surgical microscope Ultrasonic aspirator	IOM (MEP/SSEP) Ultrasonic bone scalpel Ultrasound Surgical microscope Ultrasonic aspirator Craniofacial mini plates Dural substitute Fibrin glue	IOM (MEP/SSEP, D-wave) Ultrasonic bone scalpel Ultrasound Surgical microscope Nerve stimulator
Medications	Steroids	Steroids	Steroids, MAP > 85	Steroids, MAP > 80
Anatomical considerations	Spinal cord	Spinal cord (midline dorsal median sulcus)	Dorsal columns, corticospinal tracts, midline dorsal raphe	Dorsal columns, corticospinal tracts, nontumor perforators from anterior spinal artery
Complications feared with approach chosen	Spinal cord injury	Injury to corticospinal tract and dorsal columns	CSF leak, pseudomeningocele	Injury to corticospinal tract, anterior spinal artery injury
Intraoperative				
Anesthesia	General	General	General	General
Exposure	T11–12	T11–12	T11–12	T11–12
Levels decompressed	T11–12	T11–12	None	T11–12
Levels fused	None	None	None	None

(continued on next page)

	Diego F Gómez MD MSc. Neurosurgery Fundación Santafe de Bogotá Bogota, Colombia	George I. Jallo, MD Neurosurgery Johns Hopkins All Children's Tampa, Florida, United States	Allan D. Levi, MD, PhD Meng Huang, MD Neurosurgery University of Miami Miami, Florida, United States	Sheng-Fu Lo, MD Neurosurgery Johns Hopkins Baltimore, Maryland, United States
Surgical narrative	Position prone, fluoroscopy to localize level, posterior midline incision, subperiosteal dissection exposing posterior elements, two-level laminoplasty using ultrasonic bone cutter after fluoroscopy, midline dural opening and tenting sutures, ultrasound to locate tumor and guide midline myelotomy, identify tumor and send for pathology, complete gross tumor removal if planes are identifiable with no SSEP/MEP changes, watertight dural closure with fibrin sealant, laminoplasty with titanium plates, layered closure with no drain	Position prone, baseline IOM, x-ray to confirm appropriate levels, two- to three-level laminectomy or laminoplasty, ultrasound to confirm sufficient tumor exposure, open dura and visualize tumor, midline myelotomy to identify tumor, investigate to see if there is a tumor plane/capsule, attempt en bloc, obtain frozen pathology to see if pathology consistent with planes, work inside-out if no planes and debulk as much as possible, resection guided by MEP and SSEP, watertight dura closure, multilayer closure with laminoplasty if available	Position prone on Jackson table, fluoroscopy localization, standard bilateral en bloc laminectomy with ultrasonic bone scalpel spanning level of tumor, ultrasound to confirm tumor location, microscope and dural opening with tenting sutures, identification of midline raphe, perform myelotomy with microdissection of tumor/cord interface with microsurgical instruments, frozen section, internal debulking of tumor with ultrasonic aspirator and fold tumor onto itself with gross total resection if not too adherent, watertight closure with 5-0 prolene/dural substitute/fibrin glue, reconstruction of lamina with craniofacial mini plates, layered closure with subfascial drain to gravity after 6 hours of suctioning	Position prone on Jackson table, lateral x-ray to localize levels, baseline IOM, subperiosteal dissection from T11–12 while avoiding facet joint violations, laminoplasty with bone scalpel, intraoperative ultrasound to confirm exposure and tumor anatomy, place rostral and caudal epidural leads for D-wave monitoring, open dura and tent dura up with stitches, visually identify median sulcus with microscope by identifying dorsal medullary veins entering into the sulcus and translucent pia from tumor expansion, antidromic SSEP stimulation for dorsal column mapping to help identify sulcus, dissect tumor from spinal cord, identify rostral and caudal tumor ends and dissect ventral surface, minimize traction on spinal cord and electrocautery, remove tumor en bloc and protect subarachnoid spaces with cottonoids, repeat ultrasound to evaluate resection
Complication avoidance	Laminoplasty, ultrasound to confirm opening and guide myelotomy, resection guided by planes and SSEP/MEP	Ultrasound to confirm exposure and tumor location, inspect for tumor planes, attempt en bloc, work inside-out if no planes, resection guided by MEP/SSEP, possible laminoplasty	En-bloc laminectomy with bone scalpel, ultrasound to localize tumor, identify midline raphe, internal debulking and folding in tumor, laminoplasty	Laminoplasty while avoiding facet joint violation, intraoperative ultrasound to confirm exposure and tumor anatomy, D-wave monitoring, identify median sulcus with entry of dorsal medullary veins, posterior column mapping, minimize traction on spinal cord and electrocautery, en bloc tumor removal
Postoperative				
Admission	ICU	ICU	ICU	ICU
Postoperative complications feared	Motor deficit, sensory deficit	CSF leak, motor deficit, sensory deficit	CSF leak, pseudomeningocele	Motor deficit, spinal cord stroke
Anticipated length of stay	2 days	3–4 days	3–4 days	3 days
Follow-up testing	MRI T-spine within 48 hours after surgery Oncology evaluation	MRI T-spine within 48 hours after surgery	None	MRI T-spine within 48 hours after surgery

	Diego F Gómez MD MSc. Neurosurgery Fundación Santafe de Bogotá Bogota, Colombia	George I. Jallo, MD Neurosurgery Johns Hopkins All Children's Tampa, Florida, United States	Allan D. Levi, MD, PhD Meng Huang, MD Neurosurgery University of Miami Miami, Florida, United States	Sheng-Fu Lo, MD Neurosurgery Johns Hopkins Baltimore, Maryland, United States
Bracing	None	None	None	None
Follow-up visits	2 weeks after surgery	10–14 days after surgery Oncology evaluation	2 weeks after surgery with nurse visit, 6 weeks with AP/lateral x-rays, 12 weeks/6 months/12 months MRI, followed by yearly MRI Neuro oncology evaluation Radiation oncology evaluation	2 weeks after surgery

AP, Anteroposterior; *CISS*, constructive interference in steady state; *CT*, computed tomography; *DTI*, diffusion tensor imaging; *EMG*, electromyography; *ICU*, intensive care unit; *IOM*, intraoperative monitoring; *MAP*, mean arterial pressure; *MEP*, motor evoked potentials; *MRI*, magnetic resonance imaging; *NCS*, nerve conduction study; *SSEP*, somatosensory evoked potential.

Differential diagnosis and actual diagnosis

- Glial tumor
- Spinal cord infection (abscess)
- Spinal cord infarction
- Multiple sclerosis (demyelination)
- Transverse myelitis
- Syrinx associated to Chiari malformation
- Spinal cord hemorrhage
- Tuberculoma
- Sarcoidosis

Important anatomical and preoperative considerations

The spinal cord is composed of neuronal structures and myelinated motor and sensory axons. White and gray matter are macroscopically arranged in a "butterfly" or "H" pattern and the gray matter is surrounded by the axons in the axial plane.[7] Anatomically, white matter axons can be divided into ventral, lateral, and dorsal funiculi. Ventral funiculi contain ascending sensory and descending motor axons, dorsal funiculi carry ascending sensory input, and lateral funiculi possess descending motor information through corticospinal and pain-temperature within lateral spinothalamic tract.[7] An understanding of the posterior median septum (PMS) is of critical importance for the resection of intramedullary lesions. PMS is a thin sheet of pia/arachnoid mater that separates the dorsal funiculi and is a safe entry of spinal cord and is consistent throughout the spinal cord but is less obvious in the thoracic region with the shallowest area is T4 and T6[8] and about 10% of cords do not have a well-defined sulcus. The tortuous posterior spinal vein runs over the septum so the convergence of blood vessels toward the midline can facilitate its identification when the sulcus is not readily identifiable.[8, 9] The anterior spinal artery and the posterior spinal arteries arise from the intracranial portion of the vertebral artery and descend continuously down the cord. The anterior spinal often becomes narrow in the midthoracic area and is widest at the level it meets the artery of Adamkiewicz (T9-T12).[10] The posterior spinal arteries are paired blood vessels running along the posterior aspect of the cord. These parallel arteries are commonly referred as the posterior plexiform channel. The posterior spinal arteries are widest in the cervical and lumbar areas and narrowest in the thoracic region.[10] They anastomose with the anterior spinal artery near the level of the conus medullaris. The intramedullary arteries supply the neural structures within the cord, where they originate from the anterior spinal artery, the two posterior spinal arteries and the plexus interconnecting them.[10]

The main goals are to resect the neoplasm and infiltrated cord while preserving neurological function. Severe complications like autonomic dysreflexia can result from the disruption or ischemia of eloquent tissue. Klekamp classified spinal intramedullary tumors into three groups based on its relationship with the surrounding neural tissue.[11] Tumors were categorized as displacing tumors, infiltrative tumors, and nonproliferative tumors. As aforementioned, ependymoma represents the most common intramedullary neoplasm in the thoracic region and is also the most common displacing tumor, where these lesions often possess a distinct cleavage plane and are often feasible for gross total resection (GTR).[4, 11] Most of the vascularization of the ependymomas comes from small branches of the anterior spinal cord artery.[11] Astrocytomas and gangliogliomas are infiltrative tumors, where historically, aggressive resection has been limited in order to avoid permanent and severe morbidity especially in the thoracic region. Radical resection cannot typically be achieved without risking damage to the spinal cord.[11] State of the art spine imaging is continuously improving the ability to understand whether an intramedullary lesion is infiltrating or displacing the cord tissue, although this bestows a certain predictive value before planning a GTR as this remains an intraoperative decision for the majority of surgeons.[11]

What was actually done

This patient with a preoperative diagnosis consistent with a T11-T12 IMSCT presented with bilateral loss of sensation and motor weakness in lower extremities. After MRI of the brain and spine were performed to rule out any other lesions, a T11-T12 laminectomy for IMSCT resection with continuous intraoperative monitoring was recommended. The patient was taken to the operating room and general anesthesia was provided. The patient was then placed in prone position, and neuromonitoring was done with somatosensory evoked potential (SSEP) and motor evoked potential (MEP) and D-waves were established before and throughout the procedure. Before the procedure started, the patient already had diminished MEPs in the left lower extremity. An incision was made in the avascular plane to expose from T10 to part of L1. After levels were confirmed by intraoperative fluoroscopy, the spinous process and lamina of T11 and T12, as well as the bottom of T10, were removed. Intraoperative ultrasound was used to confirm adequate exposure. The microscope was brought into the surgical field and the dura opened. The spinal cord was mapped with a Kartooch stimulator in order to identify the safest point for corticectomy. The median sulcus was identified, and a corticectomy was done. The lesion was identified, and the dissection plane was difficult to identify. Frozen pathology came back as infiltrating glioma. The tumor was debulked, but during the dissection, the SSEPs diminished to <50% in the left lower extremity. The tumor was then internally debulked. The MEP remained intact. The mean arterial pressures were elevated to maximize perfusion of the spinal cord. After continued debulking and because of a lack of distinct margins, resection was stopped when there was continued decrease in the SSEP in the left lower extremity and the MEP also decreased. This was corroborated with the D-wave. The dura was closed in a watertight fashion and the muscles in layers. The patient was extubated in the operating room with diminished left lower extremity sensation and decreased strength in the left iliopsoas 4–5 and was transferred to the intensive care unit in stable condition. The patient was discharged at postoperative day 5 with stable left leg weakness. At follow-up, she was clinically improving with improved but persistent left lower extremity weakness 4+/5 in the iliopsoas. The patient was diagnosed with a diffuse glioma

World Health Organization (WHO) IV. Postoperative MRI showed subtotal resection and decompression of the spinal cord (Fig. 52.2). The patient was administered temozolomide chemotherapy and radiation therapy.

Commonalities among the experts

Most of the surgeons chose to perform a MRI of the brain and the entire spine to evaluate for additional lesions. All would achieve intramedullary tumor resection by means of a laminectomy/laminoplasty. The majority directed their treatment for a complete tumor excision with preservation of neurological function. All were aware of the risk of spinal cord injury during the procedure. The most feared complication was damage to the corticospinal tract and/or the dorsal columns. Removal of the tumor was attained with fluoroscopy, intraoperative monitoring, ultrasound, and microscope. Steroids were recommended as a perioperative medical therapy by all the surgeons. All shared the use of intraoperative ultrasound to confirm tumor location and guide myelotomy, as well as the employment of SSEP/MEP for resection guidance. Following surgical intervention, all continued observation of their patients in the intensive care unit, and the majority requested MRI within 48 hours to evaluate for extent of tumor resection and for possible complications. Follow-up was scheduled 2 weeks after surgery by all the physicians.

SUMMARY OF QUALITY OF EVIDENCE TO GUIDE SPECIFIC INTERVENTIONS FOR THIS CASE

- Surgery for intramedullary lesions should be aimed to preserve neurological function and complete excision of the neoplasm: level III
- Perioperative steroid therapy as part of the management of intramedullary tumors: level III

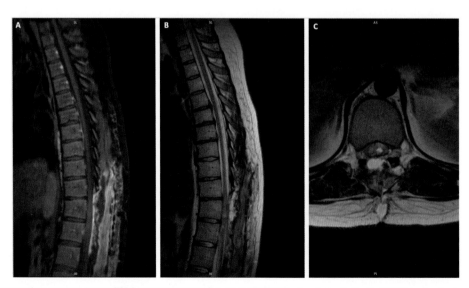

Fig. 52.2. Postoperative magnetic resonance image (MRI) of the thoracic spine. (A) Sagittal T1 imaging demonstrating the T10-T2 laminectomies with debulking of the infiltrating spinal cord tumor. (B) Sagittal and (C) axial T2 images demonstrate significant decrease in size of abnormality intrinsic to the thoracic cord from T10 to T12 but with persistent abnormal T2 signal intensity and subtle amorphic enhancement.

REFERENCES

1. Duong LM, McCarthy BJ, McLendon RE, et al. Descriptive epidemiology of malignant and nonmalignant primary spinal cord, spinal meninges, and cauda equina tumors, United States, 2004-2007. *Cancer.* 2012;118(17):4220–4227.
2. Kane PJ, el-Mahdy W, Singh A, Powell MP, Crockard HA. Spinal intradural tumours: Part II-Intramedullary. *Br J Neurosurg.* 1999;13(6):558–563.
3. Samartzis D, Gillis CC, Shih P, O'Toole JE, Fessler RG. Intramedullary Spinal Cord Tumors: Part I-Epidemiology, Pathophysiology, and Diagnosis. *Global Spine J.* 2015;5(5):425–435.
4. Alizada O, Kemerdere R, Ulu MO, et al. Surgical management of spinal intramedullary tumors: Ten-year experience in a single institution. *J Clin Neurosci.* 2020;73:201–208.
5. Khalid S, Kelly R, Carlton A, et al. Adult intradural intramedullary astrocytomas: a multicenter analysis. *J Spine Surg.* 2019;5(1):19–30.
6. Tobin MK, Geraghty JR, Engelhard HH, Linninger AA, Mehta AI. Intramedullary spinal cord tumors: a review of current and future treatment strategies. *Neurosurg Focus.* 2015;39(2):E14.
7. Hendrix P, Griessenauer CJ, Cohen-Adad J, et al. Spinal diffusion tensor imaging: a comprehensive review with emphasis on spinal cord anatomy and clinical applications. *Clin Anat.* 2015;28(1):88–95.
8. Turkoglu E, Kertmen H, Uluc K, et al. Microsurgical anatomy of the posterior median septum of the human spinal cord. *Clin Anat.* 2015;28(1):45–51.
9. Brotchi J. Intrinsic spinal cord tumor resection. *Neurosurgery.* 2002;50(5):1059–1063.
10. Bosmia AN, Hogan E, Loukas M, Tubbs RS, Cohen-Gadol AA. Blood supply to the human spinal cord: part I. Anatomy and hemodynamics. *Clin Anat.* 2015;28(1):52–64.
11. Klekamp J. Treatment of intramedullary tumors: analysis of surgical morbidity and long-term results. *J Neurosurg Spine.* 2013;19(1):12–26.

53

Thoracolumbar intradural lesion

Jaime L. Martínez Santos, MD

Introduction

Spinal tumors account for up to 15% of all tumors in the neuroaxis.[1,2] Based on their anatomical location, the spinal tumors are classified as extradural, intradural extramedullary, or intradural intramedullary (spinal cord tumors). Intradural tumors account for 3% of primary central nervous system (CNS) tumors,[3] and the most common histological types are meningiomas and nerve sheath tumors (NSTs). Microsurgical resection plays an essential role since the large majority of primary spinal intradural tumors are benign and encapsulated and a complete surgical resection is curative.[4] In this chapter, we utilize an example case to illustrate the key clinical and radiographic features as well as the surgical management of intradural extramedullary tumors in the thoracolumbar region.

Example case

Chief Complaint: leg pain
History of present illness: A 55-year-old female with a 6-week history of pain in her legs when walking and/or standing

and increased urinary frequency. She denies any weakness. She underwent imaging which was concerning for an intradural extramedullary spinal cord tumor (Fig. 53.1).
Medications: none
Allergies: no known drug allergies
Past medical history: none
Past surgical history: none
Family history: none
Social history: none
Physical examination: awake, alert, and oriented to person, place, and time; cranial nerves II–XII intact; motor and sensory intact
Laboratories: complete blood count (CBC) and basic metabolic panel (BMP) within normal limits
Lumbar spine MRI: intradural extramedullary T2 hyperintense lesion with heterogeneous gadolinium enhancement at the T11–12 level displacing the conus medullaris to the left

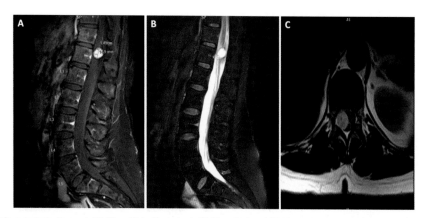

Fig. 53.1 Preoperative magnetic resonance images. (A) T1 sagittal with contrast, (B) T2 sagittal, and (C) T1 axial with contrast demonstrating a T11–12 intradural extramedullary spinal cord tumor.

	Mark H. Bilsky, MD Neurosurgery Memorial Sloan Kettering Cancer Center New York, New York, United States	Hazem Eltahawy, MD Neurosurgery St. Mary Mercy Hospital Ain Shams University Livonia, Michigan, United States	Davide Nasi, MD Neurosurgery Polytechnic University of Marche, Umberto Ancona, Italy	Daniel M. Sciubba, MD Jeffrey Ehresman, BS Neurosurgery Johns Hopkins Baltimore, Maryland, United States
Preoperative				
Additional tests requested	MRI brain and complete spine Neurogenic bladder evaluation Bilateral lower extremity dopplers	EMG bilateral lower extremities Urodynamic testing	Neurophysiological evaluation (MEP, SSEP, EMG)	CT thoracic spine
Surgical approach selected	T11–12 laminectomy with resection of tumor	T11–12 right hemilaminectomy and excision of tumor	T11–12 right hemilaminectomy and excision of tumor	T11–12 laminectomy, resection of tumor, T12 laminoplasty
Goal of surgery	Diagnosis, gross total resection of tumor	Diagnosis, gross total resection, decompression of conus	Gross total resection, preservation of neurological function	Gross total resection, prevent progression of neurological symptoms
Perioperative				
Positioning	Prone in pins	Prone	Prone	Prone on Jackson table, no pins
Surgical equipment	IOM (MEP/SSEP/EMG) Fluoroscopy Irrigating microtip bipolar Surgical microscope Nerve stimulator Ultrasound Ultrasonic aspirator	IOM Fluoroscopy Ultrasound Surgical microscope Ultrasonic aspirator	IOM (MEP/SSEP/EMG including sphincter) Fluoroscopy Surgical microscope	IOM (MEP/SSEP) Ultrasonic bone scalpel Ultrasound Surgical microscope
Medications	Steroids	MAP >80	Steroids, maintain MAP	None
Anatomical considerations	Conus medullaris	Spinal cord, vasculature	Cauda equina, conus	Spinal cord, posterior spinal artery
Complications feared with approach chosen	CSF leak, spinal cord injury	CSF leak, spinal cord injury	CSF leak, spinal cord injury	CSF leak, spinal cord injury, vascular injury
Intraoperative				
Anesthesia	General	General	General	General
Exposure	T11–12	T11–12	T11–12	T11-T12
Levels decompressed	T11–12	T11–12	T11–12	T11–12
Levels fused	None	None	None	T12
Surgical narrative	Position prone in pins, IOM, fluoroscopy to confirm levels based on rib count, incision, subperiosteal dissection of paraspinal muscles from spinous process and laminae to identify pars interarticularis and medial joint, fluoroscopy to confirm levels, match stick used to resect through base of spinous process and cerebellar retractor used to displace interspinous ligament to the left, complete partial laminectomies at T11 and T12 with dill and Kerrison punch, ultrasound to confirm extent of laminectomies and exposure of tumor, operative microscope brought into view,	Position prone on gel rolls, plan incision used AP and lateral x-rays to localize level with AP counting from last rib and lateral x-rays from L5 to S1, midline skin incision and subperiosteal muscle dissection on right side, place self-retaining William's retractors, confirm level with x-ray, right T11–12 laminectomy across midline and partial facetectomy using drill and Kerrison rongeurs, confirm exposure with ultrasound, open dura preserving arachnoid under microscopic visualization, dural stay sutures, open arachnoid around mass with scissors, control proximal	Position prone, identify T12 with K-wire and x-ray, 5–6 cm midline skin incision, muscular dissection only on right side, right T11–12 hemilaminectomy with drill and Kerrison rongeur under microscope, undercut base of spinous process for more midline exposure, midline dural opening, identify tumor and check relationship with conus/nerve roots/filum, dissect arachnoid from tumor and nerve roots, continuous IOM	Position prone, plan incision using intraoperative x-ray, midline incision from T11 to 12, subperiosteal dissection, x-ray to confirm levels, ultrasonic bone scalpel to perform T11-T12 laminectomy, ultrasound to confirm exposure, dura opened over tumor and tacked back, surgical microscope brought in and arachnoid incised and held to dura using vascular clips, IOM to identify and dissect motor and sensory branches

	Mark H. Bilsky, MD Neurosurgery Memorial Sloan Kettering Cancer Center New York, New York, United States	Hazem Eltahawy, MD Neurosurgery St. Mary Mercy Hospital Ain Shams University Livonia, Michigan, United States	Davide Nasi, MD Neurosurgery Polytechnic University of Marche, Umberto Ancona, Italy	Daniel M. Sciubba, MD Jeffrey Ehresman, BS Neurosurgery Johns Hopkins Baltimore, Maryland, United States
	dura opened and tacked back, arachnoid opened sharply, stimulate dorsal aspect of tumor with positive control and sequential reduction to 0.1 mA, capsule cauterized and opened sharply, intralesional debulking with ultrasonic aspirator, manipulate capsule to identify fascicles giving rise to tumors, fascicles stimulated with nerve stimulator and cut if no motor response, dural closure with running nonlocking suture, drain placed in epidural space	CSF flow with Gelfoam and cottonoids, bipolar surface vessels, send specimen to pathology, internally debulk tumor with ultrasonic aspirator, dissect mass circumferentially with extra attention to medial dissection from spinal cord, identify nerve root from which mass is originating, stimulate to confirm absence of function, cut nerve proximally and distal to mass, dissect mass from dura if meningioma, watertight dural and fascial closure, layered closure, flat in bed for 12–24 hours	and change surgical strategy if change in signals, en bloc resection, watertight dural closure with autologous fat and fibrin glue, layered closure	with goal of preserving motor branches, lesion completely resected, dura closed in watertight fashion and multiple Valsalva maneuvers performed, fibrin sealant patch over dural closure, T12 replaced with titanium plates, layered closure, bedrest overnight
Complication avoidance	Preserve interspinous ligament, nerve stimulator, intralesional debulking to identify fascicles giving rise to tumor	AP and lateral x-rays for identifying surgical level, right hemilaminectomy, ultrasound to confirm exposure, extra attention when dissecting from spinal cord, stimulate nerve to confirm nonfunctioning before removing	Right hemilaminectomy, undercut spinous process for more medial exposure, continuous IOM and change surgical strategy if chance in signals, en bloc resection, autologous fat for closure	T12 laminoplasty, ultrasound to confirm exposure, ION to determine whether sensory or motor nerve roots involved, Valsalva to test dura closure
Postoperative				
Admission	ICU	Floor	Floor	Floor
Postoperative complications feared	CSF leak	CSF leak, neurological deficit, residual tumor	CSF leak, neurological deficit	CSF leak, new neurological deficit
Anticipated length of stay	2–3 days	2 days	5–7 days	2 days
Follow-up testing	MRI T-L spine within 72 hours of surgery	MRI T-spine within 24 hours of surgery	MRI T-spine 3 months after surgery	MRI T-spine within 72 hours, then 3 months, 6 months, and annually after surgery
Bracing	None	None	None	None
Follow-up visits	3 weeks after surgery	2 weeks, 6 weeks, 3 months after surgery	2 weeks, 3 months after surgery	3 weeks after surgery

AP, Anteroposterior; *CSF*, cerebrospinal fluid; *CT*, computed tomography; *EMG*, electromyography; *ICU*, intensive care unit; *IOM*, intraoperative monitoring; *MAP*, mean arterial pressure; *MEP*, motor evoked potential; *MRI*, magnetic resonance imaging; *SSEP*, somatosensory evoked potential.

Differential diagnosis

- Schwannoma
- Meningioma
- Myxopapillary ependymoma
- Metastasis
- Solitary fibrous tumor
- Neuroendocrine tumor or paraganglioma

Important anatomical and preoperative considerations

Spinal tumors account for 5% to 15% of all tumors of the CNS and its coverings,[1,2] and unlike cranial tumors, approximately 60% of primary spinal tumors are benign and encapsulated.[5] Therefore, in most cases, a complete surgical resection is curative. Spinal tumors are extradural in 60%, intradural extramedullary in 30%, and intradural intramedullary in 10%.[1]

Meningiomas are the most common primary extramedullary tumor and account for >30% of all intradural spinal tumors.[2] Neurofibromas and schwannomas are benign peripheral NSTs of Schwann cell origin and account for 25% of all intradural spinal tumors. NSTs usually originate from the dorsal or posterior (sensory) root or rootless in the intradural extramedullary spine compartment and have a tendency to grow along the nerve, exit through the intervertebral foramen (sometimes expanding it), and have a paraspinal component (in 10%–15%), thus commonly acquiring a dumbbell or hourglass shape.[6] NST are more frequently located in the thoracic spine (44%) and lumbar spine (35%).[7] Schwannomas are benign, World Health Organization (WHO) grade I, and slow growing tumors that are usually solitary (>95%) but could be multiple in the setting of neurofibromatosis (type II > type I) or schwannomatosis.[1,2,6]

The gold standard management of spinal schwannomas is with an early complete microsurgical resection, which is curative in patients without neurofibromatosis or schwannomatosis. Fernandes et al. in a 30-patient series, reported a gross total resection (GTR) rate of 96.6% and a recurrence rate of 3%.[8] These tumors can continue to grow, compressing and displacing the spinal cord or cauda equina, and ultimately reducing it to a very thin delicate strip of neural tissue, which increases surgical morbidity.[5] Important considerations for surgical planning include tumor size, spinal segment involved, location (posterolateral or ventral), foraminal involvement, and presence of a paraspinal component. For instance, large tumors involving the thoracic spine (narrower spinal canal) with far lateral or ventral location and foraminal involvement might require a more extensive approach including bony removal and thus spinal stabilization. Clear indications for performing spinal instrumented fusions have not been established and should be considered on an individual basis. Some recommendations for fusion include patients with preexisting spine deformity, scoliosis, or spondylolisthesis; tumors causing extensive bony erosion or requiring extensive bony removal during surgery (facetectomy or pediculectomy); tumors located in the vulnerable cervicothoracic junction; and malignancy.[9–11]

As a general rule, the selected approach should expose the tumor attachment (or rootless of origin) and also allow for circumferential dissection with minimal spinal cord manipulation. Most NSTs can be approached posteriorly with an open a hemilaminotomy, laminectomy, or laminoplasty. A minimally invasive tubular muscle-splitting approach could be a suitable option for smaller tumors (best if <3 cm craniocaudally) in the lumbar spine,[12,13] but bear in mind that microdissection and dural closure is more challenging. Tumors located ventrally and laterally in the cervical or thoracic spine may require additional bony removal (i.e., facetectomies) for creating a surgical corridor around the spinal cord or toward the neural foramina. A medial one-third facetectomy will usually suffice for exposing most NSTs. Spinal stabilization should be considered if a more aggressive bony removal is undertaken.

NSTs usually originate from a posterior sensory root, which usually becomes nonfunctional and can be safely sacrificed without significant neurological sequela.[8] En passage nerve roots should be preserved. The tumor is then devascularized circumferentially keeping in mind that the major vascular pedicles usually run through the filum or through a nerve root.[4] Tumors of large size and ventral location often require an initial debulking prior to circumferential dissection. The dentate ligaments can be sectioned near their arachnoid attachment and used to very gently and minimally rotate the spinal cord if needed.

What was actually done

The patient was taken to the operating room and position prone on a Jackson table. The T12 level was localized using fluoroscopy and a two-level T11–12 laminectomy was performed. Adequate tumor exposure was confirmed with intraoperative ultrasound.[4,14] The dura and arachnoid membranes were open and tacked up with suture. The nerve root of origin was easily identified blending with the tumor capsule. This root was stimulated and did not elicit an electromyogram response, and therefore the lesion was safely bipolar electrocoagulated and divided. A passing nerve root was carefully dissected off the tumor capsule and preserved. The tumor capsule was stimulated with negative response, and the tumor was entered, internally debulked, and removed completely. The dura was closed using 6-0 Prolene in a running fashion and dural sealant applied to the closure. A layered closure ensued with a watertight fascial closure. The patient was placed on bedrest for 24 hours and discharged home on

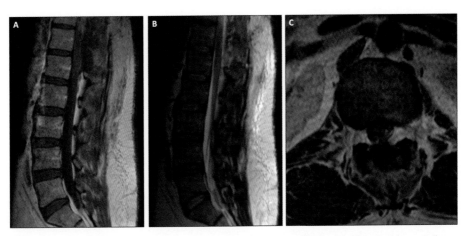

Fig. 53.2 Postoperative magnetic resonance images. (A), T1 sagittal with contrast, (B), T2 sagittal, and (C), T1 axial with contrast demonstrating gross total resection of the intradural extramedullary spinal cord tumor.

postoperative day 3. Histopathology returned as schwannoma. She was seen back in clinic 1 month after surgery and reported complete symptom resolution and her incision had healed well. Postoperative imaging showed GTR of the lesion (Fig. 53.2).

Commonalities among the experts

Most opted for a two-level T11–12 right-sided hemilaminotomy and one surgeon preferred a laminoplasty. All aimed for GTR. Surgery was generally pursued using fluoroscopy (to localize the spine level), intraoperative monitoring (to identify and protect motor nerve roots), ultrasound (to confirm exposure), operative microscope, and an ultrasonic aspirator for tumor debulking. All surgeons would stimulate the tumor prior to entering its capsule and also stimulate the sensory root (of tumor origin) prior to dividing it while preserving all motor roots. All emphasized a watertight dural closure and a layered wound closure, and half advocated using a fibrin sealant to reenforce the dural closure. The most feared complications were spinal cord injury with neurological deficit and cerebrospinal fluid leak. Most surgeons felt that fusion was not needed in this case and only one surgeon proposed a T12 single level instrumentation. Following surgery, half advocated for 12 to 24 hours of bedrest. Most would obtain a postoperative MRI within 72 hours and schedule outpatient follow-up within 2–3 weeks.

SUMMARY OF QUALITY OF EVIDENCE TO GUIDE SPECIFIC INTERVENTIONS FOR THIS CASE

- Surgery is recommended for symptomatic intradural extramedullary spinal tumors to achieve histopathologic diagnosis and neurological decompression: level IB
- Intraoperative neurophysiologic monitoring is recommended for all intradural extramedullary spinal tumors: level IB
- Intraoperative ultrasound is suggested for all intradural tumors: level III

REFERENCES

1. Ottenhausen M, Ntoulias G, Bodhinayake I, et al. Intradural spinal tumors in adults-update on management and outcome. *Neurosurg Rev.* 2019;42(2):371–388.
2. Koeller KK, Shih RY. Intradural Extramedullary Spinal Neoplasms: Radiologic-Pathologic Correlation. *Radiographics.* 2019; 39(2):468–490.
3. Ostrom QT, Gittleman H, Xu J, et al. CBTRUS Statistical Report: Primary Brain and Other Central Nervous System Tumors Diagnosed in the United States in 2009-2013. *Neuro Oncol.* 2016;18(suppl_5):v1–v75.
4. Martinez Santos JL WJE, Kalhorn SP. Microsurgical Management of a Primary Neuroendocrine Tumor of the Filum Terminale: A Surgical Technique. *Cureus.* 2020;12(8):e10080.
5. Parsa AT, Lee J, Parney IF, Weinstein P, McCormick PC, Ames C. Spinal cord and intradural-extraparenchymal spinal tumors: current best care practices and strategies. *J Neurooncol.* 2004;69(1-3):291–318.
6. Karsy M, Guan J, Sivakumar W, Neil JA, Schmidt MH, Mahan MA. The genetic basis of intradural spinal tumors and its impact on clinical treatment. *Neurosurg Focus.* 2015;39(2):E3.
7. Bhimani AD, Denyer S, Esfahani DR, Zakrzewski J, Aguilar TM, Mehta AI. Surgical Complications in Intradural Extramedullary Spinal Cord Tumors - An ACS-NSQIP Analysis of Spinal Cord Level and Malignancy. *World Neurosurg.* 2018;117:e290–e299.
8. Fernandes RL, Lynch JC, Welling L, et al. Complete removal of the spinal nerve sheath tumors. Surgical technics and results from a series of 30 patients. *Arq Neuropsiquiatr.* 2014;72(4):312–317.
9. Safaee M, Oh T, Barbaro NM, et al. Results of Spinal Fusion After Spinal Nerve Sheath Tumor Resection. *World Neurosurg.* 2016;90:6–13.
10. Ahmad FU, Frenkel MB, Levi AD. Spinal stability after resection of nerve sheath tumors. *J Neurosurg Sci.* 2017;61(4):355–364.
11. Sebai MA, Kerezoudis P, Alvi MA, Yoon JW, Spinner RJ, Bydon M. Need for arthrodesis following facetectomy for spinal peripheral nerve sheath tumors: an institutional experience and review of the current literature. *J Neurosurg Spine.* 2019;31(1):112-122.
12. Lee SE, Jahng TA, Kim HJ. Different Surgical Approaches for Spinal Schwannoma: A Single Surgeon's Experience with 49 Consecutive Cases. *World Neurosurg.* 2015;84(6):1894–1902.
13. Thavara BD, Kidangan GS, Rajagopalawarrier B. Analysis of the Surgical Technique and Outcome of the Thoracic and Lumbar Intradural Spinal Tumor Excision Using Minimally Invasive Tubular Retractor System. *Asian J Neurosurg.* 2019;14(2):453–460.
14. Martinez Santos JL, Alshareef M, Kalhorn SP. Back Pain and Radiculopathy from Non-Steroidal Anti-Inflammatory Drug-induced Dorsal Epidural Haematoma. *BMJ Case Rep..* 2019;12(3).

54

Cervico-medullary junction lesion

Fidel Valero-Moreno, MD and Henry Ruiz-Garcia, MD

Introduction

Intramedullary spinal cord lesions represent a diagnostic challenge.[1] Lesions occupying the cervico-medullary junction are rare entities, and the actual prevalence has not been reported. Patients who present with myelopathic symptoms and findings on magnetic resonance imaging (MRI) typically exhaust conservative measures before undergoing open biopsy for histological diagnosis and/or resection due to the associated neurological morbidity of the procedure.[2] The location of the lesion with respect to the spinal cord cross section may assist in narrowing the differential diagnosis, as certain conditions preferentially affect certain areas of the spinal cord.[3] In addition, lesions that affect multiple spinal cord segments in a rostral to caudal direction may also narrow the differential diagnosis with respect to possible causes.[4, 5] Open biopsy is reserved as a last diagnostic resort, and resection may be performed if intraoperative pathology demonstrates neoplastic tissue.[5] The extent of resection is limited by the type of tumor, location, and results of intraoperative monitoring. In this chapter, we present a case of a young patient with a history of walk instability and lack of coordination in both upper extremities.

Example case

Chief complaint: neck pain and weakness
History of present illness:
A 29-year-old female with a 2-month history of difficulty walking and coordination in her arms. She has been having progressive difficulty writing her name and holding items in her right hand. She has a history of recent travel to the Caribbean where she regularly performs work. She has not had any constitutional symptoms. She has had multiple MRIs, which have shown progression of an enhancing lesion at the cervico-medullary junction (Figs. 54.1–54.2).

Medications: antidepressants
Allergies: no known drug allergies
Past medical and surgical history: depression, anxiety
Family history: noncontributory
Social history: none
Physical examination: awake, alert, and oriented to person, place, and time; cranial nerves II–XII intact; bilateral deltoids/triceps/biceps 5/5; interossei 5/5; iliopsoas/knee flexion/knee extension/dorsi, and plantar flexion 5/5
Reflexes: 3+ in bilateral biceps/triceps/brachioradialis with positive Hoffman; 3+ in bilateral patella/ankle; no clonus or Babinski; sensation intact to light touch

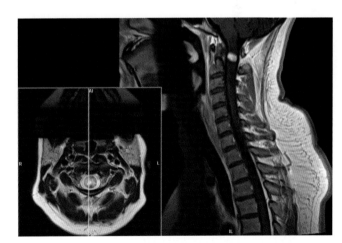

Fig. 54.1 Preoperative magnetic resonance T1 with contrast images. (A) Sagittal view demonstrating a hyperintense rounded lesion at the cervicomedullary junction surrounded by a hypointense signal extending from the medulla to the C2-C3 level. The caliber of the cord appears increased at the level of the lesion. (B) Axial view demonstrating the lesion spans most of the cross-sectional area of the spine.

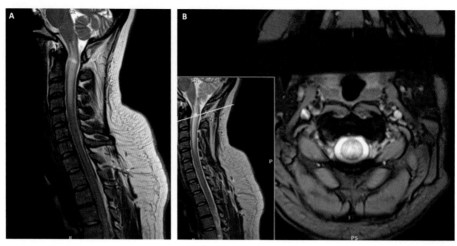

Fig. 54.2 Preoperative magnetic resonance T2 images. (A) Sagittal view demonstrating abnormal enhancement extending from the upper medulla to approximately the C6 level. (B) Axial view demonstrating a diffuse high T2 signal spanning most of the cross-sectional area of the spine.

	Maziyar A. Kalani, MD Neurosurgery Mayo Clinic Phoenix, Arizona, United States	Jorge Navarro Bonnet, MD Neurosurgery Medica Sur, Mexico City, Mexico	Rodrigo Navarro-Ramirez, MD Neurosurgery McGill University Montreal, Quebec, Canada	Jean-Paul Wolinsky, MD Neurosurgery Northwestern University Chicago, Illinois, United States
Preoperative				
Additional tests requested	MRI brain and complete spine Ophthalmology evaluation CT abdomen/pelvis Genetic evaluation for VHL	NCS/EMG/SSEP MRI complete spine Antiaquaporin antibody test Neurology evaluation	CT C-spine	Neurology evaluation, possible repeat CSF studies Spinal angiogram MRI STIR C spine PET Follow-up MRI to assess growth
Surgical approach selected	C1-2 laminectomy and resection of intramedullary spinal cord tumor	C1 laminectomy and C2 laminoplasty and resection of intramedullary spinal cord tumor	C1-2 laminectomy and resection of intramedullary spinal cord tumor	Pending workup, C1-3 laminectomy vs. laminoplasty and resection of intramedullary spinal cord tumor
Goal of surgery	Spinal cord decompression, diagnosis, tumor resection	Spinal cord decompression, diagnosis, restoration of CSF flow	Tumor resection	Gross total resection, preservation of neurological function
Perioperative				
Positioning	Prone, in Mayfield pins	Prone, in Mayfield pins	Prone on Jackson table, in Mayfield pins	Prone, in Mayfield pins
Surgical equipment	IOM (MEP/SSEP/spinal cord mapping) Fluoroscopy Ultrasound	IOM (lower cranial nerve monitoring) Ultrasonic bone scalpel Surgical microscope Ultrasonic aspirator	IOM (MEP/SSEP) Surgical microscope Ultrasound	IOM (MEP/SSEP/D-wave) Ultrasonic bone scalpel Surgical microscope Ultrasound
Medications	Steroids, MAP >85	Maintain MAP	MAP >90	Steroids, MAP >80
Anatomical considerations	Vertebral arteries	Posterior median sulcus, central canal	Spinal cord	Spinal cord, spinal cord vasculature
Complications feared with approach chosen	Ondine's curse, posterior column injury, pseudomeningocele, wound dehiscence	Spinal cord injury, namely posterior columns	Spinal cord injury	Spinal cord injury, spinal cord stroke

	Maziyar A. Kalani, MD Neurosurgery Mayo Clinic Phoenix, Arizona, United States	Jorge Navarro Bonnet, MD Neurosurgery Medica Sur, Mexico City, Mexico	Rodrigo Navarro-Ramirez, MD Neurosurgery McGill University Montreal, Quebec, Canada	Jean-Paul Wolinsky, MD Neurosurgery Northwestern University Chicago, Illinois, United States
Intraoperative				
Anesthesia	General	General	General	General
Exposure	Occiput-C3	C1-2	C1-2	C1-3
Levels decompressed	C1-2	C1-2	C1-2	C1-3
Levels fused	None	None	None	None
Surgical narrative	Position prone, incision planned based on palpation of first bifid process or preoperative x-ray, subperiosteal dissection from base of skull to C3, avoid dissecting more than 1 cm lateral to posterior tubercle of arch of C1 to avoid vertebral artery injury, piecemeal C1 laminectomy and en bloc C2 laminectomy for possible laminoplasty, intraoperative ultrasound to confirm exposure, dural opening, tack dura up with arachnoid, bipolar neuromonitoring probe to identify midline or by identifying confluence of veins, midline myelotomy, send small specimen to pathology to assess goals of surgery, remove lesion via circumferential dissection leaving draining vein for last if identified, dural closure with Gore-tex suture, Valsalva to assess for leakage, fibrin glue, potential laminoplasty of C2, layered closure with subfascial drain to half suction gravity, head at 30 degrees	Position prone, IOM baseline, midline skin incision following avascular line to expose C1-2, remove C1 posterior arch, C2 laminotomy with bone scalpel, linear dura openings, open posterior median sulcus under microscopic visualization, send samples for histopathological diagnosis, continue lesion resection attempting maximal safe resection guided by IOM, careful hemostasis with mild compression, dural closure reinforced with dural substitute, C2 laminoplasty, closure in layers	Position prone with slight flexion, midline incision from C1-2, subperiosteal dissection of muscles from C1 posterior arch and spinous process of C2, leave muscles attach to C3, subperiosteal dissection of C1 and C2 lamina with curette, C1-2 laminectomy with Kerrison rongeur preserving C1-2 and C2-3 joints, resect ligamentum flavum, ultrasound to confirm exposure and if laminectomy needed for more lateral exposure or if more rostral/caudal extension is needed, right paramedian dural opening and tacked up, myelotomy over most translucent area, sequential clockwise resection with limiting bipolar cautery under constant communication with IOM, watertight dural closure, layered closure with subfascial drain off suction, keep head elevated postop for 24 hours	Preflip IOM, midline incision from C1-3, subperiosteal exposure of posterior arch of C1 and spinous processes and lamina of C2-C3, C1-3 laminectomies with ultrasonic bone scalpel, intraoperative ultrasound to confirm sufficient exposure at both rostral and caudal ends, placement of caudal epidural electrode under C4 to establish baseline D-wave monitoring capability, midline dural opening keeping arachnoid intact, tack dura up laterally, open and dissect arachnoid under microscope, open pia at tumor-spinal cord interface, identify arterial feeders and venous drainage, dissection of tumor capsule from spinal cord, deliver tumor, hemostasis with gentle irrigation, dural closure with fibrin glue, laminoplasty, layered closure with subfascial drain, skin closure with skin glue
Complication avoidance	Avoid dissecting more than 1 cm lateral to posterior tubercle of arch of C1 to avoid vertebral artery injury, en bloc C2 laminectomy for laminoplasty, intraoperative ultrasound to confirm exposure, spinal cord mapping to identify midline, intraoperative pathology to determine goals of surgery	Bone scalpel to perform laminotomy, identify posterior median sulcus, send frozen, resection guided by IOM, C2 laminoplasty	Leave muscles attach to C3, preserve joints, ultrasound to confirm exposure, myelotomy over most translucent area, sequential clockwise resection with limiting bipolar cautery under constant communication with IOM	Preflip IOM, ultrasound to assess exposure, D-wave assessments, attempt to keep arachnoid intact to minimize CSF loss and decrease epidural bleeding, attempt to work tumor capsule, laminoplasty
Postoperative				
Admission	ICU	Intermediate care	ICU	ICU
Postoperative complications feared	Ondine's curse, posterior column injury, pseudomeningocele, wound dehiscence	Posterior column injury, edema, expansion of syrinx, dysphagia, respiratory issues	Weakness/paralysis, sensory deficit, spinal cord edema, CSF leak	Weakness/paralysis, CSF leak, wound infection, cervical kyphosis

(continued on next page)

	Maziyar A. Kalani, MD Neurosurgery Mayo Clinic Phoenix, Arizona, United States	Jorge Navarro Bonnet, MD Neurosurgery Medica Sur, Mexico City, Mexico	Rodrigo Navarro-Ramirez, MD Neurosurgery McGill University Montreal, Quebec, Canada	Jean-Paul Wolinsky, MD Neurosurgery Northwestern University Chicago, Illinois, United States
Anticipated length of stay	2–3 days	2 days	7–10 days	7 days
Follow-up testing	MRI C-spine 3 months after surgery	MRI within 48 hours of surgery	MRI C-spine prior to discharge	MRI C-spine 6 weeks after surgery (<48 hours if subtotal resection), 6 months, 12 months, 24 months, 36 months after surgery
Bracing	None	None	None	None
Follow-up visits	2 weeks, 6 weeks, 3 months after surgery	2 weeks after surgery	2 weeks, 1 month, 3 months after surgery	2 weeks, 6 weeks, 3 months, 6 months, 12 months, and annually after surgery

CSF, Cerebrospinal fluid; *CT*, computed tomography; *EMG*, electromyography; *ICU*, intensive care unit; *IOM*, intraoperative monitoring; *MAP*, mean arterial pressure; *MEP*, motor evoked potential; *MRI*, magnetic resonance imaging; *NCS*, nerve conduction study; *PET*, positron emission tomography; *SSEP*, somatosensory evoked potential; *STIR*, short T1 inversion recovery; *VHL*, von-Hippel Lindau.

Differential diagnosis

- Demyelinating disease
- Intrinsic glial spinal cord tumor
- Metastatic lesion
- Neurosarcoidosis
- Hemangioblastoma
- Lipoma

Important anatomical and preoperative considerations

The cervico-medullary junction is a relatively small area with a high-density of functional tissue. Compression and disruption affecting this structure will result in motor, sensory, and/or autonomic manifestations such as quadriparesis, cardiovascular instability, loss of involuntary respiratory function, neurogenic hypertension, and cranial neuropathy.[6–8] Intramedullary ependymomas and metastasis show predilection for this area and cervical astrocytomas are second in frequency just after the thoracic region.[4] The classical strategy for resection of intramedullary cervical lesions is through a posterior midline approach with laminectomy spanning the tumor levels. Myelotomy is ideally done after identifying the posterior median sulcus; however, it is rarely recognized in the upper cervical cord and therefore visualization of the posterior spinal arteries can serve as a reliable landmark.[9, 10] The most common morbidity in some series was posterior column dysfunction, which is likely related to the myelotomy.[10] Ependymomas and hemangioblastomas are well defined lesions and usually offer a good plane cleavage between the neoplasm and the cord tissue.[10] Conversely, astrocytomas and metastasis are less favorable for their surgical resection due to their diffuse involvement of the cord and unclear margins.[10, 11] Avoiding prolonged retraction of pial and neural structures by means of central debulking of the tumor and utilization of neurophysiological monitoring are paramount to preserving function and maximize the extent of resection in this area.[10–12]

Surgical resection remains the optimal treatment modality for these lesions, while radiation and chemotherapy should be reserved for patients suffering from high-grade tumors or neoplasms for whom surgery will be limited to subtotal resection or biopsy.[10, 11]

What was actually done

The patient underwent lumbar puncture, laboratory studies, and serial radiological examinations, which were inconclusive but demonstrated progression of the lesion on MRI. Therefore the patient was consented to open spinal cord biopsy and potential resection. Neuromonitoring with motor evoked potential (MEP) and somatosensory evoked potential (SSEP) were baselined and monitored throughout the entire procedure. The patient was placed prone in pinions and a midline incision was made to expose to C1-C2, and after subperiosteal dissection the posterior elements of C1 and C2 were removed. The microscope was brought to the surgical field and the ultrasound confirmed sufficient access to the lesion. The dura was opened in the midline. The posterior columns of the spinal cord were mapped to identify the safest entry point in the midline. Small pieces of tissue were taken from a nonfunctional region and sent for frozen and permanent pathology. MEP remained intact throughout the entire procedure, but SSEP showed a decrease. The resection was stopped and the dura was closed in a watertight fashion. The muscles were closed in layers. Postoperatively, the patient remained neurologically stable. Final pathology was consistent with a pilocytic astrocytoma. Because of the low-grade diagnosis, the lesion was continued to be followed. At 1-year follow-up, the lesion remained stable (Fig. 54.3) and the patient had significantly improved neurological examination.

Commonalities among the experts

Half of the physicians requested a total spine MRI and neurological examination as part of the preoperative assessment. However, preoperative tests choices greatly varied among surgeons. All would perform surgery mainly through a C1-C2

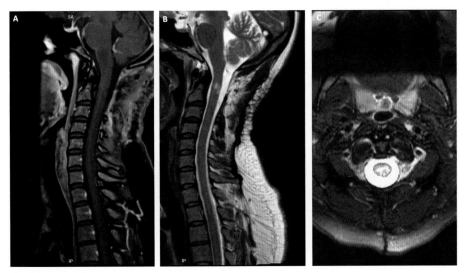

Fig. 54.3 Postoperative magnetic resonance images. (A) Sagittal T1 with contrast, (B) sagittal T2, and (C) axial T2 images demonstrating significantly decreased extent of amorphous T2 hyperintensity and associated enhancement within the cervical cord at the level of C1-C2. No new lesions are evident.

laminectomy/laminoplasty and resection of the intramedullary neoplasm. Complete tumor removal was the main goal of surgical intervention for most of the surgeons. Half of the physicians highlighted the importance of spinal cord decompression as one of the key objectives of the surgery. Most emphasized the importance of the anatomical relationships with the spinal cord, together with its tracts and vasculature. The complication of major concern among the surgeons was injury to the spinal cord. Surgical resection was generally assisted by intraoperative monitoring, ultrasound, and microscope. In terms of medical perioperative management, all the surgeons advocated for control and maintenance of a normal mean arterial pressure during the procedure. Half of the physicians recommended steroid administration perioperatively. Surgical nuances slightly varied; however, most of the physicians remarked the importance of identifying and preserving critical neurological structures through intraoperative monitoring. Subsequently after surgery, most admitted their patients to the intensive care unit for close observation. Postoperative follow-up testing was different among the experts. Some advocated for a MRI prior to discharge, and some recommended a cervical MRI within 6 to 12 weeks after surgery. All suggested a clinical follow-up 2 weeks after the surgical intervention.

SUMMARY OF QUALITY OF EVIDENCE TO GUIDE SPECIFIC INTERVENTIONS FOR THIS CASE

- Maintenance of a normal mean arterial pressure before surgical excision of an intramedullary spinal cord tumor: level III

REFERENCES

1. Diaz E, Morales H. Spinal Cord Anatomy and Clinical Syndromes. *Semin Ultrasound CT MR*. 2016;37(5):360–371.
2. Peh W. CT-guided percutaneous biopsy of spinal lesions. *Biomed Imaging Interv J*. 2006;2(3):e25.
3. Li HF, Ji XJ. The Diagnostic, Prognostic, and differential value of enhanced MR imaging in Guillain-Barre syndrome. *AJNR Am J Neuroradiol*. 2011;32(7). E140; author reply E141.
4. Mohajeri Moghaddam S, Bhatt AA. Location, length, and enhancement: systematic approach to differentiating intramedullary spinal cord lesions. *Insights Imaging*. 2018;9(4):511–526.
5. Samartzis D, Gillis CC, Shih P, O'Toole JE, Fessler RG. Intramedullary Spinal Cord Tumors: Part I-Epidemiology, Pathophysiology, and Diagnosis. *Global Spine J*. 2015;5(5):425–435.
6. Bhagwati SN, Deopujari CE, Parulekar GD. Trauma in congenital atlanto-axial dislocation. *Childs Nerv Syst*. 1998;14(12):719–721.
7. Sanford RA, Smith RA. Hemangioblastoma of the cervicomedullary junction. Report of three cases. *J Neurosurg*. 1986;64(2):317–321.
8. Yates C, Sheen J, Ma N, Naushahi M, Chaseling R. Chiari I malformation with significant motor and autonomic dysfunction in an infant. *J Clin Neurosci*. 2018;57:180–182.
9. Nauta HJ, Dolan E, Yasargil MG. Microsurgical anatomy of spinal subarachnoid space. *Surg Neurol*. 1983;19(5):431–437.
10. Rashad S, Elwany A, Farhoud A. Surgery for spinal intramedullary tumors: technique, outcome and factors affecting resectability. *Neurosurg Rev*. 2018;41(2):503–511.
11. Alizada O, Kemerdere R, Ulu MO, et al. Surgical management of spinal intramedullary tumors: Ten-year experience in a single institution. *J Clin Neurosci*. 2020;73:201–208.
12. Klimov VS, Kel'makov VV, Chishchina NV, Evsyukov AV. [Effectiveness of intraoperative monitoring of motor evoked potentials for predicting changes in the neurological status of patients with cervical spinal cord tumors in the early postoperative period]. *Zh Vopr Neirokhir Im N N Burdenko*. 2018;82(1):22–32.

55

Metastatic lesion to the cervico-thoracic junction

Fidel Valero-Moreno, MD and Henry Ruiz-Garcia, MD

Introduction

The cervical spine is the least common site affected by metastatic tumors of the vertebral column, but despite this, the presence of space occupying lesions in this region may cause severe symptomatology and morbidity.[1] Additional involvement of the upper thoracic segment often leads to instability.[2] Metastatic tumors are more common than primary tumors in this region.[2] The surgical management of metastatic lesions to the cervico-thoracic junction (CTJ) is widely variable among providers and institutions. The anatomy of the upper thoracic spine presents a challenge for anterior access, often requiring median sternotomy for complete exposure and added morbidity.[3] The biomechanics of the CTJ are also dependent on the posterior tension band provided by the paraspinal musculature and ligamentous complex, which is often disrupted by tumor and must be removed in order to complete the resection.[4,5] Tumor localization at the lower cervical segment is more frequent, and lesions on this region are related to a higher risk of instability due to its mobility.[6] Aggressive surgical resection of metastatic lesions in this area may confer a survival benefit; however, it can have considerable morbidity.[7–9] Moreover, surgical resection has shown superiority in relieving compression, controlling pain, and improving function. The most common approach for metastatic lesions involving the cervico-thoracic region involves posterior or posterolateral resection and decompression involving laminectomy and supplemented by posterior fixation to avoid instability. An exclusive anterior approach is typically not sufficient to achieve stabilization in most cases.[2] In this chapter, we present a case of a 79-year-old man who began complaining of neck pain after radiation for thyroid cancer and has a lesion involving the cervico-thoracic region.

Example case

Chief complaint: neck pain and upper and lower extremity weakness
History of present illness: This is a 79-year-old male patient with a history of thyroid cancer status post thyroidectomy and radiation who presented with a 3-week history of neck pain and rapidly progressive weakness. He was unable to ambulate or feed and dress himself. He was independent with his activities of daily living until 3 weeks ago before consultation. He also had new urinary incontinence. The patient underwent a cervical magnetic resonance image that showed a space occupying lesion at the level of the cervico-thoracic junction (Figs. 55.1–55.2).

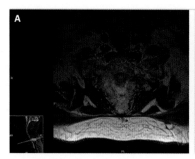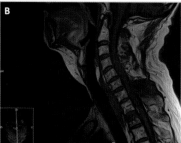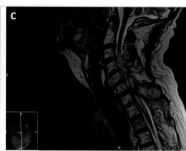

Fig. 55.1 Preoperative magnetic resonance images. (A) Axial T1 with contrast demonstrating an enhancing heterogeneous lesion extending from the posterior aspect of the vertebral arch anteriorly and laterally more on the right side. **(B)** Sagittal T1 demonstrating an abnormal hypointense lesion spanning the entire C7 spinous process. **(C)** Sagittal T2 demonstrating a hyperintense lesion at the C7 spinous process, extending anteriorly and compressing the spinal cord. There is also an extensive syrinx extending from C3 to T2. There appears to be an extradural mass right behind the C5 vertebral body.

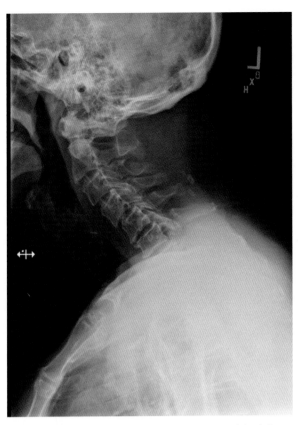

Medications: aspirin 325 mg

Allergies: no known drug allergies

Past medical and surgical history: thyroid cancer, previous transient ischemic attacks, coronary artery disease, thyroidectomy

Family history: none

Social history: none

Physical examination: awake, alert, and oriented to person, place, and time; cranial nerves II–XII intact; bilateral deltoids/triceps/biceps 3/5; interossei 2/5; iliopsoas 3/5; knee flexion/knee extension/dorsi, and plantar flexion 2/5

Reflexes: 3+ in bilateral biceps/triceps/brachioradialis with positive Hoffman; 3+ in bilateral patella/ankle; bilateral Babinski; sensation decreased to light touch

Fig. 55.2 Preoperative lateral cervico-throacic spine x-rays. Lateral view demonstrating erosion of the C7 posterior elements by a soft tissue mass. Vertebral body heights are maintained. Anterolisthesis of C4 on C5 and C5 on C6. Multilevel degenerative disc disease and facet osteoarthritis are also seen.

	Anas Abdallah, MD Neurosurgery Osmaniye State Hospital Osmaniye, Turkey	Benjamin D. Elder, MD, PhD Neurosurgery Mayo Clinic Rochester, Minnesota, United States	Aron Lazary, MD, PhD Orthopaedic Surgery Buda Health Center Semmelweis University Budapest, Hungary	Praveen Mummaneni, MD Brenton Pennicooke, MD Neurosurgery University of California at San Francisco San Francisco, California, United States
Preoperative				
Additional tests requested	CT brain and complete spine CT cervical spine Cervical x-rays PET Oncology evaluation Anesthesia evaluation	CT-guided biopsy of C7 spinous process CT neck with contrast CT chest/abdomen/pelvis Otolaryngology evaluation Possible preoperative embolization	CT C-spine	CTA C-spine PET Preoperative embolization
Surgical approach selected	If survival > 12 weeks, C7 laminectomy and excisional biopsy	Pending pathology, C5 corpectomy and posterior C3-T1 laminectomy and C2-T4 instrumented fusion	C6-T1 decompression and C5-T3 posterior fusion	C3-T2 posterior fusion and C3-T1 laminectomy
Goal of surgery	Diagnosis, decompression of spinal cord	Decompress spinal cord and nerve roots, stabilize spine	Decompress spinal cord, tumor debulking, stabilize spine	Decompress spinal cord
Perioperative				
Positioning	Prone with Mayfield pins	Stage 1: supine with gel donut and Garner-Wells tongs Stage 2: prone on Jackson table with pins	Prone, with pins	Prone on Jackson table, with Mayfield pins

	Anas Abdallah, MD Neurosurgery Osmaniye State Hospital Osmaniye, Turkey	Benjamin D. Elder, MD, PhD Neurosurgery Mayo Clinic Rochester, Minnesota, United States	Aron Lazary, MD, PhD Orthopaedic Surgery Buda Health Center Semmelweis University Budapest, Hungary	Praveen Mummaneni, MD Brenton Pennicooke, MD Neurosurgery University of California at San Francisco San Francisco, California, United States
Surgical equipment	IOM Fluoroscopy Surgical microscope	Otolaryngology exposure Fluoroscopy IOM (MEP, SSEP) Surgical microscope Bone scalpel Ultrasound O-arm	Fluoroscopy Surgical navigation	IOM (MEP/SSEP/EMG) Fluoroscopy Surgical navigation Intraoperative CT
Medications	Steroids, maintain MAP	Steroids	Steroids	None
Anatomical considerations	Spinal cord, nerve roots, dura	Stage 1: carotid sheath, recurrent laryngeal nerve, esophagus, vertebral arteries Stage 2: vertebral arteries, spinal cord, nerve roots	Dorsal muscles, lamina, spinal canal, lateral masses	Spinal cord, vertebral arteries
Complications feared with approach chosen	Instability, motor deficit, CSF leak	Worsening spinal cord compression, paralysis		Spinal cord injury
Intraoperative				
Anesthesia	General	General	General	General
Exposure	C7	C2-T4	C4-T3	C3-T2
Levels decompressed	C7	C3-T1	C6-T1	C3-T1
Levels fused	None	C2-T4	C4-T3	C3-T2
Surgical narrative	Position prone with head in Mayfield pins, slight flexion, vertical midline posterior incision from C6-T1, central splitting at midline down C7 spinous process, subperiosteal dissection of paraspinal muscles, confirm C7 level with fluoroscopy, bilateral C7 laminectomy with high-speed drill and Kerrison rongeurs, open along lamina-facet interface down to ligamentum flavum, ligament cut transversely at upper and lower ends, lamina elevated, medial portions of facet are removed to decompress existing nerve roots, biopsy specimen, layered closure with drain	Stage 1: Position supine on flat Jackson table with gel axillary roll transversely across shoulders with 10 lb of traction, localization with fluoroscopy, incision over C5 vertebral body in neck crease, transverse neck incision contralateral to area of worst compression, mobilize esophagus medially and carotid sheath laterally, place distraction pin in vertebral body for localizing x-ray, mobilize longus colli off vertebral bodies, place retractor system and 144 mm distraction pins in C4 and C6, complete C4-5 and C5-6 discectomies, remove C5 vertebral body with rongeurs taking care to not laterally injury vertebral arteries, open PLL and resect ventral epidural tumor, size and place titanium mesh cage packed with morcellized allograft, place anterior plate from C4-C6, obtain final x-rays, leave drain in retropharyngeal space, flip for stage 2 Stage 2: Position prone on Jackson table with head in neutral position with pins,	Position prone, standard posterior midline approach from C4-T3, place bilateral lateral mass screws from C4-C6 and pedicle screws from T1-T3 under navigation if available, cement T3 if bone quality poor, remove tumor-involved lamina from C6-T1, laminectomy C6-T1 and C7 foramens, lock screws with transient rods, layered closure with two deep drains	Position prone, lateral x-ray to plan incision, expose C3-T2, place navigation array on T2 spinous process, intraoperative CT and register with navigation system, plan/decorticate entry points/place T1-T2 pedicle screws with navigation, decorticate entry points/place C3-6 lateral mass screws, C3-T1 laminectomy and resection of posterior aspect of tumor, run MEP after completing laminectomies, place rods connecting screws from C3-T2, obtain intraoperative CT to confirm hardware location, final tighten caps, place allograft along decorticated lateral masses and transverse processes, layered wound closure with subfascial drains

	Anas Abdallah, MD Neurosurgery Osmaniye State Hospital Osmaniye, Turkey	Benjamin D. Elder, MD, PhD Neurosurgery Mayo Clinic Rochester, Minnesota, United States	Aron Lazary, MD, PhD Orthopaedic Surgery Buda Health Center Semmelweis University Budapest, Hungary	Praveen Mummaneni, MD Brenton Pennicooke, MD Neurosurgery University of California at San Francisco San Francisco, California, United States
		expose from C2 to T4 with preservation of C1-2 muscle/ligament insertion and distal ligaments, localizing x-ray, cannulate 14–16 mm tracts for lateral mass screws from C3-6 using normal anatomy, cannulate and place T1-4 pedicle screws, complete laminectomy from inferior aspect of C3 to superior aspect of T1, intraoperative ultrasound to confirm adequate decompression of spinal cord, cannulate C2 pedicles using anatomical landmarks and place C2 pedicle screws, intraoperative O-arm spin to confirm adequate screw position, place from C2-T4 tapered titanium rods, decortication of posterior elements, place morcellized allograft, place subfascial drains, layered closure		
Complication avoidance	Minimize opening to one level, decompress nerve roots	Preoperative embolization increase neck extension with gel axillary roll, approach contralateral to area of worse compression, distraction pin in vertebral body for localization, preserve C1-2 muscle/ligament insertion and distal ligaments, extend fusion to T4 because of T2 involvement, intraoperative ultrasound to assess decompression, O-arm to confirm screw placement, tapered titanium rods	Surgical navigation if available, cement T3 if bone quality poor	Preoperative embolization, debulk posterior aspect of tumor, repeat CT to confirm hardware location
Postoperative				
Admission	ICU	ICU	ICU	ICU
Postoperative complications feared	Hematoma, CSF leak, nerve palsy, neck pain, neuropathic pain, cervical instability, vascular injury, delayed wound recovery	Swallowing dysfunction, hoarseness, neck hematoma, C5 palsy	Wound infection	C5 palsy
Anticipated length of stay	2 days	4–5 days	5–7 days	5 days
Follow-up testing	CT cervical spine within 24 hours of surgery Oncology evaluation	Medical oncology evaluation Radiation oncology evaluation AP/lateral x-rays 6 weeks, 3 months, 6 months, 1 year after surgery	C-T spine x-ray after drain removal Oncology evaluation	AP and lateral C-spine x-ray prior to discharge Radiation oncology evaluation Radiation therapy 3 weeks after surgery
Bracing	Rigid neck collar for 3–4 weeks	Miami J with thoracic extension when out of bed	None	Miami J for 6 weeks

	Anas Abdallah, MD Neurosurgery Osmaniye State Hospital Osmaniye, Turkey	Benjamin D. Elder, MD, PhD Neurosurgery Mayo Clinic Rochester, Minnesota, United States	Aron Lazary, MD, PhD Orthopaedic Surgery Buda Health Center Semmelweis University Budapest, Hungary	Praveen Mummaneni, MD Brenton Pennicooke, MD Neurosurgery University of California at San Francisco San Francisco, California, United States
Follow-up visits	2 weeks, 6 weeks, every 3 months after surgery	2 weeks, 6 weeks, 3 months, 6 months, 1 year after surgery	3 months, 6 months, 12 months, 24 months after surgery	3 weeks after surgery

AP, Anteroposterior; *CSF*, cerebrospinal fluid; *CT*, computed tomography; *CTA*, computed tomography angiography; *DEXA*, dual-energy x-ray absorptiometry; *ICU*, intensive care unit; *IOM*, intraoperative monitoring; *MAP*, mean arterial pressure; *MEP*, motor evoked potentials; *PET*, positron emission tomography; *PLL*, posterior longitudinal ligament; *SSEP*, somatosensory evoked potentials

Differential diagnosis

- Degenerative cervical or thoracic stenosis
- Herniated cervical or thoracic disc
- Transverse myelitis
- Spinal cord infarction
- Metastatic spinal disease

Important anatomical and preoperative considerations

The CTJ is widely defined as the area spanning from C7 to T3.[2,10] The biomechanical properties of the CTJ make this area unique and prone to instability. The CTJ is a transition segment comprising the mobile, lordotic cervical spine and the rigid, kyphotic spine.[10,11] Neoplastic disruption of these structures and extensive laminectomy/facetectomy across this segment are invariably related to instability.[2,10] Moreover, the CTJ is characterized by a narrower canal size and a more fragile blood supply, thus, predisposing this area to neurological injury.[10]

Treatment for CTJ metastatic lesions should be centered on achieving neural decompression, immediate stabilization, and restoration of normal aligment.[2,10] The surgical strategy hinges upon the overall status of the patient, type of tumor, and structures involved.[2] Metastasis affecting the vertebral body require a ventral approach in most of the cases due to its deep location resulting from the normal thoracic kyphosis.[2] Resection goals may vary from palliative decompression to more aggressive en bloc curative resection attempts. If a short life expectancy is anticipated, solid bony fusion may not be indicated.[10]

Anterior approaches are divided into low cervical approach, transmanubrial/transsternal approach and thoracotomy.[2] A particular ventral approach selection is mainly directed by the level of the lesion.[2] The cervical approach yields access to the C7 level and in most cases the T1-T2 segment is reachable if necessary. The transmanubrial/transsternal approach is needed if the tumor affects or extends to the T3 level. A tumor stretching below the T4 level should be approached thorough a thoracotomy.[2] Anterior-only approaches are not enough to provide stabilization, and fixation and hardware failures are common and may represent a biomechanical disadvantage if not combined with a posterior instrumentation.[2,10]

A classical midline posterior approach is practical for decompression and resection of tumors located in the posterior columns. A transpedicular and costotransversectomy variations may be useful for limited access to more ventrally located lesions.[2] Posterior laminectomy and tumor resection should be followed by fusion of the CTJ due to instability.[2,10,11] Posterior instrumentation can provide stabilization to the CTJ either for palliative or curative procedures. Despite this, fusion and stabilization of the CTJ implies a technical challenge because of the transition from cervical lordosis to thoracic kyphosis and produces a loading shift from the posterior to the anterior structures resulting in increased stressed at this level.[2,10,11] Nevertheless, facet screw fixation in the cervical segment and transpedicular thoracic screw fixation confer good stabilization even in cases with high postoperative instability.[11]

What was actually done

This patient, with previous history of thyroid cancer presenting with new onset neck pain and weakness, had undergone imaging that revealed a compressive extradural lesion dorsal to the spinal cord at the C7 level. The patient was advised to undergo surgery to remove the tumor, decompress the cord, and establish pathological diagnosis. Resection of the anterior C5 lesion was not included in this approach. After the patient was completely worked with systemic imaging, they were taken to the operating room for a cervical decompressive laminectomy for degenerative spinal stenosis C3-C7 and tumor debulking from C6 through T1. Once general anesthesia was provided, normal baseline motor evoked and somatosensory evoked potential were obtained. The patient was positioned prone on the Jackson table. A posterior cervical-upper thoracic incision was made and the posterior elements from C2 to T1 were exposed bilaterally in a subperiosteal fashion. The tumor was identified at the C7 level, and the intraoperative pathology confirmed a metastatic lesion. Thereafter, decompressive laminectomies for degenerative stenosis were performed from C3 to C6, as well as bilateral medial facetectomies from C3-C4 to C6-C7. Another laminectomy was also performed at the T1 level. Consequently, maximal tumor resection and decompression were achieved working from C6 to T1; however, residual tumor was left behind, especially on the right side extending out into the region of the nerve roots and vertebral artery to minimize potential morbidity. The patient awoke without complications and was transferred to the intensive care unit. Imaging showed good decompression (Fig. 55.3). He remained stable and was discharged on

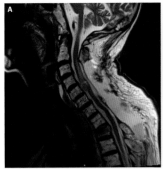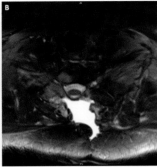

Fig. 55.3 Postoperative magnetic resonance images. (A) Sagittal and **(B)** axial T2 images demonstrating postoperative changes from decompressive laminectomy and tumor debulking with residual tumor within the right C7-T1 articular pillar extending into the right C7 vertebral body. There is also an overall decrease in the amount of cord edema. The intradural metastasis at C5 is minimally increased in size with persistent compression of the cord.

postoperative day 3 and underwent adjuvant radiation therapy 2 weeks after surgery.

Commonalities among the experts

All of the surgeons considered a cervical computed tomography scan as an important preoperative tool for evaluation of bony anatomy. Most would pursue surgery through a posterior cervico-thoracic laminectomy and instrumented fusion. The main goals of the surgery were spinal decompression and stabilization. Fluoroscopy was the only intraoperative equipment employed by all the surgeons. In addition, most advocated for intraoperative monitoring and navigation system. Most surgeons recommended perioperative steroid administration. Physicians were mindful of the spinal cord and neurovascular structures. The most feared complication was cord injury with neurological deficit. Levels of decompression and fusion slightly varied among surgeons; however, most decided to include an area between C2 and T4. Postoperatively, all admitted their patients to the intensive care unit, and most ordered imaging studies prior to discharge. Feared morbidities after surgery greatly varied. All the surgeons highlighted the importance of oncological evaluation after surgery for continued treatment of residual disease.

SUMMARY OF QUALITY OF EVIDENCE TO GUIDE SPECIFIC INTERVENTIONS FOR THIS CASE

- Posterior cervico-thoracic decompression and fusion to obtain a precise diagnosis, release cord compression, and provide stabilization: level III
- Perioperative steroid therapy for the management of metastasis to the cervico-thoracic junction: level III

REFERENCES

1. Lei M, Liu Y, Yan L, Tang C, Liu S, Zhou S. Posterior decompression and spine stabilization for metastatic spinal cord compression in the cervical spine. A matched pair analysis. *Eur J Surg Oncol.* 2015;41(12):1691–1698.
2. Wang VY, Chou D. The cervicothoracic junction. *Neurosurg Clin N Am.* 2007;18(2):365–371.
3. Howell EP, Williamson T, Karikari I, et al. Total en bloc resection of primary and metastatic spine tumors. *Ann Transl Med.* 2019;7(10):226.
4. Fayed I, Toscano DT, Triano MJ, et al. Crossing the Cervicothoracic Junction During Posterior Cervical Decompression and Fusion: Is It Necessary? *Neurosurgery.* 2020;86(6):E544–e550.
5. Goyal A, Akhras A, Wahood W, Alvi MA, Nassr A, Bydon M. Should Multilevel Posterior Cervical Fusions Involving C7 Cross the Cervicothoracic Junction? A Systematic Review and Meta-Analysis. *World Neurosurg.* 2019;127 588-595.e585.
6. Mazel C, Balabaud L, Bennis S, Hansen S. Cervical and thoracic spine tumor management: surgical indications, techniques, and outcomes. *Orthop Clin North Am.* 2009;40(1):75–92. vi-vii.
7. Klimo Jr. P, Dailey AT, Fessler RG. Posterior surgical approaches and outcomes in metastatic spine-disease. *Neurosurg Clin N Am.* 2004;15(4):425–435.
8. Petteys RJ, Spitz SM, Goodwin CR, et al. Factors associated with improved survival following surgery for renal cell carcinoma spinal metastases. *Neurosurg Focus.* 2016;41(2):E13.
9. Tatsui CE, Suki D, Rao G, et al. Factors affecting survival in 267 consecutive patients undergoing surgery for spinal metastasis from renal cell carcinoma. *J Neurosurg Spine.* 2014;20(1):108–116.
10. Le H, Balabhadra R, Park J, Kim D. Surgical treatment of tumors involving the cervicothoracic junction. *Neurosurg Focus.* 2003;15(5):E3.
11. Mazel C, Hoffmann E, Antonietti P, Grunenwald D, Henry M, Williams J. Posterior cervicothoracic instrumentation in spine tumors. *Spine (Phila Pa 1976).* 2004;29(11):1246–1253.

56

Glioblastoma

Fidel Valero-Moreno, MD

Introduction

Primary glioblastoma (GBM) of the spinal cord is a rare condition that contributes to just 1.5% of all spinal tumors.[1] This neoplasm most commonly affects the cervical spine or the cervico-thoracic junction in at least 60% of the cases[2] and usually occurs during the second decade of life.[3] Treatment approaches emulate protocols for intracranial high-grade lesions.[1,3,4] Leptomeningeal spread is a marker of poor prognosis and usually manifests as patchy lesions in the caudal cord or intracranially.[3–5] Secondary spinal cord tumors are extremely rare and may occur after radiation exposure to the spine or surrounding soft tissue structures.[6] Currently, there is limited data supporting a standardized treatment of these lesions.[7] Due to the infiltrative nature of these tumors, and the high eloquence of the cervical cord, the extent of resection is usually limited. Thus the goals of surgery are also variable depending on the location of the tumor and the patient's starting neurological status.[8] Aggressive resection of malignant spinal cord tumors has been debated on conferring a benefit to survival and carries significant neurological morbidity.[6,9,10] Moreover, degree of survival improvement after resection followed by radiotherapy alone or with chemotherapy remains controversial.[1,3] In this chapter, we present the case of a patient with a cervical cord malignancy after exposure to radiotherapy.

Example case

Chief complaint: weakness and numbness

History of present illness: This is a 45-year-old male patient with a history of multiple myeloma and plasmacytoma diagnosed in 2010. He underwent radiotherapy. He underwent treatment of an additional lesion in 2016, and at that time received radiation and bone marrow transplant. Additionally, he was started on Revlimid. He presented with 4 months of worsening weakness and numbness. He has thrombocytopenia with a platelet count of 50,000. As part of this workup, the patient underwent a magnetic resonance of the cervical spine that showed an intraaxial lesion of the cervical cord with associated mass effect (Fig. 56.1).

Medications: dexamethasone, pantorpazole, gabapentin

Allergies: no known drug allergies

Past medical and surgical history: plasmacytoma, multiple myeloma, tumor resection, bone marrow transplant

Family history: noncontributory

Social history: retired engineer, no smoking, no alcohol use

Physical examination: awake, alert, and oriented to person, place, and time; cranial nerves II–XII intact; bilateral deltoids/triceps/biceps 3/5; interossei 2/5; iliopsoas/knee flexion/knee extension/dorsi, and plantar flexion 5/5

Reflexes: 3+ in bilateral biceps/triceps/brachioradialis with negative Hoffman; 2+ in bilateral patella/ankle; no clonus or Babinski; sensation decreased in left hemibody

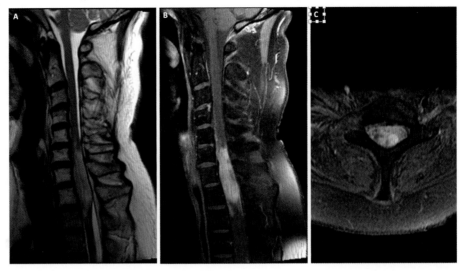

Fig. 56.1 Preoperative magnetic resonance image (MRI) of the cervical spine. (A) Sagittal T2 image demonstrating an intramedullary lesion extending from C6 to T2 levels that has a high signal intensity and is causing a diffuse spinal cord expansion. This is more pronounced at the C7-T1 level and associated with mild tumor-related edema spreading inferiorly (T2). **(B)** Sagittal and **(C)** axial T1 with contrast images demonstrating an intramedullary space-occupying mass with avid enhancement. The lesion is slightly heterogenous and displays ill-defined borders.

	Ignacio Barrenechea, MD Neurosurgery Grupo Gamma Rosario, Santa Fe, Argentina	George I. Jallo, MD Neurosurgery Johns Hopkins All Children's Tampa, Florida, United States	Jorge Navarro Bonnet, MD Neurosurgery Medica Sur, Mexico City, Mexico	Nicholas Theodore, MD A. Karim Ahmed, MD Ann Liu, MD Neurosurgery Johns Hopkins University Baltimore, Maryland, United States
Preoperative				
Additional tests requested	MRI brain and complete spine SSEP Cardiology evaluation Infectious disease evaluation	CT chest/abdomen/pelvis MRI brain and complete spine Lumbar puncture for CSF analysis Flexion-extension cervical spine x-rays	CT C-spine PET Swallowing evaluation NCS/EMG/SSEP	CT C- and T-spine PET Obtain prior medical records
Surgical approach selected	C5-T2 laminoplasty for resection of intramedullary tumor	C6-T1 laminectomy or laminoplasty for resection of tumor	C6-T1 laminectomy for resection of tumor with C6-T1 posterior fusion	C6-T1 laminectomy for resection of tumor and C5-T2 posterior fusion
Goal of surgery	Gross total resection if possible, preservation of neurological function, spinal instability	Establish diagnosis, debulk tumor	Establish diagnosis, spinal cord decompression	Establish diagnosis, prevent further neurological decline
Perioperative				
Positioning	Prone with pins	Prone with pins	Prone with no pins	Prone with pins
Surgical equipment	IOM (MEP/SSEP) Surgical microscope Ultrasonic aspirator Ultrasound	IOM (MEP/SSEP/D-wave) Fluoroscopy Surgical microscope Ultrasonic aspirator	IOM Ultrasonic bone scalpel Surgical microscope Ultrasonic aspirator O-arm	IOM (MEP/SSEP/D-wave) Ultrasonic bone scalpel Surgical microscope
Medications	Steroids, maintain MAP	Steroids	None	Steroids, maintain MAP >85
Anatomical considerations	Spinal cord anatomy (posterior median sulcus for myelotomy), spinal cord arteries	Spinal cord anatomy (posterior median sulcus for myelotomy)	Spinal cord anatomy (posterior median sulcus for myelotomy), pedicles	Spinal cord
Complications feared with approach chosen	Neurological injury, CSF leak, instability, epidural scarring	Injury to corticospinal tract and dorsal columns	Spinal cord injury, bleeding	Neurological injury, poor wound healing, CSF leak, adjacent segment disease

(continued on next page)

	Ignacio Barrenechea, MD Neurosurgery Grupo Gamma Rosario, Santa Fe, Argentina	George I. Jallo, MD Neurosurgery Johns Hopkins All Children's Tampa, Florida, United States	Jorge Navarro Bonnet, MD Neurosurgery Medica Sur, Mexico City, Mexico	Nicholas Theodore, MD A. Karim Ahmed, MD Ann Liu, MD Neurosurgery Johns Hopkins University Baltimore, Maryland, United States
Intraoperative				
Anesthesia	General	General	General	General
Exposure	C5-T2	C6-T1	C6-T1	C5-T2
Levels decompressed	C5-T2	C6-T1	C6-T1	C6-T1
Levels fused	None	None	C6-T1	C5-T2
Surgical narrative	Position prone, posterior longitudinal skin incision, expose posterior superficial cervical fascia for a few centimeters bilaterally, dissection along nuchal ligament, skeletonize attachments of cervical muscles to spinous process and lamina, expose lamina and part of lateral masses, laminotomy using high-speed drill, cut lamina caudal to cranial following a line between each spinous process and zygapophyseal joint, cut interspinous ligaments at rostral and caudal-most levels, store osteoligamentous complex in saline and gentamicin, open dura under loupe magnification, tack dura, peel arachnoid membrane off pia under microscopic magnification, identify posterior median sulcus with IOM, open midline and displace posterior columns up and down with bipolar forces to completely expose tumor, resect tumor slowly with ultrasonic aspirator, work cleavage plane between tumor and posterior columns with bipolar cautery, care taken to avoid injuring anterior spinal artery and branches, use IOM to guide resection if no cleavage plane identified, watertight dural closure with fibrin glue, laminoplasty, layered closure	Position prone, obtain IOM baseline, x-ray to confirm levels, perform three- to four-level laminectomy or laminoplasty, ultrasound to confirm tumor exposure, open dura and visualize tumor, perform midline myelotomy to identify tumor unless comes to surface, obtain frozen pathology to assess if planes are present based on histology, work inside-out if no tumor planes and debulk as much as possible, utilize MEP and SSEP to guide resection, avoid cauterizing if possible, watertight dural closure, multilayer closure with possible laminoplasty	Preflip IOM, position prone, posterior midline incision from C6-T1, linear fascia opening, subperiosteal dissection, lateral extension to expose pedicle/facet articular professes for instrumentation, C6-T1 laminotomy with ultrasonic bone scalpel, midline dural opening with microscope, open midline posterior sulcus to avoid posterior columns, biopsy lesion for histopathological diagnosis, safe maximal resection with IOM if pathology shows oncologic features, C6-T1 transpedicular screw fixation with O-arm with bone graft if needed, layered closure	Position prone with Mayfield pins, posterior midline incision from C5-T2, subperiosteal dissection, placement of C5–6 lateral mass screws and T1 and T2 pedicle screws, x-ray to evaluate position of screws, ultrasonic bone scalpel or drill to perform C6-T1 laminectomies, microsurgical intradural exploration, midline myelotomy if there is no exophytic component, aim for exophytic component or else midline myelotomy to enter cord, biopsy and/or resect lesion depending on consistency and ease of resection, watertight dural closure, rods and caps are placed, decorticate facets, place demineralized bone matrix or autograft on bone surfaces, irrigation of wound, vancomycin in cavity, layered closure with drain

	Ignacio Barrenechea, MD Neurosurgery Grupo Gamma Rosario, Santa Fe, Argentina	George I. Jallo, MD Neurosurgery Johns Hopkins All Children's Tampa, Florida, United States	Jorge Navarro Bonnet, MD Neurosurgery Medica Sur, Mexico City, Mexico	Nicholas Theodore, MD A. Karim Ahmed, MD Ann Liu, MD Neurosurgery Johns Hopkins University Baltimore, Maryland, United States
Complication avoidance	Laminoplasty, preserve articular capsule during laminoplasty, identify posterior median sulcus with IOM, completely open posterior columns to expose tumor, care taken to avoid injuring anterior spinal artery, use IOM to guide resection if no cleavage plane identified	Laminectomy or laminoplasty, ultrasound to confirm exposure, valuate if comes to surface or else midline myelotomy, inside-out debulking if no planes, resection guided by monitoring, avoid cauterizing	Preflip IOM, access lesion through midline posterior sulcus to preserve dorsal columns, biopsy to guide further resection, O-arm for instrumentation	Excisional biopsy, D-wave IOM, access exophytic component or perform midline myelotomy, resection based on ease of resection
Postoperative				
Admission	ICU	ICU	Floor	ICU
Postoperative complications feared	Neurological injury, CSF leak, instability, wound infection	CSF leak, motor or sensory deficit, spinal deformity	Hematoma, spinal cord edema	Neurological injury, CSF leak, adjacent segment disease, infection poor wound healing
Anticipated length of stay	5 days	3–4 days	2 days	4–5 days
Follow-up testing	MRI C-T spine within 24 hours, 2 months, 6 months, yearly after surgery C-spine sitting x-rays prior to discharge, 3 months after surgery	MRI C-spine within 48 hours of surgery	MRI C-spine within 48 hours of surgery C and T-spine x-rays 6 weeks after surgery	CT within 24 hours of surgery C- and T-spine x-rays 6 weeks after surgery MRI C-spine 3 months after surgery
Bracing	None	None	None	None
Follow-up visits	2 weeks, 1 month, 3 months, 6 months, 1 year after surgery	10–14 days after surgery Oncology evaluation	2 weeks after surgery	2 weeks and 6 weeks after surgery

CSF, cerebrospinal fluid; *CT*, computed tomography; *EMG*, electromyogram; *ICU*, intensive care unit; *IOM*, intraoperative monitoring; *MAP*, mean arterial pressure; *MEP*, motor evoked potential; *MRI*, magnetic resonance imaging; *NCS*, nerve conduction study; *PET*, positron emission tomography; *SSEP*, somatosensory evoked potential.

Differential diagnosis

- Primary intramedullary spinal cord tumor
- Secondary intramedullary spinal cord tumor
- Demyelinating disease
- Radiation necrosis
- Leptomeningeal disease

Important anatomical and preoperative considerations

When there is concern of an intramedullary spinal cord tumor,[4] tumor localization and neurological status are crucial factors to take into consideration before resection planning. Absence of a distinct plane between the tumor and the normal cord tissue is seen in most cases and gross total resection is rarely achieved.[11,12] However, wide resections have not demonstrated longer survivals.[11,12] An aggressive approach of a GBM of the spinal cord exposes the subarachnoid space to the tumoral cells and constitutes a feasible mechanism of leptomeningeal or intracranial dissemination.[4] In accord with this, the extent of resection has been an unreliable factor to predict survival. There have been reports of good outcomes following cordectomy when tumors confined to the lumbar and sacral regions; however, this approach is associated with complete neurological deficit.[12,13] Neurological function, cervical and upper thoracic localization, holocord involvement, and diffuse spreading represent contraindications to this approach.[13]

What was actually done

The patient was admitted to the hospital and a C5-T2 laminectomy with biopsy possible resection was planned. The patient was brough to the operating room and induced under general anesthesia. The patient was placed in Mayfield pin and positioned prone on the Jackson table. Neuromonitoring in the form of somatosensory and motor evoked potentials was utilized. A midline exposure was performed, subperiosteal dissection was performed, fluoroscopy confirmed the levels, and the posterior elements of C5-T2 were removed. The ultrasound was used to confirm exposure. The dura was opened in the midline, and the lesion was easily identified on the dorsal aspect of the cord. A small midline myelotomy was performed over the tumor, and tissue was sent for frozen section. The intraoperative pathology showed strong evidence of high-grade glioma, and thus further resection was stopped in order to preserve neurological function. A duraplasty was performed with bovine pericardium dura substitute, and the wound was closed in anatomical layers. The patient awoke without complications and was brought to the intensive care unit for maintenance of elevated mean arterial pressures overnight. The patient remained stable and was transferred to the floor the following day and discharged on postoperative day 3 at their neurological baseline. They later underwent radiation therapy with concurrent temozolomide.

Commonalities among the experts

Positron emission tomography and computed tomography scans of the cervical spine were advocated by half of the surgeons to evaluate the extent of disease. The rest preferred a magnetic resonance imaging including the brain and complete spine. All would perform a posterior laminectomy/laminoplasty of the involved segments to attain tumor excision, and half would combine it with a posterior fusion at the cervico-thoracic region. The main goals of surgery were to establish diagnosis and provide spinal cord decompression. All of the surgeons emphasized the awareness of the posterior median sulcus and dorsal columns before attempting myelotomy and resection. Approach-related complications that raised special concern were spinal cord injury and cerebrospinal fluid leak. Surgery was mostly accomplished with intraoperative monitoring, microscope, and ultrasonic aspirator, with steroids as the perioperative medication of choice. Although surgical techniques varied, all of the physicians prioritized safe maximal resection with intraoperative monitoring guidance in order to preserve spinal cord integrity. Most admitted their patients to the intensive care unit and most requested magnetic imaging within the first 48 postoperative hours to assess for extent of resection and potential complications. All recommended follow-up 2 weeks after surgery.

SUMMARY OF QUALITY OF EVIDENCE TO GUIDE SPECIFIC INTERVENTIONS FOR THIS CASE

- Safe maximal resection guided by intraoperative monitoring to reduce neurological morbidities for infiltrating gliomas of the spine: level III

REFERENCES

1. Moinuddin FM, Alvi MA, Kerezoudis P, et al. Variation in management of spinal gliobastoma multiforme: results from a national cancer registry. *J Neurooncol*. 2019;141(2):441–447.
2. Morais N, Mascarenhas L, Soares-Fernandes JP, Silva A, Magalhães Z, Costa JA. Primary spinal glioblastoma: A case report and review of the literature. *Oncol Lett*. 2013;5(3):992–996.
3. Konar SK, Maiti TK, Bir SC, Kalakoti P, Bollam P, Nanda A. Predictive Factors Determining the Overall Outcome of Primary Spinal Glioblastoma Multiforme: An Integrative Survival Analysis. *World Neurosurg*. 2016;86:341–348. e341-343.
4. Purkayastha A, Sharma N, Sridhar MS, Abhishek D. Intramedullary Glioblastoma Multiforme of Spine with Intracranial Supratentorial Metastasis: Progressive Disease with a Multifocal Picture. *Asian J Neurosurg*. 2018;13(4):1209–1212.
5. Mayer RR, Warmouth GM, Troxell M, Adesina AM, Kass JS. Glioblastoma multiforme of the conus medullaris in a 28-year-old female: a case report and review of the literature. *Clin Neurol Neurosurg*. 2012;114(3):275–277.
6. Ng C, Fairhall J, Rathmalgoda C, Stening W, Smee R. Spinal cord glioblastoma multiforme induced by radiation after treatment for Hodgkin disease. Case report. *J Neurosurg Spine*. 2007;6(4):364–367.
7. Cohen AR, Wisoff JH, Allen JC, Epstein F. Malignant astrocytomas of the spinal cord. *J Neurosurg*. 1989;70(1):50–54.
8. McGirt MJ, Goldstein IM, Chaichana KL, Tobias ME, Kothbauer KF, Jallo GI. Extent of surgical resection of malignant astrocytomas of the spinal cord: outcome analysis of 35 patients. *Neurosurgery*. 2008;63(1):55–60. discussion 60-51.
9. Alvisi C, Cerisoli M, Giulioni M. Intramedullary spinal gliomas: long-term results of surgical treatments. *Acta Neurochir (Wien)*. 1984;70(3-4):169–179.
10. Marchan EM, Sekula RF, Jr., Jannetta PJ, Quigley MR. Long-term survival enhanced by cordectomy in a patient with a spinal glioblastoma multiforme and paraplegia. Case report. *J Neurosurg Spine*. 2007;7(6):656–659.
11. Mori K, Imai S, Shimizu J, Taga T, Ishida M, Matsusue Y. Spinal glioblastoma multiforme of the conus medullaris with holocordal and intracranial spread in a child: a case report and review of the literature. *Spine J*. 2012;12(1):e1–6.
12. Shen CX, Wu JF, Zhao W, Cai ZW, Cai RZ, Chen CM. Primary spinal glioblastoma multiforme: A case report and review of the literature. *Medicine (Baltimore)*. 2017;96(16):e6634.
13. Viljoen S, Hitchon PW, Ahmed R, Kirby PA. Cordectomy for intramedullary spinal cord glioblastoma with a 12-year survival. *Surg Neurol Int*. 2014;5:101.

57

Foramen magnum meningioma

Fidel Valero-Moreno, MD and Henry Ruiz-Garcia, MD

Introduction

Foramen magnum meningiomas comprise a rare group of neoplasms that affect primarily the lower cranial nerves and cervico-medullary junction.[1] Meningiomas located on this region represent 1.8%–3.2 % of all meningiomas[2,3] and 8.6 % of all spinal meningiomas.[1] Although infrequent, extradural extension is seen in 10% of the cases.[3] These tumors are more frequently found during the fifth and sixth decades of life.[2] The onset of symptoms is subtle and typically progresses in a "clock-like" fashion, affecting the ipsilateral lower extremity and then rotating along the contralateral arm and leg due to the location of the corticospinal fibers within the spinal cord. These lesions often involve the vertebral arteries and lower cranial nerves, and present a considerable challenge in preserving these structures during tumor resection.[4, 5] Damage to the lower cranial nerves may result in prolonged intubation, dysphagia, and/or other respiratory/gastrointestinal complications. Anterior and anterolateral localizations carry a greater risk of morbidity and mortality.[2] The extent of bony removal is dependent on the tumor location and the involvement of the surrounding neurovascular structures.[4,5]

Example case

Chief complaint: increasing falls and worsening headache and neck pain

History of present illness: This is a 61-year-old female patient with a history of anxiety, depression, fibromyalgia, scoliosis, seizures, and a known cervical medullary lesion consistent with meningioma. The patient had been suffering from worsening myelopathic symptoms and recurrent falls for the past several months. She also complains of decreased dexterity in her hands, neck pain, and worsening headaches (Fig. 57.1).

Medications: Prozac, indomethacin

Allergies: no known drug allergies

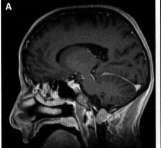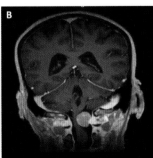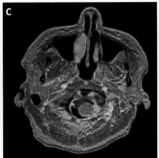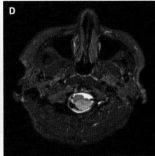

Fig. 57.1 Preoperative magnetic resonance images of the brain and cranio-cervical junction. (A) Sagittal, **(B)** coronal, and **(C)** axial T1 with contrast views demonstrating a hyperintense rounded lesion located on the left aspect of the foramen magnum, with an apparent dural tail. The lesion compresses the cervico-medullary junction with a shift to the right. **(D)** Axial T2 image demonstrating a hyperintense lesion with significant compression and displacement of the cervico-medullary junction.

Past medical and surgical history: anxiety, depression, fibromyalgia, scoliosis, seizures

Family history: noncontributory

Social history: current smoker

Physical examination: awake, alert, and oriented to person, place, and time; cranial nerves II–XII intact; bilateral deltoids/ triceps/biceps 5/5; right interossei 5/5 left interossei 4+/5; iliopsoas/knee flexion/knee extension/dorsi, and plantar flexion 5/5

Reflexes: 3+ in bilateral biceps/triceps/brachioradialis with negative Hoffman; 3+ in bilateral patella/ankle; no clonus or Babinski; sensation intact to light touch

	Andres Almendral, MD Neurosurgery Clinica Hospital San Fernando Panama City, Panama	Mohamad Bydon, MD Neurosurgery Mayo Clinic Rochester, Minnesota, United States	Daniel J. Hoh, MD Neurosurgery University of Florida Gainesville, Florida, United States	Jorge Navarro Bonnet, MD Neurosurgery Medica Sur, Mexico City, Mexico
Preoperative				
Additional tests requested	CTA or MRA CT chest Neurology evaluation	CTA	CTA	CTA
Surgical approach selected	Midline suboccipital craniectomy and C1 laminectomy for resection of tumor	Right far lateral craniotomy and C1 laminectomy for resection of tumor	Occipital, C1, C2 laminectomy for resection of tumor	Left suboccipital, C1 laminectomy with tubular retractor for resection of tumor
Goal of surgery	Gross total resection	Maximal safe tumor resection	Diagnosis, gross total resection	Diagnosis, gross total resection, spinal cord decompression
Perioperative				
Positioning	Prone, with pins	Right lateral park bench, with pins	Prone, with pins	Prone, with pins
Surgical equipment	IOM (MEP/SSEP)	TEE Central linel OM (cranial nerve EMG) Surgical microscope Ultrasonic aspirator Lumbar drain	IOM (MEP/SSEP) Surgical microscope	Tubular retractor system Fluoroscopy surgical microscope
Medications	Maintain MAP	None	Steroids, Ketorolac for 48 hours after surgery	None
Anatomical considerations	Vertebral artery, PICA, lower cranial nerves	Left vertebral artery, spinal arteries, spinal cord, brainstem	Vertebral artery (intradural portion), lower cranial nerves, upper cervical rootlets	Craniocervical junction, left vertebral artery, left C1 nerve root, arachnoid plane
Complications feared with approach chosen	Lower cranial nerve injury, stroke, bleeding	Spinal cord or brainstem injury, arterial injury, CSF leak	CSF leak, spinal instability, vertebral artery injury, cranial nerve or nerve root injury	Vertebral artery injury, C1 nerve root injury
Intraoperative				
Anesthesia	General	General	General	General
Exposure	Occiput-C1	Left occiput to C2	Occiput to C2	Occiput to C1
Levels decompressed	Occiput-C1	Left C1 hemilaminectomy	Occipital bone, C1–2	Occiput to C1
Levels fused	None	None	None	None
Surgical narrative	Preposition IOM, position prone, postposition IOM to confirm stability, neck flexed slightly, midline skin incision made from above the inion to C2 spinous process, suboccipital craniectomy 3–4 cm from foramen magnum making sure enough bone is removed to completely decompress posterior	Left retrosigmoid far lateral hockey stick incision down to C2, subperiosteal dissection, left C1 hemilaminectomy, expose but not skeletonize left vertebral artery, wide left retrosigmoid craniotomy to expose transverse and sigmoid sinuses, circumlinear dural	Position prone with Mayfield pins, vertical midline incision from occiput to C2, limited occipital craniectomy over foramen magnum and C1–2 laminectomy, midline vertical dural opening, microscope-assisted lysis of arachnoid, drainage of CSF for relaxation, identify	Position prone with Mayfield pins, 3 cm vertical linear incision 2 cm lateral to midline under fluoroscopic guidance, dissection of subcutaneous tissue, fascia is opened, placement of tubular system dilators to expose the outer table of the occipital bone and

	Andres Almendral, MD Neurosurgery Clinica Hospital San Fernando Panama City, Panama	Mohamad Bydon, MD Neurosurgery Mayo Clinic Rochester, Minnesota, United States	Daniel J. Hoh, MD Neurosurgery University of Florida Gainesville, Florida, United States	Jorge Navarro Bonnet, MD Neurosurgery Medica Sur, Mexico City, Mexico
	surface of cerebellar tonsils and 2.5–3.0 cm from side to side, remove posterior arch of C1 after separating muscles attached to it, maintain muscle attachments to C2, midline durotomy at C1 and carried superiorly to create a Y-shaped dural opening above foramen magnum, dura retracted, incise arachnoid and dissect PICA from tumor, separate vertebral artery and lower cranial nerves from tumor, resect tumor and internal debulking if needed with low gently bipolar cautery, watertight dural closure, perform Valsalva to confirm no CSF leak seen, layered closure	opening over tumor, expose tumor using cotton balls, debulk tumor with ultrasonic aspirator, identify cranial nerves with stimulation, watertight dural closure, replace craniotomy flap, anatomical closure	tumor, bipolar lateral dural attachment, internally debulk tumor, roll tumor capsule away from cord from medial to lateral, peel tumor inferiorly away from intradural vertebral artery and lower cranial nerves, resect tumor capsule, inspect ventrolateral dura and curette any residual, bipolar residual dural, close dura in water tight fashion with fibrin glue, close in layers, horizontal mattress sutures on skin	posterolateral arch of the atlas, small suboccipital craniectomy and lateral portion of the posterior arch of the atlas with 4 mm diamond drill, dura coagulated, resect any evident lesion infiltration, sample tissue and intratumor debulking, dissect lesion from surrounding structures with special care of left vertebral artery and C1 spinal nerve, closure with dural graft, layered closure
Complication avoidance	Preposition IOM, maintain muscle attachments to C2, early dissection of PICA from the tumor, debulk tumor with low gentle bipolar cautery, perform Valsalva to confirm no CSF leak seen	Identify vertebral artery, wide suboccipital craniectomy, cranial nerve identification	Midline approach, relax CSF, early coagulation of dural attachment, internal tumor debulking, peel tumor away from artery and nerves last, fibrin glue	Minimally invasive approach, tubular retractor system, intratumor debulking
Postoperative				
Admission	ICU	ICU	Floor	Floor
Postoperative complications feared	Lower cranial nerve injury, stroke, bleeding	CSF leak, neurological deficit	CSF leak, nerve root palsy, pain, urinary retention, paralytic ileus	Vertebral artery injury, C1 nerve root injury
Anticipated length of stay	4–5 days	4–6 days	2–4 days	2 days
Follow-up testing	CT within 24 hours of surgery MRI 1 month after surgery	Swallow evaluation, pulmonary function test, EMG, MRI 3 months after surgery	MRI within 3 months and annually for at least 5 years after surgery	MRI within 48 hours of surgery
Bracing	None	None	None	None
Follow-up visits	1 week, 1 month after surgery	3 months after surgery	3 weeks, 6 weeks and 3 months after surgery	2 weeks after surgery

CSF, Cerebrospinal fluid; *CT*, computed tomography; *EMG*, electromyography; *ESI*, epidural spinal injections; *ICU*, intensive care unit; *IOM*, intraoperative monitoring; *MAP*, mean arterial pressure; *MIS*, minimally invasive surgery; *MRA*, magnetic resonance angiography; *MRI*, magnetic resonance imaging; *PICA*, posterior inferior cerebellar artery; *SSEP*, somatosensory evoked potential; *TEE*, transesophageal echogram.

Differential diagnosis

- Dermoid tumor
- Lipoma
- Teratoma
- Hemangioblastoma
- Cavernoma
- Metastatic disease
- Meningioma

Important anatomical and preoperative considerations

Anatomical limits of the foramen magnum are required for tumor classification. Three borders define its area, with an anterior border formed by the basal portion of the clivus and the upper edge of C2, the posterior border by the squamosal part of the occipital bone and C2 spinous process and lateral border by the jugular tubercles and the upper aspect of C2 laminae. The occipital condyles connect the squamosal and clival parts and then articulate with the atlas, where the hypoglossal canal is located above the condyles.[3, 6] The average anteroposterior length of the foramen magnum is 34.5 mm and the transverse diameter is 29 mm.[6] The vertebral artery (VA) is the most important vascular structure related to the foramen magnum. The extradural course of the VA is divided into three parts, the third segment (V3 or suboccipital segment) runs from the C2 transverse process to the foramen magnum dura mater behind the occipital condyles and is in close relationship to the foramen magnum.[3] Three different portions of V3 can be identified, a vertical portion running on the transverse processes of atlas and axis, a horizontal portion on the posterior arch of the atlas, and a curved portion that leaves this structure in the depth of the suboccipital triangle up to the dura mater.[3] The VA pierces the dural ring just inferior to the lateral edge of the foramen magnum,[7] where on imaging evaluation this portion of the vessel can appear smaller in caliber due to a periosteal sheath surrounding it.[3] Once intradural, the artery can be divided into lateral and anterior medullary segments.[7] The lateral medullary segment starts at the dural piercing and extends to the preolivary sulcus. The anterior segment rests on the clivus and includes the area between the preolivary sulcus and the junction close to the pontomedullary sulcus. The hypoglossal rootlets have intimate relationships with this area.[7] The posterior spinal, anterior spinal, posterior inferior cerebellar artery, and the anterior and posterior meningeal arteries are branches originated during this trajectory.[7] PICA is the largest branch, and, although rare, may originate from the extradural segment. Several critical neural structures are localized within the limits of the foramen magnum and include the caudal medulla oblongata, cerebellar vermis and tonsils, fourth ventricle, upper spinal cord, and lower cranial nerves (9th–12th), which all pose potential surgery-related risks.[1] A thoughtful examination of the lower cranial nerves is mandatory before surgery. Intraoperative monitoring is crucial to preserve function.[8]

Tumors in the foramen magnum can be resected through anterior, lateral, and posterior approaches.[9] Anterior approaches are not frequently used for intradural lesions primarily because of difficulty in dural repair and high risk for cerebrospinal fluid (CSF) leak and infection.[1] Suboccipital craniotomy and transcondylar approach are frequently preferred to treat most of the lesions in this region, where the latter requires drilling of the condyle.[8] Suboccipital craniotomy, or craniectomy, is usually indicated for the resection of posterior meningiomas with or without extradural extension. This approach provides a good visualization of the VA and typically provides adequate proximal vascular control. In addition, this technique offers rapid identification of the brainstem and cranial nerves.[8] The transcondylar approach, or posterolateral, addresses lesions located more laterally and anteriorly. Two variations are usually described: the far lateral approach in which excision of the foramen magnum rim close to the condyle and removal of the ipsilateral atlantal arch are required, and the transcondylar approach with partial or total excision of the occipital condyle.[3, 8–10] The far lateral approach is a variation of the suboccipital approach and has been associated to a higher neurological morbidity in comparison to the suboccipital median approach.[2]

What was actually done

The patient was consented for a left suboccipital craniectomy and C1 laminectomy and resection of the tumor. The patient was brought to the operating room, induced under general anesthesia, and then placed in the prone position in pinions. Neuromonitoring in the form of somatosensory and motor evoked potentials and cranial nerve monitoring was performed. Navigation system was used to trace the transverse sinus as well as the location of the lesion below the foramen magnum. A midline incision was made from above the inion to the spinous process of C2. A subperiosteal exposure was performed and the arch of C1 was identified. The foramen magnum, as well as the suboccipital bone, was exposed. The exposure was carried laterally on the left side to the sulcus arteriosus. The posterior arch of C1 was removed, the top of C2 was undercut, and a suboccipital craniectomy was performed. The dura was opened in the midline and curved to the left side over the cerebellar hemisphere. The dural was tacked laterally, and the V4 segment of the VA was identified. The microscope was brought in. The tumor margins were visualized, and the area was stimulated to identify and confirm the presence of cranial nerve 11. The tumor was then dissected from the underlying cervico-medullary junction, and internal debulking was achieved. The VA was protected and the tumor removed with assistance from an ultrasonic aspirator. The tumor capsule was dissected away from the surrounding neurovascular structures, and the dural attachment was bipolared. The dura was primarily closed, and the wound closed in anatomical layers. Postoperatively, the patient was extubated and had mild dysphagia that improved over the course of several days. Pathology was consistent with meningioma. At follow-up the patient reported pain reduction and minimal complaints. Postoperative imaging showed gross total resection of the lesion (Fig. 57.2).

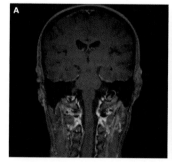
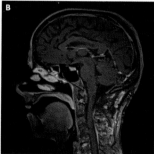

Fig. 57.2 Postoperative T1 with contrast magnetic resonance images of the brain and cranio-cervical junction. (A) Sagittal and **(B)** coronal images demonstrating gross total resection of the previously described extraaxial lesion at the cervico-medullary junction.

Commonalities among the experts

All of the surgeons selected a computed tomography angiography to better assess the vascular structures involved. The majority conducted a suboccipital craniectomy and C1 laminectomy, with certain variations. Most aimed for a gross total resection. All were aware of the VAs, lower cranial nerves, and upper cervical rootlets. The most feared complications were VA injury, nerve injury, and CSF leak. Surgery was performed with intraoperative monitoring and surgical microscope in most cases. No specific preoperative medical therapy was recommended. Surgical strategies varied but all shared the concept of decompression spanning from the occiput to at least C1 level and the importance of an early identification and dissection of crucial vascular structures. Following intervention, half admitted their patients to the intensive care unit, and half continued observation in the floor. Immediate postoperative follow-up testing significantly varied; however, most of the surgeons opted for a magnetic resonance imaging after discharge to evaluate extent of resection.

SUMMARY OF QUALITY OF EVIDENCE TO GUIDE SPECIFIC INTERVENTIONS FOR THIS CASE

- Gross total resection for meningiomas affecting the foramen magnum: level III

REFERENCES

1. Hajhouji F, Lmejjati M, Aniba K, Laghmari M, Ghannane H, Benali SA. Foramen magnum meningioma's management: the experience of the department of neurosurgery in Marrakesh. *Pan Afr Med J*. 2017;26:42.
2. Bilgin E, Çavus G, Açik V, et al. Our surgical experience in foramen magnum meningiomas: clinical series of 11 cases. *Pan Afr Med J*. 2019;34:5.
3. Bruneau M, George B. Foramen magnum meningiomas: detailed surgical approaches and technical aspects at Lariboisière Hospital and review of the literature. *Neurosurg Rev*. 2008;31(1):19–32; discussion 32-13.
4. Srinivas D, Sarma P, Deora H, et al. "Tailored" far lateral approach to anterior foramen magnum meningiomas - The importance of condylar preservation. *Neurol India*. 2019;67(1):142–148.
5. Wu Z, Hao S, Zhang J, et al. Foramen magnum meningiomas: experiences in 114 patients at a single institute over 15 years. *Surg Neurol*. 2009;72(4):376–382. discussion 382.
6. Avci E, Dagtekin A, Ozturk AH, et al. Anatomical variations of the foramen magnum, occipital condyle and jugular tubercle. *Turk Neurosurg*. 2011;21(2):181–190.
7. de Oliveira E, Rhoton AL, Jr.,Peace D. Microsurgical anatomy of the region of the foramen magnum. *Surg Neurol*. 1985; 24(3):293–352.
8. Boulton MR, Cusimano MD. Foramen magnum meningiomas: concepts, classifications, and nuances. *Neurosurg Focus*. 2003; 14(6):e10.
9. Flores BC, Boudreaux BP, Klinger DR, Mickey BE, Barnett SL. The far-lateral approach for foramen magnum meningiomas. *Neurosurg Focus*. 2013;35(6):E12.
10. Bernard F, Lemee JM, Delion M, Fournier HD. Lower third clivus and foramen magnum intradural tumor removal: The plea for a simple posterolateral approach. *Neurochirurgie*. 2016;62(2):86–93.

58

Thoracic intradural extramedullary lesion

Fidel Valero-Moreno, MD and Henry Ruiz-Garcia, MD

Introduction

Intradural extramedullary thoracic spinal cord tumors are rare entities that cause thoracic myelopathy and occasionally radiculopathy.[1] These tumors occur in 5 to 10 per 100,000 persons.[2] The two most common intradural extramedullary pathological diagnoses are schwannomas and meningiomas.[2,3] Schwannomas are usually solitary lesions and multiple schwannomas occur in patients with neurofibromatosis type 2. Ninety percent of spinal meningiomas are located in the thoracic spine and 95% of the cases are World Health Organization (WHO) grade I.[4] Less common tumors include neurofibroma and hemangiopericytoma. While schwannomas typically arise from a thoracic sensory rootlet, meningiomas have a dural attachment and are often located ventral to the spinal cord.[3,5] The surgical removal of these lesions often requires working in a tight corridor, as the diameter of the spinal canal in the thoracic levels is the smaller compared with the lumbar and cervical levels.[6] Complete removal of a ventrolateral or ventral lesion may require removal of the rib head or pedicle for adequate exposure without cord manipulation.[7] On the other hand, most of the spinal schwannomas and meningiomas are noninfiltrative and often can be completely resected.[8] In the present chapter, we describe a case of a patient with a benign tumor involving the intradural extramedullary compartment of the thoracic spine.

Example case

Chief complaint: difficulty walking

History of present illness: This 44-year-old male with a history of back pain and buttock pain. This has been going on for approximately 8 months. Patient also developed gait difficulties, as well as numbness in his bilateral lower extremities. He reports some urinary urgency but denies any incontinence. This has progressively worsened over the last few months. He underwent imaging and this revealed a thoracic intradural extramedullary lesion (Fig. 58.1).

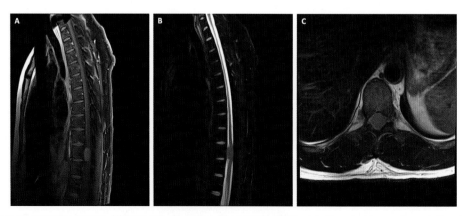

Fig. 58.1 Preoperative magnetic resonance images. (A) Sagittal T1 with contrast, **(B)** sagittal T2, **(C)** T1 axial with contrast images demonstrating a homogeneously enhancing extraaxial mass filling the spinal canal at the level of T10 measuring 1.5 × 1.8 × 2.2 cm, causing severe mass effect on the spinal cord, displacing/flattening it posteriorly and to the right. Associated T2 hyperintensity within the cord is consistent with compressive myelopathy.

Medications: fluoxetine, indomethacin
Allergies: no known drug allergies
Past medical and surgical history: none
Family history: none
Social history: none
Physical examination: awake, alert, and oriented to person, place, and time; cranial nerves II–XII intact; bilateral deltoids/triceps/biceps 5/5; interossei 5/5; iliopsoas/knee flexion/

knee extension/dorsi, and plantar flexion 5/5
Reflexes: 2+ in bilateral biceps/triceps/brachioradialis with negative Hoffman; 3+ in bilateral patella/ankle; 2 beats of clonus; diminished sensation intact to light touch in bilateral lower extremities

	Eyal Itshayek, MD Neurosurgery Hadassah Medical Center Jerusalem, Israel	Alugolu Rajesh, MD Neurosurgery Nizam's Institute of Medical Sciences Punjagutta, Hyderabad, India	Justin S. Smith, MD, PhD Neurosurgery University of Virginia Charlottesville, Virginia, United States	Anand Veeravagu, MD Neurosurgery Stanford University Palo Alto, California, United States
Preoperative				
Additional tests requested	CT T-spine Anesthesia evaluation	MRI brain and complete spine MRI spine tractography Anesthesiology evaluation	MRI brain and complete spine CT T-spine Long cassette x-ray for rib counting for intraoperative localization	CT chest/abdomen/pelvis CT T-spine
Surgical approach selected	T10 right hemilaminectomy, T10 right pediculectomy, excision of intradural extramedullary tumor and T9-T11 fusion	T9-11 laminectomy and resection of the lesion	T9-11 instrumented arthrodesis with T9-11 laminectomy, T10 pedicle and rib head resection	T9-11 laminectomy for resection of intradural mass with possible transpedicular or costotransversectomy
Goal of surgery	Gross total resection, preservation of neurological function	Resection of lesion, decompression of spinal cord	Resection of lesion, diagnosis, decompression of spinal cord	Resect mass, decompress spinal cord, stabilize thoracic spine
Perioperative				
Positioning	Prone on Jackson table	Prone	Prone on Jackson table	Prone on Jackson table, no pins
Surgical equipment	IOM Fluoroscopy Surgical microscope Ultrasonic aspirator	IOM (MEP) Fluoroscopy Ultrasonic bone scalpel Surgical microscope Ultrasonic aspirator	IOM (MEP/SSEP) Fluoroscopy Surgical microscope Micro instruments Dural sealant	IOM (SSEP/MEP) Fluoroscopy Surgical microscope Surgical navigation Ultrasound Ultrasonic aspirator
Medications	MAP >80	Steroids	None	Steroids
Anatomical considerations	Lamina, transverse process, pedicle	Spinal cord, nerve roots, dentate ligament	Spinal cord, confirmation of spinal level	Appropriate level, central canal, spinal cord
Complications feared with approach chosen	Spinal cord injury	Spinal cord injury	Neurological deficit	Spinal cord injury
Intraoperative				
Anesthesia	General	General	General	General
Exposure	T9-11	T9-11	T9-11	T9-11
Levels decompressed	T10	T9-11	T9-11	T9-11
Levels fused	T9-11	None	T9-11	None

(continued on next page)

	Eyal Itshayek, MD Neurosurgery Hadassah Medical Center Jerusalem, Israel	Alugolu Rajesh, MD Neurosurgery Nizam's Institute of Medical Sciences Punjagutta, Hyderabad, India	Justin S. Smith, MD, PhD Neurosurgery University of Virginia Charlottesville, Virginia, United States	Anand Veeravagu, MD Neurosurgery Stanford University Palo Alto, California, United States
Surgical narrative	Preflip IOM baseline, position prone onto Jackson table, localize surgical level with fluoroscopy in AP position counting ribs, midline skin incision, subperiosteal dissection exposing bilateral spinous processes/laminas/transverse processes, place left T9-T11 and right T9 and T11 pedicle screws with titanium rod on left, right T11 hemilaminectomy and the ascending and descending facets, complete hemilaminectomy with Kerrison, right T9-10 and T10-11 facetectomy, remove T10 pedicle to level of vertebral body, identify T9-10 nerve roots, open dura with paramidline incision under microscopic visualization right T11 nerve root, retract dura with Prolene, identify tumor, cut dentate ligament and nerve root if needed, sharply dissect arachnoid defining plane surrounding tumor, identify planes, coagulate tumor capsule, open capsule and internally decompress with ultrasonic aspirator, dissect tumor capsule from arachnoid plane from spinal cord, coagulate insertion area on dura and resect any remnants from dura, watertight dural closure with TachoSil patch, connect right T9-T11 pedicle screws with titanium rod, layered closure, lumbar drain if dura unable to be closed	Position prone, skin incision planning using x-ray, midline skin incision one level above and one level lower than incision, subperiosteal dissection of paraspinal muscles until facet joints, laminectomy one level above and below lesion and more on right side, dural opening starting at cranial aspect, dura tacked up, lesion identified and arachnoid peeled over the while length until capsule is removed under microscope, intratumoral decompression using ultrasonic aspirator after biopsy, remaining capsule dissected off and making to spare adherent nerve roots after adequate decompression, small rootlet entering tumor is sacrificed, watertight dural closure, layered closure with drain	Position prone on Jackson table, fluoroscopy to mark incision from T9 to 11, expose T9-11 and confirmation of levels with fluoroscopy once exposed, place T9-11 pedicle screws excluding right T10, T9-11 laminectomies, removal of right T10 pedicle and rib head, open dura under microscopic visualization off to right side, tack up dural edges, use micro instruments to dissect and remove tumor, likely release dentate ligaments to facilitate tumor removal, goal is gross total removal, close dura, dural sealant, places rods spanning T9-11 along with graft for arthrodesis, two subfascial drains layered wound closure	Obtain prepositioning IOM, position prone, AP fluoro for localizing level, expose and two-level laminectomy centered on the mass, intraoperative ultrasound to ensure dural exposure is sufficient, dural opening on side of tumor origin under microscope, tumor biopsy and intraoperative pathology, resect tumor with ultrasonic aspirator, dissect tumor off surface of spinal cord to resect completely, resect dural attachment and bipolar depending on location, close with Gore-tex suture and fibrin flue
Complication avoidance	Preflip IOM baseline, localize surgical level with fluoroscopy in AP position counting ribs, cut dentate ligament and nerve root if needed, internally debulk tumor, lumbar drain if dura unable to be closed	More laminectomy on right side, peel arachnoid over entire length of lesion, internal debulking of tumor before removing off nerve roots	Removing pedicle and rib head to allow more lateral access and less spinal cord manipulation, paramedian dural opening eccentric to side of tumor, release dentate ligaments to decrease cord manipulation, dural sealant with closure	Prepositioning IOM, AP fluoroscopy for localization, intraoperative ultrasound to assess exposure, transpedicular or costotranversectomy if needed for exposing, Gore-tex suture

	Eyal Itshayek, MD Neurosurgery Hadassah Medical Center Jerusalem, Israel	Alugolu Rajesh, MD Neurosurgery Nizam's Institute of Medical Sciences Punjagutta, Hyderabad, India	Justin S. Smith, MD, PhD Neurosurgery University of Virginia Charlottesville, Virginia, United States	Anand Veeravagu, MD Neurosurgery Stanford University Palo Alto, California, United States
Postoperative				
Admission	ICU	Floor	ICU	Floor
Postoperative complications feared	Spinal cord injury, CSF leak	Neurological deficit, CSF leak	Hematoma, CSF leak	Worsening thoracic myelopathy, CSF leak
Anticipated length of stay	3 days	1–2 days	4 days	4 days
Follow-up testing	MRI T-spine 3 months after surgery	None if gross total resection achieved	MRI T-spine 6 weeks, 1 year, 3 years after surgery Spine x-rays 6 weeks, 6 months, 1 year, 2 years after surgery	MRI T-spine 1 month, 6 months, 12 months, and annually after surgery
Bracing	None	None	None	None
Follow-up visits	6 weeks, 3 months after surgery	4 weeks after surgery	10–14 days, 6 weeks, 1 year, 2 years after surgery	2 weeks, 1 month, 3 months, 6 months after surgery

AP, Anteroposterior; *APP*, advanced practice provider; *BAERs*, brainstem auditory evoked responses; *CSF*, cerebrospinal fluid; *CT*, computed tomography; *DEXA*, dual-energy x-ray absorptiometry; *IOM*, intraoperative monitoring; *MAP*, mean arterial pressure; *MEP*, motor evoked potentials; *MRI*, magnetic resonance imaging; *PLL*, posterior longitudinal ligament; *PSIS*, posterior superior iliac spine; *SSEP*, somatosensory evoked potential.

Differential diagnosis

- Meningioma
- Schwannoma
- Other spinal cord tumor

Important anatomical and preoperative considerations

Although the majority of intradural extramedullary tumors are noninvasive lesions and are suitable for total resection, the anatomical features of the dorsal spine constitute a surgical challenge. The thoracic spinal canal is narrower in comparison to the rest of the spine,[6] and its rib attachments could limit the exposure of ventrally located neoplasms.[7] Open surgical resection represents the primary treatment for intradural extramedullary lesions.[9] Most of the intradural extramedullary lesions are treated using a posterior midline approach. Some authors recommend a limited hemilaminectomy and facet preservation in order to avoid kyphosis and maintain structural stability.[6,8] The posterolateral approach is a feasible alternative for the resection of ventrally located tumors or dumbbell tumors with paraspinal invasion and may require a facetectomy for sufficient exposure.[10] Surgical instrumentation may be required in the setting of large tumors involving destruction of the vertebral body (one-third), facet compromise, multilevel laminectomies, or destruction of the posterior tension band.[6] Recurrence is not frequently reported after complete resection of tumors[9]; however, certain conditions such as significant calcification, en plaque lesions, and lesions surrounding nerve roots can make resection challenging.

What was actually done

Due to the progressive myelopathy and compression of the spinal cord, the patient was taken to the operating room. A T9–T11 laminoplasty and resection of the intradural as planned. The patient was placed in prone position on an OSI table (ProAxis® Spinal Surgery Table). Neuromonitoring was performed in the form of somatosensory and motor evoked potential throughout the entire procedure. After x-ray localization of the correct levels, a midline incision was made and the subperiosteal exposure was performed. A laminectomy was achieved after confirmation of the T9–T11 level with intraoperative fluoroscopy, and the dura was opened in the midline after confirming tumor location by intraoperative ultrasound. The microscope was brought into the surgical field and the lesion was approached laterally. After initial microdissection, an ultrasonic aspirator was used to debulk the tumor until it was possible to lateralize the tumor to proceed with a piecemeal dissection, roll the capsule onto itself, and completely remove the lesion from the operative field. Vancomycin powder was placed within the wound after the dura was closed in a watertight fashion. The wound was closed in anatomical layers. The patient tolerated the procedure well without any immediate postoperative complication and was taken to the intensive care unit for recovery. He was discharged to rehabilitation on postoperative day 4. He returned to neurological baseline 1 year after follow-up. Postoperative imaging showed gross total resection of the lesion (Fig. 58.2).

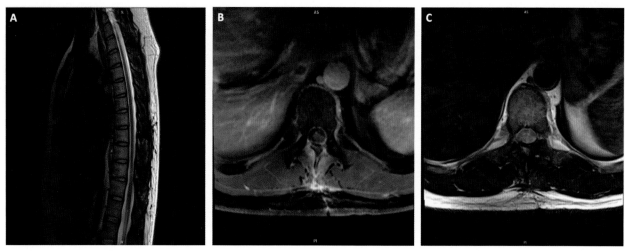

Fig. 58.2 Postoperative magnetic resonance image. (A) T2 sagittal demonstrating complete resection of the lesion with mild myelomalacia in the thoracic spinal cord at T10 level is noted. **(B)** Axial T1 postgadolinium and **(C)** T2 image of the T10 level demonstrating optimal decompression of the spinal cord.

Commonalities among the experts

Most opted for computed tomography scan of the thoracic spine, and half recommended brain and complete spine MRI as part of their preoperative evaluation. Most approached the lesion through T9-T11 laminectomy, and half would combine this approach would instrumented fusion. The main goal of surgical intervention was decompression of the spinal cord. Most were mindful of the spinal cord anatomy. Neurological deficit due to damage to the spinal cord was the most feared complication associated with the selected approach. Surgery was facilitated by the use of intraoperative monitoring, microscope, fluoroscopy, and ultrasonic aspirator, and half advocated for perioperative steroids. Surgical schemes varied, but all shared the notion of minimizing spinal cord manipulation to preserve critical function. After surgery, half admitted their patients to the intensive care unit. Most recommended postoperative magnetic resonance imaging for the evaluation of removal extent. Timing for imaging follow-up significantly varied among physicians.

SUMMARY OF QUALITY OF EVIDENCE TO GUIDE SPECIFIC INTERVENTIONS FOR THIS CASE

- Maximal safe resection to decompress neural structures and preserve function: level III

REFERENCES

1. Yang I, Paik E, Huh NG, Parsa AT, Ames CP. Giant thoracic schwannoma presenting with abrupt onset of abdominal pain: a case report. *J Med Case Rep.* 2009;3:88.
2. Wong AP, Lall RR, Dahdaleh NS, et al. Comparison of open and minimally invasive surgery for intradural-extramedullary spine tumors. *Neurosurg Focus.* 2015;39(2):E11.
3. Liu WC, Choi G, Lee SH, et al. Radiological findings of spinal schwannomas and meningiomas: focus on discrimination of two disease entities. *Eur Radiol.* 2009;19(11):2707–2715.
4. Merhemic Z, Stosic-Opincal T, Thurnher MM. Neuroimaging of Spinal Tumors. *Magn Reson Imaging Clin N Am.* 2016;24(3):563–579.
5. Sridhar K, Ramamurthi R, Vasudevan MC, Ramamurthi B. Giant invasive spinal schwannomas: definition and surgical management. *J Neurosurg.* 2001;94(2 Suppl):210–215.
6. Valle-Giler EP, Garces J, Smith RD, Sulaiman WA. One-stage resection of giant invasive thoracic schwannoma: case report and review of literature. *Ochsner J.* 2014;14(1):135–140.
7. Lee MT, Panbehchi S, Sinha P, Rao J, Chiverton N, Ivanov M. Giant spinal nerve sheath tumours - Surgical challenges: case series and literature review. *Br J Neurosurg.* 2019;33(5):541–549.
8. Tumialán LM, Theodore N, Narayanan M, Marciano FF, Nakaji P. Anatomic Basis for Minimally Invasive Resection of Intradural Extramedullary Lesions in Thoracic Spine. *World Neurosurg.* 2018;109:e770–e777.
9. Gerszten PC, Quader M, Novotny J, Jr. Flickinger JC. Radiosurgery for benign tumors of the spine: clinical experience and current trends. *Technol Cancer Res Treat.* 2012;11(2):133–139.
10. Steck JC, Dietze DD, Fessler RG. Posterolateral approach to intradural extramedullary thoracic tumors. *J Neurosurg.* 1994;81(2):202–205.

59

Cervical chordoma

Fidel Valero-Moreno, MD and Henry Ruiz-Garcia, MD

Introduction

Chordomas are uncommon malignant neoplasms of the bone that can arise anywhere along the central nervous system.[1–3] These tumors originate from persisting remnants of the notochord,[2,3] and their behavior is aggressive due to their invasiveness and high recurrence rates.[4] Distant metastases are not unusual, and sacral and vertebral chordomas are more prone to metastasize.[2,5,6] Chordomas most often metastasize to the lung, followed by the lymph nodes and bone.[2] This entity represents 1% to 4% of all primary malignant bone tumors.[1,3,4] They show predilection for the sacrococcygeal region (49% of the cases), followed by the clival area (36%) and the mobile spine (15%).[4] Interestingly, chordomas in the cervical spine account for only 6% of the cases.[7] Vertebral chordomas occur in the following order of frequency: lumbar, cervical, and thoracic regions.[6] Cervical chordomas affect males and females evenly and appear one decade earlier than other locations.[2] Patients typically present with cervical pain, progressive dysphagia or dysphonia, and the tumor is locally advanced by the time of diagnosis.[7,8] Posterior growth can lead to radicular symptoms or even myelopathy.[8] Complete surgical resection with or without radiation therapy remains the mainstay of treatment.[1–4,7,9] However, local recurrence affects more than 50% of patients after total resection with or without radiation.[10] In this chapter, we present a case of a patient with right upper extremity weakness due to recurrent C2 chordoma.

Example case

Chief complaint: progressive right upper extremity weakness

History of present illness: This is a 70-year-old male with a history of C2 chordoma status post resection in 2011 followed by occipital to T2 fusion and radiation therapy, reflux disease, glaucoma, and hypertension, who presents with progressive right upper extremity weakness. In 2011, he presented with swallowing dysfunction and was found to have a large C2 chordoma and underwent transoral C2 corpectomy and partial resection with C2 laminectomy and C1-C4 fusion. He later developed instability and underwent occipital to T2 fusion. He underwent postoperative fractionated radiation therapy and imatinib chemotherapy. He presented with 6 months of right upper extremity intrinsic hand weakness. The patient underwent a magnetic resonance imaging of the cervical spine that demonstrated the presence of a large lobulated recurrent tumor at the level of the upper cervical segment (Fig. 59.1).

Medications: atenolol, amlodipine, ranitidine, latanoprost

Allergies: no known drug allergies

Past medical and surgical history: C2 corpectomy and C1–4 fusion in 2011, occipital to T2 fusion in 2012

Family history: noncontributory

Social history: retired, no smoking, no alcohol

Physical examination: awake, alert, and oriented to person, place, and time; cranial nerves II–XII intact; bilateral deltoids/triceps/biceps 5/5; right interossei 4/5, left interossei 5/5; iliopsoas/knee flexion/knee extension/dorsi, and plantar flexion 5/5

Reflexes: 3+ in bilateral biceps/triceps/brachioradialis with positive Hoffman; 3+ in bilateral patella/ankle; three beats of ankle clonus and positive Babinski; sensation intact to light touch

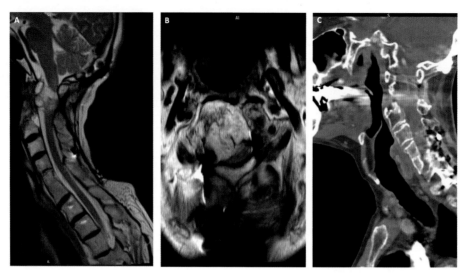

Fig. 59.1 Preoperative cervical spine images. (A) Sagittal T2 and **(B)** axial T1 with contrast magnetic resonance images demonstrating a large lobulated recurrent tumor involving the C2 corpectomy bed and affects the residual nonresected left lateral mass and odontoid process, the medial portion of the right C1 arch, and the right occipital condyle. There is also a large lobulated extension into the cervical medullary junction on the right, and the left ventral lateral epidural space. Severe compression of the cervicomedullary junction is evident. **(C)** Sagittal computed tomography scan demonstrating postsurgical changes after craniospinal fusion. Residual chordoma centered at the cranio-cervical junction with surrounding osseous involvement is seen.

	Ziya L. Gokaslan, MD Tianyi Niu. MD Neurosurgery Brown University Providence, Rhode Island, United States	Tong Meng, MD Orthopaedic Surgery Shanghai General Hospital Shanghai Jiao Tong University Shanghai, China	Jorge Navarro Bonnet, MD Neurosurgery Medica Sur, Mexico City, Mexico	Meic H. Schmidt, MD, MBA Neurosurgery University of New Mexico Albuquerque, New Mexico, United States
Preoperative				
Additional tests requested	Cerebral angiogram with right vertebral occlusion evaluation Sacrifice right vertebral artery if able to tolerate	C-spine x-ray CT angiography Cerebral angiogram with right vertebral occlusion evaluation	C-spine flexion-extension x-rays Electrophysiological evaluation (SSEP, NCS, EMG)	Swallow study Vocal cord function Chest/abdomen/pelvis CT Cerebral angiogram with possible left vertebral artery embolization
Surgical approach selected	C1-3 laminectomy and tumor debulking with occipital-C3 fusion	Stage 1: C1-3 posterior decompression Stage 2: anterolateral retropharyngeal transcervical resection and C1-3 cage	Anterior C1-5 tumor debulking and decompression	Left far lateral transcondylar resection of C2
Goal of surgery	Palliative neurological function preservation	Palliative spinal cord decompression	Safe maximal resection, spinal cord decompression	Palliative spinal cord decompression
Perioperative				
Positioning	Prone on Jackson table, with pins	Stage 1: prone Stage 2: supine with head rotated to left 30 degrees	Supine, with Mayfield pins	Lateral, with Mayfield pins
Surgical equipment	IOM (MEP/SSEP) Surgical navigation Surgical microscope Ultrasonic aspirator Dural sealant Ultrasound	Ultrasonic bone scalpel	IOM Fluoroscopy Ultrasonic aspirator O-arm	IOM Surgical microscope
Medications	Steroids, maintain MAP >85	Steroids	Steroids	Steroids

	Ziya L. Gokaslan, MD Tianyi Niu. MD Neurosurgery Brown University Providence, Rhode Island, United States	Tong Meng, MD Orthopaedic Surgery Shanghai General Hospital Shanghai Jiao Tong University Shanghai, China	Jorge Navarro Bonnet, MD Neurosurgery Medica Sur, Mexico City, Mexico	Meic H. Schmidt, MD, MBA Neurosurgery University of New Mexico Albuquerque, New Mexico, United States
Anatomical considerations	Right vertebral artery, spinal cord	Anterior C1 arch, right vertebral artery	Right vertebral artery, lower cranial nerves, anterolateral spinal cord	C1 tubercle, C2 nerve roots
Complications feared with approach chosen	Spinal cord injury, vertebral artery injury, CSF leak	Injury to right vertebral artery/carotid artery/laryngeal vessels and nerve/submandibular duct/hypoglossal nerve	Injury to right vertebral artery, lower cranial nerve injury, spinal cord injury, bleeding	Spinal cord injury, CSF leak
Intraoperative				
Anesthesia	General	General	General	General
Exposure	Occiput-C3	C1-3	C1-5	Skull base, C1, C2
Levels decompressed	C1-3	C1-3	C1-5	C1-2
Levels fused	Occiput-C3	C1-3	None	None
Surgical narrative	Intubated, positioned prone, midline incision with hock stick toward right, dissect down to expose posterior bony elements and previous hardware, free suboccipital muscles from bony element to expose suboccipital bone/C1-3 lateral mass on right, perform suboccipital craniectomy and C1-3 laminectomy, remove previous right-sided rod, remove previous right C1 lateral mass and C2 screws, place navigation reference array, obtain intraoperative images, visualize tumor, tumor debulked until sufficient spinal cord decompression with microscopic visualization, resect C1 and C2 lateral masses if necessary, ensure right vertebral artery sacrificed by placing aneurysm clip, intraoperative ultrasound to ensure adequate decompression, assess residual lateral masses and reinstrument, can use occipital condyle screws as salvage if occipital plate not sufficient	Intubated, positioned prone, posterior midline longitudinal incision, remove posterior arch of C1 and lamina of C3 with ultrasonic bone scalpel, position supine with head rotated 30 degrees to left and slightly extended, anterolateral retropharyngeal transcervical approach, incision made from midline below the chine and toward the body of the mandible to the mastoid, incision curved downward and medially along posterior border of sternocleidomastoid, open platysma, develop fascial plane between pharyngeal and prevertebral musculature, separate carotid sheath laterally from esophagus and trachea medially, identify hypoglossal nerve by locating posterior digastric muscle and stylohyoid, expose external carotid branches and superior laryngeal nerve, palpate anterior arch of C1, open posterior pharyngeal tissue, expose C1-3, remove as much tumor as possible, reconstruct with titanium mesh filled with allograft, confirm hardware location with x-ray, closure in layers	Position supine with mild elevation of head and slight neck extension, fluoroscopy/O-arm to plan incision aiming for C5, displace carotid-jugular vessels laterally and trachea/esophagus medially, internally debulk tumor with coagulation and ultrasonic aspiration, avoid going too lateral to right vertebral artery as well as too deep for lower cranial nerves and spinal cord, support with hemostatic agents if needed, duraplasty with dural graft and sealant if CSF leak encountered, review surgical bed for esophageal injury with water and infuse air through nasogastric tube, layered closure	Intubated with reinforced ET tube, lateral decubitus position with left side up, lazy S-incision, muscles dissected down to C1/C2/base of skull, resect embolized vertebral artery, ligate both C1 and C2 nerve roots, resect tumor as much as possible, no reconstruction

(continued on next page)

	Ziya L. Gokaslan, MD Tianyi Niu. MD Neurosurgery Brown University Providence, Rhode Island, United States	Tong Meng, MD Orthopaedic Surgery Shanghai General Hospital Shanghai Jiao Tong University Shanghai, China	Jorge Navarro Bonnet, MD Neurosurgery Medica Sur, Mexico City, Mexico	Meic H. Schmidt, MD, MBA Neurosurgery University of New Mexico Albuquerque, New Mexico, United States
Complication avoidance	Sacrifice right vertebral artery if possible, surgical navigation, decompress spinal cord, remove hardware for improved access, intraoperative ultrasound to assess decompression, occipital condyle screws as salvage if necessary, new rods placed and secured, closure in layers	Two-staged approach, decompress posteriorly, preserve hypoglossal nerve, palliative debulking	Anterior approach, avoid going too far right to avoid injury to vertebral artery and too deep for lower cranial nerves, duraplasty if CSF leak encountered, evaluate for esophageal injury	Vertebral artery embolization, ligation of C1-2 nerve roots
Postoperative				
Admission	ICU	ICU	ICU	ICU
Postoperative complications feared	CSF leak, spinal cord injury, hardware failure	Neurological deficit, spinal instability	Hematoma, lower cranial neuropathy	Spinal cord injury, CSF leak
Anticipated length of stay	4–5 days	10 days	4–5 days	4–5 days
Follow-up testing	MRI C-spine prior to radiation therapy Standing AP/lateral cervical x-rays prior to discharge	C-spine x-ray 1 day after surgery CT and MRI 3 days after surgery, 3 months, 6 months, 6 month intervals for 2 years, then annually	MRI C-spine within 48 hours of surgery	MRI and CT while inpatient
Bracing	None	Cervicothoracic brace for 3–6 months	None	None
Follow-up visits	2 weeks and 3 months after surgery	3 months, 6 months, 6 month intervals for 2 years, then annually	2 weeks after surgery	2 weeks after surgery
Radiation therapy for STR	Proton beam	Proton beam	Radiosurgery	Proton beam
Radiation therapy for GTR	Proton beam	Proton beam	Observation	Proton beam

AP, Anteroposterior; *CSF*, cerebrospinal fluid; *CT*, computed tomography; *EMG*, electromyography; *GTR*, gross total resection; *ICU*, intensive care unit; *IOM*, intraoperative monitoring; *MAP*, mean arterial pressure; *MEP*, motor evoked potential; *MIS*, minimally invasive surgery; *MRI*, magnetic resonance imaging; *NCS*, nerve conduction study; *SSEP*, somatosensory evoked potential; *STR*, subtotal resection.

Differential diagnosis

- Chordoma
- Chondrosarcoma
- Meningioma
- Myoepithelioma/myoepithelial carcinoma
- Glioma
- Metastatic tumor (mucinous adenocarcinoma and clear cell renal cell carcinoma)

Important anatomical and preoperative considerations

Chordomas found in the cervical spine are rare and entail a challenge for neurosurgeons due to the complexity of this region.[4] Chordomas in this spine segment are in close relationship with vertebral arteries, nerve roots, and the spinal cord.[4, 11] In the mobile spine, chordoma occurs mostly from the vertebral body and extend to the whole vertebra.[12] By the time these lesions are detected, most of the chordomas have extended to the epidural and paravertebral space, encasing nerves and the vascular structures.[4–7, 11] Chordomas have a significant tendency for recurrence, especially after subtotal removal.[4, 7] En bloc resection with wide negative margins is commonly advocated as the first treatment modality for conventional chordoma.[1, 7] Despite this, a piecemeal resection is often used for cervical chordomas given the risk of neurological compromise.[5, 6] The extent of local disease must be established utilizing contrast-enhanced MRI.[10] Tumor extension is the main factor that impedes resection and leads to poorer prognosis.[12] As can be expected, success of a radical resection at time of recurrence is less likely.[12]

Although the appearance of chordoma on MRI is characteristic, a percutaneous biopsy can be done to guide the treatment and the prognosis in certain cases.[7] The ideal management of chordomas in the cervical spine consists of radical excision and stabilization, complemented by adjuvant therapy.[6, 12] Boriani et al. extensively reviewed a large series of chordomas of the mobile spine and found the only treatment strategy associated with disease control longer than 5 years, performed on a tumor not previously approached, is margin-free en bloc resection.[6, 12] Inadequate tumor margin and tumor rupture are the main factors associated with negative prognosis and seeding of the tumor, respectively.[10, 12] This implies that gross total resection is insufficient if the capsule is violated.[12, 13] Moreover, the rate of recurrence after intralesional excision or biopsy, even if combined with conventional radiotherapy, is higher and earlier.[12, 13] Nevertheless, a margin-free resection of a chordoma in the cervical spine requires the tumor to be confined to the vertebral body.[6, 14] When approaching a large tumor that invades the paravertebral soft tissue, it is very challenging to expose the tumor-free margins of the lesion, and therefore these require intralesional resection.[14] Thus a lesion extending beyond the limits of the vertebral column represents a high risk of morbidity for the patient if en bloc resection is attempted.[6] Even when the paravertebral muscles, vertebral artery or the upper cervical nerve roots (C1-C2) are sacrificed, en bloc resection can be limited by the irregular invasion of the tumor,[4, 6, 15] which makes confirmation of negative surgical margins extremely challenging.[6, 7] Special attention should be paid to avoid spillage of the tumor to surrounding tissues.[8, 13]

The operative approach to treat cervical chordomas hinges on the specific characteristics of the tumor, especially location, and the surgical team expertise.[11, 15] The transoral approach provides the most direct corridor to midline lesions in the craniocervical junction.[11] Inferior extent of this exposure reaches the C2-C3 intervertebral space and spans 2 cm laterally from the midline.[15] This approach is limited by the tongue volume.[11] An extended transoral approach implies mandible and tongue splitting, yielding access down to the C4 vertebral body. However, if the mass stretches laterally out of the transverse process, a radical excision is unlikely.[15] Moreover, this extension is associated with severe postoperative complications.[11] The high cervical retropharyngeal approach allows visualization of the lower clivus down to the C3-C4 intervertebral level. Furthermore, this exposure provides access to lateral structures, such as the C2-C3 and C3-C4 intervertebral foramina and vertebral arteries.[11] The main advantage is the avoidance of oropharynx opening.[11, 15] An important structure

encountered in this approach is the superior laryngeal nerve, where this nerve must be properly identified and retracted for optimal visualization.[11] Reconstruction and stabilization of the cervical spine should be performed as required based on the extent of resection. Anterior instrumentation alone is often insufficient to provide stability if more than two cervical levels are resected, and thus posterior instrumentation and fusion is usually needed.[7]

In the setting of local recurrence, a biopsy should be considered in specific scenarios. Pathological confirmation is required in the case of diagnostic hesitancy or suspicion of tumor dedifferentiation.[10] Salvage treatment can include surgery and/or radiotherapy.[10] Reresection should be aimed at achieving en bloc excision with negative margins when feasible.[10] Currently, there is no specific data to support surgery alone or surgery with radiotherapy. Debulking surgery is unlikely to prolong survival.[10] Traditionally, chordomas are not sensitive to chemotherapy.[2]

What was actually done

Due to the recurrent invasive mass and the presence of progressive symptoms, surgical intervention was recommended for palliative debulking. The patient induced under general anesthesia and the patient was positioned on the surgical table. Baseline motor and somatosensory evoked potentials were performed. The neck was then prepped and draped in usual fashion as well as the right leg in preparation for a fascia lata graft. Incision was planned using the previous scar as reference. The skin was incised. Monopolar cautery was used to dissect out the previous posterior instrumentation from the occiput to the thoracic spine. The fusion mass was inspected and found to be solidly fused with intact hardware. The posterior arch of C1 was identified, and dissection was carried out laterally on the right side all the way to the sulcus arteriosus. Set screws were then removed from the right side of the construct. The right C1 lateral mass screw was also removed in order to make room for the decompression. A combination of bipolar cautery and micro instruments were used to expose the V3 segment of the vertebral artery in the sulcus arteriosus. A C1 laminectomy was then performed with a high-speed drill and a rongeur. The entire posterior arch of C1 was removed. Extensive tumor was seen in the lateral and ventral aspect of the dura which appeared to be extradural. Decompression outside the dura was done and was continued inferiorly all the way down to C4 level. Surgical microscope was brought into the field. At the right lateral and ventral aspect of the spinal canal, the tumor was seen to invade the dura. Removal of tumor revealed scar and arachnoid. A combination of micro instruments, bipolar cautery, and suction was used to remove the chordoma that was seen to arise from the ventral aspect of the spinal canal. This was carefully dissected off the ventral aspect of the spinal cord. Tumor removal was carried all the way up to the foramen magnum. Adequate decompression of the ventral spinal canal was achieved. Then, a fascia lata graft was obtained from the right leg. The fascia lata graft was tacked to the dural edges and was tucked underneath the ventral aspect of the spinal canal. A circumferential covering was obtained. A piece of muscle tissue was placed superiorly and inferiorly on the decompressed aspects of the spinal canal. A Valsalva maneuver indicated no cerebrospinal fluid

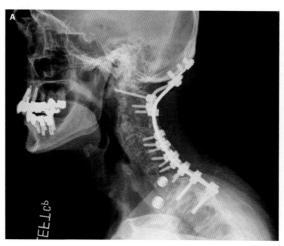
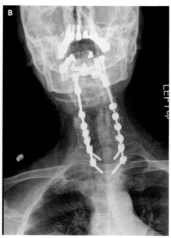

Fig. 59.2 **Postoperative cervical spine x-rays. (A)** Lateral and **(B)** anteroposterior x-rays demonstrating excellent alignment of the hardware. Unchanged vertebral body heights and alignment.

leakage. A new cobalt chrome rod was cut and contoured to the appropriate length and placed within the set screw heads. All set screws were placed and tightened. Hemostasis was achieved. The wound was then closed in anatomical layers. Prolene sutures were used in the skin due to the patient's previous radiation and multiple surgeries. There were no changes in the motor and somatosensory evoked potential tracings throughout the procedure. The patient was rotated off the operating table and awoke in stable fashion. Then he was taken to the intensive care unit for recovery. Upper extremity weakness improved postoperatively. Postoperative radiographs showed excellent hardware alignment (Fig. 59.2).

Commonalities among the experts

Most of the surgeons advocated for a CT angiography for a better understanding of the vascular anatomy. Half remarked the necessity of a right vertebral artery occlusion evaluation. All recommended surgical resection, but specific approaches considerably varied among surgeons. All directed their treatment to obtaining decompression of the neural elements and preventing further functional decline. Most of the surgeons centered their focus on the right vertebral artery and the spinal cord. Right vertebral artery injury and disruption of neural structures were potential complications that raised concern among all the experts. Surgery was usually pursued with intraoperative monitoring, microscope, and ultrasonic aspirator. Although surgical technique varied, all advocated for pursuing an upper cervical decompression and half would perform an instrumented fusion afterward. Following the procedure, all admitted their patients to the intensive care unit, and all requested MRI imaging before discharge. The majority would pursue proton beam therapy for either subtotal or gross total resection.

SUMMARY OF QUALITY OF EVIDENCE TO GUIDE SPECIFIC INTERVENTIONS FOR THIS CASE

- Palliative spinal cord decompression for the treatment of cervical chordoma: level III
- Proton beam therapy after resection of cervical chordoma: level III

REFERENCES

1. Shih AR, Cote GM, Chebib I, et al. Clinicopathologic characteristics of poorly differentiated chordoma. *Mod Pathol.* 2018; 31(8):1237–1245.
2. Wasserman JK, Gravel D, Purgina B. Chordoma of the Head and Neck: A Review. *Head Neck Pathol.* 2018;12(2):261–268.
3. Zhang J, Gao CP, Liu XJ, Xu WJ. Intradural cervical chordoma with diffuse spinal leptomeningeal spread: case report and review of the literature. *Eur Spine J.* 2018;27(Suppl 3):440–445.
4. Zhong N, Yang X, Yang J, et al. Surgical Consideration for Adolescents and Young Adults With Cervical Chordoma. *Spine (Phila Pa 1976).* 2017;42(10):E609–e616.
5. Choi GH, Yang MS, Yoon DH, et al. Pediatric cervical chordoma: report of two cases and a review of the current literature. *Childs Nerv Syst.* 2010;26(6):835–840.
6. Barrenechea IJ, Perin NI, Triana A, Lesser J, Costantino P, Sen C. Surgical management of chordomas of the cervical spine. *J Neurosurg Spine.* 2007;6(5):398–406.
7. Aoun SG, Elguindy M, Barrie U, et al. Four-Level Vertebrectomy for En Bloc Resection of a Cervical Chordoma. *World Neurosurg.* 2018;118:316–323.
8. D'Haen B, De Jaegere T, Goffin J, Dom R, Demaerel P, Plets C. Chordoma of the lower cervical spine. *Clin Neurol Neurosurg.* 1995;97(3):245–248.
9. Baumann BC, Lustig RA, Mazzoni S, et al. A prospective clinical trial of proton therapy for chordoma and chondrosarcoma: Feasibility assessment. *J Surg Oncol.* 2019;120(2):200–205.
10. Stacchiotti S, Gronchi A, Fossati P, et al. Best practices for the management of local-regional recurrent chordoma: a position paper by the Chordoma Global Consensus Group. *Ann Oncol.* 2017;28(6):1230–1242.
11. Ito K, Nakamura T, Aoyama T, Horiuchi T, Hongo K. A Case of Laterally Extended High-Positioned Chordoma Treated Using the High Cervical Retropharyngeal Approach. *World Neurosurg.* 2017;105: 1043.e1015-1043.e1019.
12. Boriani S, Bandiera S, Biagini R, et al. Chordoma of the mobile spine: fifty years of experience. *Spine (Phila Pa 1976).* 2006;31(4):493–503.
13. Yamazaki T, McLoughlin GS, Patel S, Rhines LD, Fourney DR. Feasibility and safety of en bloc resection for primary spine tumors: a systematic review by the Spine Oncology Study Group. *Spine (Phila Pa 1976).* 2009;34(22 Suppl):S31–38.
14. Zhou H, Yang X, Jiang L, Wei F, Liu X, Liu Z. Radiofrequency ablation in gross total excision of cervical chordoma: ideas and technique. *Eur Spine J.* 2018;27(12):3113–3117.
15. Jiang L, Liu ZJ, Liu XG, et al. Upper cervical spine chordoma of C2-C3. *Eur Spine J.* 2009;18(3):293–298. discussion 298–300.

60

Sacral chordoma

Fidel Valero-Moreno, MD

Introduction

Chordoma is a malignant tumor of the bone and should be always considered when a midline tumor of the axial skeleton is found.[1,2] The majority of chordomas affect the sacral region, representing 49% of all the cases.[2-4] There is a modest male prevalence and a peak incidence between the fifth and seventh decades of life.[1,2] Chordomas follow a slow progressive course, with aggressive local invasion and metastasis.[1] Patients usually present with an advanced disease, and the symptoms usually result from neurological compression or invasion to adjacent organs.[5] Perineal pain and neurological deficits are often reported. Other symptoms include constipation, urinary incontinence, and rectal bleeding.[6] The best strategy to reduce recurrence and improve long-term prognosis is total resection with wide margins spanning surrounding healthy tissue.[1,7-9] However, the close proximity to neural and pelvic structures decreases the feasibility for obtaining negative margins without serious morbidity, such as sexual dysfunction and bowel incontinence.[1,8-10] High-dose radiotherapy (60–70 Gy) can be used as either adjuvant therapy or main treatment when operative management is not possible.[9] Despite this, chordomas exhibit significant resistance to radiotherapy and chemotherapy, and recurrence occurs in virtually all cases.[1,5] Complete surgical resection for local sacral recurrences is recommended in the literature.[1,5,7,8,10,11] In this chapter, we discuss the case of a middle aged man with a history of bilateral posterior thigh pain whose symptoms originated from a large anterior sacral space occupying lesion.

Example case

Chief complaint: leg pain and urinary incontinence

History of present illness: This is a 57-year-old male patient with a history of hypertension and coronary artery disease who presented with bilateral posterior thigh pain for 3 to 4 months and new urinary incontinence. The patient underwent a magnetic resonance image of the lumbosacral spine that showed a large mass occupying the upper sacral segment with soft tissue involvement. (Fig. 60.1).

Medications: amlodipine, aspirin

Allergies: no known drug allergies

Past medical and surgical history: hypertension, coronary artery disease

Family history: noncontributory

Social history: no smoking or alcohol

Physical examination: awake, alert, and oriented to person, place, and time; cranial nerves II–XII intact; bilateral deltoids/triceps/biceps 5/5; interossei 5/5; iliopsoas/knee flexion/knee extension/dorsi, and plantar flexion 5/5

Reflexes: 2+ in bilateral biceps/triceps/brachioradialis with negative Hoffman; 2+ in bilateral patella/ankle; no clonus or Babinski; sensation diminished in perianal area

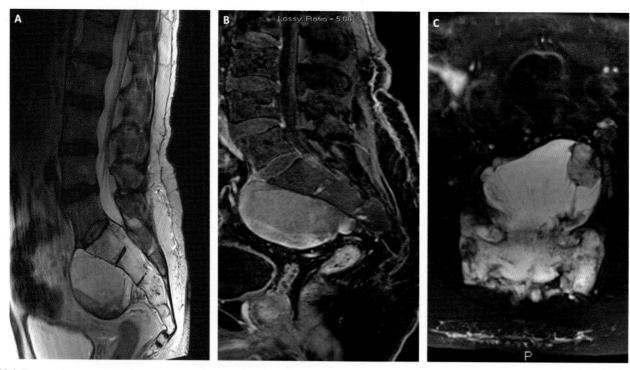

Fig. 60.1 Preoperative magnetic resonance image (MRI) of the lumbosacral spine. (A) Sagittal T2 image demonstrating a voluminous sacral chordoma arising from the upper sacrum. **(B)** Sagittal T1 with contrast image demonstrating the mass with significant mass effect on the pelvic organs and involving the intervertebral discs. **(C)** Axial short tau inversion recovery image demonstrating a large hyperintense and heterogenous mass invading the sacrum and adjacent muscles.

	Stefano Boriani, MD Orthopaedic Surgery IRCCS Istituto Ortopedico Galeazzi, Milan, Italy	Ziya L. Gokaslan, MD Tianyi Niu, MD Neurosurgery Brown University Providence, Rhode Island, United States	Sheng-Fu Lo, MD Neurosurgery Johns Hopkins Baltimore, Maryland, United States	Claudio Yampolsky, MD Neurosurgery Hospital Italiano de Buenos Aires Buenos Aires, Argentina
Preoperative				
Additional tests requested	CT-guided biopsy confirming chordoma	CT sacrum and pelvis	CT chest/abdomen/pelvis CTA abdomen/pelvis Upright scoliosis x-rays CT-guided biopsy with guarded needle	CT L-spine MRI L-spine STIR CTA abdomen/pelvis Angiogram and potential embolization CT-guided biopsy
Surgical approach selected	En bloc resection or carbon ion therapy; for surgery: Stage 1: anterior midline laparotomy and L5 transverse osteotomy Stage 2: posterior L2-sacrum fusion	Stage 1: anterior L5-S1 discectomy with colostomy Stage 2: L2-pelvic instrumentation, L5-S1 complete facetectomy, sacrectomy, hemipelvectomy	Stage 1: anterior midline laparotomy, presacral tumor dissection, L5 transverse osteotomy, VRAM flap elevation Stage 2: posterior L4-5 laminectomy with thecal sac ligation, L5 transverse vertebral body and lateral sagittal osteotomy, L5 hemivertebrectomy and total sacrectomy for en bloc removal of tumor, L3-pelvis fusion, pelvic ring reconstruction, VRAM flap closure	Transabdominal L5 and sacral transverse osteotomy and sacrectomy with L3-iliac fusion
Goal of surgery	En bloc resection with negative margins	En bloc resection, reconstruction/stabilization of spine	En bloc resection with negative margins	En bloc resection with negative margins, fixation

	Stefano Boriani, MD Orthopaedic Surgery IRCCS Istituto Ortopedico Galeazzi, Milan, Italy	Ziya L. Gokaslan, MD Tianyi Niu, MD Neurosurgery Brown University Providence, Rhode Island, United States	Sheng-Fu Lo, MD Neurosurgery Johns Hopkins Baltimore, Maryland, United States	Claudio Yampolsky, MD Neurosurgery Hospital Italiano de Buenos Aires Buenos Aires, Argentina
Perioperative				
Positioning	Stage 1: supine Stage 2: prone	Stage 1: supine Stage 2: prone on Jackson table	Stage 1: supine Stage 2: prone on Jackson table, with pins	Stage 1: supine Stage 2: prone
Surgical equipment	Stage 1: vascular and abdominal surgeon	Stage 1: IOM (MEP/SSEP/ EMG), surgical navigation, silastic sheath Stage 2: IOM (including sphincter), navigation, ultrasonic bone scalpel	IOM (EMG) Ultrasonic bone scalpel Surgical navigation	IOM Fluoroscopy Surgical navigation
Medications	None	None	Tranexamic acid	None
Anatomical considerations	Dural sac, aorta and inferior vena cava bifurcation, hypogastric arteries and veins, piriformis, rectum	Stage 1: great vessels, peritoneal contents, iliac vessels, lumbosacral plexus Stage 2: thecal sac, bilateral L5 nerve roots	Iliac vessels, middle sacral vessels, superior gluteal vessels, rectum, descending colon, ureters, L5 nerve roots	Sacrum, pelvis, pars lateralis, ventral ligamentous complex, aorta, iliac arteries, sacral middle artery, lateral sacral arteries, sacral plexus
Complications feared with approach chosen	CSF leak, arterial or venous bleeding, tumor breach, rectal perforation	Tumor breach, injury to vascular structures, unintended injury to nerves, CSF leak	Catastrophic bleeding, colonic perforation, ureteral injury	Vascular injury, nerve root injury
Intraoperative				
Anesthesia	General	General	General	General
Exposure	Stage 1: L5/iliac Stage 2: L2-sacrum	Stage 1: L5-S1 Stage 2: L2-sacrum	Stage 1: L5-sacrum Stage 2: L3-pelvis	L5-sacrum
Levels decompressed	Stage 1: L5 Stage 2: L4-5	Stage 1: L5-S1 Stage 2: L2-L5	Stage 1: L5 Stage 2: L4-5	L5-S1
Levels fused	Stage 1: none Stage 2: L2-sacrum	Stage 1: none Stage 2: L2-sacrum	Stage 1: none Stage 2: L3-pelvis	L3-iliac
Surgical narrative	Stage 1: vascular surgeon and abdominal surgeon, midline laparotomy, vascular surgery to free great vessels/iliac vessels, ligate both hypogastric arteries and veins, anterior L5 osteotomy and start bilateral iliac osteotomies Stage 2 (same day): prone position, Mercedes-like incision, subperiosteal dissection, L4–5 laminectomy, ligate thecal sac at L4–5 level and transect above L5 nerve roots, full tumor release making sure to leave healthy tissue all around, cut piriformis muscle bilaterally as far as possible, cut the ligament from the coccyx and the sacrospinous and sacrotuberous ligaments, complete osteotomies of L5 and iliac wings, en bloc removal, Varga-type	Stage 1: position supine, IOM baseline, midline laparotomy, vascular surgery to free great vessels/iliac vessels and expose lower lumbar spine and anterior sacral pelvis, plastics to harvest VRAM, colorectal surgery performs colectomy, attach surgical navigation and perform intraoperative CT, dissect bilateral L5 nerve roots to lumbosacral plexus, dissect medial to psoas muscles bilaterally and free up L4 and L5 contribution to plexus, L5-S1 anterior annulotomy and discectomy making sure to disconnect lateral annula, score medial pelvis just lateral to SI joints, place silastic sheath to protect vessels and nerves from tumor, VRAM placed into pelvis and incision closed Stage 2 (2 days	Preoperative placement of ureteral stents, bowel prep, IVC filter Stage 1: position supine, anterior midline laparotomy by vascular surgery down to presacral space and lumbosacral junction, mobilize aortic and IVC bifurcation / middle sacral vessels/bilateral internal iliac vessels/external iliac vessel down to pelvis, identify L5 nerve roots and dissect off of tumor, dissect mesorectum and descending colon off of of tumor with colorectal surgery with possible diverting colostomy if tumor adherent/infiltrative or cannot obtain adequate exposure, transverse cut into L5 vertebral body above tumor through ALL and down to PLL, place silastic sheath between tumor and external iliac	Stage 1: GI or general surgeon to perform transabdominal incision via an infraumbilical incision, mobilize aorta and IVC as well as middle and lateral sacral vessels, expose L5 and sacrum, osteotomy guided by surgical navigation through L5 and sacrum, complete radical resection, placement of pedicle screws and L3–5 with iliac screws, place rods for L3-iliac fusion

| Stefano Boriani, MD Orthopaedic Surgery IRCCS Istituto Ortopedico Galeazzi, Milan, Italy | Ziya L. Gokaslan, MD Tianyi Niu, MD Neurosurgery Brown University Providence, Rhode Island, United States | Sheng-Fu Lo, MD Neurosurgery Johns Hopkins Baltimore, Maryland, United States | Claudio Yampolsky, MD Neurosurgery Hospital Italiano de Buenos Aires Buenos Aires, Argentina |

reconstruction, place pedicle screws at L2-4, connect pedicle screws to U-bend rod fixed by double screw in each iliac wing, femoral shaft allograft combined with titanium cage interposed between iliac wings and L5 or possible 3D printed titanium prosthesis, layered closure

later): position prone, baseline IOM, expose L2- sacrum, intraoperative navigation and CT scan that is fused to preoperative MRI, place bilateral L2-4 pedicle screws and pelvis screws, cannulate and tap L5 pedicle screws, L5 laminectomy and facetectomy, complete posterior L5-S1 discectomy, thecal sac tied off at L5-S1 with silk ties and divided, drill the pelvis just lateral to the SI joint using navigation, complete bony disconnection with osteotome, dissect sacrum down to the most inferior aspect and disconnect muscle attachments, rotate specimen to deliver it, protect L4 and L5 contribution to the plexus, remove specimen en bloc, inspect the specimen to ensure there is no breach, remove silastic sheath, place L5 pedicle screws, femur shaft sized in placed with ilium-femur-ilium screw at normal sacral promontory position, fibula grafts are sized and placed in effect and anchored between inferior aspect of L5 vertebral body and medial remaining pelvis and secure in place with screws in a V-shape, four-rod construct is placed with each of the rods secured using pelvic screws and multiple side-to-side connectors, place horizontal cross rod between left and right pelvic screws, VRAM is pulled out to fill defect, decorticate and place allograft on all bony surfaces, plastics surgery to close in anatomical layers with drains

vessels and L5 nerve roots, elevation of epithelialized VRAM by plastic surgery to close off dead space, plastic surgery closure of wound
Stage 2 (next day): position prone, midline posterior incision, subperiosteal dissection L3-5 and sacrum and leave gluteal muscles attached to sacrum, expose PSIS and ilium, L4-5 laminectomy and L5 inferior facetectomy, skeletonize L5 nerve roots proximally, ligate thecal sac below L5, attach navigation array and intraoperative CT scan, CT-guided sagittal cuts lateral to SI joints and tumor bilaterally through ilium using bone scalpel, identify transverse osteotomy across L5 from stage 1, complete osteotomy through PLL and lateral vertebral body to disconnect L5, detach pyriformis muscle lateral to tumor and ligaments while avoiding injury to underlying viscera/gluteal vessels/sciatic nerve, rotate tumor specimen with laminar spreader, bluntly dissect mesorectum and colon away from tumor making sure to preserve tumor capsule, detach coccygeus muscle inferior to tumor and anococcygeal ligament, deliver tumor en bloc, examination of specimen and resection cavity to ensure R0 resection, floor surgical field with sterile water to lyse tumor, lateral x-ray to confirm detachment and alignment, reposition pelvis using bolsters to match preoperative lumbosacral pelvic parameters on scoliosis x-rays, confirm with x-ray, place bilateral L3-5 pelvic screws and

	Stefano Boriani, MD Orthopaedic Surgery IRCCS Istituto Ortopedico Galeazzi, Milan, Italy	Ziya L. Gokaslan, MD Tianyi Niu, MD Neurosurgery Brown University Providence, Rhode Island, United States	Sheng-Fu Lo, MD Neurosurgery Johns Hopkins Baltimore, Maryland, United States	Claudio Yampolsky, MD Neurosurgery Hospital Italiano de Buenos Aires Buenos Aires, Argentina
			double iliac screws, fashion structural femoral allograft to wedge against lateral osteotomies for pelvic ring reconstruction, horizontal rods across iliac screws with double vertical rods up to L3 with cross connectors for four-rod reconstruction, cable femoral structural allograft to horizontal rods across ilium, examine for CSF leak, decorticate exposed bone surfaces and place morselized allograft, identify VRAM from stage 1 and obliterate sacral dead space to prevent bowel herniation, plastic surgery closure	
Complication avoidance	Multidisciplinary team approach, free anterior border to tumor before posterior, ligate thecal sac above L5 nerve roots, en bloc resection, Varga-type reconstruction, femoral shaft allograft with titanium cage to reconstruct defect	Multidisciplinary team approach, silastic sheath to protect nerves and vessels, VRAM to fill dead space, surgical navigation tow staged approach, en bloc resection, four-rod construct, plastics surgery closure	Preoperative placement of ureteral stents/bowel prep/IVC filter, staged procedure, multidisciplinary care, preserve L5 nerve roots, silastic sheath to protect vessels for posterior portion of surgery, VRAM flap to close dead space, surgical navigation, flood field with water to lyse microtumor cells,	Preoperative angiogram and possible embolization, general surgery to perform the approach, surgical navigation
Postoperative				
Admission	ICU	ICU	ICU	ICU
Postoperative complications feared	CSF leak, wound dehiscence, hematoma, wound infection	CSF leak, wound dehiscence, wound infection, hardware failure	CSF leak, wound dehiscence, L5 nerve root injury, medical complications, lower extremity vascular insufficiency	Vascular injury, nerve root injury
Anticipated length of stay	12–14 days	7 days	5–7 days	4–5 days
Follow-up testing	MRI every 6 months for 5 years	Non-weight bearing for 6 weeks MRI sacrum/pelvis prior to discharge Standing x-rays 3 months after surgery	CT L-spine within 48 hours of surgery MRI L-spine within 48 hours of surgery Bilateral lower extremity Dopplers	CT L-spine within 48 hours of surgery MRI L-spine within 48 hours of surgery
Bracing	None	None	None	None
Follow-up visits	2 weeks and 6 months after surgery	2 weeks and 3 months after surgery	2 weeks after surgery	7 days and 2 weeks after surgery

	Stefano Boriani, MD Orthopaedic Surgery IRCCS Istituto Ortopedico Galeazzi, Milan, Italy	Ziya L. Gokaslan, MD Tianyi Niu, MD Neurosurgery Brown University Providence, Rhode Island, United States	Sheng-Fu Lo, MD Neurosurgery Johns Hopkins Baltimore, Maryland, United States	Claudio Yampolsky, MD Neurosurgery Hospital Italiano de Buenos Aires Buenos Aires, Argentina
Radiation therapy for STR	Carbon ion	Proton beam	Proton beam or stereotactic radiosurgery	External beam radiation
Radiation therapy for GTR	Observation	Observation	Proton beam or stereotactic radiosurgery	Observation

CSF, Cerebrospinal fluid; *CT,* computed tomography; *CTA,* computed tomography angiography; *EMG,* electromyography; *GTR,* gross total resection; *ICU,* intensive care unit; *IOM,* intraoperative monitoring; *IVC,* inferior vena cava; *MEP,* motor evoked potential; *MRI,* magnetic resonance imaging; *PSIS,* psoterior superior iliac spine; *SI,* sacroiliac; *SSEP,* somatosensory evoked potential; *STIR,* short tau inversion recovery; *STR,* subtotal resection; *VRAM,* vertical rectus abdominis myocutaneous.

Differential diagnosis

- Chordoma
- Chondrosarcoma
- Giant cell tumor
- Plasmacytoma
- Glioma
- Metastatic tumor
- Ewing sarcoma
- Chronic infections (tuberculosis, fungus)

Important anatomical and preoperative considerations

Despite being a rare entity, chordoma is the most common primary neoplasm found in the sacrum.[12] Surgical intervention of the sacrum is challenging and complex due to the risk of neurovascular injury.[12,13] The sacrum is a triangular structure consisting mainly of cancellous bone[14] formed by five vertebrae, fusing along with the intervertebral discs.[15] The sacrum articulates with the vertebra above through a disc space and facet joint complex, with the coccyx below by ligamentous structures and on each side with the ilium via the sacroiliac joint.[15] The sacrum has a concave ventral surface, a convex dorsal surface, and an apex that projects posteriorly and increases the size of the pelvic cavity. The sacral promontory or sacrovertebral angle is evident in the sagittal plane and represents a landmark for anterior lumbosacral approaches.[13,15] This angle increases with age and measures 70 degrees in adulthood.[15] On the inner surface, the neural foraminae are oriented in an anterolateral direction and contain their respective sacral nerves and arteries before passing to the pelvis.[13,15] The lateral masses of the sacrum are located lateral to the foraminae.[15] The dorsal aspect of the sacrum is convex, where the initial three or four vertebrae are marked by a prominent longitudinal crest that is formed by the rudimentary spinous processes.[13,15] The fused lamina are lateral to the rudimentary spinous processes.[15] The lamina of the fifth sacral segment is not fused, but instead it forms an opening called the sacral hiatus.[13,15] The fused articular processes are located lateral to the laminae and form a paired longitudinal crest.[13,15] Lateral to the crest are the four pairs of neural foramina that create an important landmark for spinal instrumentation.[15]

Important midline structures in the sacral area include the middle sacral artery (MSA) and the intestine.[16] The MSA branches from the abdominal aorta, just before the aortic bifurcation. The MSA descends posteriorly to the iliac vessel, and courses along the anterior aspect of the sacrum and sometimes provides a branch for the rectum.[17] The vessel runs caudally over the coccyx and ends at the coccygeal gland.[16–18] Despite the MSA being a relatively small vessel (2.3–2.8 mm in diameter),[16] it represents a potentially significant source of bleeding and often is sacrificed, especially during anterior approaches.[18] The lateral regions of the sacrum contain the internal iliac artery (IIA), its branch the lateral sacral artery (LSA), the internal iliac vein (IIV), and the sympathetic trunk.[14,16] The IIA has a close relationship with the sacroiliac joint. The presence of presacral anastomoses between medial and lateral veins contributes to the complexity of the anterior approach.[16] Thus the most fear and prevalent complication in anterior approaches to the sacrum is vascular injury.[16, 18]

The location of the chordoma often dictates whether an anterior, posterior, or combined approach is required.[5] As expected, MRI and meticulous planning are essential before any surgical strategy is established.[12] The posterior approach is mainly used when tumors are caudal to the third sacral vertebra. The opposite is true for the anteroposterior approach, which is preferred for lesions above this segment.[5] The main advantages of the posterior approach are the shorter operating time and lesser invasiveness.[5,19] However, the likelihood of iatrogenic injury of abdominopelvic viscera and vessels when the tumor extends ventrally is the main factor limiting the use of posterior approaches.[19] Anteroposterior approach is a safer strategy when the ventral part of the tumor is in close relationship with pelvic structures, such as the rectum, iliac artery, and iliac veins.[19] This approach allows the tumor to be dissected from hollow viscera and would protect them as well during osteotomies.[5,19] The mainstay of sacral chordoma treatment is radical resection with an unruptured capsule and preservation of as much function as possible.[12] Therefore, protection of neural structures, when possible, plays a fundamental role for optimizing quality of life for patients.[12,19] When feasible, one nerve root at each level should be preserved. Resections including the S1 root (even single root) are invariably related to sexual dysfunction and motor deficits.[12,19] Sacrectomies with neural amputation below the S3 level preserve sphincter control with minimal perineal anesthesia.[12,19] As large and radical resection of sacral chordomas is the only management associated with local control, spinopelvic stability must be evaluated and addressed. Instrumented spinopelvic reconstruction is required for most sacral chordomas resection.[19]

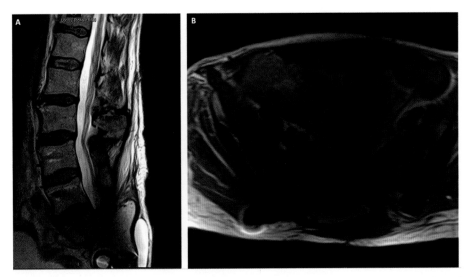

Fig. 60.2 Postoperative magnetic resonance image (MRI) of the lumbosacral spine. (A) T2 sagittal image demonstrating sacrectomy and complete tumor resection of the tumor. **(B)** T2-axial image demonstrating gross total resection.

What was actually done

The patient was taken to the operating room for a staged procedure. In the first stage, the patient was taken to the operating room and positioned supine. The patient was induced under general anesthesia. Baseline somatosensory and motor evoked potentials were obtained. A midline laparotomy was performed and then vascular surgery proceeded with the identification and mobilization of aorta and inferior vena cava bifurcation, great iliac vessels, and middle sacral vessels for the exposure of the anterior lumbar and sacral spine. Surgical navigation was brought in. General surgery dissected the colon off of tumor. L5 roots to lumbosacral plexus were identified and dissect from the tumor. L5-S1 anterior annulotomy and discectomy with disconnection of lateral annula was then done. A silastic sheath was placed between the external iliac vessels, the L5 roots, and the tumor. A vertical rectus abdominis musculocutaneous (VRAM) flap was harvested by plastic surgery and placed into the pelvis. The incision was closed. Stage 2 was done two days after the first stage. The patient was brought back to the operating room and positioned prone on the operating table after induction of general anesthesia. Baseline intraoperative neuromonitoring was obtained. Incision was done from L2 to the sacrum followed by the subperiosteal dissection. Intraoperative navigation, using fused preoperative MRI and CT scans, was set. Pedicle screws were placed bilaterally from L2 to L4 pedicle as well as pelvic screws. A laminectomy and facetectomy was done at L4-5 and complete posterior L5-S1 discectomy. The thecal sac was tied off at L5-S1 and divided. Using navigation, the pelvis was drilled lateral to the sacroiliac joint, complete bony disconnection was achieved with an osteotome, and resection of muscle attachments. The silastic sheath was then removed allowing en bloc removal of the tumor. L5 pedicle screws were then placed. L2-pelvis instrumentation was completed. Horizontal cross rod between left and right pelvic screws were placed. VRAM to cover sacral dead space and closure in anatomical layers was done by plastic surgery. The patient was transferred in stable condition to the intensive care unit. Postoperative MRI demonstrated gross total resection (Fig. 60.2). Radiation was held in the postoperative period.

Commonalities among the experts

Most of the surgeons requested a computed tomography (CT)-guided biopsy to confirm the presence of chordoma. Half considered CT angiogram of the abdomen and pelvis for surgery planning. Although several technique differences were described, all would achieve resection primarily through an anterior transabdominal approach. All would perform surgery in conjunction with a multidisciplinary team, including general surgeons and vascular surgeons. All the experts considered en bloc resection with negative margins the best option for the patient. Vascular structures, including aorta, inferior vena cava (IVC) bifurcation, iliac arteries, and sacral vessels, attracted special attention from all the surgeons. The most feared complications were vascular injury, tumor breach, and perforation of hollow viscera. Surgery was carried out with intraoperative monitoring, surgical navigation, and ultrasonic bone scalpel. No special perioperative medications were recommended by most of the surgeons. Although surgical details varied among experts, all shared the concept of multidisciplinary approach for the adequate manipulation of nonneural elements and complex vascular structures. Since the aim of the surgery was a large radical resection, all the surgeons pursued a posterior instrumented fusion. Half recommended a L2-sacrum fusion and the rest preferred either a L3-pelvis or a L3-iliac fusion. Postoperatively, wound infection/dehiscence and cerebrospinal fluid leak were the most feared complications. Following surgery, all the surgeons admitted their patients to the intensive care unit, and the majority requested a lumbosacral MRI study before discharge to assess extent of resection and rule out potential complications. In addition, half also requested a CT scan of the lumbar spine to assess hardware placement. Most advocated for proton beam therapy if subtotal resection was achieved, and most would observe patients who underwent gross total resection.

SUMMARY OF QUALITY OF EVIDENCE TO GUIDE SPECIFIC INTERVENTIONS FOR THIS CASE

- *En bloc* radical resection is the treatment of choice for sacral chordoma: level II-1
- Complete surgical resection for local sacral recurrences: level II-1
- Instrumented posterior lumbosacral or lumbopelvic fusion, if the aim of the surgery is local control of the disease: level III
- Complementary proton beam therapy if STR was achieved: level III

REFERENCES

1. Lim JBT, Soeharno H, Tan MH. Sacral chordoma: clinical experience of a series of 11 patients over 18 years. *Eur J Orthop Surg Traumatol.* 2019;29(1):9–15.
2. Shih AR, Cote GM, Chebib I, et al. Clinicopathologic characteristics of poorly differentiated chordoma. *Mod Pathol.* 2018;31(8):1237–1245.
3. van Wulfften Palthe ODR, Tromp I, Ferreira A, et al. Sacral chordoma: a clinical review of 101 cases with 30-year experience in a single institution. *Spine J.* 2019;19(5):869–879.
4. Zhong N, Yang X, Yang J, et al. Surgical Consideration for Adolescents and Young Adults With Cervical Chordoma. *Spine (Phila Pa 1976).* 2017;42(10):E609–e616.
5. Kayani B, Hanna SA, Sewell MD, Saifuddin A, Molloy S, Briggs TW. A review of the surgical management of sacral chordoma. *Eur J Surg Oncol.* 2014;40(11):1412–1420.
6. Gleghorn K, Goodwin B, Sanchez R. Cutaneous Metastasis From Sacral Chordoma. *Am J Dermatopathol.* 2017;39(4):e54–e57.
7. Xie C, Whalley N, Adasonla K, Grimer R, Jeys L. Can local recurrence of a sacral chordoma be treated by further surgery? *Bone Joint J.* 2015;97-b(5):711–715.
8. Yang Y, Li Y, Liu W, Xu H, Niu X. The clinical outcome of recurrent sacral chordoma with further surgical treatment. *Medicine (Baltimore).* 2018;97(52):e13730.
9. Yolcu Y, Wahood W, Alvi MA, et al. Evaluating the Role of Adjuvant Radiotherapy in the Management of Sacral and Vertebral Chordoma: Results from a National Database. *World Neurosurg.* 2019;127:e1137–e1144.
10. Chen KW, Yang HL, Kandimalla Y, Liu JY, Wang GL. Review of current treatment of sacral chordoma. *Orthop Surg.* 2009;1(3):238–244.
11. Ailon T, Torabi R, Fisher CG, et al. Management of Locally Recurrent Chordoma of the Mobile Spine and Sacrum: A Systematic Review. *Spine (Phila Pa 1976).* 2016;41 Suppl 20 (Suppl 20):S193–s198.
12. Pillai S, Govender S. Sacral chordoma: A review of literature. *J Orthop.* 2018;15(2):679–684.
13. Xu R, Ebraheim NA, Gove NK. Surgical anatomy of the sacrum. *Am J Orthop (Belle Mead NJ).* 2008;37(10):E177–181.
14. Ergur I, Akcali O, Kiray A, Kosay C, Tayefi H. Neurovascular risks of sacral screws with bicortical purchase: an anatomical study. *Eur Spine J.* 2007;16(9):1519–1523.
15. Cheng JS, Song JK. Anatomy of the sacrum. *Neurosurg Focus.* 2003;15(2):E3.
16. Güvençer M, Dalbayrak S, Tayefi H, et al. Surgical anatomy of the presacral area. *Surg Radiol Anat.* 2009;31(4):251–257.
17. Gailloud P. Spinal Vascular Anatomy. *Neuroimaging Clin N Am.* 2019;29(4):615–633.
18. Sae-Jung S, Khamanarong K, Woraputtaporn W, Amarttayakong P. Awareness of the median sacral artery during lumbosacral spinal surgery: an anatomic cadaveric study of its relationship to the lumbosacral spine. *Eur Spine J.* 2015;24(11):2520–2524.
19. Stephens M, Gunasekaran A, Elswick C, Laryea JA, Pait TG, Kazemi N. Neurosurgical Management of Sacral Tumors: Review of the Literature and Operative Nuances. *World Neurosurg.* 2018;116:362–369.

61

Spontaneous CSF leak

Fidel Valero-Moreno, MD and Jaime L. Martinez Santos, MD

Introduction

Spontaneous intracranial hypotension is often caused by structural defects in the dura within the spinal canal or along the nerve root sleeve.[1] Although rare, cerebrospinal fluid (CSF) venous fistula has also been recognized recently as a cause of spontaneous intracranial hypotension.[2] This condition has an estimated annual incidence of 5 per 100,000 persons,[2,3] has a female predilection,[2] and can occur in any region along the spine, but most often occurs in the thoracic levels.[3] Symptoms classically include orthostatic headaches that improve with recumbency; however, the headache symptoms may be variable in location, onset, and quality.[3–6] Cranial imaging typically demonstrates enhancement of the dura mater, empty sella, sagging of the cerebellar tonsils, and, in more severe cases, subdural hematomas.[3,7] A computed tomography (CT) myelogram may be useful in pinpointing the exact location of a spontaneous leak. In many cases, there are multiple offending locations. CSF opening pressure is not a reliable diagnostic tool because most of the patients show pressures within the normal range.[2] Autologous epidural blood patching may be employed as a first-line treatment and can be repeated if necessary.[2] Persistent symptoms with identified leaks may require surgical intervention and direct closure. In this chapter, we present a case of a male patient presenting with the classic symptoms of spontaneous intracranial hypotension.

Example Case

Chief complaint: postural headaches

History of present illness: This is a 50-year-old male nonobese patient with a 3-month history of worsening postural headaches. He has not had any spinal procedures. Magnetic resonance image (MRI) of the thoracic spine showed epidural fluid collection consistent with spontaneous CSF leak (Fig. 61.1).

Medications: none

Allergies: no known drug allergies

Past medical and surgical history: none

Family history: noncontributory

Social history: lawyer, no smoking, occasional alcohol

Physical examination: awake, alert, and oriented to person, place, and time; cranial nerves II–XII intact; bilateral deltoids/ triceps/biceps 5/5; interossei 5/5; iliopsoas/knee flexion/ knee extension/dorsi, and plantar flexion 5/5

Reflexes: 2+ in bilateral biceps/triceps/brachioradialis with negative Hoffman; 2+ in bilateral patella/ankle; no clonus or Babinski; sensation intact to light touch

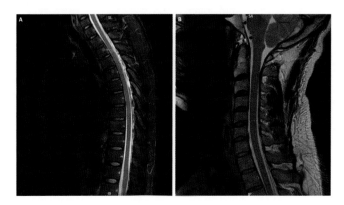

Fig. 61.1 Preoperative magnetic resonance imaging (MRI). (A) Sagittal T2 thoracic MRI demonstrating a dorsal cervicothoracic epidural collection of cerebrospinal fluid (CSF) intensity with flow voids (possibly from enlarged internal vertebral venous plexus of Batson) and ventral displacement of the spinal cord. **(B)** Sagittal T2 cervical MRI demonstrating absence of cerebellar tonsil ectopia (no Chiari malformation). There is no evidence of a nerve root cyst, pseudomeningocele, intervertebral disc herniation, or transdural osteophyte.

	Ignacio Barrenechea, MD Neurosurgery Grupo Gamma Rosario, Santa Fe, Argentina	Selby Chen, MD Neurosurgery Mayo Clinic Jacksonville, Florida, United States	Fernando Hakim, MD Hospital Universitario Fundacion Santafe de Bogota Bogota, Colombia	Daniel C. Liu, MD, PhD Neurosurgery University of California at Los Angeles Los Angeles, California, United States
Preoperative				
Additional tests requested	MRI brain CT myelogram Anesthesia evaluation Interventional radiology for blood patch	CT myelogram	MRI brain CT myelogram Interventional radiology for blood patch	MRI brain CT myelogram Interventional radiology for blood patch
Surgical approach selected	If blood patch did not work, thoracic laminectomy and repair of CSF leak	Thoracic laminectomy and repair of CSF leak	If blood patch did not work, thoracic laminectomy and repair of CSF leak	If blood patch did not work, thoracic laminectomy and repair of CSF leak
Goal of surgery	Repair CSF leak	Repair CSF leak, improve postural headaches	Repair CSF leak	Repair CSF leak
Perioperative				
Positioning	Prone on Wilson frame	Prone	Prone on gel rolls, no pins	Prone on Jackson table, no pins
Surgical equipment	Fluoroscopy Surgical microscope Tubular retractor	Fluoroscopy Surgical microscope Castro-Viejo needle driver	Fluoroscopy Piezoelectric drill Ultrasound Surgical microscope	Fluoroscopy IOM (MEP/SSEP) Surgical navigation Lumbar drain
Medications	None	None	Maintain MAP	Fluorescein
Anatomical considerations	Thoracic facet joint, ligamentum flavum, dura, spinal cord	Thecal sac, spinal cord	Nerve roots	Spinal cord, facets
Complications feared with approach chosen	Spinal cord injury, CSF leak, spinal instability	Spinal cord injury	Recurrence of CSF leak	Spinal cord injury, recurrence of CSF leak
Intraoperative				
Anesthesia	General	General	General	General
Exposure	One level above and below area of CSF leak on myelogram	One level above and below area of CSF leak on myelogram	Hemilaminectomy at area of CSF leak on myelogram	One level above and below area of CSF leak on myelogram
Levels decompressed	Level of leak on myelogram	Level of leak on myelogram	Level of leak on myelogram	Level of leak on myelogram
Levels fused	None	None	None	Only if needed
Surgical narrative	Position prone, x-ray to plan incision with true PA levels, incision made between upper and lower pedicular line of target level, fascia incision and opened under skin edge with monopolar cautery, sequential dilation with tubular retractors, dock 25 mm tube and secure to table, monopolar cautery to remove remaining muscle and soft tissue attached to the bone inside the tube, bring surgical microscope in, hemilaminotomy with drill, keep ligamentum flavum until bone work is done to protect the dura, resect ligamentum with Kerrison rongeurs, dissect dura and locate site of CSF	Position prone, midline incision over target level after confirmation with fluoroscopy, dissect down to level of spinous process, localize level with fluoroscopy, insert retractors, dissect soft tissue off of lamina, laminectomy with high-speed bur and rongeurs, yellow ligament resected with curette and Kerrison rongeurs, site of CSF leak identified, dural defect repaired under microscope with 6-0 Prolene, muscle pledget if defect large,	Position prone, fluoroscopy to localize level, midline long incision where neuroradiologist identified leakage, subperiosteal dissection exposing posterior elements, hemilaminectomy at level selected, expose dura, Valsalva to confirm area of leakage, attempted primary repair of defect under microscopic visualization, also use muscle patch and fibrin sealant, Valsalva to confirm proper closure, layered closure, upright in bed for 24 hours	Position prone, fluoroscopy to localize level based on rib counting in AP view, mark midline incision, posterior midline incision, dissect to posterior elements, x-ray to confirm level, laminectomy or laminectomies over relevant level, identify CSF leak and can inject intrathecal fluorescein with small-gauge needle if needed or intraoperative myelogram with x-ray or CT, primary closure of leak if possible with dural sealant, dural substitute and sandwich closure if cannot primary repair, can use muscle to help

	Ignacio Barrenechea, MD Neurosurgery Grupo Gamma Rosario, Santa Fe, Argentina	Selby Chen, MD Neurosurgery Mayo Clinic Jacksonville, Florida, United States	Fernando Hakim, MD Hospital Universitario Fundacion Santafe de Bogota Bogota, Colombia	Daniel C. Liu, MD, PhD Neurosurgery University of California at Los Angeles Los Angeles, California, United States
	leak, ligate if clear leak seen, Valsalva to identify leak if not clearly seen, if no leak seen then fat and fibrin glue, remove tube, layered closure	Surgery on dural repair site, wound closed in anatomical layers with absorbable sutures		closure, multilayer closure with subfascial drain to gravity, vancomycin powder epifascially, head of bed at 0 degrees for at least 24 hours, fusion if concern of instability
Complication avoidance	Minimally invasive tubular retractor, keep ligamentum flavum until bone work is done to protect the dura, Valsalva to identify leak, pack with fat and fibrin glue if no leak seen	Myelogram to confirm leak, muscle pledget if needed	Myelogram to confirm leak, hemilaminectomy, confirm presence and repair with Valsalva maneuver	Rib counting to determine level, intraoperative fluorescein or myelogram to identify CSF leak, attempt primary repair
Postoperative				
Admission	Floor	Floor	Floor	Floor
Postoperative complications feared	CSF leak, spinal instability	CSF leak, neurological injury	CSF leak	CSF leak
Anticipated length of stay	2 days	3 days	2 days	2–5 days
Follow-up testing	MRI brain and complete spine within 48 hours, 2 months, 6 months, 12 months after surgery	None	None	None
Bracing	None	None	None	None
Follow-up visits	2 weeks, 6 weeks, 3 months, 6 months, 12 months after surgery	4–6 weeks after surgery	2 weeks after surgery	2 weeks, 6 weeks after surgery

AP, Anteroposterior; *CSF*, cerebrospinal fluid; *CT*, computed tomography; *IOM*, intraoperative monitoring; *MAP*, mean arterial pressure; *MEP*, motor evoked potential; *MRI*, magnetic resonance imaging; *PA*, posteroanterior; *SSEP*, somatosensory evoked potential.

Differential diagnosis

- Traumatic chronic subdural hematoma
- Aseptic meningitis
- Ventriculoperitoneal shunt (overshunting)
- Abnormalities of connective tissue
- Meningeal diverticula
- CSF leak

Important anatomical and preoperative considerations

In the recumbent position, pressures in the lumbar, cisternal, intracranial regions, and vertex are believed to be equal, ranging from 60 to 250 mm H_2O. In the vertical position, pressure in the vertex tends to be negative.[8] Three mechanisms are known to cause CSF leakage in the spinal cord: dural mechanical weakness causing tears along the spinal cord or meningeal diverticula affecting mostly nerve sleeves,[2,9] dural tears related to disc herniations (ventrally located) or osteophytic spurs, and CSF venous fistulas.[2] Dural weakness and certain arachnoid configurations (septations) cause protrusion of the arachnoid layer, whereby diverticula are formed and are vulnerable to rupture, especially within the thoracic and upper lumbar spine.[2,8] Dural tears originated due to calcified discs or osteophytes are most frequently located in the thoracic and lower cervical spine and can produce rapid leakage and a large volume epidural fluid on imaging.[2] CSF venous fistulas are mainly located in the lower half of the thoracic spine, and in most cases an epidural leak cannot be identified.[10]

The most common treatment modality utilized for either localized or nonlocalized CSF leakage is the nontargeted epidural blood patching (EBP). Targeted EBP can be technically challenging and limited by a lack of precise knowledge of the location of the leaking site. The utilization of EBP was found to be superior compared with conservative treatment of postural headaches.[11,12] There is no consensus regarding the most appropriate volume of injected blood.[11] Patients with refractory symptoms after EBP treatment and localized lesions may benefit from surgical intervention, which is especially true in the setting of dural tears due to calcified discs and osteophyte protrusion.[2]

What was actually done

The patient underwent a CT myelogram, which demonstrated a ventral CSF fistula at the T8-T9 level consistent with spontaneous CSF leakage and intracranial hypotension. The patient then underwent a trial of autologous EBP. The patient was placed in the lateral position under local anesthesia. A needle was introduced into the epidural space, ultrasound showed good needle localization, then a blood volume of 25 mL was slowly introduced. After the procedure, the patient continued observation in the recovery room. At 2-week and 3-month follow-up, the patient reported complete resolution of his symptoms.

Commonalities among the experts

All of the experts requested a CT myelogram for an appropriate preoperative assessment. In addition, most of the surgeons would complement it with a magnetic resonance image of the brain. The majority would perform blood patching before attempted surgical intervention. All would attain CSF leak repair through a thoracic laminectomy. The main goals of surgical treatment were resolution of CSF leak and prevention of recurrence. Most of the physicians were aware of the spinal cord, thecal sac, and thoracic facet joints. The most feared approach-associated complications were spinal cord injury and worsening of CSF leak. Surgery was generally facilitated by fluoroscopy and surgical microscope. Most of the surgeons would not recommend special perioperative medications. Surgical strategy was similar among all surgeons, where exposure would span one level above and one below the area defined by myelogram. Most would employ muscle or fibrin sealant to complement primary closure. Following operation, all would admit their patients to the floor for continued observation. The greatest postoperative concern was recurrence of CSF leak. Most would not request any specific postoperative test.

SUMMARY OF QUALITY OF EVIDENCE TO GUIDE SPECIFIC INTERVENTIONS FOR THIS CASE

- Initial treatment of spinal spontaneous CSF leak is blood patch defect sealing: class II-2

- Epidural blood patch effectiveness for postdural puncture headache relief is superior to conservative management: level I.

REFERENCES

1. Albes G, Weng H, Horvath D, Musahl C, Bäzner H, Henkes H. Detection and treatment of spinal CSF leaks in idiopathic intracranial hypotension. *Neuroradiology*. 2012;54(12):1367–1373.
2. Kranz PG, Malinzak MD, Amrhein TJ, Gray L. Update on the Diagnosis and Treatment of Spontaneous Intracranial Hypotension. *Curr Pain Headache Rep*. 2017;21(8):37.
3. Schievink WI, Maya MM, Moser F, Tourje J, Torbati S. Frequency of spontaneous intracranial hypotension in the emergency department. *J Headache Pain*. 2007;8(6):325–328.
4. Sencakova D, Mokri B, McClelland RL. The efficacy of epidural blood patch in spontaneous CSF leaks. *Neurology*. 2001; 57(10):1921–1923.
5. Mokri B, Aksamit AJ, Atkinson JL. Paradoxical postural headaches in cerebrospinal fluid leaks. *Cephalalgia*. 2004;24(10):883–887.
6. Schievink WI. Spontaneous spinal cerebrospinal fluid leaks: a review. *Neurosurg Focus*. 2000;9(1):e8.
7. Schievink WI, Maya MM, Jean-Pierre S, Nuño M, Prasad RS, Moser FG. A classification system of spontaneous spinal CSF leaks. *Neurology*. 2016;87(7):673–679.
8. Nauta HJ, Dolan E, Yasargil MG. Microsurgical anatomy of spinal subarachnoid space. *Surg Neurol*. 1983;19(5):431–437.
9. Ferrante E, Trimboli M, Rubino F. Spontaneous intracranial hypotension: review and expert opinion. *Acta Neurol Belg*. 2020;120(1):9–18.
10. Kranz PG, Amrhein TJ, Gray L. CSF Venous Fistulas in Spontaneous Intracranial Hypotension: Imaging Characteristics on Dynamic and CT Myelography. *AJR Am J Roentgenol*. 2017;209(6):1360–1366.
11. Kapoor SG, Ahmed S. Cervical epidural blood patch-A literature review. *Pain Med*. 2015;16(10):1897–1904.
12. Boonmak P, Boonmak S. Epidural blood patching for preventing and treating post-dural puncture headache. *Cochrane Database Syst Rev*. 2010(1):Cd001791.

62

Lumbar osteomyelitis and discitis

Fidel Valero-Moreno, MD and Jaime L. Martinez Santos, MD

Introduction

The incidence of vertebral osteomyelitis is approximately 1 per 100,000 per year worldwide[1]; however, this incidence increases with age up to 6.5 per 100,000 among persons older than 70 years of age.[2] Overall, vertebral infections represent 1% of all the skeletal infections.[3] *Staphylococcus aureus* is the most common pathogen implicated.[2] The primary route of spread is hematogenous,[2] usually from the urinary tract.[3] It primarily affects the vertebral bodies, with only a small percentage of cases affecting the posterior elements.[4] Posterior elements infection is associated with advanced disease.[5] The complete spectrum of pyogenic vertebral osteomyelitis comprises spondylitis, discitis, spondylodiscitis, osteomyelitis, and epidural abscesses.[6] The most common presenting symptom is back pain, which is reported in 86% of the cases.[2] Fever occurs in less than 50% of patients at presentation. The most common spinal segments affected are the lumbar vertebrae, followed by the thoracic and cervical spine.[2,3] Most cases resolve with prolonged medical therapy (i.e., antibiotics); however, surgical intervention may be employed for patients who have progressive neurological deficits, failure of adequate conservative treatment, or intractable radicular pain from epidural extension of the infection.[4,7] Delayed surgical treatment may be associated with higher rates of sepsis and impaired neurological status.[5] Spinal instrumentation may or may not be used and depends on the stability of the affected spinal segments or the presence of deformity.[7] Currently, there is a gap in the literature describing high levels of evidence for surgical versus nonsurgical intervention. Thus surgical indications and modalities are still controversial.[6]

Herein, we describe the case of a 60-year-old immunosuppressed woman who presented with nonspecific back pain and left dorsiflexion weakness and imaging concerning for lumbar osteomyelitis.

Example case

Chief complaint: back pain, weakness

History of present illness: A 60-year-old female patient with progressive back pain and left dorsiflexion weakness. She is immunosuppressed from a previous renal transplant and has no other constitutional symptoms. She also reports left greater than right leg pain when ambulating. The patient underwent a magnetic resonance (Fig. 62.1) and a computed tomography of the lumbar spine (Fig. 62.2) that showed the presence of vertebral osteomyelitis associated with discitis and ventral epidural collection.

Medications: immunosuppressants

Allergies: no known drug allergies

Past medical and surgical history: renal failure, immunosuppression, renal transplantation

Family history: none

Social history: none

Physical examination: awake, alert, and oriented to person, place, and time; cranial nerves II–XII intact; bilateral deltoids/triceps/biceps 5/5; interossei 5/5; iliopsoas/knee flexion/knee extension/plantar flexion 5/5; left dorsiflexion 4/5.

Reflexes: 2+ in bilateral biceps/triceps/brachioradialis with negative Hoffman; 2+ in bilateral patella/ankle; no clonus or Babinski; sensation intact to light touch

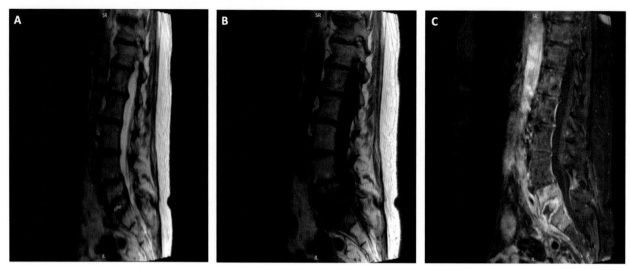

Fig. 62.1 Preoperative sagittal magnetic resonance image of the lumbar spine. (A) T2 sagittal image demonstrating high signal intensity in the disc space (suggestive of infectious fluid), L5 and S1 vertebral bodies (suggestive of marrow edema), and paraspinal soft tissue (suggestive of paraspinal infectious fluid or abscess). **(B)** T1 sagittal image demonstrating low signal intensity in the disc space, L5 and S1 vertebral bodies, and paraspinal soft tissue. **(C)** T1 postgadolinium image confirming L5-S1 spondylodiscitis with peripheral contrast enhancement around the disc space fluid collection. Additionally, it shows disc space narrowing and abnormal contrast enhancement of L5, S1, and paraspinal extension anteriorly and posteriorly resulting in a ventral epidural abscess.

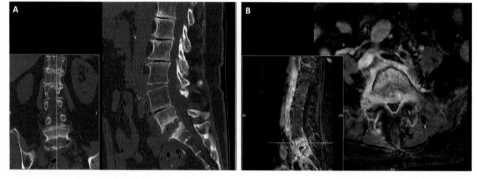

Fig. 62.2 Preoperative computed tomography scans. (A) Coronal and sagittal images demonstrating erosion of the caudal L5 and cranial S1 endplates and narrowing of the L4-5 disc space. **(B)** Sagittal and axial images demonstrating ventral epidural abscess causing moderate spinal canal stenosis and bilateral neuroforaminal stenosis.

	John H. Chi, MD, MPH Neurosurgery Brigham and Women's Hospital Boston, Massachusetts, United States	Luis Rodrigo Diaz Iniguez, MD Orthopaedic Surgery Hospital Angeles Lindavista Mexico City, Mexico	Juan Fernando Ramon, MD Neurosurgery University Hospital Fundacion Santa Fe de Bogata Bogota, Columbia	Anand Veeravagu, MD Neurosurgery Stanford University Palo Alto, California, United States
Preoperative				
Additional tests requested	Blood cultures Interventional radiology for biopsy	L-spine x-ray Infectious disease evaluation CBC/ESR/CRP Febrile antigen panel, BCG test	Infectious disease evaluation CBC/ESR/CRP	Standing flexion-extension lumbar x-rays
Surgical approach selected	If infection persistent after treatment and/or worsening symptoms, MIS L5-S1 TLIF and posterior percutaneous L4-5 fusion	Lumbar wound incision and drainage and biopsy of L5-S1 disc space	After antibiotics, L2-iliac posterior fusion	L4-S1 (possible S2) decompression and fusion

	John H. Chi, MD, MPH Neurosurgery Brigham and Women's Hospital Boston, Massachusetts, United States	Luis Rodrigo Diaz Iniguez, MD Orthopaedic Surgery Hospital Angeles Lindavista Mexico City, Mexico	Juan Fernando Ramon, MD Neurosurgery University Hospital Fundacion Santa Fe de Bogata Bogota, Columbia	Anand Veeravagu, MD Neurosurgery Stanford University Palo Alto, California, United States
Goal of surgery	Decompression, stabilization, debridement of infection	Drainage and washing, bacterial cultures, biopsy	Stabilization	Sample infection, debride L5-S1 level, stabilization
Perioperative				
Positioning	Prone	Prone	Prone	Prone on Jackson table
Surgical equipment	Fluoroscopy O-arm Surgical navigation Surgical microscope	Fluoroscopy	Fluoroscopy O-arm	IOM (SSEP/MEP) Surgical navigation
Medications	Liposomal bupivacaine	Hold antibiotics until sampling	None	Hold antibiotics until sampling
Anatomical considerations	Thecal sac, pedicles, disc space	Thecal sac, nerve root, intervertebral disc	Pedicles, transverse processes, facets	L5 nerve roots
Complications feared with approach chosen	Wound issues	Wound complication, progressive infection	Reinfection, CSF leak	Wound complication
Intraoperative				
Anesthesia	General	General	General	General
Exposure	L4-5	L5-sacrum	L2-sacrum	L4-S1
Levels decompressed	L4-5	L5	None	L4-S1
Levels fused	L4-5	None	L2-iliac	L4-S1
Surgical narrative	Position prone, place reference array on iliac crest, O-arm spin and navigation acquisition, bilateral paramedian incisions, place percutaneous MIS pedicle screws at L5-S1, dock MIS tubular retractor over L5-S1 facet joint for TLIF, facetectomy under microscope, TLIF and cage placement, swab disc space, irrigate with antibiotics, place vancomycin powder, place auto and allograft, place rods, standard closure	Position prone, midline incision L5-sacrum, dissect in surgical layers until reaching space between L5 lamina and sacrum, cut yellow ligament, protect thecal sac and nerve roots, take cultures, biopsy disc space, wash with antiseptic solution, place Garacoll if available, layered closure	Position prone, linear incision from L2-sacrum, dissection of paravertebral muscles, identify facets and transverse processes, locate pedicle insertion sites, placement of pedicle screws with fluoroscopic verification, verify pedicle integrity, insert screws from L2 to S1, locate iliac bone, wedge excision on iliac bone after dissection of iliac, iliac tunneling, iliac screw placement, layered closure with drain	Position prone on Jackson table, localizing x-ray, midline incision, insert pedicle screws L4-S1 using navigation, L5-S1 laminectomy with discectomy, send samples from disc space, irrigate with 3 L of vancomycin and gentamycin, insert rods, perform fusion with allograft from L4 to S1, close with subfascial drain, PICC line for antibiotics
Complication avoidance	MIS, percutaneous pedicle screws, indirect decompression of nerve roots	Aim for disc space, protect neural structures when biopsy disc, place Garacoll if possible	Anatomical placement of pedicle screws	Hold antibiotics until samples obtained, surgical navigation
Postoperative				
Admission	Floor	Floor	ICU	Floor
Postoperative complications feared	Persistent infection	Progress infection, neurological injury	Reinfection, neurological injury, CSF leak	Failure of fusion, wound breakdown
Anticipated length of stay	3–4 days	7 days	3 days	4–5 days

(continued on next page)

	John H. Chi, MD, MPH Neurosurgery Brigham and Women's Hospital Boston, Massachusetts, United States	Luis Rodrigo Diaz Iniguez, MD Orthopaedic Surgery Hospital Angeles Lindavista Mexico City, Mexico	Juan Fernando Ramon, MD Neurosurgery University Hospital Fundacion Santa Fe de Bogata Bogota, Columbia	Anand Veeravagu, MD Neurosurgery Stanford University Palo Alto, California, United States
Follow-up testing	Infectious disease follow-up L-spine x-ray 4 weeks after surgery MRI L-spine 3 months after surgery CT L-spine 3 months after surgery	CBC/ESR/CRP 48 hours after surgery	L-spine x-ray within 24 hours, and 1 month, 3 months, 6 months after surgery Monthly CBC/ESR/CRP	MRI L-spine 6 weeks after surgery Lumbar spine x-rays at 1 month, 3 months, 6 months, 12 months after surgery
Bracing	None	None	None	None
Follow-up visits	4 weeks, 3 months, 6 months after surgery	1 week after surgery	10 days, 1 month, 3 months, 6 months after surgery	2 weeks, 1 month, 3 months, 6 months, 1 year after surgery

BCG, Bacille Calmette–Guérin; *CBC*, complete blood count; *CRP*, C-reactive protein; *CSF*, cerebrospinal fluid; *CT*, computed tomography; *ESR*, erythrocyte sedimentation rate; *IOM*, intraoperative monitoring; *MEP*, motor evoked potential; *MIS*, minimally invasive surgery; *MRI*, magnetic resonance imaging; *SSEP*, somatosensory evoked potential; *TLIF*, transforaminal lumbar interbody fusion.

Differential diagnosis

- Vertebral osteomyelitis/discitis
- Malignancy
- Retroperitoneal infection
- Spondylosis
- Vertebral body and pars interarticularis fracture

Important anatomical and preoperative considerations

The metaphyseal region of the vertebrae has been described as the site of initial innoculation in cases of osteomyelitis.[8] Spinal arteries get access to the canal through the intervertebral foramen. The posterior central and prelaminar branches originate from this vessel and supply neural, meningeal, and epidural structures. Branches of the spinal artery ascend and descend between adjacent vertebral bodies above and below involving also the periphery of the intervertebral disc. Bacteria can spread hematogenously through these anastomoses and also by destruction of the nucleus pulposus toward the avascular disc.[8]

As aforementioned, most of the patients can be treated successfully with prolonged pharmacological therapy, especially if *S. aureus* is involved.[3,9] Antibiotics should be started just after susceptibility studies and there is no consensus regarding the appropriate length of the treatment. The majority of patients are treated between 4 and 6 weeks.[3] Patients harboring methicillin-resistant *Staphylococcus* frequently require surgical intervention for debridement.[10] A computed tomography (CT)-guided or open biopsy should be performed in cases with a pathogen that cannot be identified, poor response to medical treatment, and suspicion of polymicrobial infection.[3] Surgery is recommended for patients with symptoms of cord compression, radicular neurological deficit, deformity, or intractable pain.[3] Additionally, surgical intervention is always required in the case of infection associated with a spinal implant.[2,11]

What was actually done

This patient presented with progressive back pain and new-onset left dorsiflexion weakness, as well as MRI- and CT-proven vertebral osteomyelitis, discitis, and ventral epidural collection leading to complete spine instability. The patient first underwent a CT-guided biopsy, which did not yield any culture, probably due to the previous antibiotic treatment received at another institution. Due to the spine instability and radicular pain, the patient was offered instrumentation and discectomy at L5-S1 for culture and interbody fusion with the use of autograft. Once the patient was taken to the operative room and general anesthesia was provided, they were placed in the prone position and an incision was made from L2 to the pelvis. After the subperiosteal dissection from L2 to the pelvis was completed, the intraoperative O-arm was brought to the surgical field, and together with the stealth neuro navigation helped to verify the accuracy of the instrumentation. Screws were placed bilaterally from L2 to S1, including iliac bolts after iliac crest harvesting. Bilateral L5-S1 facetectomies were created, and the existing nerve roots were decompressed at the same level. Then, an L5-S1 discectomy was done, and debridement of the disc space and interbody fusion using the autograft obtained from both iliac crests. Additionally, disc material was obtained and sent for culture. A titanium rod and autograft obtained from the transverse and spinous processes were used to complete the L2-S1 fusion. Two Hemovac drains were placed after fluoroscopy confirmed adequate instrumentation. Vancomycin powder was used during wound closure. Postoperative x-rays demonstrated adequate hardware placement (Fig. 62.3). The patient was then placed on long-course IV antibiotics for 6 weeks and discharged to a rehabilitation facility on postoperative day 4, with a brace when out of bed. Follow-up evaluation showed remarkable improvement of previous symptoms.

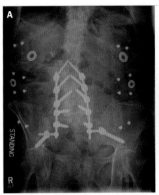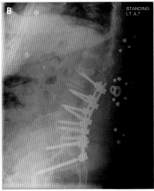

Fig. 62.3 Postoperative lumbar x-rays. (A) Anteroposterior and **(B)** lateral x-rays demonstrating adequate posterior fixation of the lumbar spine with rods and screws extending from the L2 through the sacrum with sacropelvic fusion.

Commonalities among the experts

Preoperative test assessment varied considerably with half opting for infectious disease evaluation and blood inflammation biomarkers. The majority advocated for a posterior lumbosacral or lumboiliac fusion. Half would pursue antibiotic therapy before surgical intervention. Goals of surgery were debridement and stabilization. Most were aware of the thecal sac, nerve roots, and pedicles. The most feared complication related to the surgical approach was the development of wound-related issues, such as reinfection. Surgery was completed with fluoroscopy, O-arm, and surgical navigation. Half recommended to hold antibiotics before sampling. Surgical approaches varied but the majority shared the concept of irrigation with antibiotics or antiseptic solution and provide stabilization. Following surgery, most admitted their patients to the floor to continue observation. Reinfection or persistent infection were the most common postoperative concerns. Follow-up image testing greatly varied with most recommending lumbar x-rays within the first postoperative month.

SUMMARY OF QUALITY OF EVIDENCE TO GUIDE SPECIFIC INTERVENTIONS FOR THIS CASE

- Antibiotic therapy just after debridement or biopsy: level II-2
- Posterior instrumented fusion provides stabilization in cases of osteomyelitis/discitis: level III
- Surgical intervention in cases of concomitant infection and spinal implants: level I

REFERENCES

1. Issa K, Diebo BG, Faloon M, et al. The Epidemiology of Vertebral Osteomyelitis in the United States From 1998 to 2013. *Clin Spine Surg.* 2018;31(2):E102–E108.
2. Zimmerli W. Clinical practice. Vertebral osteomyelitis. *N Engl J Med.* 2010;362(11):1022–1029.
3. Mylona E, Samarkos M, Kakalou E, Fanourgiakis P, Skoutelis A. Pyogenic vertebral osteomyelitis: a systematic review of clinical characteristics. *Semin Arthritis Rheum.* 2009;39(1):10–17.
4. Park KH, Cho OH, Lee YM, et al. Therapeutic outcomes of hematogenous vertebral osteomyelitis with instrumented surgery. *Clin Infect Dis.* 2015;60(9):1330–1338.
5. Segreto FA, Beyer GA, Grieco P, et al. Vertebral Osteomyelitis: A Comparison of Associated Outcomes in Early Versus Delayed Surgical Treatment. *Int J Spine Surg.* 2018;12(6):703–712.
6. Canouï E, Zarrouk V, Canouï-Poitrine F, et al. Surgery is safe and effective when indicated in the acute phase of hematogenous pyogenic vertebral osteomyelitis. *Infect Dis (Lond).* 2019;51(4):268–276.
7. Berbari EF, Kanj SS, Kowalski TJ, et al. 2015 Infectious Diseases Society of America (IDSA) Clinical Practice Guidelines for the Diagnosis and Treatment of Native Vertebral Osteomyelitis in Adults. *Clin Infect Dis.* 2015;61(6):e26–e46.
8. Wiley AM, Trueta J. The vascular anatomy of the spine and its relationship to pyogenic vertebral osteomyelitis. *J Bone Joint Surg Br.* 1959;41-b:796–809.
9. Chen WH, Jiang LS, Dai LY. Surgical treatment of pyogenic vertebral osteomyelitis with spinal instrumentation. *Eur Spine J.* 2007;16(9):1307–1316.
10. Shoji H, Urakawa T, Watanabe K, et al. Clinical features, outcomes, and survival factor in patients with vertebral osteomyelitis infected by methicillin-resistant staphylococci. *J Orthop Sci.* 2016;21(3):282–286.
11. Kowalski TJ, Berbari EF, Huddleston PM, Steckelberg JM, Mandrekar JN, Osmon DR. The management and outcome of spinal implant infections: contemporary retrospective cohort study. *Clin Infect Dis.* 2007;44(7):913–920.

63

Adult basilar invagination

Henry Ruiz-Garcia, MD and Fidel Valero-Moreno, MD

Introduction

Basilar invagination (BI) is among the common pathological conditions afflicting the cranio-cervical junction.[1] Primary development is associated with syndromic conditions such as trisomy 21, Ehlers-Danlos syndrome, and Marfan syndrome; secondary development is associated with inflammatory conditions such as rheumatoid arthritis[2] and bony abnormalities such as cervical-vertebral body fusions.[3] Other associated conditions include Chiari malformation, platybasia, and atlanto-axial (AA) instability.[1] BI is a dynamic condition characterized by progressive caudal displacement of the cervico-medullary junction that can be related to untreated odontoid displacement into the skull base.[4] The majority of patients present with occipital pain and gait ataxia[4] as a result of bulbomedullary compression and instability.[5,6] No management guidelines have been established for patients with BI thus far. The surgical management of BI is complex and must be tailored based on the inciting pathology, patient condition, and stability of the craniocervical junction and AA joints.[5] Patients may require prolonged traction before surgical fixation. A posterior-only approach may be employed, as the majority of cases involving a pannus from AA instability resolve after fusion. Other cases with a significantly retroflexed odontoid process may require a combined anterior/posterior approach with anterior odontoid resection.[1,2,4–8] In this chapter, we present the case of a patient with progressive quadriparesis and associated rheumatoid arthritis.

Example case

Chief complaint: progressive upper and lower extremity weakness

History of present illness: This is a 65-year-old female with a history of rheumatoid arthritis, hypothyroidism, and cervical stenosis status post C4–7 anterior cervical decompression and fusion (ACDF) in 2009 with progressive upper and lower extremity weakness. Approximately 6 months prior, she developed bilateral upper extremity weakness that

has progressed to her legs, and she is now wheelchair bound. She also presented with dysphagia and urinary incontinence since a month ago. She underwent computed tomography and magnetic resonance imaging demonstrating compression of the cervico-medullary junction (Fig. 63.1).

Medications: levothyroxine

Allergies: no known drug allergies

Past medical and surgical history: rheumatoid arthritis, hypothyroidism, cervical stenosis, anterior cervical decompression and fusion 10 years prior

Family history: none

Social history: healthcare worker, no smoking, occasional alcohol

Physical examination: awake, alert, and oriented to person, place, and time; cranial nerves II–XII intact; bilateral deltoids/triceps/biceps 5/5; interossei 5/5; iliopsoas/knee flexion/knee extension/dorsi, and plantar flexion 5/5

Reflexes: 3+ in bilateral biceps/triceps/brachioradialis with positive Hoffman; 3+ in bilateral patella/ankle; two beats of clonus; positive Babinski

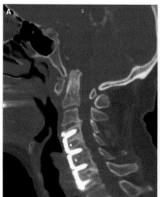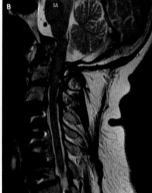

Fig. 63.1 Preoperative imaging. (A) Cervical sagittal computed tomography scan demonstrating basilar invagination with the dens projecting 15 mm above the Chamberlain line, and an atlas-dens interval was 4 mm. **(B)** Sagittal T2 magnetic resonance imaging confirming basilar invagination, with compression of the spinal cord at the C2 level and restriction of the cerebrospinal fluid circulation.

	Fabio Cofano, MD Neurosurgery University of Turin Turin, Italy	Eyal Itshayek, MD Neurosurgery Hadassah Medical Center Jerusalem, Israel	K. Daniel Riew, MD Orthopaedic Surgery Columbia University New York, New York, United States	Jean-Paul Wolinsky, MD Neurosurgery Northwestern University Chicago, Illinois, United States
Preoperative				
Additional tests requested	CTA Neurophysiological evaluation (MEP/SSEP)	CT craniocervical junction with flexion-extension CTA ENT evaluation of lower cranial nerves Anesthesia evaluation Preoperative traction using body weight for 3 days	CTA DEXA MRI T- and L-spine	Parasagittal CT to evaluate articulation of the occipital condyles to C1
Surgical approach selected	Endoscopic endonasal odontoidectomy with C1 arch preservation	C1-3 laminectomy, occipital-C5 fusion	Posterior occiput to C6 fusion, C1 laminectomy, distraction C1-2 with possible staged odontoidectomy	Stage 1: posterior C1-5 fusion, C1-2 laminectomy, attempted reduction of C1-2 subluxation Stage 2 (if stage 1 unsuccessful): anterior transcervical endoscopic odontoidectomy
Goal of surgery	Decompress cervico-medullary junction	Decompress cervico-medullary junction, stabilize spine	Decompress cervico-medullary junction, stabilize spine	Decompress cervico-medullary junction, stabilize spine
Perioperative				
Positioning	Supine with pins	Prone, with halo-ring	Prone, with Gardner-Wells tongs	Stage 1: prone, with Mayfield pins Stage 2: supine, with Mayfield frame
Surgical equipment	Surgical navigation Intraoperative CT 3D endoscopes IOM Laser Ultrasonic aspirator	IOM Fluoroscopy	Fluoroscopy Surgical microscope	Stage 1: IOM (MEP/SSEP) Fluoroscopy Ultrasound Ultrasonic bone scalpel Stage 2: IOM (MEP/SSEP) Angled endoscope Beveled tubular retractor Rotating Kerrison rongeurs Surgical navigation Ultrasonic aspirator
Medications	None	MAP >80	None	MAP >80
Anatomical considerations	Nasal cavities, nasopharynx, clivus, atlas, dens, cranio-cervical junction ligaments, internal carotid artery, vertebral artery, dura	Inion, posterior arch of C1, bifid spinous process of C2, C1-2 joint	Vertebral arteries, spinal cord	Vertebral arteries, spinal cord hypoglossal nerve, carotid arteries, pharynx, recurrent laryngeal nerve, dura
Complications feared with approach chosen	CSF leak, vessel injury, dysphagia	Brainstem/spinal cord injury, vertebral artery injury, CSF leak	Hematoma, infection, instrumentation failure with pull-out, loss of fixation	Inability to reduce, dysphagia, meningitis, CSF leak, instability
Intraoperative				
Anesthesia	General	General	General	General
Exposure	C2	Occiput-C5	Occiput-C6	Stage 1: C1-5 Stage 2: C1-2
Levels decompressed	C2	C1-3	C1	Stage 1: C1-2 Stage 2: C2
Levels fused	None	Occiput-C5	Occiput-C6	Stage 1: C1-5 Stage 2: none

	Fabio Cofano, MD Neurosurgery University of Turin Turin, Italy	Eyal Itshayek, MD Neurosurgery Hadassah Medical Center Jerusalem, Israel	K. Daniel Riew, MD Orthopaedic Surgery Columbia University New York, New York, United States	Jean-Paul Wolinsky, MD Neurosurgery Northwestern University Chicago, Illinois, United States
Surgical narrative	Position supine with head slightly tilted to left and flexed, navigation acquisition after intraoperative CT, find inferior margin of middle turbinate/nasopharynx and eustachian tubes and use as anatomical landmarks, displace inferior turbinates laterally, access nasopharyngeal cavity, remove posterior third of nasal septum, form a U-shaped nasopharyngeal mucosal and muscular layer flap with the laser from the inferior third of the clivus to the inferior edge of the C2 vertebral body, expose lateral masses of C1, subperiosteal skeletonization of anterior arch of C1 and odontoid process, resection of ALL and full exposure of atlanto-axial articulation, removal of lower clivus, removal of upper portion of anterior arch of C1, removal of tip and base of odontoid using ultrasonic curette, leave a residual shell to carefully dissect and section apical and alar ligaments, remove other adhesions, expose dura of the pontomedullary junction after excision of inflammatory tissue, use navigation to help with location, intraoperative CT to confirm adequacy of decompression, put U-shaped nasopharyngeal flap with fibrin glue, place foley catheter for 3 days to compress mucosal flap and allow its adhesion	CT immediately preoperative, awake transnasal endoscopic intubation, preoperative IOM baseline, positioned prone with maintaining traction, midline linear incision from inion to C5 spinous process, subperiosteal dissection, expose occipital bone/posterior arch of C1/spinous processes and lamina and lateral masses of C2-5, place C2 pedicle and C3-5 lateral mass screw holes, place occipital plates, C1-3 laminectomy, decorticate C1-2 articular surfaces, widen C1-2 joint space and place small cage filled with bone chips, place screws, bend titanium rods to fit into plate and screws connecting occipital plate down to lateral mass screws, decorticate bone lateral and caudal to occipital plate and lateral to screws, apply bone graft, layered closure with drain	Fiberoptic or awake intubation, placement in Garner-Wells tongs, position prone, obtain immediate fluoroscopy images to confirm no spinal malalignment, expose occiput to C6 using subperiosteal dissection, C1 laminectomy, instrument occiput and then C2 pedicles and then lateral mass C3-6, distract across C1-2 joint, add bone or cage into C1-2 joint to keep it distracted, fluoroscopy to evaluate amount of distraction, add structural allograft with BMP or take autograft, intraoperative CT, layered closure with subfascial drain; if neurologically not improved after 3-4 weeks, then anterior odontoidectomy	Stage 1: position prone, midline incision from C1-5, subperiosteal dissection of posterior arch of C1 and spinous processes/lamina of C2-5, dissection and mobilization of bilateral C2 nerve roots, ligate and section C2 nerve roots proximal to dorsal root ganglion if needed to access C1 lateral mass, expose and remove C1-2 joint, place pilot holes for C1 and C3-5 lateral mass instrumentation, C1-2 laminectomy, place lateral mass at C1 and C3-5 bilaterally, contour rods to span from C1-5 with extra length to allow distraction and reduction of deformity, attempt reduction by distracting C1-2 joints bilaterally with small laminar spreaders across joint, attempt reduction if prior did not work by fixing rods from C3-5 with locked locking nuts and loose locking nuts at C1, distract between C1 and C3 lateral mass screws and nuts locked down if reduction is achieved, continuous MEP and spinal cord visualization with ultrasound, reduce reduction if MEP changes, confirm reduction with O-arm and lateral x-rays, apply cross-link between C1 instrumentation, decorticate and apply autograft to joints, posterior arch can be used as a structural autograft if there is a large space from the distraction, layered closure with subfascial drain Stage 2 (same day): head fixed and secured in halo, attach array for surgical navigation, intraoperative O-arm and registered, incision made on prior side of previous ACDF ideally at C4-5 level staying above previous approach, standard ACDF approach, blunt dissection in loose areolar tissue to the level of anterior tubercle of C1, place beveled tubular retractor with lip sitting on anterior tubercle of C1 and opening of bevel over C2-C3 body, 30-degree endoscope inserted down fixed retractor, ventral surface of the mid portion of C3 and C2 body are removed with ultrasonic aspirator, continue to work toward tip of odontoid under C1 anterior arch, width of resection is width of odontoid estimated by resecting bone aided by navigation between medial aspect of bilateral C1-2 articulation, resect odontoid in top down fashion, caudal extent based on preoperative MRI and CT, remove transverse and apical ligaments with Kerrison, O-arm spin to confirm adequacy of decompression, layered closure

(continued on next page)

	Fabio Cofano, MD Neurosurgery University of Turin Turin, Italy	Eyal Itshayek, MD Neurosurgery Hadassah Medical Center Jerusalem, Israel	K. Daniel Riew, MD Orthopaedic Surgery Columbia University New York, New York, United States	Jean-Paul Wolinsky, MD Neurosurgery Northwestern University Chicago, Illinois, United States
Complication avoidance	Use middle turbinate/nasopharynx/eustachian tubes as anatomical landmarks, laser to form nasopharyngeal and muscle flap, preserve lower portion of anterior arch of C1, leave a shell of bone to help with dissecting ligaments, surgical navigation to help check position, intraoperative CT to evaluate decompression, foley catheter to place against flap to promote adhesion	Preop traction, preflip IOM, open C1-2 joint to promote fusion, C1-3 laminectomy	Attempt at only prone approach, avoid odontoidectomy if possible, place bone in C1-2 joint to keep it distracted, BMP to promote fusion	Avoid incorporating occiput into fusion to minimize dysphagia, section C2 nerve roots if necessary for instrumentation, longer rods to allow for attempted distraction and reduction of deformity, continuous MEP and ultrasound of spinal cord during attempted reductions, ventral approach rostral to previous ACDF, beveled tubular retractor, preserve C1 anterior arch, resect odontoid in top down fashion, resection aided by navigation, O-arm to confirm adequacy of decompression
Postoperative				
Admission	ICU	ICU	Floor	ICU
Postoperative complications feared	CSF leak, dysphagia, C1-2 instability	Pseudoarthrosis, new neurological deficit	Hematoma, infection, instrumentation failure with pull-out, loss of fixation	Stage 1: pseudoarthrosis, instrumentation failure, infection, inability to reduce compression, spinal cord injury Stage 2: CSF leak, dysphagia
Anticipated length of stay	4–5 days	3–5 days	3 days	4–5 days
Follow-up testing	Dynamic CT 1 months after surgery	CT craniocervical junction within 24 hours, 3 months after surgery C-spine AP/lateral x-rays 6 weeks after surgery MRI craniocervical junction 3 months after surgery	Cervical x-rays within 48 hours of surgery, 6 weeks, 6 months, 12 months after surgery	Cervical x-rays 2 weeks, 6 weeks, 3 months, 6 months, 1 year after surgery
Bracing	Philadelphia collar for 1 month	Rigid collar for 6–12 weeks	Hard collar for 6 weeks	None
Follow-up visits	1 month, 3 months, 6 months, 12 months after surgery	6 weeks, 3 months after surgery	6 weeks, 6 months, 12 months after surgery	2 weeks, 6 weeks, 3 months, 6 months, 1 year after surgery

ACDF, Anterior cervical decompression and fusion; *AP*, anteroposterior; *ALL*, anterior longitudinal ligament; *BMP*, bone morphogenic protein; *CSF*, cerebrospinal fluid; *CT*, computed tomography; *CTA*, computed tomography angiography; *DEXA*, dual-energy x-ray absorptiometry; *ENT*, ear, nose and throat; *ICU*, intensive care unit; *IOM*, intraoperative monitoring; *MAP*, mean arterial pressure; *MEP*, motor evoked potential; *SSEP*, somatosensory evoked potential.

Differential diagnosis

- Basilar invagination
- Atlanto-axial instability
- Platybasia
- Chiari malformation
- Occipital condyle hypoplasia
- Cranio-cervical junction tumor

Important anatomical and preoperative considerations

Stability and proper function of the cranio-cervical junction hinge on complex ligamentous and bony structures that confer most of the rotation and flexion-extension movements of the head and neck.[5] In symptomatic patients, crossing of the Chamberlain line is commonly used to determine the diagnosis of BI.[9,10] The Chamberlain line extends from the posterior tip of the hard palate to the posterior rim of the foramen magnum.[10] The degree of odontoid invagination ranges from 4 mm to more than 20 mm. BI should be considered severe when the tip of the odontoid process is more than 10 mm above the Chamberlain line.[10]

BI has been classified by several authors in two groups: BI with AA joint instability and BI without instability.[9,10] AA instability is determined by an increase in the atlantodental or clivodental interval.[10] For patients without cranial nerve abnormalities (which suggests low-level ventral compression),[6] and AA instability, craniovertebral realignment, stabilization, and subsequent posterior instrumentation and fusion can be the optimal surgical intervention.[6,10] Alignment can be attained with preoperative traction through a halo or intraoperative traction.[6,11] When BI is reducible via cervical traction, a posterior-only approach may be feasible.[11] In the setting of nonreducible BI, moderate to severe high ventral compression and cranial nerve deficits, an anterior decompression may be required, regardless of posterior complex stability. Moreover, an anterior approach is necessary when the C1-C2 complex is fused or the posterior distraction has failed to achieve appropriate ventral decompression.[6] A major disadvantage of the anterior approach is that odontoidectomy can precipitate cervical instability, especially when there is ligamentous laxity. In these cases, posterior instrumentation is necessary.[6]

What was actually done

Due to the severe compressive myelopathy and progressive quadriparesis, the decision was made to perform a staged anterior-posterior approach. In order to select the anterior approach, anatomical considerations were evaluated in the sagittal and coronal view of a preoperative computed tomography angiogram, which also allowed for evaluation of the surrounding vasculature (see Fig. 63.1). As the compression was located above the palatine line, an endonasal endoscopic odontoidectomy was performed in the first stage,[12] followed by a posterior decompression and occiput-C6 fusion. Transoral and transcervical approaches were also evaluated as potential options but not preferred. During the first approach, the patient was positioned supine, with the head fixed in neutral position. A septoplastic and low posterior septectomy was performed. Once the posterior nasopharynx was clearly identified, the bilateral carotids, location were confirmed by navigation and intraoperative Doppler. After this, a long U-shaped incision was made, and the soft palate was retracted using an 8-0 rubber catheter. The C1 arch and the lower third of the clivus were identified and drilled using a combination of a high-speed drill and an ultrasonic aspirator. Once the C2 dens were identified, the bone was drilled internally and eggshelled and outfractured. A 30-degree endoscope allowed for inferior and superior visualization during the drilling. The wound was irrigated with a vancomycin-impregnated saline solution, and fat was placed in the epidural space to reinforce the area. Closure was done by reapproximating the pharyngeal mucosa with dural sealant. Postoperative computed tomography scan confirmed good decompression (Fig. 63.2). The following day the patient underwent the posterior decompression and occiput-C6 fusion. A midline incision was made, followed

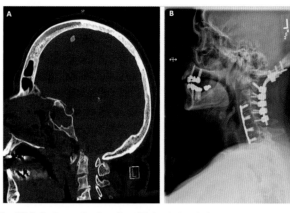

Fig. 63.2 Postoperative imaging. (A) Cervical sagittal computed tomography scan showing removal of the inferior clivus, anterior C1 arch, and tip of the dens with anterior decompression of the cervico-medullary junction. **(B)** Lateral cervical x-ray demonstrating occiput through C6 instrumented fusion. Anterior cervical fusion C4-C7 performed years prior is also appreciated.

by subperiosteal dissection. An occipital plate, C2 pedicle, and C3-6 lateral mass screws were placed with a C1-2 laminectomy. The fusion was supplemented with iliac crest bone grafts, demineralized bone matrix, and bone morphogenic protein (BMP). There were no complications, and the patient was discharged to rehabilitation at postoperative day 5. At 10 months' follow-up, the patient showed excellent improvement and was able to carry out her activities of daily living. Postoperative x-rays showed good location of the instrumentation (see Fig. 63.2).

Commonalities among the experts

Most requested a computed tomography angiogram of the craniocervical junction to better evaluate the vascular structures involved, namely the vertebral arteries. The other recommended tests varied and included lower cranial nerves evaluation, neurophysiological evaluation, and bone density scans. Most would attain surgery primarily through a posterior laminectomy, ranging from C1 to C3, depending on the surgeon preference. The main purpose of surgery was to decompress the cervico-medullary junction and to stabilize the spine. Instrumented fusion from the occipital bone to at least the level of C5 was advocated by the majority. Most were cognizant of the vertebral and carotid arteries, spinal cord, and bony landmarks. Approach-related most feared complications were vascular injury, neural elements damage, cerebrospinal fluid leak, and infection. Surgery was assisted by intraoperative monitoring, microscope, ultrasound, and endoscope. No special medications were recommended preoperatively. Surgical nuances varied but the majority highlighted the importance of occipito-cervical fusion with instrumentation of lateral masses in order to allow distraction and reduction of the deformity. Most of the physicians admitted their patients to the intensive care unit after surgery. Follow-up testing preferences also varied. Most advocated for rigid collar use, and close follow-up with imaging during the first postoperative year.

SUMMARY OF QUALITY OF EVIDENCE TO GUIDE SPECIFIC INTERVENTIONS FOR THIS CASE

- Posterior occipito-cervical fusion for distraction and reduction of cranio-cervical junction deformity: level III
- Postoperative use of rigid collar after surgical reduction of basilar invagination: level III
- Anterior versus posterior approaches for cervico-medullary compression: level III

REFERENCES

1. Goel A. Basilar invagination, syringomyelia and Chiari formation and their relationship with atlantoaxial instability. *Neurol India.* 2018;66(4):940–942.
2. Ferrante A, Ciccia F, Giammalva GR, et al. The Craniovertebral Junction in Rheumatoid Arthritis: State of the Art. *Acta Neurochir Suppl.* 2019;125:79–86.
3. Goel A. Cervical Fusion as a Protective Response to Craniovertebral Junction Instability: A Novel Concept. *Neurospine.* 2018;15(4):323–328.
4. Klekamp J. Treatment of basilar invagination. *Eur Spine J.* 2014;23(8):1656–1665.
5. Joaquim AF, Ghizoni E, Giacomini LA, Tedeschi H, Patel AA. Basilar invagination: Surgical results. *J Craniovertebr Junction Spine.* 2014;5(2):78–84.
6. Chaudhry NS, Ozpinar A, Bi WL, Chavakula V, Chi JH, Dunn IF. Basilar Invagination: Case Report and Literature Review. *World Neurosurg.* 2015;83(6). 1180.e1187–1111.
7. Chibbaro S, Ganau M, Cebula H, et al. The Endonasal Endoscopic Approach to Pathologies of the Anterior Craniocervical Junction: Analytical Review of Cases Treated at Four European Neurosurgical Centres. *Acta Neurochir Suppl.* 2019;125:187–195.
8. Kahilogullari G, Eroglu U, Yakar F, Beton S, Meco C, Caglar YS. Endoscopic Endonasal Approaches to Craniovertebral Junction Pathologies: A Single-Center Experience. *Turk Neurosurg.* 2018; 29(4):486–492.
9. Botelho RV, Ferreira JA, Zandonadi Ferreira ED. Basilar Invagination: A Craniocervical Kyphosis. *World Neurosurg.* 2018;117:e180–e186.
10. Goel A, Jain S, Shah A. Radiological Evaluation of 510 Cases of Basilar Invagination with Evidence of Atlantoaxial Instability (Group A Basilar Invagination). *World Neurosurg.* 2018;110:533–543.
11. Pinter NK, McVige J, Mechtler L. Basilar Invagination, Basilar Impression, and Platybasia: Clinical and Imaging Aspects. *Curr Pain Headache Rep.* 2016;20(8):49.
12. Ruiz-Garcia H, Gassie K, Marenco-Hillembrand L, Donaldson AM, Chaichana KL. *Endoscopic endonasal odontoidectomy for the treatment of basilar invagination.* 2020;3(1):V3.

64

Spinal type I AVF

Fidel Valero-Moreno, MD and Henry Ruiz-Garcia, MD

Introduction

Spinal dural arteriovenous fistulas (dAVFs) are the most common vascular lesion of the spinal cord, and they account for 70% of all AV shunts of the spine.[1–3] Type I dAVFs are defined as an abnormal intradural low flow communication between a radiculomeningeal artery and a radicular vein (radiculomedullary vein) draining into the intradural venous plexus.[1,2,4] In general, spinal vascular malformations encompass 3% to 4% of all intradural spinal cord masses. Men are affected five times more often than women, and the fistulous abnormality usually occupies the thoracolumbar region (80%).[2,5] The mean age at the time of diagnosis is 55 to 60 years.[2,4] This condition is usually underdiagnosed, in part because of its insidious neurological decline, which can cause acute, subacute, or chronic cord dysfunction, and also due to its challenging diagnosis.[1,6] Congestion of the venous outflow of the spinal cord leads to mass effect and ischemia, resulting in progressive myelopathy that often mimics an anterior horn neurological disorder.[4] Patients typically present with lower-extremity weakness (75%), pain (52%), and sensory disturbances (60%).[7,8] Most of the patients will develop a stepwise progressive neurological deterioration.[7] Spinal cord hemorrhage due to a dural AVF is a rare occurrence.[9] Initial diagnosis is attained with magnetic resonance imaging (MRI) and MR angiography (MRA); however, definitive diagnosis requires spinal digital subtraction angiography (DSA) to appropriately categorize the condition and establish the extent of the disease.[2] The progressive nature of the disorder and the necessity to halt and reverse the gradual neurological deterioration undoubtedly require timely intervention.[1,2,6,7] Treatment should attain complete occlusion of the shunting zone and restore normal spinal cord perfusion and intravascular pressures.[2,6] This can be achieved by either surgical obliteration or endovascular embolization.[1,2,6]

Example case

Chief complaint: lower limb weakness and urinary incontinence

History of present illness: This is a 55-year-old male with progressive lower extremity weakness and new-onset urinary incontinence. He was referred after receiving a magnetic resonance imaging (MRI) report showing tortuous dorsal venous structures. Additionally, spinal angiogram demonstrated a feeding vessel from the left sacral artery (Fig. 64.1).

Medications: none

Allergies: not known

Past medical and surgical history: none

Family history: none

Social history: none

Physical examination: awake, alert, and oriented to person, place, and time; cranial nerves II–XII intact; bilateral deltoids/triceps/biceps 5/5; interossei 5/5; iliopsoas/knee flexion/knee extension 3/5, and dorsi and plantar flexion 4/5

Reflexes: 2+ in bilateral biceps/triceps/brachioradialis with negative Hoffman; 3+ in bilateral patella/ankle; two beats of clonus and positive Babinski; decreased sensation to light touch diffusely throughout bilateral lower extremities

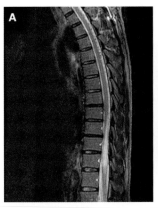
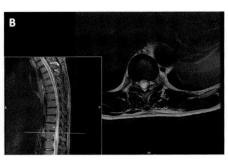
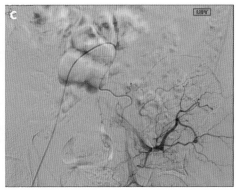

Fig. 64.1 Preoperative imaging. (A) Sagittal T2 image demonstrating abnormal vascularity extending along the thoracic and lumbar spinal canal with mild expansion with increased T2 signal and patchy enhancement in the distal thoracic cord extending from the inferior aspect of T8 to the conus. **(B)** Axial T2 image demonstrating cross-sectional increased T2 signal at the T10-T11 level. **(C)** Spinal angiogram showing dural arteriovenous fistula at the T11 segmental level, feeding vessel was a branch of the lateral sacral artery entering the left T10 neural foramen.

	Nicolas Dea, MD, MSc Neurosurgery Vancouver Spine Surgery Institute Vancouver, Canada	Diego F Gómez MD MSc. Neurosurgery Fundación Santafe de Bogotá Bogota, Colombia	Michael T. Lawton, MD Fabio Frisoli, MD Harrison Farber, MD Neurosurgery Barrow Neurological Institute Phoenix, Arizona, United States	Jang Yoon, MD Neurosurgery University of Pennsylvania Philadelphia, Pennsylvania, United States
Preoperative				
Additional tests requested	Anesthesia evaluation	EMG/NCS/SSEP Anesthesia evaluation	Complete spinal angiogram Urological evaluation MRI L-spine	MRI C- and L-spine Spinal angiogram if edema present in cervical or lumbar spine
Surgical approach selected	T10-T11 laminectomy and obliteration of spinal AV fistula	T10-11 laminoplasty for obliteration of spinal AV fistula	T10-11 laminectomy for obliteration of spinal AV fistula	T10-11 laminectomy for obliteration of spinal AV fistula
Goal of surgery	Disconnect fistula	Disconnect fistula, eliminate venous congestion	Disconnect fistula	Disconnect fistula
Perioperative				
Positioning	Prone on Jackson table with pins	Prone, no pins	Prone on Jackson table	Prone on Wilson frame on Jackson table
Surgical equipment	Endovascular Fluoroscopy. Surgical microscope. IOM (MEP/SSEP) if cord feeder involved. Temporary clip.	IOM (MEP/SSEP) Fluoroscopy Ultrasound Surgical microscope Miniclips	IOM (MEP/SSEP) Fluoroscopy Surgical microscope with ICG	IOM (MEP/SSEP) Fluoroscopy Surgical microscope with ICG Dural sealant
Medications	None	Steroids, Maintain MAP	Steroids, Maintain MAP >75	None
Anatomical considerations	Spinal cord feeders	Spinal cord, veins	Spinal cord, nerve roots, posterior spinal artery, artery of Adamkiewicz, dentate ligaments	Thoracic spinal cord, en passage spinal arteries and veins
Complications feared with approach chosen	Spinal cord infarct	Spinal cord infarct, hemorrhage	Spinal cord injury, nerve root injury, spinal cord infarct	Incomplete disconnection, presence of multiple fistulas
Intraoperative				
Anesthesia	General	General	General	General
Exposure	T10-T11	T10-11	T10-T11	T10-T11
Levels decompressed	T10-T11	T10-11	T10-T11	T10-T11
Levels fused	None	None	None	None

(continued on next page)

	Nicolas Dea, MD, MSc Neurosurgery Vancouver Spine Surgery Institute Vancouver, Canada	Diego F Gómez MD MSc. Neurosurgery Fundación Santafe de Bogotá Bogota, Colombia	Michael T. Lawton, MD Fabio Frisoli, MD Harrison Farber, MD Neurosurgery Barrow Neurological Institute Phoenix, Arizona, United States	Jang Yoon, MD Neurosurgery University of Pennsylvania Philadelphia, Pennsylvania, United States
Surgical narrative	Position prone, xray localisation. midline incision. T10-t11 laminectomy centered on the t10 foramen. midline durotomy and tenting sutures. identify culprit vessels. if doubt about cord feeder use IOM and temporary clip. Temporary decrease MAP and monitor for any change. If pre-op angio confirms that there is no spinal cord feeder involved then just localised abnormal vessel. Then take vessel at its intradural entrance. Note change of color of arterialized veins. Watertight dural closure. No drain. Bed rest × 24h.	Position prone, 3D fluoroscopy to localize level, midline incision where neuroradiology demarcated shunt, subperiosteal dissection exposing posterior elements, two-level laminoplasty, ultrasound to identify tortuous vein, midline dural opening and tenting sutures, identify arterialized medullar vein under microscope usually near the entrance of the dorsal root, disconnect fistula immediate at entrance using min-clips, monitor SSEP/MEP if clip reversal is needed, pay attention to the change in color of arterialized vein, watertight dural closure with fibrin sealant, laminoplasty with titanium plates, layered closure with no drain	Position prone, skin incision localized with fluoroscopy, surgical dissection carried out in the midline, expose lamina of correct level and confirm with fluoroscopy, laminectomy, dura is opened and tacked up under microscopic visualization, dorsal nerve roots followed to the root sleeve to identify the radiculomedullary artery, dentate ligaments may be cut to gently rotate the spinal cord, ICG videoangiography and microdissection to identify fistulous point, place clip on vein as close to the fistula as possible, fistula is cauterized and then divided sharply, ICG used to confirm obliteration of the fistula and preservation of normal vasculature, dura is closed with dural sealant, closure in layers	Position prone, confirm fistulous location on spinal angiogram, count levels in both anterior-posterior and lateral, midline incision from T10 to T11, expose posterior elements, preserve posterior tension band and facet complexes, reconfirm level with fluoroscopy, open dura, tack up dura, identify fistulous point with surgical microscope, confirm location with ICG injected intravenously, place aneurysm clip on abnormal arterial feeder near fistulous point, look for change in color in venous drainage, confirm obliteration with ICG, disconnect fistulous point with bipolar and microscissors, final ICG, watertight dural closure with dural sealant, closure in layers, bed rest until next day
Complication avoidance	Ensure good level with fluoroscopy. Alternatively, radiology can leave a coil for localisation during diagnostic spinal angiogram. Ensure no spinal cord feeder involved in the fistula. If any doubt use temporary clip and IOM. Ensure only one vessel contributing to the fistula. Watertight closure with dural sealant.	3D fluoroscopy to help localize level, laminoplasty, ultrasound to identify tortuous vein, disconnect fistula at dural entrance, monitor SSEP/MEP if clip reversal is needed, pay attention to the change in color of arterialized vein	Follow nerve roots to the root sleeve to identify radiculomedullary artery, cut dentate ligaments to rotate spinal cord, ICG video angiography, place clip on vein as close to fistula as possible to avoid venous aneurysm	Count in both anteroposterior and lateral, preserve posterior tension brand and facet complexes, ICG to evaluate fistula and confirm disconnection
Postoperative				
Admission	Floor	ICU	ICU	ICU
Postoperative complications feared	Spinal cord infarct. CSF leak. Epidural hematoma.	Spinal cord/nerve root injury	Spinal cord/nerve root injury, spinal infarct, CSF leak	Residual fistula, pseudomeningocele, wrong level surgery
Anticipated length of stay	2-3 days	2 days	2–3 days	3–5 days
Follow-up testing	Intraprocedural angiogram MRI 2 month post-op. If residual tortuous vein, no change in cord signal change or no clinical improvement: follow-up angiogram.	Spinal angiogram within 48 hours	Spinal angiogram during hospitalization after surgery MRI T-spine 6 months after surgery	Standing T- and L-spine x-rays 6 weeks after surgery MRI T- and L-spine 12 weeks, 1 year, 2 years after surgery Repeat spinal angiogram if needed
Bracing	None	None	None	None
Follow-up visits	2 months after surgery	2 weeks after surgery	10–14 days, 6 weeks, 6 months after surgery	2 weeks, 6 weeks, 3 months, 6 months, 12 months, 24 months after surgery

AV, Arteriovenous; *CSF*, cerebrospinal fluid; *EMG*, electromyogram; *ICG*, indocyanine green; *ICU*, intensive care unit; *IOM*, intraoperative monitoring; *MAP*, mean arterial pressure; *MEP*, motor evoked potential; *MRI*, magnetic resonance imaging; *NCS*, nerve conduction study; *SSEP*, somatosensory evoked potential.

Differential diagnosis

- Radicular arteriovenous malformations
- Epidural arteriovenous shunts
- Polyneuropathy
- Degenerative disk disease
- Spinal tumors

Important anatomical and preoperative considerations

As aforementioned in this book, the anterior spinal artery derives from the two vertebral arteries, while the paired posterolateral spinal arteries originate from the preatlantal part of the vertebral artery and occasionally from the posteroinferior cerebellar artery.[3,10] The three vessels form a longitudinal axis from the level of the basilar artery to the filum terminale. However, they do not supply blood to the entire spinal cord.[2,3] Segmental arteries arise from the vertebral-subclavian arteries, the thoracoabdominal aorta, and the internal iliac arteries.[10] The segmental arteries supply the spine, including the vertebral bodies, paraspinal muscles, dura, nerve roots, and the spinal cord.[2,3,10] Each segmental artery gives rise to a dorsospinal branch, which is also called the spinal radicular artery. The radicular artery branches into ventral, middle, and dorsal branches in the intervertebral foramen.[3,10] The ventral and dorsal branches supply the dura mater and vertebral bone. The middle division (radiculomeningeal artery) supplies the dura mater and the nerve root at each segment and is contiguous with the intervertebral foramen. Moreover, from this division (middle), the radiculomedullary and radiculopial arteries branch. The radiculomedullary artery supplies the spinal cord and the radiculopial artery reaches the surface of the cord.[10]

The venous anatomy of the spinal cord is divided into intrinsic and extrinsic systems.[10] The spinal cord is drained intrinsically by the radial perforation veins, which in turn connect to a pial venous network on the spinal cord surface. The anterior sulcal vein runs ventrally in the anterior median sulcus. The posterior counterpart, the posterior sulcal vein, occupies the posterior median sulcus. Eventually, the vessels drain into the anterior spinal vein and posterior spinal vein, respectively.[10] The pial venous plexus, as well as the anterior and posterior spinal veins, configurate to form the external venous drainage of the spine. The pial venous plexus (coronal venous plexus) is a longitudinal and axially anastomosed plexus on the cord surface. These superficial venous elements are drained by the radiculomedullary vein (radicular vein). In the intervertebral foramen, the radicular veins join the epidural veins and form the internal vertebral plexus, which establish the segmental communications with the external vertebral plexus. This plexus, in turn, joins the caval system through the innominate veins at the cervical level, the azygos vein at the thoracic level, and the ascending lumbar vein at lumbar level.[10]

A dAVF is situated between the outer and inner layers of the dura mater, close to the nerve root at the intervertebral foramen. Classically, this condition is defined as an arteriovenous communication linking the dural branch of the radicular artery with the radiculomedullary vein. Sometimes, the fistula may be supplied by multiple feeders.[11] Consequently, dilated and tortuous veins appear on the surface of the spinal cord, causing retrograde flow of shunted blood, resulting in venous congestion and mass effect.[2,3,10] This occurrence leads to chronic hypoxia and progressive myelopathy.[3] On magnetic imaging, dAVFs are characterized by cord edema and perimedullary dilated vessels. T2-weighted images can demonstrate swelling of the spinal cord with a centrally located hyperintensity, as well as a hypointense flow void dorsal to the cord, which may indicate enlarged and tortuous veins.[3,4,12] Even though MRI is an essential tool for the initial diagnosis of dAVFs, which can identify these abnormalities in 67% to 100% of patients, angiography is still the gold standard for the diagnosis. It is also critical for determining the exact location (height) of the fistula and its angio-architecture.[4,9] The angio-architecture is important to understand because if the dAVF feeder is a segmental medullary artery, it will entail a high risk of spinal cord ischemia if embolized, and therefore open surgical treatment is preferred in these situations.[4]

The treatment of spinal dAVF hinges on surgical occlusion and endovascular therapy.[3,4,9] Due to its minimal invasiveness and the ability to diagnose and treat in a single procedure, endovascular therapy is considered the first option in some centers.[9,11] However, success rates of endovascular therapy broadly varied, ranging between 25% and 75%.[3,9] Several factors may affect the effectiveness of this treatment modality including the use of particles such as polyvinyl alcohol (PVA) and liquid cyanoacrylates,[11] endovascular techniques including filling of the fistula itself without embolization of the draining vein and when there is arterial wall dissection of the feeding vessels during catheterization,[4] and when the fistula is made up of several small feeding arteries.[4,9] For the treatment to be efficient, the embolic agent should occlude the fistula site, including the proximal draining vein.[4,9] Those patients in whom endovascular treatment have failed require prompt surgical intervention.[3,11] A meta-analysis of the literature demonstrated a complete obliteration rate of 98% with surgical occlusion of the fistula.[9,11] Surgery was associated to improvement or stabilization of symptoms within 12 months of follow-up, but long-term outcomes remain unclear.[11] Surgical treatment is typically done through a laminectomy or laminoplasty with interruption of the draining vein. The two main complications associated with surgical approaches are pseudomeningoceles and instability after laminectomy.[11]

What was actually done

The patient presented with a symptomatic dAVF. This was located near the midline at the S1 segmental level and was supplied by a branch of the lateral sacral artery entering the left L3 neural foramen based on angiography (Fig. 64.1). A transarterial therapeutic embolization was attempted, but it was not possible because of the difficulty in navigating the feeding branch. The next day the patient was taken to the operating room in order to perform a T10-T11 laminectomy and ligation of the spinal dAVF. The patient was placed in the prone position on the Jackson table, and after a lumbosacral midline incision, a T10-T11 laminectomy was done. Under microscopic visualization, the arterial feeding vessel was identified running over the dorsal aspect of the dural sac that ran toward the midline, until the arterialized vein emerged at the level of the attachment of the filum terminale. The dura was opened in the midline and the arterialized vein was followed rostrally to confirm it was the correct target. The vein was coagulated and disconnected, and the feeding vessel was

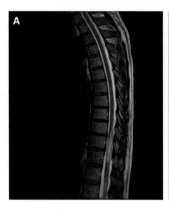
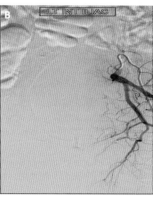

Fig. 64.2 Postoperative follow-up images. (A) Sagittal T2 image showing confluent T2 hyperintensity involving the distal thoracic cord, which is now better demarcated from adjacent cord parenchyma, less longitudinally extensive (spanning T9-T11 compared with T8-T12 on prior imaging), and less expansile. **(B)** Left internal iliac artery spinal angiogram with no evidence of arteriovenous shunting or other spinal vascular abnormality.

occluded. The dura was then closed in a watertight fashion. Intraoperative somatosensory and motor-evoked potentials were used and were unchanged during the entire procedure. Immediate postoperative angiogram showed resolution of the treated fistula and postoperative MRI showed decreased T2 signal in spinal cord (Fig. 64.2).

Commonalities among the experts

Half of the surgeons advocated for a spinal angiogram and additional MRI of the cervical and lumbar spine. The majority would perform surgery as the initial treatment through a laminectomy. One surgeon opted for endovascular obliteration. All agreed the goal of surgical intervention was disconnection of the fistula. Most were aware of the spinal cord and vascular structures such as cord feeders. The most feared complication was spinal cord injury in the form of either infarction or hemorrhage. Surgery was generally conducted with intraoperative monitoring, fluoroscopy, and surgical microscope. Half recommended perioperative steroids. Following surgery, the majority would admit their patients to the intensive care unit. Half advocated for a postoperative spinal angiogram during hospitalization to confirm fistula occlusion. Additionally, most requested a thoracic magnetic resonance imaging 3 to 6 months after intervention.

SUMMARY OF QUALITY OF EVIDENCE TO GUIDE SPECIFIC INTERVENTIONS FOR THIS CASE

- Surgical occlusion of the fistula has shown a complete obliteration rate of 98%: level I
- Prompt surgical obliteration for residual disease after attempted endovascular embolization: level II.2

REFERENCES

1. Adeeb N, Moore JM, Alturki AY, et al. Type I Spinal Arteriovenous Fistula with Ventral Intradural Venous Drainage: A Proposal of a Modified Classification. *Asian J Neurosurg.* 2018;13(4):1048–1052.
2. Krings T, Geibprasert S. Spinal dural arteriovenous fistulas. *AJNR Am J Neuroradiol.* 2009;30(4):639–648.
3. Krings T, Lasjaunias PL, Hans FJ, et al. Imaging in spinal vascular disease. *Neuroimaging Clin N Am.* 2007;17(1):57–72.
4. Jellema K, Tijssen CC, van Gijn J. Spinal dural arteriovenous fistulas: a congestive myelopathy that initially mimics a peripheral nerve disorder. *Brain.* 2006;129(Pt 12):3150–3164.
5. Li J, Li G, Bian L, et al. Concomitant Lumbosacral Perimedullary Arteriovenous Fistula and Spinal Dural Arteriovenous Fistula. *World Neurosurg.* 2017;105 1041.e1047-1041.e1014.
6. Flores BC, Klinger DR, White JA, Batjer HH. Spinal vascular malformations: treatment strategies and outcome. *Neurosurg Rev.* 2017;40(1):15–28.
7. Rangel-Castilla L, Russin JJ, Zaidi HA, et al. Contemporary management of spinal AVFs and AVMs: lessons learned from 110 cases. *Neurosurg Focus.* 2014;37(3):E14.
8. Ropper AE, Gross BA, Du R. Surgical treatment of Type I spinal dural arteriovenous fistulas. *Neurosurg Focus.* 2012;32(5):E3.
9. Chaudhary N, Pandey AS, Gemmete JJ. Endovascular treatment of adult spinal arteriovenous lesions. *Neuroimaging Clin N Am.* 2013;23(4):729–747.
10. Miyasaka K, Asano T, Ushikoshi S, Hida K, Koyanagi I. Vascular anatomy of the spinal cord and classification of spinal arteriovenous malformations. *Interv Neuroradiol.* 2000;6 Suppl 1(Suppl 1):195–198.
11. Steinmetz MP, Chow MM, Krishnaney AA, et al. Outcome after the treatment of spinal dural arteriovenous fistulae: a contemporary single-institution series and meta-analysis. *Neurosurgery.* 2004;55(1):77–87. discussion 87-78.
12. Hurst RW, Grossman RI. Peripheral spinal cord hypointensity on T2-weighted MR images: a reliable imaging sign of venous hypertensive myelopathy. *AJNR Am J Neuroradiol.* 2000; 21(4):781–786.

65

Cavernous malformation

Fidel Valero-Moreno, MD and Henry Ruiz-Garcia, MD

Introduction

Cavernous malformations (CMs) rarely occur in the spinal cord and account for less than 10% of all CMs.[1] However, since the broad use of high-resolution magnetic scans, CMs of the spinal cord are found more often and currently represent 20% of all the intramedullary spinal tumors.[2] They generally present in younger populations (second and third decade) and do not appear to have a sex predilection. CMs represent low flow vascular malformations but may have hemorrhagic events leading to neurological injury. The annual hemorrhage rate appears to be approximately 1% to 3% and is comparable to intracranial lesions, but this metric is difficult to assess and is reliant on the appearance of new or worsened patient symptoms. CMs may be managed with conservative observation or surgical intervention.[3] The natural history of spinal cord CMs is not well defined, and the neurological outcomes after surgical intervention are not well understood.[3–5] In this chapter, we present the case of a young female patient with a spinal CM with mild symptomatology and no evidence of spinal cord hemorrhage.

Example case

Chief complaint: bilateral upper extremity paresthesias
History of present illness: This is a 38-year-old female with a 4-week history of sudden onset numbness and tingling in her bilateral upper extremities. She describes an event that occurred 1 month prior in which she had sudden onset of weakness in her bilateral upper extremities that had improved, but since that time she has had persistent paresthesias. A magnetic resonance image was advocated as part of her evaluation for her current condition. The study demonstrated an intramedullary lesion at the level of C5 (Fig. 65.1).

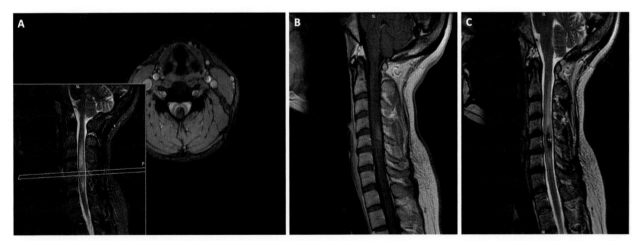

Fig. 65.1 Preoperative magnetic resonance images of the cervical spine. (A) Sagittal and axial T2-weighted images demonstrating an intramedullary cavernous malformation in the central part of the cord at the C5 level. **(B)** Sagittal T1 with contrast image demonstrating a hypointense intramedullary mass with minimal enhancement. **(C)** Sagittal T2-weighted image demonstrating the classic hyperintense core and a hypointense surrounding rim characteristic of an intramedullary cavernomas. Some cord edema is evident.

Medications: oral contraceptives
Allergies: no known drug allergies
Past medical and surgical history: none
Family history: none
Social history: none
Physical examination: awake, alert, and oriented to person, place, and time; cranial nerves II–XII intact; bilateral deltoids/

triceps/biceps 5/5; interossei 5/5; iliopsoas/knee flexion/knee extension/dorsi, and plantar flexion 5/5
Reflexes: 3+ in bilateral biceps/triceps/brachioradialis with negative Hoffman; 3+ in bilateral patella/ankle; clonus in bilateral feet, positive Babinski; sensation decreased in both upper and lower extremities

	John H. Chi, MD, MPH Neurosurgery Brigham and Women's Hospital Boston, Massachusetts, United States	Fernando Hakim, MD Hospital Universitario Fundacion Santafe de Bogota Bogota, Colombia	Michael T. Lawton, MD Fabio Frisoli, MD Harrison Farber, MD Neurosurgery Barrow Neurological Institute Phoenix, Arizona, United States	Davide Nasi, MD Neurosurgery Polytechnic University of Marche, Umberto Ancona, Italy
Preoperative				
Additional tests requested	None	Spinal angiogram MRI brain Anesthesiology evaluation Neurophysiological testing (MEP/SSEP)	MRI C-spine with contrast C-spine flexion-extension x-rays	Spinal angiogram MRI C-spine tractography Neurophysiological testing (MEP/SSEP)
Surgical approach selected	C4-5 laminectomy for resection of cavernous malformation	C4-5 laminoplasty for resection of cavernous malformation	C4-5 laminectomy for resection of cavernous malformation	C4-5 laminectomy for resection of cavernous malformation
Goal of surgery	Gross total resection	Gross total resection	Gross total resection, preservation of neurological function	Lesion removal with resolution of syrinx
Perioperative				
Positioning	Prone with Mayfield pins	Prone with Mayfield pins	Prone with Mayfield pins in Jackson table	Prone with Mayfield pins
Surgical equipment	Fluoroscopy IOM (MEP/SSEP) Surgical microscope	Fluoroscopy IOM (MEP/SSEP) Piezoelectric drill Ultrasound Surgical microscope	Fluoroscopy IOM (MEP/SSEP) Surgical microscope	Fluoroscopy IOM (MEP/SSEP) Ultrasound Surgical microscope
Medications	Steroids	Mannitol, maintain MAP	Steroids, maintain MAP >75	Steroids, MAP >100
Anatomical considerations	Spinal cord, dorsal midline	Spinal cord	Rexed lamina of spinal cord, midline dorsal raphe between dorsal columns	Spinal cord
Complications feared with approach chosen	Spinal cord injury	Spinal cord injury, spinal instability	Spinal cord injury	Spinal cord injury, CSF leak
Intraoperative				
Anesthesia	General	General	General	General
Exposure	C4-5	C4-5	C4-5	C4-5
Levels decompressed	C4-5	C4-5	C4-5	C4-5
Levels fused	None	None	None	None

	John H. Chi, MD, MPH Neurosurgery Brigham and Women's Hospital Boston, Massachusetts, United States	Fernando Hakim, MD Hospital Universitario Fundacion Santafe de Bogota Bogota, Colombia	Michael T. Lawton, MD Fabio Frisoli, MD Harrison Farber, MD Neurosurgery Barrow Neurological Institute Phoenix, Arizona, United States	Davide Nasi, MD Neurosurgery Polytechnic University of Marche, Umberto Ancona, Italy
Surgical narrative	Position prone, IOM, posterior midline incision, C4-5 laminectomy, dural opening and tack up, under microscope identify midline with anatomy, careful midline myelotomy with micro dissectors, resection of tumor, dural closure, layered closure	Position prone on transverse rolls, fluoroscopy to identify level, midline incision, subperiosteal dissection exposing posterior elements, laminoplasty at C4-5 using piezoelectric drill after x-ray confirmation, midline durotomy with tenting sutures, ultrasound to locate malformation and to guide midline myelotomy, midline myelotomy, identify malformation and gliotic plane, evacuate hematoma and resect malformation under microscopic visualization, gross total resection dependent on cleavage plane and SSEP/MEP change, watertight dural closure with fibrin sealant, laminoplasty with titanium plates, layered closure	Position prone on Mayfield with slight flexion, skin incision localized with fluoroscopy, dissection carried in the midline avascular plane, lamina exposed and correct level confirmed with fluoroscopy, standard laminectomy, microscope brought into the field, dura opened and tacked up, point of entry most superficial to the dorsal surface, midline myelotomy if not superficial, dorsal column separated until lesion encountered, capsule dissected from surrounding tissue, lesion removed in piecemeal, cavity inspected for complete removal, dura closed with fibrin glue, layered closure	Position prone, standard laminectomy minimizing removal of articular processes, open dura, dissect arachnoid, inspect spinal cord to see if there are any exophytic components, dissection from extramedullary toward intramedullary portion if there is an exophytic component, look for presence or absence of hemosiderin ring to guide entry, ultrasound to guide entry if no visual area to enter based on lesion or hemorrhage, perform midline myelotomy under IOM if no clear entry seen, careful dissection, spatula to remove lesion from white matter, watertight dural closure, layered closure
Complication avoidance	Identify the midline based on anatomy, enter into the cord through the dorsal midline	Laminoplasty, ultrasound to locate malformation and to guide midline myelotomy, resection guided by availability of plane and IOM changes	Point of entry most superficial to the dorsal surface, midline myelotomy if not superficial, lesion removed in piecemeal	Minimize removal of articular processes, attempt to enter spinal cord through exophytic component, ultrasound to guide entry if no visual area to enter
Postoperative				
Admission	ICU	ICU	ICU	ICU
Postoperative complications feared	Spinal cord injury	Spinal cord injury	Spinal cord injury, CSF leak, infection, cervical instability	Spinal cord injury
Anticipated length of stay	4–7 days	2 days	2–3 days	7 days
Follow-up testing	MRI C-spine 6 weeks after surgery	MRI C-spine within 48 hours of surgery	Maintain MAP >75 MRI C-spine before discharge and 6 months after surgery	MRI C-spine 3 months after surgery
Bracing	None	None	None	None
Follow-up visits	4 weeks, 3 months, 12 months after surgery	2 weeks after surgery	10–14 days, 6 weeks, 6 months after surgery	2 weeks, 3 months after surgery

CSF, Cerebrospinal fluid; *ICU*, intensive care unit; *IOM*, intraoperative monitoring; *VHL*, von-Hippel Lindau; *MAP*, mean arterial pressure; *MEP*, motor evoked potential; *MRI*, magnetic resonance imaging; *SSEP*, somatosensory evoked potential.

Differential diagnosis

- Cavernous malformation
- Spinal cord AVM
- Intramedullary spinal cord tumor
- Spinal cord infarction

Important anatomical and preoperative considerations

Spinal cord CMs are most frequently located in the thoracic spine followed by cervical and lumbar levels.[2] Clinical presentation is widely variable and includes sensorimotor deficits, radiculopathy, and myelopathy.[6] Onset of neurological symptoms ranges from a slow and stepwise deterioration to a rapid progressive decline.[7,8] Neurological impairment depends on the level affected, anatomical location, mass effect, and presence of intramedullary bleeding.[2,7,8] Acute onset of neurological deficits is often related to hemorrhage.[2] Whether extraaxial cavernomas have a higher rate of bleeding than intramedullary lesions remains unclear. Interestingly, extramedullary lesions seem to show a faster growth pattern.[6]

Spinal cavernomas have an increased tendency to bleed in comparison to their supratentorial counterparts. The risk of hemorrhage was estimated ranging from 3.1% to 4.5% per patient-year.[9–11] Moreover, the risk of rebleeding was determined to be 66% per patient-year.[9] Interestingly, triggering factors for bleeding occurrence such as pregnancy, trauma, and strenuous activity have been described in the literature.[9,12] Knowledge regarding the natural course of untreated intramedullary spinal cord CMs is scarce. In a retrospective study by Kharkar et al., nonsurgically treated patients were followed for a combined period of 66.8 patient-years. During this time, none of these patients had an acute intramedullary hemorrhage. Nonhemorrhagic clinical deterioration was infrequent and was usually caused by mass effect secondary to gliosis.[13] This review contributes to the understanding of the natural history of the disease and suggests that conservative management is feasible. Conservative management of spinal cavernomas might be considered a safe alternative for asymptomatic patients, even those harboring exophytic lesions and for masses without progression over time.[2,7] However, due to the narrow space of the spinal canal and the low tolerance of the spinal cord to mass effect, conservative treatment carries the risk of potential sudden clinical deterioration.[14]

Currently, a standardized surgical rationale has not been established for spinal cavernomas and the majority of surgeons advocate for resection in symptomatic patients with exophytic lesions or with deep lesions when progressive or severe symptoms are present.[2,6,7] As aforementioned in previous chapters, the spinal cord is a highly functional tissue and the approach to these lesions implies both a surgical challenge and a high risk of morbidity especially with intraaxial masses and those located in the anterior compartment[14]; thus somatosensory evoked potentials (SEPs), motor evoked potentials (MEPs), and D-wave should be intraoperatively monitored.[7] The posterior approach provides a good corridor for most of these malformations.[7] Before attempting removal, an ultrasonographic evaluation is recommended in order to delimit the extension of the malformation and tailor the dural opening.[2,7] Complete resection can be attempted after disconnection of arterial feeders and draining veins. The goal of surgery for CMs is gross total removal; partial resection is associated with an increased risk of bleeding.[14] Removing of the hemosiderin layer is not recommended because it increases the risk of cord damage and has not shown any benefit.[7] Meticulous hemostasis is paramount.[2,7]

What was actually done

This case involves a young patient with sudden onset of sensory symptoms few days before evaluation. Although the strength was intact in the physical examination, the sensation was affected in lower and upper extremities. Spine MRI showed a hemorrhagic intramedullary lesion compatible with a CMs. Therefore a nonurgent surgical intervention was recommended. After discussing risks, benefits, and alternatives, the patient was taken to the operating room. General anesthesia was provided, and neuromonitoring with MEPs and SSEPs was established. After the Mayfield head frame was affixed, the patient was placed in the prone position on the

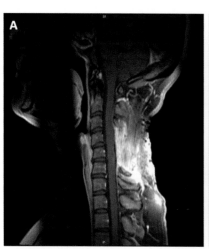 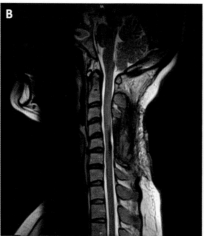 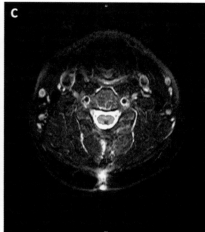

Fig. 65.2 Postoperative magnetic resonance images of the cervical spine. (A) Sagittal postcontrast T1-weighted image, **(B)** sagittal T2, and **(C)** axial T2-weighted images demonstrating C4-C6 laminectomy and gross total resection with expected residual hemosiderin staining and focal atrophy of the posterior cord.

operating room table. The initial incision was made, and the dissection proceeded until finding the spinous process of C4, which was confirmed with intraoperative fluoroscopy. Then subperiosteal dissection was done in the usual fashion from C4 down to C6. The laminectomy was performed from the bottom of C4 to the top of C6. The intraoperative ultrasound was brought to assess the extent of the lesion before opening the dura, which led us to complete the C4 laminectomy. The microscope was taken into the surgical field, the dura was opened in the midline, and the arachnoid was opened and sutured to the dura. A midline myelotomy was performed and the hematoma was immediately encountered within the spinal cord. The hematoma was dissected following a decent plane in all levels. An aggregate of abnormal vessels was dissected and sent to pathology. After inspecting around the surgical cavity, no grossly abnormal tissue was appreciated, and the resection was stopped to avoid neurological complications. The dura was closed in a watertight fashion with a running Prolene suture and a dural sealant. The wound was then closed in anatomical layers. Neuromonitoring remained stable throughout the entire case. There were no complications. Postoperative MRI showed no evidence of residual malformation or bleeding (Fig. 65.2).

Commonalities among the experts

Half of the experts advocated for spinal angiogram, MRI of the cervical spine, and neurophysiological evaluation as part of the additional preoperative testing. All would perform surgical resection of the CMs through a C4-C5 laminectomy. The majority would aim for gross total resection as the main goal of surgery. All were focused on avoiding the potential morbidities associated to spinal cord manipulation during the approach and excision. The most feared complication was damage to the cervical cord. All performed surgical resection with fluoroscopy, intraoperative monitoring, and microscope, with steroids as perioperative medication. Surgical approaches were comparable, and all shared the notion of a meticulous dorsal myelotomy and cleavage from surrounding neural tissue to minimize damage to the cord. Following surgery, all admitted their patients to the intensive care unit for further observation. Half would request cervical MRI before discharge, and half within a period of 6 months after intervention.

SUMMARY OF QUALITY OF EVIDENCE TO GUIDE SPECIFIC INTERVENTIONS FOR THIS CASE

- Gross total resection for symptomatic spinal CMs: level III

REFERENCES

1. Gross BA, Du R, Popp AJ, Day AL. Intramedullary spinal cord cavernous malformations. *Neurosurg Focus.* 2010;29(3):E14.
2. Velz J, Bozinov O, Sarnthein J, Regli L, Bellut D. The current management of spinal cord cavernoma. *J Neurosurg Sci.* 2018;62(4):383–396.
3. Badhiwala JH, Farrokhyar F, Alhazzani W, et al. Surgical outcomes and natural history of intramedullary spinal cord cavernous malformations: a single-center series and meta-analysis of individual patient data: Clinic article. *J Neurosurg Spine.* 2014;21(4):662–676.
4. Kim DS, Park YG, Choi JU, Chung SS, Lee KC. An analysis of the natural history of cavernous malformations. *Surg Neurol.* 1997;48(1):9–17. discussion 17-18.
5. Liang JT, Bao YH, Zhang HQ, Huo LR, Wang ZY, Ling F. Management and prognosis of symptomatic patients with intramedullary spinal cord cavernoma: clinical article. *J Neurosurg Spine.* 2011;15(4):447–456.
6. Kivelev J, Niemelä M, Hernesniemi J. Outcome after microsurgery in 14 patients with spinal cavernomas and review of the literature. *J Neurosurg Spine.* 2010;13(4):524–534.
7. Giammattei L, Messerer M, Prada F, DiMeco F. Intramedullary cavernoma: A surgical resection technique. *Neurochirurgie.* 2017;63(5):426–429.
8. Otten M, McCormick P. Natural history of spinal cavernous malformations. *Handb Clin Neurol.* 2017;143:233–239.
9. Kivelev J, Niemelä M, Hernesniemi J. Characteristics of cavernomas of the brain and spine. *J Clin Neurosci.* 2012;19(5):643–648.
10. Sandalcioglu IE, Wiedemayer H, Gasser T, Asgari S, Engelhorn T, Stolke D. Intramedullary spinal cord cavernous malformations: clinical features and risk of hemorrhage. *Neurosurg Rev.* 2003;26(4):253–256.
11. Bian LG, Bertalanffy H, Sun QF, Shen JK. Intramedullary cavernous malformations: clinical features and surgical technique via hemilaminectomy. *Clin Neurol Neurosurg.* 2009;111(6):511–517.
12. Labauge P, Bouly S, Parker F, et al. Outcome in 53 patients with spinal cord cavernomas. *Surg Neurol.* 2008;70(2):176–181. discussion 181.
13. Kharkar S, Shuck J, Conway J, Rigamonti D. The natural history of conservatively managed symptomatic intramedullary spinal cord cavernomas. *Neurosurgery.* 2007;60(5):865–872. discussion 865-872.
14. Kivelev J, Niemelä M, Hernesniemi J. Treatment strategies in cavernomas of the brain and spine. *J Clin Neurosci.* 2012;19(4):491–497.

66

Spinal hemangioblastoma

Fidel Valero-Moreno, MD

Introduction

Hemangioblastoma of the spine is an infrequent, benign (World Health Organization [WHO] I), and highly vascularized tumor accounting for about 3% of all intramedullary spinal tumors and 2% to 15% of all the spinal cord neoplasms.[1–3] Among the intramedullary tumors of the spinal cord, hemangioblastomas come third in frequency, just after ependymomas and astrocytomas.[2] Sporadic neoplasms represent the majority of cases (70%–80%), whereas those associated to von Hippel Lindau disease (VHL) account for a third of the cases (20%–30%).[1,3] Most of the patients become affected during the fourth decade of life, and it has a predilection for the male population.[3–5] VHL is characterized by early onset of diagnosis and/or presence of multiple lesions.[4,6] Sporadic lesions are often extraspinal tumors, specifically in the cerebellum.[7] Despite these differences, hemangioblastomas of the spine share identical clinical and histological features.[8] Overall, most of the spinal hemangioblastomas originate in the cervical and thoracic segments.[6,9] Moreover, the majority of symptomatic lesions are found in the cervical spine.[10] The most common associated findings are a tumor cyst or a syrinx, which can be found in up to 90% of the occurrences.[8,11] Mass effect causes most symptoms including pain and sensory disturbances.[7,8] A rapid progression of symptoms is not uncommon.[3] Surgical resection is the definitive and curative treatment for symptomatic lesions.[8] However, preferred treatment of asymptomatic, sporadic, or multiple lesions is less clear.[8,12] In this chapter, we present the case of a young female patient with a history of VHL disease and sensory disturbances in both lower extremities.

Example case

Chief complaint: bilateral lower extremity paresthesias
History of present illness: This is a 20-year-old female patient with a known family history of VHL disease who presents with numbness and tingling of her bilateral lower extremities for 1 month. This has progressively worsened and she also

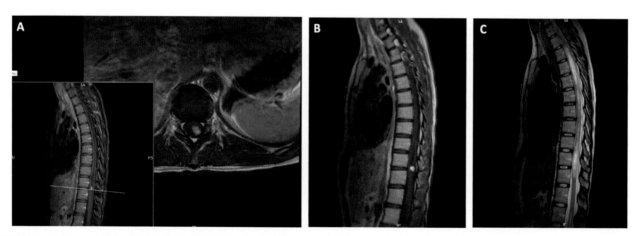

Fig. 66.1 Preoperative magnetic resonance image (MRI) of the thoracic spine. (A) T1 with contrast sagittal and axial image demonstrating an intramedullary mass with significant enhancement at the level of T8-T9, corresponding to hemangioblastoma. **(B)** T1 sagittal with gadolinium image demonstrating a hyperintense intramedullary mass exerting mass effect on the cord. **(C)** T2 sagittal image demonstrating the aforementioned mass with associated surrounding edema and an extensive proximal syrinx.

complains of some dyscoordination when exercising. As part of her evaluation, the patient underwent a magnetic resonance image of the thoracic spine, which demonstrated an intramedullary lesion exerting mass effect at the level of T8-T9 (Fig. 66.1).

Medications: none

Allergies: no known drug allergies

Past medical and surgical history: none

Family history: von Hippel Lindau disease

Social history: college student, no smoking, no alcohol

Physical examination: awake, alert, and oriented to person, place, and time; cranial nerves II–XII intact; bilateral deltoids/triceps/biceps 5/5; interossei 5/5; iliopsoas/knee flexion/knee extension/dorsi, and plantar flexion 5/5

Reflexes: 2+ in bilateral biceps/triceps/brachioradialis with negative Hoffman; 3+ in bilateral patella/ankle; left foot clonus, bilateral Babinski; sensation diminished in both lower extremities with a sensory level at T10

	Anas Abdallah, MD Neurosurgery Osmaniye State Hospital Osmaniye, Turkey	Amro F. Al-Habib, MD, MPH Neurosurgery King Khalid University Hospital King Saud University Riyadh, Saudi Arabia	Ilya Laufer, MD Neurosurgery Memorial Sloan Kettering New York, New York, United States	Michael T. Lawton, MD Fabio Frisoli, MD Harrison Farber, MD Neurosurgery Barrow Neurological Institute Phoenix, Arizona, United States
Preoperative				
Additional tests requested	MRI brain and spine Cerebral angiogram Whole spine x-rays Genetics, ophthalmology, abdominal CT, metanephrines evaluations Anesthesia evaluation	MRI brain and cervical spine CT chest/abdomen/pelvis Ophthalmology evaluation Genetics evaluation	MRI brain and complete spine	MRI brain and spine Genetic evaluation for VHL CT abdomen Urine/plasma metanephrines Possible angiogram
Surgical approach selected	T9 laminoplasty and gross-total resection	T8-9 laminectomy and tumor resection	T8-9 laminectomy and hemangioblastoma resection	T8-9 laminectomy and hemangioblastoma resection
Goal of surgery	Gross total resection, preservation of neurological function, diagnosis, spinal cord decompression	Tumor resection	Gross total resection	Gross total resection
Perioperative				
Positioning	Prone, no pins	Prone on Jackson table, no pins	Prone	Prone on Jackson table, no pins
Surgical equipment	IOM (SSEP/MEP) Fluoroscopy Ultrasound Surgical microscope Laminoplasty plates	IOM (SSEP/MEP) Fluoroscopy Ultrasound Surgical microscope	IOM (SSEP/MEP) Fluoroscopy Ultrasound Surgical microscope	IOM (SSEP/MEP) Fluoroscopy Surgical microscope
Medications	Steroids, maintain MAP	Steroids, MAP >80	Steroids, maintain MAP	Steroids, maintain MAP > 75
Anatomical considerations	Posterior columns of spinal cord, surface vasculature	Midline spinal cord structures (midline artery, posterior sulcus)	Hemangioblastoma vasculature, dorsal root associated with hemangioblastoma	Ascending and descending motor and sensory tracts
Complications feared with approach chosen	Paraparesis, paraplegia, urinary/fecal incontinence/retention	Spinal cord injury, neurological worsening	Spinal instability, CSF leak	Spinal cord injury
Intraoperative				
Anesthesia	General	General	General	General
Exposure	T9	T8-9	T8-9	T8-9
Levels decompressed	T9	T8-9	T8-9	T8-9
Levels fused	T9	None	None	None

(continued on next page)

	Anas Abdallah, MD Neurosurgery Osmaniye State Hospital Osmaniye, Turkey	Amro F. Al-Habib, MD, MPH Neurosurgery King Khalid University Hospital King Saud University Riyadh, Saudi Arabia	Ilya Laufer, MD Neurosurgery Memorial Sloan Kettering New York, New York, United States	Michael T. Lawton, MD Fabio Frisoli, MD Harrison Farber, MD Neurosurgery Barrow Neurological Institute Phoenix, Arizona, United States
Surgical narrative	Position prone, vertical midline posterior incision one level above and below level of interest down to spinous processes, dissection of paraspinal muscles, confirm level with fluoroscopy, bilateral laminotomy to span level with high-speed drills, remove ligamentum flavum and adipose tissue, surgical microscope brought into field, confirm lesion with ultrasound, study dorsal midline to identify median raphe with ultrasound, dura opened and tacked open, dorsal midline myelotomy, use IOM probe to help identify neural tissue, save dorsal vascular tissues by dissecting and rotating, coagulate feeding arteries, lesion removed en bloc if possible, intraoperative ultrasound to confirm extent of resection, watertight dural closure and fibrin glue, laminoplasty with plate and screws, nonabsorbable sutures to fix lamina to cranial and caudal interspinal ligaments and paraspinal muscles, layered closure with drain	Position prone on Jackson table, mark levels using anatomical landmarks and intraoperative fluoroscopy, laminectomy intraoperative ultrasound to confirm level and assess spinal cord compression, midline dural opening, baseline MEP, examine dorsal surface of spinal cord to identify midline and lateral side for possible entry into the tumor where it reaches the surface of the spinal cord, expose tumor and stay out of lesion, try to go around the lesion to achieve a complete resection, serial MEP throughout, send tissue for pathology examination, another ultrasound view to determine decompression of spinal cord, watertight dural closure, application of fibrin glue, closure in layers	Position prone, x-ray for level verification, midline subperiosteal dissection, laminectomy over enhancing nodule, ½ level above and ½ level below, ultrasound to confirm correct level and adequate exposure, midline dural incision, tack dura to muscle, arachnoid dissection under microscope visualization, identify orange surface of hemangioblastoma, dissect and coagulate feeding surface vessels, sharp dissection of normal pia from pia of hemangioblastoma, extend myelotomy as needed to identify rostral and caudal poles, extracapsular dissection from gliotic spinal cord, coagulate and ligate vessels, coagulate and ligate draining vein last, en bloc removal, dural closure with compressed Gelfoam and fibrin glue, layered closure	Position prone, skin incision localized with fluoroscopy, lamina are exposed and correct level confirmed with fluoroscopy, standard laminectomy, microscope brought into field, dura opened and tacked up, myelotomy where lesion comes closest to dorsal surface and eccentric on left, en bloc resection, dura closed with suture and fibrin glue, layered closure
Complication avoidance	One-level laminotomy, ultrasound to confirm exposure, identify median raphe, IOM probe to identify neural tissue, save dorsal vascular structures, en bloc resection, fibrin glue	Surgical navigation, intraoperative ultrasound, examine for midline, enter tumor at most superficial aspect, stay out of lesion, continuous MEP, fibrin glue	Intraoperative ultrasound, sharp dissection, extracapsular dissection, coagulate and ligate draining vein last, en bloc resection	Myelotomy at most superficial aspect, en bloc resection, fibrin glue
Postoperative				
Admission	ICU	Stepdown unit	ICU	ICU
Postoperative complications feared	Hematoma, CSF leak, neurological injury, vascular injury, urinary/fecal incontinence, neuropathic pain, sensory loss	Neurological compromise, CSF leak	CSF leak, neurological deficit, subtotal removal	Spinal cord injury, CSF leak, infection
Anticipated length of stay	3–4 days	7 days	3–4 days	2–3 days
Follow-up testing	CT T-spine within 24 hours of surgery MRI T-spine within 24 hours of surgery	Physical therapy MRI 48 hours after surgery if worsening deficit, 3 months after surgery	MRI within 48 hours of surgery	Maintain MAP >75 for 24 hours MRI T-spine before discharge and 1 year after surgery

	Anas Abdallah, MD Neurosurgery Osmaniye State Hospital Osmaniye, Turkey	Amro F. Al-Habib, MD, MPH Neurosurgery King Khalid University Hospital King Saud University Riyadh, Saudi Arabia	Ilya Laufer, MD Neurosurgery Memorial Sloan Kettering New York, New York, United States	Michael T. Lawton, MD Fabio Frisoli, MD Harrison Farber, MD Neurosurgery Barrow Neurological Institute Phoenix, Arizona, United States
Bracing	Thoracolumbar brace for 6 weeks	None	None	None
Follow-up visits	2 weeks, 6 weeks, 3 months, 6 months, 12 months after surgery	1 month after surgery	3–4 weeks, 3–4 months, 1 year after surgery	10–14 days, 6 weeks, 1 year after surgery

CSF, Cerebrospinal fluid; *CT*, computed tomography; *ICU*, intensive care unit; *IOM*, intraoperative monitoring; *VHL*, von-Hippel Lindau; *MAP*, mean arterial pressure; *MEP*, motor evoked potential; *MRI*, magnetic resonance imaging; *SSEP*, somatosensory evoked potential.

Differential diagnosis

- Ependymoma
- Astrocytoma
- Simplex syringomyelia
- Arteriovenous malformation

Important anatomical and preoperative considerations

Hemangioblastomas are most commonly found in the cervical and thoracic segments. Interestingly, most of the symptomatic lesions occupy the cervical spine.[6,9,10] The vast majority of hemangioblastomas are located on the dorsal aspect of the spinal cord and develop under the pia mater.[2,5,8,11] As reported in the literature, these lesions affect the posterior aspect of the denticulate ligament in around 93% to 95% of the cases, where two-thirds of these tumors arise from the posterior root entry zone.[8,11] A T1 with gadolinium and T2-weighted magnetic resonance are best for precisely delineating the location of the tumor and its extension.[8,12] Hemangioblastomas are isointense lesions on T1-weighted images and hyperintense on T2. Small tumors are commonly associated with the presence of surrounding edema and the formation of a syrinx, while larger lesions are associated with a high vascularity pattern and characterized by flow voids on magnetic imaging studies.[8] Hemorrhage is uncommon, but when present usually does so as subarachnoid bleeding. Angiographic identification of the feeding artery and draining vessels may be an important tool for surgical planning; however, embolization of the lesion is rarely employed.[8,11]

The definitive treatment for spinal hemangioblastomas is surgical extirpation. For symptomatic patients harboring sporadic lesions or enlarging masses, particularly those associated with edema and syrinx, surgical excision should be the primary treatment option.[8,11–13] For asymptomatic patients with small and nondynamic tumors, conservative treatment is justified.[11] Currently, there is no consensus regarding invasive treatment in the setting of asymptomatic or/and multiple lesions related to VHL disease. Traditionally, conservative management and close follow-up is encouraged for multiple tumors due to the difficulty of correlating a particular lesion to specific neurological symptoms.[13,14] However, some authors emphasize the importance of timely surgical removal before the tumor exceeds a diameter of 10 mm (500 mm^3), especially for dorsal neoplasms and evidence of radiological progression. This is based on the observation that lesions larger than 10 mm typically develop neurological symptoms.[14–16]

The surgical approach for spinal hemangioblastoma is determined by the position of the tumor within the spinal cord. As anticipated, the majority of lesions are resected via a posterior approach, which is the logical choice for tumors occupying a posterior or lateral situation.[8,13] Hemangioblastomas located anterior to the dentate ligament are typically accessed via an anterior or anterolateral approach through corpectomy.[8,10] In general, en bloc excision with meticulous dissection of pial attachments is recommended due to the high risk of bleeding with a subtotal resection.[12,13,17] Laminectomies typically provide adequate exposure of the dura above and below the tumor, and a margin of at least 1 cm beyond the cranial and caudal limits is preferred.[10,16] After opening of the dura and the pia layer, the feeding arteries and draining vessels should be identified.[12,17] Tumor blood supply is commonly originated from the ipsilateral radicular artery and the anterior spinal artery.[11] The anterior and posterior spinal arteries arise from the vertebral arteries rostrally, and along their trajectory they are joined by multiple radicular arteries that branch from the aorta and the iliac arteries.[12] The tumor is generally easily identified and a clear boundary between the lesion and the neural tissue is usually present, allowing careful circumferential dissection of the mass from the surrounding cord.[11,12,17] Disruption of the tumor itself should be avoided due to its high vascularity and consequently challenging hemostasis.[12] Once the neoplasm is dissected, it can typically be detached from its arterial supply and removed in a single piece.[12]

Stereotactic radiosurgery (SRS) represents a safe alternative in cases of hemangioblastomatosis and for lesions that carry a high risk for resection. SRS can be effectively performed either in sporadic tumors or in VHL disease-related lesions.[7,10] However, the role and the long-term value of SRS are not well-defined. Initial clinical response of benign tumors like hemangioblastoma to radiotherapy should be interpreted cautiously. Short-term control rates does not automatically correlate to long-term remission and may only overlap with a quiescent phase of the tumor.[7,10]

What was actually done

The patient was admitted to hospital and the diagnosis of a thoracic intramedullary tumor between the levels of T9, T10, and T11 was confirmed. The patient was taken to the operating room for a T9-11 laminoplasty and tumor resection. The patient was induced and was administered general anesthesia. The patient was placed prone on the operating table. The use of motor evoked potential (MEP)/somatosensory evoked potential (SSEP) was used throughout the case. Intraoperative x-rays were employed to localize the T9-T11 levels, where a laminoplasty was performed. The exact location of the tumor within the cord was confirmed with intraoperative ultrasound. A midline myelotomy was performed and extracapsular dissection with en bloc resection with assistance of visualization by the surgical microscope was achieved. Intraoperative SSEPs remained stable, while some MEPs slightly decreased in the middle of the resection. A complete excision was achieved. The patient received steroids at the end of the procedure. The patient awoke in the operating room without complications and was transferred to the intensive care unit. She remained stable and was transferred to the floor, and was discharged on postoperative day 3. She remained neurologically stable except for slight weakness (4+/5) in her left lower extremity. Follow-up imaging showed no evidence of residual or recurrent tumor or collapsing of the syrinx (Fig. 66.2).

Commonalities among the experts

All surgeons requested complete neuro-axis magnetic resonance imaging (MRI) as part of the preoperative assessment. Moreover, most of the surgeons pursued a genetics evaluation and abdominal computed tomography (CT) scan for workup of multiple hemangioblastomas. All advocated for surgical resection with the aim for a gross total resection and the majority would pursue tumor resection through a T8-T9 laminectomy. Most were aware of the vascular structures involved, as well as the spinal cord and its functional anatomical elements, such as the dorsal column and descending tracts. The most feared complication was spinal cord injury. Surgery was generally completed with intraoperative monitoring, fluoroscopy, ultrasound, and microscope. All indicated steroids as perioperative therapy. Surgical technique slightly varied, but most emphasized their preference for extracapsular dissection and complete excision. Ultrasound and intraoperative monitoring were employed to minimize the risk of neural tissue damage. After surgery, most admitted their patients to the intensive care unit. All of the experts requested a postoperative MRI before discharge, typically within 48 hours of surgery. Most recommended continued close follow-up during the first year after surgery.

SUMMARY OF QUALITY OF EVIDENCE TO GUIDE SPECIFIC INTERVENTIONS FOR THIS CASE

- Gross total resection of hemangioblastomas in symptomatic patients: level III
- Steroids for the perioperative management of spinal hemangioblastomas: level III

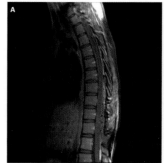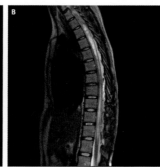

Fig. 66.2 Postoperative magnetic resonance image (MRI) of the thoracic spine. **(A)** T1 with gadolinium sagittal and **(B)** T2 sagittal images demonstrating no gross total resection of the tumor.

REFERENCES

1. Pojskic M, Arnautovic KI. Microsurgical Resection of Spinal Cord Hemangioblastoma: 2-Dimensional Operative Video. *Oper Neurosurg (Hagerstown).* 2018;15(6):E88–E89.
2. Wu TC, Guo WY, Lirng JF, et al. Spinal cord hemangioblastoma with extensive syringomyelia. *J Chin Med Assoc.* 2005;68(1):40–44.
3. Yasuda T, Hasegawa T, Yamato Y, et al. Relationship between Spinal Hemangioblastoma Location and Age. *Asian Spine J.* 2016;10(2):309–313.
4. Nguyen TH, Pham T, Strickland T, Brewer D, Belirgen M, Al-Rahawan MM. Von Hippel-Lindau with early onset of hemangioblastoma and multiple drop-metastases like spinal lesions: A case report. *Medicine (Baltimore).* 2018;97(39):e12477.
5. Wang C. Spinal hemangioblastoma: report on 68 cases. *Neurol Res.* 2008;30(6):603–609.
6. Baker KB, Moran CJ, Wippold FJ, 2nd et al. MR imaging of spinal hemangioblastoma. *AJR Am J Roentgenol.* 2000;174(2):377–382.
7. Pan J, Ho AL, D'Astous M, et al. Image-guided stereotactic radiosurgery for treatment of spinal hemangioblastoma. *Neurosurg Focus.* 2017;42(1):E12.
8. Mandigo CE, Ogden AT, Angevine PD, McCormick PC. Operative management of spinal hemangioblastoma. *Neurosurgery.* 2009;65(6):1166–1177.
9. Chu BC, Terae S, Hida K, Furukawa M, Abe S, Miyasaka K. MR findings in spinal hemangioblastoma: correlation with symptoms and with angiographic and surgical findings. *AJNR Am J Neuroradiol.* 2001;22(1):206–217.
10. Lonser RR, Oldfield EH. Spinal cord hemangioblastomas. *Neurosurg Clin N Am.* 2006;17(1):37–44.
11. Wang H, Zhang L, Wang H, Nan Y, Ma Q. Spinal hemangioblastoma: surgical procedures, outcomes and review of the literature. *Acta Neurol Belg.* 2020; 121;973–981.
12. Messerer M, Cossu G, Pralong E, Daniel RT. Intramedullary hemangioblastoma: Microsurgical resection technique. *Neurochirurgie.* 2017;63(5):376–380.
13. Oppenlander ME, Spetzler RF. Advances in spinal hemangioblastoma surgery. *World Neurosurg.* 2010;74(1):116–117.
14. Ammerman JM, Lonser RR, Dambrosia J, Butman JA, Oldfield EH. Long-term natural history of hemangioblastomas in patients with von Hippel-Lindau disease: implications for treatment. *J Neurosurg.* 2006;105(2):248–255.
15. Kanno H, Yamamoto I, Nishikawa R, et al. Spinal cord hemangioblastomas in von Hippel-Lindau disease. *Spinal Cord.* 2009;47(6):447–452.
16. Kim TY, Yoon DH, Shin HC, et al. Spinal cord hemangioblastomas in von Hippel-Lindau disease: management of asymptomatic and symptomatic tumors. *Yonsei Med J.* 2012;53(6):1073–1080.
17. Lanzino G, Morales-Valero SF, Krauss WE. Resection of spinal hemangioblastoma. *Neurosurg Focus.* 2014;37(Suppl 2):Video 15.

67

Chiari malformation

Fidel Valero-Moreno, MD

Introduction

Chiari malformations represent a class of posterior fossa disorders that stem from congenital abnormalities.[1] The Chiari I malformation is the most common type, characterized by tonsillar descent that may or may not be associated with syringomyelia. The overall prevalence of the condition in the general population is estimated to be 1%.[2,3] The chief complaint from patients with symptomatic Chiari I malformation is pain/headaches, with symptom onset during Valsalva maneuvers such as coughing.[4,5] Those cases associated with syrinx formation may also present with myelopathy. Around 70% to 80% of patients with Chiari I malformation develop a syrinx[6] and 41% develop arachnoid adhesions.[5] Surgical management is indicated in symptomatic patients and in those with progressive syringomyelia.[2] Resolution of the syrinx may occur after surgical decompression of the foramen magnum. In cases of surgical intervention that fail, revision decompression and lysis of adhesions may be warranted.[2,3,6] Not uncommonly, there is an arachnoid veil present at the obex, which may prevent cerebrospinal fluid (CSF) outflow from the fourth ventricle and lead to recurrent symptoms. In this chapter, we present a case of a young patient with worsening headaches with coughing and straining.

Example case

Chief complaint: headaches

History of present illness: This is a 44-year-old female with no significant past medical history who presents with worsening headaches over the past 6 months. She states that her headaches have worsened over the past half-year and that they worsened with coughing and straining as well as with neck extension. She also complains of decreased coordination in her nondominant left hand. The patient underwent magnetic resonance imaging of the cranio-cervical junction that demonstrated significant caudal cerebellar tonsillar displacement compatible with Chiari malformation (Fig. 67.1).

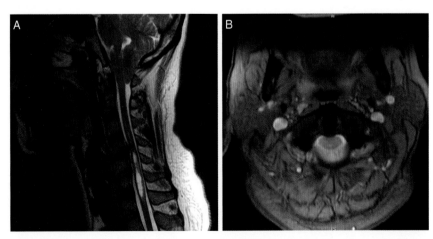

Fig. 67.1 Preoperative magnetic resonance image (MRI) of the cervical spine. (A) Sagittal and **(B)** axial T2 images demonstrating signficant cerebellar tonsil ectopia. There is caudal displacement of the tonsils into the upper cervical canal (10 mm) through the foramen magnum. There is significant compression of the cervico-medullary junction with an associated syrinx spanning from C3 to C7.

Medications: none
Allergies: no known drug allergies
Past medical and surgical history: C-section
Family history: noncontributory
Social history: accountant, no smoking or alcohol
Physical examination: awake, alert, and oriented to person, place,

and time; cranial nerves II–XII intact; bilateral deltoids/triceps/biceps 5/5; interossei 5/5; iliopsoas/knee flexion/knee extension/dorsi, and plantar flexion 5/5
Reflexes: 2+ in bilateral biceps/triceps/brachioradialis with negative Hoffman; 2+ in bilateral patella/ankle; no clonus or Babinski; sensation intact to light touch

	Andres Almendral, MD Neurosurgery Clinica Hospital San Fernando Panama City, Panama	Gordon Deen, MD Neurosurgery Mayo Clinic Jacksonville, Florida, United States	Jorge Eduardo Guzman Prenk, MD Neurosurgery Pontifica Universidad Javeriana Bogota, Colombia	Daniel J. Hoh, MD Neurosurgery University of Florida Gainesville, Florida, United States
Preoperative				
Additional tests requested	CTA Upper limb MEP/SSEP/EMG	None	Upper limb MEP/SSEP/EMG	None
Surgical approach selected	Suboccipital craniectomy, C1 laminectomy, duraplasty and C4-5 laminectomy with C4-6 fusion	Suboccipital craniectomy, C1 laminectomy, duraplasty	Suboccipital craniectomy, C1 laminectomy, duraplasty	Occipital craniectomy and C1 laminectomy
Goal of surgery	Decompress cervicomedullary junction and cervical space	Decompress cervicomedullary junction	Decompress cervicomedullary junction, tonsillar decompression, syrinx resolution	Decompress pontomedullary junction, reestablish CSF flow
Perioperative				
Positioning	Prone, with pins	Prone, with pins	Prone, Concorde, no pins	Prone, with pins
Surgical equipment	IOM (MEP/SSEP) Fluoroscopy	Surgical microscope IOM	Fluoroscopy Surgical microscope Tubular retractor	Surgical microscope
Medications	None	Maintain MAP >90	None	Ketorolac 48 hours after surgery
Anatomical considerations	Midline posterior cervical nuchal ligament, vertebral artery, PICA, cerebellar tonsils, arachnoid membrane	Spinal cord, vertebral arteries, cerebellar tonsils	C2 spinous process, lateral venous plexus, atlanto-occipital membrane	Cerebellar tonsils
Complications feared with approach chosen	CSF leak	Spinal cord injury, vertebral artery injury	Spinal instability, chronic pain	CSF leak, hydrocephalus
Intraoperative				
Anesthesia	General	General	General	General
Exposure	Occiput-C6	Occiput-C1	Occiput-C2	Occiput-C1
Levels decompressed	Occiput-C1 and C4-5	Occiput-C1	Occiput-C1	Occiput-C1
Levels fused	C4-6	None	None	None

	Andres Almendral, MD Neurosurgery Clinica Hospital San Fernando Panama City, Panama	Gordon Deen, MD Neurosurgery Mayo Clinic Jacksonville, Florida, United States	Jorge Eduardo Guzman Prenk, MD Neurosurgery Pontifica Universidad Javeriana Bogota, Colombia	Daniel J. Hoh, MD Neurosurgery University of Florida Gainesville, Florida, United States
Surgical narrative	Position prone with Mayfield pins, neck slightly flexed, midline skin incision from above inion to C7 spinous process, triangular pericranial graft is obtained from the occipital area measuring 4–5 cm in length and width, open fascia in Y-shaped incision at nuchal ligament by freeing skin margins from deep fascia, suboccipital craniectomy 3–4 cm from foramen magnum, remove enough bone to completely decompress entire posterior surface of cerebellar tonsils and 2.5–3.0 cm from side to side, remove posterior arch of C1 after separating muscles attached to it, keep muscles attached to C2 and C7, open dura in midline at C1 with care to avoid injuring arachnoid membrane and extend superiorly in Y-shaped fashion above foramen magnum, retract dura, suture pericranial autograft to durotomy margins after sizing by using a cottonoid as a guide, separate muscles from C4-6 spinous process, C4-5 laminectomy, place C4-6 lateral mass screws with fluoroscopic guidance, confirm absence of CSF leak with Valsalva maneuver, layered closure	Position prone with Mayfield pins, head and neck neutral with head slightly up, incision from inion to C4, suboccipital decompression followed by C1 decompression, microscope brought in, open dura with Y-shaped opening, free adhesions, explore floor of fourth ventricle, harvest fascia lata, duraplasty with fascia lata, close wound in layers, bedrest night of surgery	Position prone in Concorde position without pins, identify midpoint between foramen magnum and C2 spinous process under fluoroscopy, 2.5 cm median skin incision at midpoint, place tubular dilators using Seldinger's technique, remove rectus capitis posterior major and minor muscles using monopolar cautery, expose occipital midline/posterior rim of foramen magnum/C1/C2 spinous process, dock 22 mm tube on C2 spinous process and occipital midline within 1 cm of foramen magnum, decompress 1 cm of foramen magnum, angle tube upward to complete 2 cm wide plus 1 additional cm of occipital bone, remove posterior arch of C1 with drill, widen channel with high-speed drill, completely resect posterior atlanto-occipital membrane, median dural opening with preservation of arachnoid membrane, duraplasty with synthetic patch, remove tube, layered closure	Position prone with Mayfield pins, vertical midline incision, expose occiput to C2, occipital craniectomy and C1 laminectomy, midline vertical opening of dura, microscope-assisted lysis of arachnoid, elevate tonsils to confirm outflow of CSF from fourth ventricle, close dura in water tight fashion with fibrin glue, close muscle and skin in layers, approximate skin with horizontal mattress sutures
Complication avoidance	Pericranium for duraplasty, maintain muscles attachments to C2 and C7, preserve arachnoid during dural opening, cervical laminectomy and fusion over cyst	Explore floor of fourth ventricle, fascia lata for duraplasty	Minimally invasive tubular retractor, leave muscles attached to C2 spinous process, resect posterior atlanto-occipital membrane, preserve arachnoid membrane	Elevate tonsils to assess fourth ventricular CSF flow, fibrin glue
Postoperative				
Admission	ICU	ICU	ICU	Floor
Postoperative complications feared	CSF leak, vertebral and PICA injury, infection, medullary lesions	Hematoma, spinal cord/brainstem compression, infection	CSF leak, hematoma, infection	CSF leak, delayed hydrocephalus
Anticipated length of stay		2 days	2 days	2–4 days

(continued on next page)

	Andres Almendral, MD Neurosurgery Clinica Hospital San Fernando Panama City, Panama	Gordon Deen, MD Neurosurgery Mayo Clinic Jacksonville, Florida, United States	Jorge Eduardo Guzman Prenk, MD Neurosurgery Pontifica Universidad Javeriana Bogota, Colombia	Daniel J. Hoh, MD Neurosurgery University of Florida Gainesville, Florida, United States
Follow-up testing	MRI C-spine 6 months after surgery	MRI C-spine 3 months after surgery	MRI C-spine 4 months, 1 year after surgery	Head CT if needed MRI cervical spine 6 weeks after surgery if no improvement
Bracing	None	None	None	None
Follow-up visits	1 month, 3 months, 6 months, 1 year after surgery	4 weeks after surgery	2 weeks, 4 months, 1 year after surgery	3 weeks, 6 weeks surgery

CSF, cerebrospinal fluid; *CT*, computed tomography; *CTA*, computed tomography angiography; *EMG*, electromyography; *ICU*, intensive care unit; *IOM*, intraoperative monitoring; *MAP*, mean arterial pressure; *MEP*, motor evoked potentials; *MRI*, magnetic resonance imaging; *PICA*, posterior inferior cerebellar artery; *SSEP*, somatosensory evoked potential.

Differential diagnosis

- Chiari malformation
- Cranio-cervical junction tumor
- Basilar invagination
- Intracranial mass lesion causing displacement
- Dandy-Walker malformation

Important anatomical and preoperative considerations

Chiari malformation is a hindbrain congenital anomaly.[7] The caudal displacement of the cerebellar tonsils 5 mm below the foramen magnum without associated brainstem herniation is commonly accepted as diagnostic for Chiari I malformation.[2,3,6] The mismatch between the volume of the posterior fossa and its contents, cerebellum and brainstem, has an important role in the pathogenesis of this condition.[3] Clinical manifestations result from a combination of brainstem compression and altered dynamics of CSF flow at the cervico-medullary junction.[3] The impairment of normal CSF flow through the foramen magnum produces a partially entrapped spinal subarachnoid space which subsequently forms a syrinx.[2,3] The surgical rationale hinges on the presence of symptoms, neurological dysfunction, and syringomyelia.[2,3,6] Brainstem and cerebellar dysfunction, as well as typical and atypical headache, can benefit from decompressive intervention.[2,6] Surgical treatment must focus on achieving the following: decompression of the cervico-medullary junction, reestablishing adequate CSF circulation, and resolving the syrinx.[6] The classical approach includes bony decompression by means of suboccipital craniectomy, excision of the posterior arch of C1, and sometimes laminectomy of C2. In addition, bony decompression is complemented with duraplasty.[2,6] Most neurosurgeons advocate for this technique, which is supported by good functional outcomes[2,6]; however, some authors recommend the incorporation of tonsil resection or coagulation for optimal decompression of the craniocervical region.[8] Conservative management should be reserved for asymptomatic patients without syringomyelia, especially those with incidental findings. Patients managed conservatively may be followed with clinical examinations and serial imaging.[3]

What was actually done

This patient presented with a significant Chiari malformation with caudal cerebellar ectopia of more than 10 mm and an associated syrinx. Due to the presence of symptoms and radiological evidence of CSF flow disruption, surgical intervention was advised. The patient was brought to the operating room. Anesthesia conducted intubation per routine. After intubation, the patient was placed in a Mayfield head holder and placed prone on the operating table. The patient underwent motor and somatosensory evoked potential. After the surgical area was cleaned and draped, an incision was made spanning from above the inion to the C2 spinous process. Bovie cautery was used to dissect down through the subcutaneous fat in between the avascular plane in the suboccipital muscles until the occipital bone was encountered. Subperiosteal dissection was done until the superior aspect of the C2 spinous process was identified. The dissection was then extended laterally. Suboccipital craniectomy was performed and extended just lateral to the cervico-medullary junction. The C1 spinous process was dissected and drilled until the dura was identified. The ligament between C1 and the foramen magnum was removed. The dura mater was opened in a Y-shaped fashion. The microscope was brought for the remainder of the case. A 1 cm lipoma was found in the obex and was resected en bloc. The arachnoid between the tonsils was opened and dissected upward to expose the tela choroidea. The tonsils were then cauterized with bipolar to open up the cervico-medullary junction. The medial and the superficial aspects of the tonsils were cauterized until the foramen was open. A dural patch was sutured in place. Surgical wound was closed in layers. The patient was extubated and awoke at her neurological baseline. After surgery was taken to the intensive care unit for recovery. At last follow-up, the patient reported significant headache relief and resolution of coordination issues. Three-month follow-up MRI demonstrated an optimal decompression and improvement in the syrinx (Fig. 67.2).

Commonalities among the experts

Half of the surgeons requested upper limb motor and somatosensory evoked potential as well as electromyograms as additional preoperative tests. All would attain

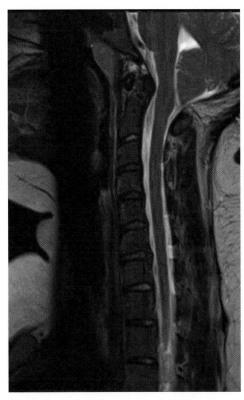

Fig. 67.2 Postoperative magnetic resonance image (MRI) of the cervical spine. T2-weighted sagittal scan of the cranio-cervical junction showing postoperative changes for treatment of a Chiari I malformation with satisfactory decompression of the posterior fossa and cervico-medullary junction and resolution of the syrinx.

bony decompression through a suboccipital craniectomy combined with a C1 laminectomy. Half would combine this with duraplasty. The goal of surgery was to decompress the cervico-medullary junction and restore normal CSF flow. Most were aware of the cerebellar tonsils, vertebral artery, and spinal cord. Half of the surgeons were concerned of CSF leak. Other feared complications were spinal cord damage,

instability and vertebral artery injury. Surgery was usually achieved with surgical microscope, intraoperative monitoring, and fluoroscopy. No perioperative medications were regularly used. Surgical nuances were similar, with half highlighting the relevance of duraplasty and preserving the arachnoid membrane. Following surgery, most admitted their patients to the intensive care unit. All recommended postoperative cervical MRI within a period ranging from 6 weeks to 6 months.

SUMMARY OF QUALITY OF EVIDENCE TO GUIDE SPECIFIC INTERVENTIONS FOR THIS CASE

- Cervico-medullary decompression for symptomatic patients, or radiological evidence of hydrocephalus and/or syrinx: level II-2

REFERENCES

1. McClugage SG, Oakes WJ. The Chiari I malformation. *J Neurosurg Pediatr*. 2019;24(3):217–226.
2. Beretta E, Vetrano IG, Curone M, et al. Chiari malformation-related headache: outcome after surgical treatment. *Neurol Sci*. 2017;38(Suppl 1):95–98.
3. Olszewski AM, Proctor MR. Headache, Chiari I malformation and foramen magnum decompression. *Curr Opin Pediatr*. 2018;30(6):786–790.
4. Strahle J, Muraszko KM, Kapurch J, Bapuraj JR, Garton HJ, Maher CO. Chiari malformation Type I and syrinx in children undergoing magnetic resonance imaging. *J Neurosurg Pediatr*. 2011;8(2):205–213.
5. Paul KS, Lye RH, Strang FA, Dutton J. Arnold-Chiari malformation. Review of 71 cases. *J Neurosurg*. 1983;58(2):183–187.
6. Zhao JL, Li MH, Wang CL, Meng W. A Systematic Review of Chiari I Malformation: Techniques and Outcomes. *World Neurosurg*. 2016;88:7–14.
7. Tubbs RS, Beckman J, Naftel RP, et al. Institutional experience with 500 cases of surgically treated pediatric Chiari malformation Type I. *J Neurosurg Pediatr*. 2011;7(3):248–256.
8. Won DJ, Nambiar U, Muszynski CA, Epstein FJ. Coagulation of herniated cerebellar tonsils for cerebrospinal fluid pathway restoration. *Pediatr Neurosurg*. 1997;27(5):272–275.

68

Chiari malformation with recurrent symptoms

Fidel Valero-Moreno, MD

Introduction

As described in Chapter 67, Chiari I malformation is a condition derived from the abnormal caudal displacement of the cerebellar tonsils through the foramen magnum into the upper cervical canal, often with intramedullary cyst formation.[1-3] Surgical treatment is advocated for symptomatic patients and for those harboring syringomyelia.[4] Currently, suboccipital bony decompression with duraplasty is the treatment of choice for restoration of adequate cerebrospinal fluid (CSF) flow and symptom relief.[4-6] However, persistent or recurrent syringomyelia after foramen magnum decompression is not uncommon, with rates ranging from 22% to 66%.[3,7] Despite adequate posterior fossa decompression and initial clinical improvement, persistent or enlarging syringomyelia and tonsillar herniation can occur.[1,3] Therefore, routine clinical and radiological follow-up is mandatory. There is some data indicating that the timing of the initial operation plays a role in influencing the need of reoperation, especially in patients undergoing primary surgery before age 5.[8] This complication is less likely when decompression is accompanied by duraplasty.[1] Contrary to the initial management of Chiari I malformations, the rationale for operative treatment is not clear in cases of failed surgery and no standard treatment has been established.[7] Despite this, persistent or enlarging symptomatic syringomyelia is an important indication for surgical intervention.[2,3] Redo posterior fossa decompression should address the reimpactation of the foramen magnum and the aberrant CSF flow through it.[2,3,9] When a large syringomyelia is present, a syringo-pleural or syringo-subarachnoid shunt should be considered.[3,7] In this chapter, we describe the case of a young female patient with recurrent tussive headaches 1 year after posterior fossa decompression and duraplasty.

Example case

Chief complaint: headaches, upper extremity paresthesias

History of present illness: This is a 42-year-old female patient with a history of previous Chiari I malformation treated with suboccipital craniotomy and C1 laminectomy/duraplasty 1 year prior. Initially her symptoms of tussive headaches improved, but in the last month, the headaches have returned. In addition, she has developed paresthesias in both upper extremities and mild gait disturbances. The patient underwent radiological evaluation that showed a large spinal cord fluid-filled cavity compatible with syringomyelia (Fig. 68.1). In addition, an obstruction at the level of the fourth ventricle was elucidated on cine magnetic resonance imaging.

Medications: antidepressants

Allergies: no known drug allergies

Past medical and surgical history: as above

Family history: none

Social history: none

Physical examination: awake, alert, and oriented to person, place, and time; cranial nerves II–XII intact; bilateral deltoids/triceps/biceps 5/5; interossei 5/5; iliopsoas/knee flexion/knee extension/dorsi, and plantar flexion 5/5

Reflexes: 3+ in bilateral biceps/triceps/brachioradialis with positive Hoffman; 3+ in bilateral patella/ankle; no bilateral feet clonus, and positive Babinski; sensation decreased in both upper (C6 and C7 distribution); mild gait instability

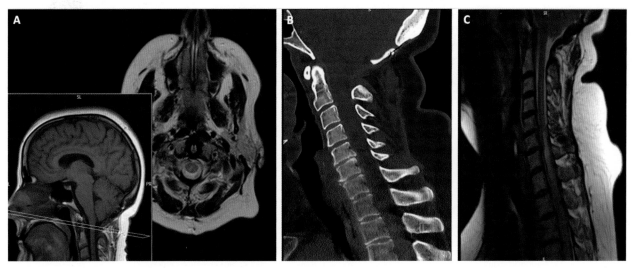

Fig. 68.1 Preoperative imaging of the craniocervical junction. (A) T1-weighted axial and sagittal magnetic resonance imaging (MRI) demonstrating absence of cerebellar tonsil caudal displacement. **(B)** Sagittal computed tomography scan (bone window) demonstrated previous suboccipital craniectomy and the absence of the C1 posterior arch. No obvious Chiari malformation was identified. **(C)** Sagittal T2 MRI demonstrating a large fluid-filled cavity compatible with the presence of a syrinx affecting from C3 to T1. The dilation of the cord is more significant at the C6-T1 levels.

	Hazem Eltahawy, MD Neurosurgery St. Mary Mercy Hospital Ain Shams University Livonia, Michigan, United States	George I. Jallo, MD Neurosurgery Johns Hopkins All Children's Tampa, Florida, United States	Sheng-Fu Lo, MD Neurosurgery Johns Hopkins Baltimore, Maryland, United States	Khoi D. Than, MD Neurosurgery Duke University Durham, North Carolina, United States
Preoperative				
Additional tests requested	MRI cine and CSF flow study	MRI C-spine flexion-extension MRI brain and complete spine EMG	MRI brain and complete spine with cine CSF flow study C-spine flexion-extension x-rays MRI C-spine flexion-extension Low volume lumbar puncture with CSF analysis Neurology evaluation	MRI brain with CSF flow study
Surgical approach selected	Revision suboccipital decompression and possible C6–7 laminectomy for syringo-pleural shut	Revision suboccipital decompression and possible C5–6 laminectomy for syringosubarachnoid shunt	Revision suboccipital craniectomy, C1 laminectomy with possible tonsillar coagulation with obex stenting	Conservative management pending flow studies
Goal of surgery	Restoration of CSF flow	Recreate CSF flow and treat syrinx	Reestablish CSF flow	Possible syringo-subarachnoid shunt if symptoms worsen
Perioperative				
Positioning	Prone, with pins	Prone, with pins	Prone on Jackson table, with pins	
Surgical equipment	Surgical microscope Ultrasound	Surgical microscope	Surgical microscope Ultrasound	
Medications	MAP >80	Steroids	Steroids	
Anatomical considerations	Vertebral arteries, PICA, medulla, cerebellum	Foramen magnum, floor of fourth ventricle	PICA branches, choroid plexus	
Complications feared with approach chosen	CSF leak, vascular or neural injuries	CSF leak, hydrocephalus, neurological deficits	PICA injury, choroid plexus bleeding, hydrocephalus	

(continued on next page)

	Hazem Eltahawy, MD Neurosurgery St. Mary Mercy Hospital Ain Shams University Livonia, Michigan, United States	George I. Jallo, MD Neurosurgery Johns Hopkins All Children's Tampa, Florida, United States	Sheng-Fu Lo, MD Neurosurgery Johns Hopkins Baltimore, Maryland, United States	Khoi D. Than, MD Neurosurgery Duke University Durham, North Carolina, United States
Intraoperative				
Anesthesia	General	General	General	
Exposure	Occiput-C1	Occiput-C1	Occiput-C1	
Levels decompressed	Occiput-C1	Occiput-C1	Occiput-C1	
Levels fused	None	None	None	
Surgical narrative	Position prone on gel rolls and Mayfield pins, midline craniocervical incision along prior incision, careful dissection down to bony edges or prior craniectomy and C1, widen bony decompression at foramen magnum and C1, excision of thickened scar on top of dural graft, assessment of flow with ultrasound, V or Y-shaped durotomy under microscope, lysis of any arachnoid bands around cerebellar tonsils and brainstem, possible shrinking of tonsils with bipolar if needed, duroplasty with dural substitute, water tight closure confirmed with Valsalva, supplement with dural sealant, reassess CSF flow with ultrasound, layered closure with antibiotic irrigation, be prepared for syringo-pleural shunt if intraoperative findings dictate, flat for 12–24 hours	Position prone with neck flexion, open old incision, identify normal anatomy, open dura, utilize microscope to inspect obex and outflow of fourth ventricle, one- to two-level cervical laminectomy if no adhesions seen, open dura, visualize spinal cord and perm midline myelotomy in the thinnest area, place syringo-subarachnoid shunt, secure stent with 8-0 Prolene, watertight dural closure	Position prone with neck flexion, subperiosteal dissection down to suboccipital bone and prior craniotomy flap, blunt dissection over cut edge of posterior arch of C1, remove prior craniotomy, intraoperative ultrasound to confirm exposure and absence of normal CSF pulsations, Y-shaped dural opening across prior graft, avoid injury to PICA while dissecting and cutting arachnoid adhesions, mobilize cerebellar tonsils to access obex and floor of fourth ventricle, possibly coagulate tonsils if needed to access obex, open up membrane to confirm CSF pulsatile flow from the fourth ventricle through the median aperture, avoid manipulation of the roof, consider stenting with shunt tubing with extra holes and anchored with pial stitch, watertight expansile duraplasty with a reverse triangle pattern, fibrin sealant, replace craniotomy flap, layered closure	
Complication avoidance	Widen bony decompression at foramen magnum and C1, assessment of flow with ultrasound, possible shrinking of tonsils with bipolar if needed, syringo-pleural shunt if intraop findings dictate	Find normal anatomy, evaluate flow of fourth ventricle, syringo-subarachnoid shunt if no adhesions in fourth ventricle, secure shunt down	Ultrasound to evaluate CSF pulsations, observe for PICA when dissecting, possible tonsillar coagulation, possible stenting to keep aperture open	
Postoperative				
Admission	ICU	ICU	ICU	
Postoperative complications feared	CSF leak, vascular or neurological injury, persistent syrinx	CSF leak, hydrocephalus, neurological deficits	Chemical meningitis, pseudomeningocele, unrecognized bleeding causing hydrocephalus, PICA injury	
Anticipated length of stay	1–2 days	4–5 days	2–3 days	
Follow-up testing	MRI C-spine prior to discharge, 3 months after surgery	MRI brain and cervical spine 3 months after surgery	MRI C-spine with CINE 4–6 weeks after surgery	CSF flow study in 6 months
Bracing	None	None	None	
Follow-up visits	2 weeks, 6 weeks, 3 months after surgery	10–14 days after surgery	2 weeks after surgery	

CSF, Cerebrospinal fluid; *EMG*, electromyography; *ICU*, intensive care unit; *IOM*, intraoperative monitoring; *MAP*, mean arterial pressure; *MEP*, motor evoked potential; *MIS*, minimally invasive surgery; *MRI*, magnetic resonance imaging; *PICA*, posterior inferior cerebellar artery; *SSEP*, somatosensory evoked potential.

Differential diagnosis

- Chiari malformation
- Basilar invagination
- Intracranial mass lesion causing displacement
- Dandy-Walker malformation

Important anatomical and preoperative considerations

Currently, there is no consensus regarding the rationale and treatment modality in cases of persistent symptoms and syringomyelia after primary Chiari I malformation surgery.[3] Nevertheless, the presence of complaints referable to a persistent syrinx and enlarging syringomyelia are considered important indications for redo surgery.[1,2] The pathophysiological mechanism for enlargement or persistence of syringomyelia is a matter of debate and has not been completely elucidated, but several factors could be involved.[9,10] The impaction of the foramen magnum is one of the most important factors causing disturbance of CSF flow dynamics.[9] Certain conditions predispose patients for inadequate bone removal during surgery and further necessitate reoperation. Individuals with syndromic cranial configurations or craniosynostosis commonly demonstrate anatomical variations or generalized skull compression, respectively. These conditions have been related to persistent cerebellar tonsillar herniation and failed foramen magnum decompression (FMD) surgery.[8,9] Another theory hypothesizes that after FMD surgery there is less support for the cerebellum, which may lead to further caudal displacement of the cerebellar tonsils and, consequently, stenosis of the subarachnoid space around the cranio-vertebral junction (CVJ).[9,10] Additionally, aberrant outflow of CSF from the fourth ventricle may be involved in the pathogenesis of persistent syrinx, especially when the foramen of Magendie is partially obstructed by arachnoid adhesions or scarring.[2] Regardless of the cause, local stenosis of the subarachnoid space can lead lead to progression of the syrinx.[10] Other postoperative conditions associated to disruption of adequate CSF flow include arachnoiditis, infections, and bleeding.[10]

As aforementioned, the treatment after failed FMD, evidenced by persistent, enlarging, or development of new syringomyelia, remains controversial.[10] On the other hand, persistent symptomatic syrinx, progressive neurological symptoms, and enlarging syringomyelia represent dynamic conditions that must be approached by means of surgical intervention.[1,3,10] Surgical options include redo FMD accompanied by a broader opening, with or without tonsillar shrinking, and syringomyelia shunting.[1-3,10] Management strategy should be case-tailored. Magnetic resonance imaging (MRI) is crucial for this purpose because anatomical and functional status of the CVJ must be thoroughly investigated.[1,3,10] In addition, different etiologies of a persistent syrinx should be ruled out, such as spine instability, tethered cord, basilar invagination, and hydrocephalus.[10] Syringomyelia associated with recurrent impaction of the foramen magnum may benefit from redo FMD with bony expansion and dura graft, with or without tonsillar shrinkage.[3,10] If the patients do not exhibit clear signs of a tightened CVJ on MRI, the benefit of a decompression is questionable.[10] In symptomatic patients presenting with an extensive and enlarging syrinx, concurrent FMD and syringo-subarachnoid shunt is indicated.[1,3,10] To avoid spinal cord damage, myelotomy should be performed in the midline or on the dorsal root entry zone at the largest segment of the syrinx.[10] Syringo-subarachnoid shunt has shown less complications than syringo-pleural and syringo-peritoneal shunts.[10]

What was actually done

Due to the presence of headaches and upper limb paresthesias, the patient underwent imaging evaluation that demonstrated the presence of a large cervical syrinx and obstruction at the level of the fourth ventricle (obex scarring). Her case was thoroughly examined and presented in our complex spine and tumor conference. After discussion, an exploration of the level of the fourth ventricle was advised for the patient with reexploration and revision of the previous suboccipital craniectomy. The patient was taken to the operating room. The patient was induced under general anesthesia and positioned prone with Mayfield pins. Somatosensory and motor evoked potentials were used throughout the case. The dural substitute from the previous surgery was identified and opened in a Y-shaped fashion. The tonsils and cerebellum came into view. The microscope was introduced. There was a dense arachnoid scar, including a web over the outlet of the fourth ventricle. This was widely opened with sharp dissection. The fourth ventricle as well as the foramen of Luschka laterally and the foramen of Magendie medially were decompressed. A dural graft was used for the duraplasty. The patient awoke with no complications. Repeat imaging showed resolution of the syrinx 3 months later (Fig. 68.2), with improvement in her upper extremity symptoms and headache remission.

Commonalities among the experts

Most requested a cine MRI scan to observe CSF flow as well as MRI of the brain. Half of the experts added a dynamic cervical spine MRI to their preoperative assessment. The majority advocated for a suboccipital craniectomy revision, and likely a lower cervical laminectomy. While all agreed the goal of surgical reintervention was restoration of CSF flow, strategies to attain this greatly varied and included syringo-pleural shunt, syringo-subarachnoid shunt, and coagulation with obex stenting. Most were aware of posterior inferior cerebellar artery (PICA), vertebral arteries, and critical neural elements such as cerebellum, fourth ventricle, and choroid plexus. Major approach-related complications feared by most surgeons were CSF leak, vascular injury, and hydrocephalus. Half recommended perioperative steroids therapy. Surgery was usually pursued with surgical microscope and ultrasound. All admitted their patients to the intensive care unit after intervention. All opted for postoperative imaging.

SUMMARY OF QUALITY OF EVIDENCE TO GUIDE SPECIFIC INTERVENTIONS FOR THIS CASE

- Suboccipital craniectomy revision for patients presenting with persistent or enlarging symptomatic syrinx: level II-2

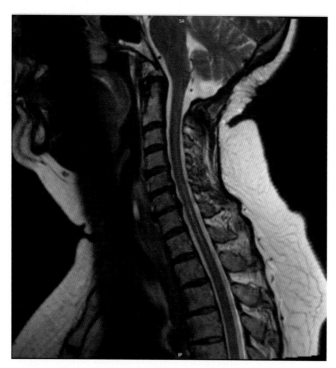

Fig. 68.2 Postoperative magnetic resonance image (MRI) of the cervical spine 3 months after revision surgery. Sagittal T2 image demonstrating postsurgical changes of prior redo suboccipital craniectomy. A mostly collapsed cervical and upper thoracic syringomyelia is evident. The cerebellar tonsils are normal in appearance without caudal displacement.

REFERENCES

1. Mazzola CA, Fried AH. Revision surgery for Chiari malformation decompression. *Neurosurg Focus.* 2003;15(3):E3.
2. Riordan CP, Scott RM. Fourth ventricle stent placement for treatment of recurrent syringomyelia in patients with type I Chiari malformations. *J Neurosurg Pediatr.* 2018;23(2):164–170.
3. Soleman J, Bartoli A, Korn A, Constantini S, Roth J. Treatment failure of syringomyelia associated with Chiari I malformation following foramen magnum decompression: how should we proceed? *Neurosurg Rev.* 2019;42(3):705–714.
4. Beretta E, Vetrano IG, Curone M, et al. Chiari malformation-related headache: outcome after surgical treatment. *Neurol Sci.* 2017; 38(Suppl 1):95–98.
5. Zhao JL, Li MH, Wang CL, Meng W. A Systematic Review of Chiari I Malformation: Techniques and Outcomes. *World Neurosurg.* 2016;88:7–14.
6. Ellenbogen RG, Armonda RA, Shaw DW, Winn HR. Toward a rational treatment of Chiari I malformation and syringomyelia. *Neurosurg Focus.* 2000;8(3):E6.
7. Schuster JM, Zhang F, Norvell DC, Hermsmeyer JT. Persistent/ Recurrent syringomyelia after Chiari decompression-natural history and management strategies: a systematic review. *Evid Based Spine Care J.* 2013;4(2):116–125.
8. Sacco D, Scott RM. Reoperation for Chiari malformations. *Pediatr Neurosurg.* 2003;39(4):171–178.
9. Gil Z, Rao S, Constantini S. Expansion of Chiari I-associated syringomyelia after posterior-fossa decompression. *Childs Nerv Syst.* 2000;16(9):555–558.
10. Soleman J, Roth J, Bartoli A, Rosenthal D, Korn A, Constantini S. Syringo-Subarachnoid Shunt for the Treatment of Persistent Syringomyelia Following Decompression for Chiari Type I Malformation: Surgical Results. *World Neurosurg.* 2017;108:836–843.

69

Tethered cord

Fidel Valero-Moreno, MD

Introduction

Tethered cord syndrome (TCS) refers to the clinical condition produced by excessive tension of the spinal cord, with its caudal part anchored by inelastic structures that restrict its vertical movement.[1,2] Inelastic structures include adipose filum terminale, tumor, myelomeningoceles, lipomyelomeningoceles, and scar formations.[2] In the vast majority of cases, the spinal cord is tethered at the lumbosacral level.[3] TCS results from the coexistence of anatomical and functional disturbances of the spinal cord.[4] The degree of cord traction and the metabolic impairment of the spinal cord are the determining factors for the development and the severity of symptoms.[1,5] The most consistent complaints are back and leg pain exacerbated by postural changes.[5,6] Onset of clinical manifestations can occur early in life or during adulthood. Patients with tethering of the spinal cord can be divided into two groups depending on the presence or absence of spinal dysraphism. Prognosis and treatment of patients with dysraphism is similar to pediatric TCS.[6] The presence of progressive symptoms or signs are indications for surgical treatment especially in patients with incontinence.[2,7] In addition, some surgeons recommend surgery when signs of dysraphism are present.[1] Around 86% of patients experience pain relief after operative treatment.[7] In this chapter, we present the case of a young female patient with urinary retention, lower limb pain, and a history of previous closed neural tube defect.

Example case

Chief complaint: urinary retention, lower limb and back pain

History of present illness: This is a 48-year-old female patient with a history of spina bifida and a spinal mass who underwent lumbar surgery more than 15 years prior. She has been stable for many years with chronic but tolerable back pain. The patient was lost to follow-up and presented recently with new urinary retention and pain in her both lower extremities when active. She does not report any weakness. As part of her evaluation, the patient underwent a lumbar spine magnetic resonance image demonstrating a tethered cord and a large cystic intradural mass at the level of L3 (Fig. 69.1).

Medications: antidepressants

Allergies: no known drug allergies

Past medical and surgical history: as above

Family history: noncontributory

Social history: none

Physical examination: awake, alert, and oriented to person, place, and time; cranial nerves II–XII intact; bilateral deltoids/triceps/biceps 5/5; interossei 5/5; iliopsoas/knee flexion/knee extension/dorsi, and plantar flexion 5/5

Reflexes: 2+ in bilateral biceps/triceps/brachioradialis with negative Hoffman; 1+ in bilateral patella/ankle; no clonus or Babinski; sensation diminished in perianal region and both lower extremities

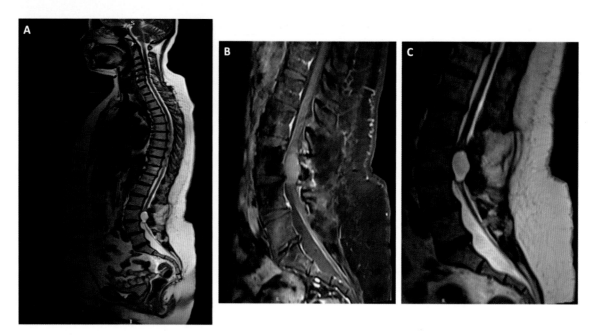

Fig. 69.1 Preoperative magnetic resonance imaging (MRI) of the lumbosacral spine. (A) Sagittal T2 MRI of the entire spine demonstrating a hyperintense cystic lesion occupying the L3 level and an apparent tethered cord with a low lying conus medullaris. The lesion is slightly heterogenous with a central hypointensity, sharply circumscribed, corresponding to an intradural adipose tissue. **(B)** Sagittal T1 with contrast and fat suppression demonstrating the lipoma as an isointense mass. **(C)** Sagittal T2 MRI of the lumbar spine demonstrating a tethered spinal cord attached to the lipoma at the L3 level. Degenerative disc changes at L4-L5 and L5-S1 are also present.

	Carlos A. Bagley, MD Neurosurgery University of Texas Southwestern Dallas, Texas, United States	Nicolas Dea, MD, MSc Neurosurgery Vancouver Spine Surgery Institute Vancouver, Canada	Fernando Hakim, MD Hospital Universitario Fundacion Santafe de Bogota Bogota, Colombia	Jang Yoon, MD Neurosurgery University of Pennsylvania Philadelphia, Pennsylvania, United States
Preoperative				
Additional tests requested	Urology evaluation with urodynamic studies Bilateral lower extremity EMG/NCS Medicine evaluation	Urology evaluation with urodynamic studies Compare previous MRI scans	MRI brain, C- and T-spine CT L-spine Urodynamic studies Neurophysiological testing (EMG, NCS, SSEP) Anesthesiology evaluation	MRI C- and T-spine Standing L-spine x-rays with flexion-extension Urology evaluation Neurology evaluation
Surgical approach selected	Revision L2-4 laminectomy and excision of intradural lipoma and release of tethered cord	Revision laminectomy, spinal lipoma resection, spinal cord untethering	Revision laminectomy, spinal lipoma resection, spinal cord untethering	Revision laminectomy, removal of intradural extramedullary lesion, spinal cord untethering
Goal of surgery	Spinal cord untethering, remove the mass, decompress neural elements	Spinal cord untethering, remove the mass, decompress neural elements	Spinal cord untethering, remove the mass	Spinal cord untethering, cord decompression, diagnosis, removal of mass, complex wound closure
Perioperative				
Positioning	Prone on Jackson table	Prone with pins	Prone, no pins	Prone in Wilson frame on flat Jackson table
Surgical equipment	IOM (MEP/SSEP/EMG) Nerve stimulator Surgical microscope Laser	IOM (MEP/SSEP/EMG) Laser Dural substitute Surgical microscope	IOM (MEP/SSEP/EMG) Surgical microscope Ultrasound Ultrasonic aspirator	IOM (MEP/SSEP/EMG) Ultrasound Nerve stimulator Surgical microscope
Medications	Steroids, pregabalin	Steroids	None	None
Anatomical considerations	Spinal cord, facet joints	Spinal cord, conus, cauda equina nerve roots	Cauda equina nerve roots	Spinal cord, conus, cauda equina nerve roots

	Carlos A. Bagley, MD Neurosurgery University of Texas Southwestern Dallas, Texas, United States	Nicolas Dea, MD, MSc Neurosurgery Vancouver Spine Surgery Institute Vancouver, Canada	Fernando Hakim, MD Hospital Universitario Fundacion Santafe de Bogota Bogota, Colombia	Jang Yoon, MD Neurosurgery University of Pennsylvania Philadelphia, Pennsylvania, United States
Complications feared with approach chosen	Spinal cord injury, CSF leak, spinal instability	Conus injury	Nerve root injury, CSF leak	Spinal cord injury, nerve root injury, retethering
Intraoperative				
Anesthesia	General	General	General	General
Exposure	L2-4	L2-5	L2-4	L1-4
Levels decompressed	L2-4	L2-4	L2-4	L1-4
Levels fused	None	None	None	None
Surgical narrative	Position prone, open previous incision from L2-4, expose remnant posterior elements as well as inferior portion of L1 and superior portion of L5, remove superficial elements from L2-L4 and partially L1 and L5 to find normal anatomy and dura using drill, define lateral edges of dural plane, widen laminectomy from L2 to 4 to obtain sufficient exposure, linear dural opening and tack dural edges using microscope, expose lipoma and normal spinal cord both rostral and caudal, shave down and remove as much lipoma as possible using laser and microdissector leaving a thin rim, use stimulator to identify any questionable neural vs. scar tissue, detether cord, watertight dural closure with Valsalva, irrigate wound, dural sealant to suture line, multilayer closure	Position prone, obtain baseline SSEP/MEP, revision laminectomy from normal to abnormal, find normal dura, expose previous durotomy, midline durotomy, localize normal anatomy, find mass and dissect off of nerve roots, potential laser to remove lipoma with constant IOM, attempt neural tube closure with pial sutures, cut filum, duraplasty with suturable patch	Position prone, fluoroscopy to localize level, midline incision, subperiosteal dissection, expose posterior elements, fluoroscopy to confirm level, scar tissue dissection under microscopic visualization, midline durotomy, ultrasound to make sure exposure is sufficient, tenting sutures, identify lipoma, debulk mass using ultrasonic aspirator, subtotal resection, cauda equina dissection under EMG monitoring, identify filum terminale, separate from surrounding cauda equina, suture placed through filum to aid in pathological examination, watertight dural closure, dural patch if necessary, fibrin sealant, layered closure	Position prone, expose normal anatomy at L1 and bottom on L4, work around the scars to expose normal lamina, preserve posterior tension band and facet complexes, remove bottom of L1 and L4 to find normal dura, work toward the scar tissue, ultrasound to identify lesion, open dura from normal toward scar, tack dura up, dissect lesion away from spinal cord under microscope, try freeing dentate ligaments or scar if present to minimize tension on spinal cord, resect filum terminale after removal of lesion, stimulate cauda equina to confirm nerves are not resected, watertight dural closure with dural sealant, closure in layers
Complication avoidance	Identify remnant posterior elements, find normal anatomy and dura cranial and caudal from previous opening, widen laminectomy to obtain sufficient exposure, leave tiny rim of lipoma, nerve stimulator	Laminectomy from normal to abnormal, locate conus and nerve roots, laser lipoma removal	Ultrasound to guide opening, aim for subtotal resection, cauda equina dissection under EMG monitoring, suture placed through filum to aid in pathological examination	Expose to find normal anatomy, preserve posterior tension band and facet complexes, dissect dentate ligaments and scar to minimize tension, nerve stimulator to avoid injury to cauda equina, dural sealant
Postoperative				
Admission	Floor	Floor	ICU	ICU
Postoperative complications feared	CSF leak, urinary retention, urinary tract infection, wound infection, medical complication	CSF leak, conus injury, retethering	CSF leak, nerve injury	Pseudomeningocele, CSF leak, retethering, instability, wound complications
Anticipated length of stay	4 days	2–5 days	2–3 days	3–5 days

(continued on next page)

	Carlos A. Bagley, MD Neurosurgery University of Texas Southwestern Dallas, Texas, United States	Nicolas Dea, MD, MSc Neurosurgery Vancouver Spine Surgery Institute Vancouver, Canada	Fernando Hakim, MD Hospital Universitario Fundacion Santafe de Bogota Bogota, Colombia	Jang Yoon, MD Neurosurgery University of Pennsylvania Philadelphia, Pennsylvania, United States
Follow-up testing	MRI L-spine within 2 days of surgery	MRI L-spine 2-3 months after surgery Urology follow-up	None	Lumbar x-rays including flexion-extension prior to discharge Physical therapy MRI L-spine 12 months after surgery
Bracing	None	None	None	None
Follow-up visits	6 weeks after surgery	2–3 months after surgery	2 weeks after surgery	2 weeks, 6 weeks, 3 months, 6 months, 12 months, 24 months after surgery

CSF, Cerebrospinal fluid; *CT*, computed tomography; *EMG*, electromyography; *ICU*, intensive care unit; *IOM*, intraoperative monitoring; *MRI*, magnetic resonance imaging; *NCS*, nerve conduction study; *SSEP*, somatosensory evoked potential.

Differential diagnosis

- Intramedullary tumor
- Intradural extramedullary tumors
- Multiple sclerosis
- Bone tumors (multiple myeloma)
- Lipoma

Important anatomical and preoperative considerations

The spinal cord is formed by neurons, neural tracts, glial tissue, vasculature, and the pia mater tightly attached to the cord. The content of elastin within the pial layer and subpial tissue confers elasticity to the spinal cord. In a similar way, collagen in the dentate ligaments, pia, and blood vessels helps to resist traction and prevent neuronal disruption.[8] Glia replaced by fibrous tissue and decreased elastin in the spinal cord are factors strongly related to the loss of viscoelasticity and thickening of the filum.[4,5] The diameter of a normal filum terminale is 1.1 to 1.2 mm,[5,9] and the minimal diameter to define a tethered cord ranges from 1 to 2 mm.[5] An inelastic filum is defined as <10% of viscoelasticity on a stretch test.[4] This manifests as elongation of the spinal cord, which, consequently, is more susceptible to caudal traction.[4] Theoretically, there is an important correlation between the extent of elongation and the degree of metabolic impairment in the spinal cord.[2] The metabolic derangement causes electrophysiological disturbances in the lumbosacral cord, which leads to neuronal and tract dysfunction.[5] The degree of cord traction is the main factor associated to onset of symptoms.[1,10]

In the supine position, the spinal cord is located anteriorly in the thoracic spine and posteriorly in the cervical and lumbar segments. In addition, the cord is situated toward the concave area of the curvature. Hence, the subarachnoid space posterior to the spinal cord and the cauda equina is narrower in the lumbosacral level.[4] In individuals with TCS, the conus and filum appear attached to the posterior arachnoid membrane, especially at the most lordotic level in order to minimize tension within the caudal cord.[4,5] Interestingly, the posterior displacement of the filum terminale is the only regular finding to suggest increased tension in the spinal cord.[2,5] This is an important protective mechanism in younger patients, which lessens the stretching process during accelerated growth.[5] Some conditions, such as trauma, physical activity, and spinal stenosis, can increase the tension and hasten the development of symptoms.[1,11]

The diagnosis of TCS must be based on a combination of functional and anatomical features. Elongation of the spinal cord and thickening of the filum are valid diagnostic tools when neurological impairment or symptoms are present.[4,12] Moreover, the presence of progressive deficits or symptoms in patients harboring these anomalies should be followed by surgical treatment, especially if certain conditions such as dysraphism or tumors are involved.[1,2] Surgical technique usually implies a skin incision and laminectomy at the level of the conus and filum junction, where the laminectomy should not disturb the facet joints.[2] Incision of the dura and arachnoid membrane is done to identify the posteriorly shifted conus or filum.[2] Intraoperative endoscopy thorough a small opening of the dura and pia arachnoid is an alternative to identify the location of the filum.[1] The filum starts just caudal to the exit of the coccygeal nerve root. Cauterization and resection of the filum between 5 mm and 10 mm long, sparing 5 mm from the conus, as well as resection of a possible tumor or mass, is advocated by most experts.[4]

What was actually done

Surgical intervention was advocated due to escalating back and bilateral leg pain with imaging showing an enlarging cystic lesion within the conus medullaris and tethered cord. The patient was brought to the operating room. The patient was induced with general anesthesia and positioned prone on the Jackson table. Baseline somatosensory and motor evoked potentials were obtained. The previous midline low lumbar surgical incision was reopened. Level was confirmed with fluoroscopy. The posterior elements from L2 to L4 were exposed bilaterally in a subperiosteal fashion. Laminectomy was done over the lower aspect of L2, redo laminectomy at L3, and superior L4. The operating microscope was introduced. The dura was opened vertically in the midline and the conus was identified. A lipoma arising from the conus was identified. Distal to the lipoma there was a cystic mass lesion with loculations. These loculations were entered and evacuated. There was a reduction in the motor evoked potentials in the right foot. Frozen samples showed no tumor. The neural

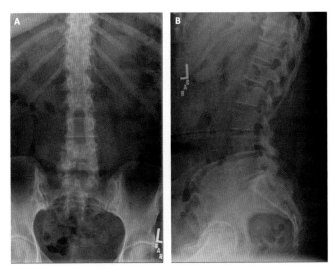

Fig. 69.2 Postoperative x-rays. (A) Anteroposterior and **(B)** lateral x-rays demonstrating normal lumbar vertebral body height, unchanged grade I anterolisthesis of L4 and L5, and posterior decompression at L3 level.

surgical microscope, and ultrasound. Half recommended perioperative steroids. Following surgery, half admitted their patients to the intensive care unit and the rest to the department. Most recommended a lumbar MRI for appropriate follow-up; however, the interval between surgery and follow-up testing greatly varied, ranging from 2 days to 12 months.

SUMMARY OF QUALITY OF EVIDENCE TO GUIDE SPECIFIC INTERVENTIONS FOR THIS CASE

- The degree of cord traction is the main factor associated to onset of symptoms: level II-2
- The presence of progressive deficits or symptoms in patients with tethered cord should be followed by surgical treatment: level II-2
- Cauterization and resection of the filum between 5 mm and 10 mm long, and resection of associated masses: level II-2
- Urodynamic studies as part of preoperative valuation of tethered cord: level III

elements were decompressed and the cystic mass was untethered form the dura. All nerve roots were intact. The dura and wound were closed in a regular fashion. The patient was taken to the recovery room in stable neurological condition. The patient reported pain improvement and was neurologically stable. The patient was discharged to home on postoperative day 3 with some right leg weakness (4+/5). Three months after surgery, leg symptoms improved about 80% but still had some numbness, with no urinary retention and no need for ambulatory aids. Postoperative lumbar radiographs were satisfactory (Fig. 69.2).

Commonalities among the experts

Although there was a broad variability in the preferred perioperative tests by the experts, most of the surgeons recommended a urodynamic study and urology evaluation to better understand the neurological status and more specifically the bladder function. Moreover, half opted for neurophysiological studies, as well as magnetic resonance imaging (MRI) of the brain and cervicothoracic spine. All agreed the main goal of surgical intervention was spinal cord untethering and removal of the mass. For this purpose, all advocated for revision laminectomy, combined with excision of intradural lipoma and cord release. The approach-associated complications feared by most surgeons were spinal cord injury, damage to nerve roots, and cerebrospinal fluid leak. Surgery was generally achieved with intraoperative monitoring,

REFERENCES

1. Hertzler 2nd DA, DePowell JJ, Stevenson CB, Mangano FT. Tethered cord syndrome: a review of the literature from embryology to adult presentation. *Neurosurg Focus*. 2010;29(1):E1.
2. Yamada S, Won DJ, Siddiqi J, Yamada SM. Tethered cord syndrome: overview of diagnosis and treatment. *Neurol Res*. 2004;26(7):719–721.
3. Agarwalla PK, Dunn IF, Scott RM, Smith ER. Tethered cord syndrome. *Neurosurg Clin N Am*. 2007;18(3):531–547.
4. Yamada S, Won DJ, Yamada SM, Hadden A, Siddiqi J. Adult tethered cord syndrome: relative to spinal cord length and filum thickness. *Neurol Res*. 2004;26(7):732–734.
5. Woods KR, Colohan AR, Yamada S, Yamada SM, Won DJ. Intrathecal endoscopy to enhance the diagnosis of tethered cord syndrome. *J Neurosurg Spine*. 2010;13(4):477–483.
6. Yamada S, Siddiqi J, Won DJ, et al. Symptomatic protocols for adult tethered cord syndrome. *Neurol Res*. 2004;26(7):741–744.
7. Gao J, Kong X, Li Z, Wang T, Li Y. Surgical treatments on adult tethered cord syndrome: A retrospective study. *Medicine (Baltimore)*. 2016;95(46):e5454.
8. Yamada S, Zinke DE, Sanders D. Pathophysiology of "tethered cord syndrome." *J Neurosurg*. 1981;54(4):494–503.
9. Yundt KD, Park TS, Kaufman BA. Normal diameter of filum terminale in children: in vivo measurement. *Pediatr Neurosurg*. 1997;27(5):257–259.
10. Pang D, Wilberger Jr. JE. Tethered cord syndrome in adults. *J Neurosurg*. 1982;57(1):32–47.
11. Yamada S, Won DJ, Yamada SM. Pathophysiology of tethered cord syndrome: correlation with symptomatology. *Neurosurg Focus*. 2004;16(2):E6.
12. Warder DE, Oakes WJ. Tethered cord syndrome and the conus in a normal position. *Neurosurgery*. 1993;33(3):374–378.

70

Chronic adhesive arachnoiditis with spinal cord dysfunction

Fidel Valero-Moreno, MD

Introduction

Arachnoiditis is an inflammatory condition of the arachnoid mater, leading to thickened leptomeninges and neurological symptoms in many cases.[1] Ninety percent of patients with arachnoiditis experience a burning type pain.[2] The most common location of spinal arachnoiditis is the thoracic segment.[3] The known causes include idiopathic, iatrogenic, foreign bodies (intrathecal pain pumps, radiographic contrast), subarachnoid hemorrhage, and infection.[4] Overall, spine surgery is the most common condition associated with arachnoiditis.[5] Spinal arachnoiditis can manifest as meningeal thickening, adhesions with cord deformity, meningeal enhancement, arachnoid cyst formation, and syrinx.[6] Chronic adhesive arachnoiditis can result from prolonged irritation of the arachnoid and lead to spinal cord or nerve root tethering. Spinal cord dysfunction and progressive syringomyelia can also occur as a result of this syndrome. In turn, spinal arachnoid cysts can cause progressive compressive myelopathy.[7] The evaluation and diagnosis of arachnoiditis can be made with magnetic resonance imaging (MRI) or myelography, which will typically demonstrate loculations of cerebrospinal fluid in one or multiple locations.[3] Increased T2 signal change within the cord can also be seen in severe cases with tethering. The main goal of arachnoiditis treatment is pain relief. Heterogeneous results have been reported for conservative and surgical modalities.[6] Despite this, surgery remains a treatment option for this condition. In this chapter, we discuss the case of a young patient with a history of meningitis who presented with progressive left hemiparesis.

Example case

Chief complaint: new weakness

History of present illness: This is a 21-year-old male patient with a history of a seizure disorder and developmental delay due to meningitis during childhood, who presented with worsening left upper and lower extremity weakness. His mother states that he has been having increased difficulty ambulating and feeding himself over the last month. He has also been experiencing urinary incontinence. The patient underwent a magnetic resonance imaging (MRI) of the cervical and thoracic spine that demonstrated the presence of an anterior intradural arachnoid cyst spanning the cervical and thoracic spine (Fig. 70.1).

Medications: Vimpat, Keppra

Allergies: no known drug allergies

Past medical and surgical history: coccidioidal meningitis, right hemispheric stroke, hydrocephalus, ventriculoperitoneal shunt placement.

Family history: none

Social history: lives with mother, dependent for activities of daily living

Physical examination: awake, alert, and oriented to person, place, and time; cranial nerves II–XII intact; right deltoids/triceps/biceps 5/5; interossei 5/5; iliopsoas/knee flexion/knee extension/dorsi, and plantar flexion 5/5. Left deltoids/triceps/biceps 3/5; interossei 3/5; iliopsoas/knee, flexion/knee, extension/dorsi, and plantar flexion 3/5

Reflexes: 3+ in bilateral biceps/triceps/brachioradialis with positive Hoffman; 3+ in bilateral patella/ankle; no clonus or Babinski; sensation normal on left hemibody

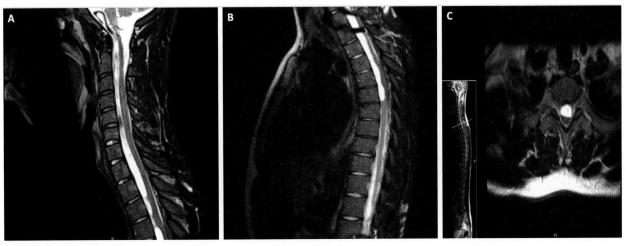

Fig. 70.1 Preoperative magnetic resonance imaging (MRI) of the cervical and thoracic spine. (A) Sagittal T2 image demonstrating the presence of a large abnormal intradural extramedullary fluid collection compatible with arachnoid cyst, where the cystic collection extends from the foramen magnum and continues enlarging caudally within the cervical and upper thoracic spine. **(B)** Sagittal T2 image demonstrating an arachnoid cyst spanning the entire thoracic spine, with loculations within the collection, most prominent at T4-T6 levels. Cerebrospinal fluid (CSF) intensity within the cyst is slightly brighter than the normal CSF. **(C)** Axial T2 image demonstrating the abnormal intradural extramedullary fluid collection ventral to the cervical and thoracic spinal cord with significant compression of the neural tissue.

	Adrian Casey, MD Neurosurgery National Hospital for Neurology and Neurosurgery Queen Square, Holborn, London, United Kingdom	Patrick C. Hsieh, MD Neurosurgery University of Southern California Los Angeles, California, United States	Daniel C. Liu, MD, PhD Neurosurgery University of California at Los Angeles Los Angeles, California, United States	Claudio Yampolsky, MD Neurosurgery Hospital Italiano de Buenos Aires Buenos Aires, Argentina
Preoperative				
Additional tests requested	MRI brain and complete spine with CISS CT C-T spine Anesthesiology evaluation +/- Mental capacity assessment	CT myelogram complete spine CSF studies	CT myelogram complete spine Interventional myelogram if T myelogram insufficient MRI brain Neurology evaluation	SSEP MRI brain with cine imaging
Surgical approach selected	T1–2 laminectomy for arachnoid cyst fenestration and lysis of adhesions (+/- shunt)	C6-T6 laminectomy for arachnoid cyst fenestration, possible extension to C3	C6-T6 laminectomy for lysis of adhesion	If flow obstruction present on imaging with medullary compression, T1–2 laminectomy and placement of arachnoid cyst-subarachnoid shunt
Goal of surgery	Spinal cord decompression, arachnoid cyst fenestration, open CSF pathways	Spinal cord decompression, excision of arachnoid cyst, minimize cyst recurrence	Lysis of adhesions, reduce mass effect	Medullary decompression, cyst drainage
Perioperative				
Positioning	Prone, with Mayfield pins	Prone on Jackson table, with Mayfield pins	Prone, with Mayfield pins	Prone
Surgical equipment	IOM Fluoroscopy Surgical microscope +/- Ultrasound Lumbar drain	IOM (MEP/SSEP) Fluoroscopy O-arm Ultrasound	IOM (MEP/SSEP) Fluoroscopy Surgical microscope Lumbar drain	IOM Fluoroscopy Surgical navigation Surgical microscope
Medications	Steroids, maintain MAP	Steroids, MAP 85	Fluorescein	None
Anatomical considerations	Spinal cord, facet joints	Spinal cord, dentate ligaments, segmental nerves, anterior spinal artery	Spinal cord, vertebral arteries	Lamina, dentate ligaments, dura, medulla
Complications feared with approach chosen	CSF leak, progressive neurological decline, recurrent arachnoiditis or arachnoid cyst	Spinal cord injury, CSF leak	Spinal cord injury, spinal instability	CSF fistula, infection, neurological deficit

(continued on next page)

	Adrian Casey, MD Neurosurgery National Hospital for Neurology and Neurosurgery Queen Square, Holborn, London, United Kingdom	Patrick C. Hsieh, MD Neurosurgery University of Southern California Los Angeles, California, United States	Daniel C. Liu, MD, PhD Neurosurgery University of California at Los Angeles Los Angeles, California, United States	Claudio Yampolsky, MD Neurosurgery Hospital Italiano de Buenos Aires Buenos Aires, Argentina
Intraoperative				
Anesthesia	General	General	General	General
Exposure	T1-2	C6-T6	C6-T6	T1-2
Levels decompressed	T1-2	C6-T6	C6-T6	T1-2
Levels fused	None	None	If needed	None
Surgical narrative	Position prone, x-ray level check, midline incision high thoracic spine, subperiosteal muscle strip to expose T1–2 laminae, laminectomy with high-speed drill, x-ray to confirm level, ultrasound to check location for cyst, midline durotomy and lateral suspension of dura under microscope, identification of cyst and drainage, section dentate ligament if needed, consider shunt, check for cord decompression proximally and distally, dural closure with clips and dural substitute with glue, layered closure	Position prone, baseline MEP/SSEP, expose from C6-T6, confirm levels with fluoroscopy, C6-T6 laminectomy without facet violation, open dura under microscopic visualization, examine spinal cord/nerves/dentate ligaments, release all arachnoid adhesions, ultrasound to visualize size and contour of arachnoid cyst to spinal cord relationship, cut dentate ligaments bilaterally between segment nerves from C6 to T6, place 6-0 Prolene stitch on medial end of cut dentate ligament, gently rotate spinal cord to examine ventral subarachnoid space, identify cyst wall and excise cyst wall, check for decompression and deflation of cyst with ultrasound, watertight dural closure, dural substitute onlay and tissel over dural closure site, drain placement in epidural space, intraoperative topic vancomycin and tobramycin, wound closure in layers	Preflip IOM, position prone, mark midline incision based on x-ray, midline posterior incision, dissect to posterior elements in avascular plane, drill bilateral troughs at cervical level overlying arachnoid cyst, separate ligamentum flavum with Kerrison rongeurs and lift lamina from dura in one piece, drill out thoracic lamina if noncommunicating arachnoid cyst extends into thoracic level, midline longitudinal durotomy and retract dural leaflets, identify isolated arachnoid cysts under microscopic visualization and fluorescein injection as needed, minimize spinal cord manipulation, expand laminectomies as needed, lyse arachnoid cysts with sharp dissection and bipolar cauterization, verify communication with the subarachnoid space using fluorescein, confirm stability/improvement with IOMN, primary dural closure with dural sealant, fusion if needed, layered closure with subfascial drain to gravity, vancomycin epifascially	Position prone, midline incision at T1–2 level, left-side laminectomy, placement of minimally invasive tubular retractor, dural opening, dissection of dentate ligament, mobilization with continuous IOM, drain collection, placement catheter and connect to subarachnoid space, layered closure
Complication avoidance	Limit exposure T1–2, ultrasound to confirm location of cyst, section dentate ligament if needed, consider shunt	Avoid facet violation, ultrasound to better delineate relationship between arachnoid cyst and spinal cord, release dentate ligaments, manipulate cord by stitching cut dentate ligament, ultrasound to evaluate decompression	Preflip IOM, en bloc laminectomy, fluorescein to help identify arachnoid cyst, minimize spinal cord manipulation, verify communication with the subarachnoid space using fluorescein	Hemilaminectomy, cut dentate ligament, cyst-subarachnoid shunt

	Adrian Casey, MD Neurosurgery National Hospital for Neurology and Neurosurgery Queen Square, Holborn, London, United Kingdom	Patrick C. Hsieh, MD Neurosurgery University of Southern California Los Angeles, California, United States	Daniel C. Liu, MD, PhD Neurosurgery University of California at Los Angeles Los Angeles, California, United States	Claudio Yampolsky, MD Neurosurgery Hospital Italiano de Buenos Aires Buenos Aires, Argentina
Postoperative				
Admission	High dependency unit	ICU	Floor	Floor
Postoperative complications feared	CSF leak, meningitis, spinal cord injury, recurrence, adhesions	New neurological deficit, CSF leak, hematoma, recurrence of cyst, cord compression	CSF leak, recurrence of adhesions	CSF leak, infection, neurological deficit
Anticipated length of stay	5–7 days	4–5 days	2–5 days	2 days
Follow-up testing	MRI prior to discharge, 3 months after surgery	MRI before discharge, 3 months after surgery	CT myelogram 3 months after surgery	MRI within 48 hours of surgery
Bracing	None	None	Hard collar	None
Follow-up visits	6 weeks, 3 months, 6 months, 12 months after surgery	2–3 weeks, 6 weeks, 3 months, 6 months, 12 months, then annually after surgery	2 weeks, 6 weeks, 3 months after surgery	7 days, 2 weeks, 4 weeks after surgery

CISS, constructive interference in steady state; *CSF*, cerebrospinal fluid; *CT*, computed tomography; *ICU*, intensive care unit; *IOM*, intraoperative monitoring; *MAP*, mean arterial pressure; *MEP*, motor evoked potential, *MRI*, magnetic resonance imaging; *SSEP*, somatosensory evoked potential.

Differential diagnosis

- Arachnoiditis
- Meningitis
- Intramedullary spinal cord tumor
- Congenital arachnoid cysts

Important anatomical and preoperative considerations

The arachnoid matter is the central layer of the meninges and is characterized for being thin and fragile.[2] The release of fibrinous exudates during an inflammatory response causes nerve roots to adhere to themselves and to the thecal sac.[1] The healing process in this location is not effective due to the lack of innervation and vascularization.[1,2] Moreover, the normal cerebrospinal fluid (CSF) dynamics interfere with the phagocytic and enzymatic functions involved in preventing scar tissue formation.[1] The physiopathological mechanism is similar to the repair process in serous membranes.[5] On magnetic imaging of the spine, the most common associated finding is the formation of arachnoid cysts, which ranges from a segmental distribution to the whole spine and usually are dorsal to the spinal cord.[8] Three characteristics on imaging evaluation have been linked steadily with arachnoiditis: nerve root thickening and clumping, empty sac appearance due to the peripheral adhesions and tethering of the nerve roots, and an inflammatory process with or without enhancement.[8] Arachnoiditis is most commonly located in the thoracolumbar spine, followed by isolated lumbar and lumbosacral, according to Anderson et al., where adhesions occur predominantly on the dorsal aspect of the cord.[8]

Although the gold of arachnoiditis management is pain relief, this is a very rare occurrence.[1,2] Pain mechanism in this condition is not well established, and the likelihood of improvement or cure is very low with either conservative management (nonsteroidal antiinflammatory drugs [NSAIDs], steroids, opioids) or surgery.[1,2] Currently, surgical intervention is considered the last option after failure of conservative therapies. Direct spinal stimulation aims for pain control through replacement of pain with paresthesia, where this method theoretically provides relief by means of synaptic inhibition.[1] Laminectomy and placement of spinal electrodes is advocated just after pain improvement is well documented.[1] A second surgical option, and the most common strategy, is laminectomy, microsurgical lysis of adhesions, and fenestration if necessary, where this procedure has offered temporal improvement in mild symptomatic patients and minimal relief in patients with severe disease.[1,2,6] This procedure is associated with neurological stabilization, and decompression can be effective for patients with paraparesis due to arachnoid cyst compression.[3] In cases of arachnoid cysts, surgical treatment should be aimed to address decompression of the spinal cord and establishment of continuous CSF flow.[9,10] A wide fenestration or partial resection of the cyst are effective to produce cyst collapse and achieve decompression.[9] Regardless, creating a normal unobstructed CSF flow is challenging. Manipulation of neural tissue should be avoided in order to prevent additional scar or adhesion formation.[9] Whereas placement of shunting devices has been advocated, cyst shunting carries the risk of arachnoid scarring, infection, and blocking of the catheter secondary to cyst collapse.[9]

What was actually done

Due to the progressive nature of the patient's symptoms, surgical intervention was advised. Special considerations of the surgery and risks were explained, and the patient consented to surgical intervention. The patient was brought to the operating room and was induced under general anesthesia. The patient was positioned prone on the operating table. Intraoperative x-rays were used to identify the proper level. A decompressive

T4-T6 laminectomy was performed with care taken to preserve as much of the facet as possible. Intraoperative ultrasound was brought into the field revealing the arachnoid cyst with loculations, finding consistent with the MRI study. The dura was opened in the midline from T4 to T6, and intradural exploration and lysis of adhesions was done. The cord was gently retracted to the right, and the arachnoid cyst was visualized and opened sharply, causing egress of CSF. Then, ultrasound was brought again into the filed demonstrating excellent decompression of the cyst. The dura was closed. Valsalva was performed and showed no sign of CSF leak. Somatosensory and motor evoked potential monitoring was utilized throughout the case and remained stable. The patient awoke from anesthesia without any complications. Postoperatively, the patient had improvement of lower extremity function and spasticity. Three months after surgery, the patient underwent imaging that showed improved mass effect but persistent residual loculation of CSF within the cervical segment (Fig. 70.2). Because of the patient's improved symptoms, serial imaging was recommended.

Commonalities among the experts

There was variability in the additional preoperative tests chosen by the experts. Half advocated for a brain MRI and half recommended a computed tomography myelogram of the complete spine. While all agreed that the goal of surgery was to alleviate spinal cord compression, half of the surgeons would attain decompression through a C6-T6 laminectomy and the rest would pursue a T1-T2 laminectomy with possible arachnoid cyst-subarachnoid shunt. Most favored drainage/excision of the arachnoid cyst. Most were cognizant of the spinal cord, vascular elements, and dentate ligaments. The most feared complications were spinal cord injury, CSF leak, and neurological decline. The majority would utilize intraoperative monitoring, fluoroscopy, and surgical microscope to perform surgery. Half would use perioperative steroids. Surgical nuances were different among experts; however, most shared the concept of compression relief while minimizing cord manipulation. Half would admit their patients to the floor. Most recommended a postoperative MRI before discharge.

SUMMARY OF QUALITY OF EVIDENCE TO GUIDE SPECIFIC INTERVENTIONS FOR THIS CASE

- Surgical intervention versus conservative management for spinal cord dysfunction in the setting of chronic arachnoiditis: level III
- Surgical treatment for arachnoiditis after failure of conservative management: level III

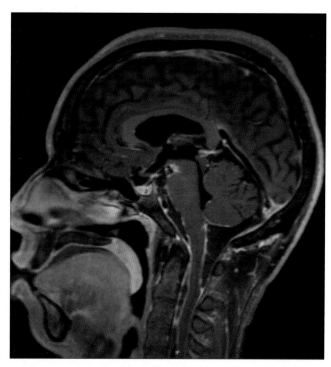

Fig. 70.2 Postoperative magnetic resonance images. Sagittal T1 with contrast demonstrating the craniocervical junction. There is persistent entrapment and loculation of CSF within the posterior fossa and the upper cervical spinal canal due to arachnoid adhesions but with improved mass effect.

REFERENCES

1. Wright MH, Denney LC. A comprehensive review of spinal arachnoiditis. *Orthop Nurs.* 2003;22(3):215–219. quiz 220-211.
2. Kalina J. Arachnoiditis. *J Pain Palliat Care Pharmacother.* 2012;26(2):176-177.
3. Basaran R, Kaksi M, Efendioglu M, Onoz M, Balkuv E, Kaner T. Spinal arachnoid cyst associated with arachnoiditis following subarachnoid haemorrhage in adult patients: A case report and literature review. *Br J Neurosurg.* 2015;29(2):285–289.
4. Guyer DW, Wiltse LL, Eskay ML, Guyer BH. The long-range prognosis of arachnoiditis. *Spine (Phila Pa 1976).* 1989;14(12):1332–1341.
5. Ribeiro C, Reis FC. [Adhesive lumbar arachnoiditis]. *Acta Med Port.* 1998;11(1):59–65.
6. Todeschi J, Chibbaro S, Gubian A, Pop R, Proust F, Cebula H. Spinal adhesive arachnoiditis following the rupture of an Adamkiewicz aneurysm: Literature review and a case illustration. *Neurochirurgie.* 2018;64(3):177–182.
7. Nath PC, Mishra SS, Deo RC, Satapathy MC. Intradural Spinal Arachnoid Cyst: A Long-Term Postlaminectomy Complication: A Case Report and Review of the Literature. *World Neurosurg.* 2016;85(367):e361–364.
8. Anderson TL, Morris JM, Wald JT, Kotsenas AL. Imaging Appearance of Advanced Chronic Adhesive Arachnoiditis: A Retrospective Review. *AJR Am J Roentgenol.* 2017;209(3):648–655.
9. Klekamp J. A New Classification for Pathologies of Spinal Meninges-Part 2: Primary and Secondary Intradural Arachnoid Cysts. *Neurosurgery.* 2017;81(2):217–229.
10. Velz J, Fierstra J, Regli L, Germans MR. Spontaneous Spinal Subarachnoid Hemorrhage with Development of an Arachnoid Cyst-A Case Report and Review of the Literature. *World Neurosurg.* 2018;119:374–380.

Index

Note: Page numbers followed by *f*, *t*, or *b* indicate figures, tables, or boxes, respectively.